FOURTH EDITION

Handbook for **Stoelting's Anesthesia and Co-Existing Di...**

ROBERT...
Nicholas M. ...
Department ...
Yale Univers...
Chief of Ane...
Yale-New Ha...
New Haven, ...

KATHERI...
Department ...
Yale Univers...
Attending A...
Yale-New Ha...
New Haven, ...

ELSEVIER
SAUNDERS

1600 John F. Kennedy Blvd.
Ste 1800
Philadelphia, PA 19103-2899

HANDBOOK FOR STOELTING'S ANESTHESIA
AND CO-EXISITING DISEASE ISBN: 978-1-4377-2866-8

Notices

Knowledge and best practice in this field are constantly changing. As new research and experience broaden our understanding, changes in research methods, professional practices, or medical treatment may become necessary.

Practitioners and researchers must always rely on their own experience and knowledge in evaluating and using any information, methods, compounds, or experiments described herein. In using such information or methods, they should be mindful of their own safety and the safety of others, including parties for whom they have a professional responsibility.

With respect to any drug or pharmaceutical products identified, readers are advised to check the most current information provided (i) on procedures featured or (ii) by the manufacturer of each product to be administered to verify the recommended dose or formula, the method and duration of administration, and contraindications. It is the responsibility of practitioners, relying on their own experience and knowledge of their patients, to make diagnoses, to determine dosages and the best treatment for each individual patient, and to take all appropriate safety precautions.

To the fullest extent of the law, neither the Publisher nor the authors, contributors, or editors assume any liability for any injury and/or damage to persons or property as a matter of products liability, negligence or otherwise, or from any use or operation of any methods, products, instructions, or ideas contained in the material herein.

Library of Congress Cataloging-in-Publication Data

Handbook for Stoelting's anesthesia and co-existing disease / [edited by] Roberta L. Hines, Katherine E. Marschall. -- 4th ed.
p. ; cm.
Companion to: Stoelting's anesthesia and co-existing disease. 6th ed. c2012.
Includes bibliographical references and index.
ISBN 978-1-4377-2866-8 (pbk. : alk. paper)
I. Stoelting, Robert K. II. Hines, Roberta L. III. Marschall, Katherine E. IV. Stoelting's anesthesia and co-existing disease.
[DNLM: 1. Anesthesia--adverse effects--Handbooks. 2. Anesthesia--adverse effects--Outlines. 3. Anesthesia--methods--Handbooks. 4. Anesthesia--methods--Outlines. 5. Anesthetics--adverse effects--Handbooks. 6. Anesthetics--adverse effects--Outlines. 7. Intraoperative Complications--Handbooks. 8. Intraoperative Complications--Outlines. WO 231]

617.9'6--dc23 2012028212

Executive Content Strategist: William Schmitt
Content Development Manager: Lucia Gunzel
Publishing Services Manager: Anne Altepeter
Senior Project Manager: Cheryl A. Abbott
Design Direction: Louis Forgione

Printed in the United States of America

Last digit is the print number: 9 8 7 6 5 4 3 2 1

CONTRIBUTORS

Shamsuddin Akhtar, MD
Associate Professor of Anesthesiology
Director, Medical Student Education
Yale University School of Medicine
New Haven, Connecticut

Brooke E. Albright, MD
Captain, U.S. Air Force
Staff Anesthesiologist
Landstuhl Regional Medical Center
Landstuhl/Kirchberg, Germany

Sharif Al-Ruzzeh, MD, PhD
Resident in Anesthesiology
Yale-New Haven Hospital
New Haven, Connecticut

Ferne R. Braveman, MD
Professor of Anesthesiology
Vice-Chair of Clinical Affairs
Chief, Division of Obstetrics Anesthesia
Department of Anesthesiology
Yale University School of Medicine
New Haven, Connecticut

Michelle W. Diu, MD, FAAP
Assistant Professor of Anesthesiology
Yale University School of Medicine
New Haven, Connecticut

Samantha A. Franco, MD
Assistant Professor of Anesthesiology
Yale University School of Medicine
New Haven, Connecticut

Loreta Grecu, MD
Assistant Professor of Anesthesiology
Yale University School of Medicine
New Haven, Connecticut

Alá Sami Haddadin, MD, FCCP
Assistant Professor, Division of Cardiothoracic Anesthesia and Adult Critical Care Medicine
Medical Director, Cardiothoracic Intensive Care Unit
Department of Anesthesiology
Yale University School of Medicine
New Haven, Connecticut

Laura L. Hammel, MD
Assistant Professor of Anesthesiology and Critical Care
University of Wisconsin Hospital and Clinics
Madison, Wisconsin

Michael Hannaman, MD
Assistant Professor, Department of Anesthesiology
University of Wisconsin School of Medicine and Public Health
Madison, Wisconsin

Antonio Hernandez Conte, MD, MBA
Assistant Professor of Anesthesiology
Co-Director, Perioperative Transesophageal Echocardiography
Cedars-Sinai Medical Center
Partner, General Anesthesia Specialists Partnership, Inc.
Los Angeles, California

Adriana Herrera, MD
Assistant Professor of Anesthesiology
Associate Residency Program Director
Department of Anesthesiology
Yale University School of Medicine
New Haven, Connecticut

Zoltan G. Hevesi, MD, MBA
Professor of Anesthesiology and Surgery
University of Wisconsin
University of Wisconsin Hospital and Clinics
Madison, Wisconsin

Roberta L. Hines, MD
Nicholas M. Greene Professor and Chairman
Department of Anesthesiology
Yale University School of Medicine
Chief of Anesthesiology
Yale-New Haven Hospital
New Haven, Connecticut

Natalie F. Holt, MD, MPH
Assistant Professor of Anesthesiology
Yale University School of Medicine
New Haven, Connecticut;
Attending Physician, West Haven Veterans Affairs Medical Center
West Haven, Connecticut

Viji Kurup, MD
Associate Professor of Anesthesiology
Yale University School of Medicine
New Haven, Connecticut

William L. Lanier, Jr., MD
Professor of Anesthesiology
College of Medicine
Mayo Clinic
Rochester, Minnesota

Thomas J. Mancuso, MD, FAAP
Associate Professor of Anesthesia
Harvard Medical School
Senior Associate in Anesthesia
Director of Medical Education
Children's Hospital of Boston
Boston, Massachusetts

Katherine E. Marschall, MD
Department of Anesthesiology
Yale University School of Medicine
Attending Anesthesiologist
Yale-New Haven Hospital
New Haven, Connecticut

Veronica A. Matei, MD
Assistant Professor of Anesthesiology
Yale University School of Medicine
New Haven, Connecticut

Raj K. Modak, MD
Assistant Professor of Cardiac and Thoracic Anesthesia
Director, Cardiac Anesthesia Fellowship Program
Department of Anesthesiology
Yale University School of Medicine
New Haven, Connecticut

Tori Myslajek, MD
Assistant Professor of Anesthesiology
Yale University School of Medicine
New Haven, Connecticut

Adriana Dana Oprea, MD
Assistant Professor of Anesthesiology
Yale University School of Medicine
New Haven, Connecticut

Jeffrey J. Pasternak, MD
Assistant Professor of Anesthesiology
College of Medicine
Mayo Clinic
Rochester, Minnesota

Wanda M. Popescu, MD
Associate Professor of Anesthesiology
Director, Thoracic Anesthesia Section
Yale University School of Medicine
New Haven, Connecticut

Ramachandran Ramani
Associate Professor of Anesthesiology
Yale University School of Medicine
New Haven, Connecticut

Robert B. Schonberger, MD, MA
Fellow of Cardiac and Thoracic Anesthesia
Department of Anesthesiology
Yale University School of Medicine
New Haven, Connecticut

Denis Snegovskikh, MD
Assistant Professor of Anesthesiology
Yale University School of Medicine
New Haven, Connecticut

Gail A. Van Norman, MD
Professor
Director, Pre-Anesthesia Clinic
Department of Anesthesiology and Pain Medicine
University of Washington
Seattle, Washington

Hossam Tantawy, MD
Assistant Professor of Anesthesiology
Yale University School of Medicine
New Haven, Connecticut

Russell T. Wall, III, MD
Vice-Chair and Program Director
Department of Anesthesiology
Georgetown University Hospital
Professor of Anesthesiology and Pharmacology
Senior Associate Dean
Georgetown University School of Medicine
Washington, DC

Kelley Teed Watson, MD
Clinical Assistant Professor
Yale University School of Medicine
New Haven, Connecticut;
Cardiothoracic Anesthesiologist
Department of Anesthesiology
Self Regional Healthcare
Greenwood, South Carolina

PREFACE

The fourth edition of the *Handbook for Stoelting's Anesthesia and Co-Existing Disease* is intended to provide a ready source of information about the impact of disease states on the management of patients in the perioperative period. The handbook uses an outline format that follows the chapters and headings that appear in the sixth edition of *Stoelting's Anesthesia and Co-Existing Disease* so readers can refer to corresponding areas in the textbook for more detailed information. The handbook thus serves as a more portable counterpart to the textbook that can be reviewed on site in the operating room or at other anesthetizing locations. Much of the information in the handbook is presented in tables, illustrations, and algorithms. This format helps with rapid access to salient aspects of particular medical conditions.

We wish to thank Dr. Gail A. Van Norman for her invaluable help in redacting the text.

Roberta L. Hines
Katherine E. Marschall

CONTENTS

CHAPTER 1

Ischemic Heart Disease

Ischemic heart disease affects approximately 30% of patients undergoing surgery in the United States. Angina pectoris, acute myocardial infarction (MI), and sudden death are often the first manifestations of this disease. Cardiac dysrhythmias are the major cause of sudden death. The two most important risk factors for the development of coronary artery atherosclerosis are male gender and increasing age (Table 1-1). Presentation of patients with ischemic heart disease can include chronic stable angina or an acute coronary syndrome (ACS). ACS can manifest as ST-elevation MI (STEMI) or unstable angina/non–ST-elevation MI (UA/NSTEMI).

I. ANGINA PECTORIS

Angina pectoris occurs when there is a mismatch of oxygen delivered to the myocardium (supply) and myocardial oxygen consumption (demand). Stable angina typically develops in the setting of partial occlusion or significant (>70%) chronic narrowing of a segment of coronary artery. When the imbalance between myocardial oxygen supply and demand becomes critical, congestive heart failure (CHF), electrical instability with dysrhythmias, and MI can result.

A. Diagnosis. The pain of angina pectoris is generally described as retrosternal chest discomfort, pain, pressure, or heaviness that often radiates to the neck, left shoulder, left arm, or jaw and occasionally to the back or down both arms. Angina may also cause epigastric discomfort resembling indigestion, chest tightness, or shortness of breath. Discomfort usually lasts several minutes and follows a crescendo-decrescendo pattern; a sharp pain lasting only a few seconds or a dull ache lasting for hours is rarely angina. *Stable* angina is unchanged in frequency or severity over 2 months or longer. *Unstable angina* (UA) is angina at rest, of new onset, or of increased severity or frequency compared with previously stable angina. Chest wall tenderness suggests a musculoskeletal origin of chest pain. Sharp retrosternal pain exacerbated by deep breathing, coughing, or change in body position suggests pericarditis. Esophageal spasm can produce discomfort similar to angina pectoris and may be similarly relieved by administration of nitroglycerin.

1. Electrocardiography

a. Standard Electrocardiography. Subendocardial ischemia is associated with ST-segment depression during anginal pain. Variant angina (angina that results from coronary vasospasm) is characterized by ST elevation during anginal pain. T-wave inversion may be present. In patients with chronic T wave inversion, ischemia may be associated with "pseudonormalization" of T waves to the upright position during episodes of ischemia.

b. Exercise Electrocardiography. Exercise electrocardiography can detect signs of myocardial ischemia in relationship to chest pain. A new murmur of mitral regurgitation or a decrease in blood pressure during exercise increases the diagnostic value of this test. Exercise testing may be contraindicated in some conditions (e.g., severe aortic stenosis, severe hypertension (HTN), acute myocarditis, uncontrolled CHF, infective endocarditis) and may not be possible in patients who cannot exercise or if other conditions interfere

TABLE 1-1 ■ Risk Factors for Development of Ischemic Heart Disease

Male gender
Increasing age
Hypercholesterolemia
Hypertension
Cigarette smoking
Diabetes mellitus
Obesity
Sedentary lifestyle
Genetic factors, family history

with interpretation of the exercise electrocardiogram (ECG) (e.g., paced rhythm, left ventricular hypertrophy, digitalis administration, or preexcitation syndrome). A minimum criterion for an abnormal ST-segment response is 1 mm or more of horizontal or downsloping ST-segment depression during or within 4 minutes after exercise.

2. **Noninvasive Imaging Tests.** Noninvasive imaging tests are recommended when exercise electrocardiography is not possible or interpretation of ST-segment changes would be difficult. Cardiac stress can be induced by administration of atropine, dobutamine, or by cardiac pacing to increase heart rate, or by administration of a coronary vasodilator such as adenosine or dipyridamole.
   a. ***Echocardiography.*** Wall motion analysis is performed immediately after stressing the heart. Ventricular wall motion abnormalities induced by stress correspond to the site of myocardial ischemia.
   b. ***Nuclear Stress Imaging.*** Nuclear stress imaging is more sensitive than exercise testing in detecting ischemia. Nuclear tracers (thallium, technetium) are injected into the bloodstream and detected over the myocardium by single-photon emission computed tomography (SPECT) techniques. Imaging is performed twice: immediately after exercise, and 4 hours later at rest. Areas of reduced tracer activity during cardiac stress that are not present at rest indicate regions of reversible ischemia.
   c. ***Stress Cardiac Myocardial Imaging.*** Pharmacologic stress imaging with stress cardiac magnetic resonance imaging (CMRI) compares favorably with other imaging modalities.
   d. ***Electron Beam Computed Tomography.*** Coronary artery calcifications can be detected by electron beam computed tomography. Sensitivity is high but specificity is low, and routine use is not recommended.
3. **Invasive Methods**
   a. ***Coronary Angiography.*** Coronary angiography provides the most information about the condition of the coronary arteries. It is indicated in patients who continue to have angina pectoris despite maximal medical therapy, in those who are being considered for coronary revascularization, and for the definitive diagnosis of coronary disease in individuals whose occupations could place others at risk (e.g., airline pilots).
      i. The most important prognostic determinants are the extent of atheromatous coronary artery disease, the stability of coronary plaque, and left ventricular function (ejection fraction).
      ii. Left main coronary artery disease is the most dangerous anatomic lesion (>50% stenosis is associated with an annual mortality of 15%).
      iii. Plaques most likely to rupture and initiate ACS, vulnerable plaques, have a thin fibrous cap and large lipid core.
      iv. Left ventricular ejection fraction of less than 40% is associated with poorer prognosis.

TABLE 1-2 ■ **Medical Treatment of Myocardial Ischemia**

CLASSIFICATION	DRUGS	COMMENTS
Antiplatelet drugs	Low-dose aspirin Adenosine diphosphate receptor blockers: clopidogrel (Plavix), ticlopidine (Ticlid) Platelet glycoprotein IIb/IIIa receptor antagonists (abciximab, eptifibatide, tirofiban)	Decrease risk of cardiac events in patients with stable or unstable angina. Particularly useful after intracoronary stent placement. • Low-dose aspirin recommended in all patients with ischemic heart disease without contraindications. • 10% to 20% of patients are hyporesponders to aspirin and clopidogrel.
β-Blockers	β_1-Blockers (atenolol, metoprolol, acebutolol, bisoprolol) β_2-Blockers (propranolol, nadolol)	Principal drug treatment for angina. Long-term use decreases risks of death and repeat MI. Used even in patients with congestive heart failure and pulmonary disease.
Calcium channel blockers (CCBs)	Long-acting: amlodipine, nicardipine, isradipine, felodipine, long-acting nifedipine Short-acting: nifedipine, verapamil, diltiazem	Long-acting CCBs are effective at relieving anginal pain; short-acting CCBs are not. Not as effective as β-blockers in reducing risk of MI. Contraindicated in CHF; use with caution in patients already taking β-blockers.
Nitrates	Sublingual nitroglycerin, isosorbide dinitrate	Decrease frequency, duration, and severity of angina. Contraindicated in obstructive cardiomyopathy and severe aortic stenosis. Must not be used within 24 hours of sildenafil (Viagra), tadalafil (Cialis), or vardenafil (Levitra), due to potential hypotension.
Angiotensin-converting enzyme inhibitors	Captopril, enalapril	Recommended for all patients with coronary artery disease, especially those with HTN, diabetes, or left ventricular dysfunction. Contraindicated in patients with renal failure and bilateral renal artery stenosis.

CHF, Congestive heart failure; *HTN,* hypertension; *MI,* myocardial infarction.

B. Treatment

1. **Lifestyle Modification.** Progression of atherosclerosis may be slowed by cessation of smoking; maintenance of an ideal body weight through a low-fat, low-cholesterol diet; regular aerobic exercise; and treatment of HTN. Lowering the low-density lipoprotein level to less than 100 mg/dL by diet and/or drugs such as statins reduces risk of cardiac death. Lowering blood pressure from hypertensive levels to normal levels decreases the risk of MI, CHF, and cerebrovascular accident.
2. **Treatment of Associated Conditions.** Associated conditions may include those that increase myocardial oxygen demand (e.g., fever, infection, tachycardia, thyrotoxicosis, heart failure, cocaine use) or decrease myocardial oxygen delivery (e.g., anemia).
3. **Medical Treatment of Myocardial Ischemia** (Table 1-2)
4. **Revascularization.** Revascularization by coronary artery bypass grafting (CABG) or percutaneous coronary intervention (PCI) with or without placement of intracoronary

stents is indicated when optimal medical therapy fails to control angina pectoris. Revascularization is also indicated for specific anatomic lesions (left main stenosis of more than 50%, combinations of two-vessel or three-vessel disease that include a proximal left anterior descending artery stenosis of more than 70%) and decreased left ventricular ejection fraction (ejection fraction < 40%). Operative mortality rates for CABG surgery are 1.5% to 2%.

II. ACUTE CORONARY SYNDROME

ACS is a hypercoagulable state caused by focal disruption of an atheromatous plaque, generation of thrombin, and partial or complete occlusion of the coronary artery. Patients with ischemic chest pain are categorized by ECG characteristics and the presence of cardiac-specific biomarkers. Patients with ST-segment elevation have STEMI. Those with ST-segment depression or nonspecific ECG changes and ischemic pain are classified as having NSTEMI when cardiac biomarkers are positive or as having UA if biomarkers are negative.

A. ST-Elevation Myocardial Infarction. Short-term mortality of patients with STEMI who receive aggressive reperfusion therapy is approximately 6.5% versus 15% to 20% in patients who do not receive reperfusion therapy. Long-term prognosis is determined by left ventricular ejection fraction (determined 2 to 3 months after MI), the degree of any residual ischemia, and the potential for malignant ventricular dysrhythmias.

1. Pathophysiology. Inflammation plays an important role in events leading to rupture of atherosclerotic plaque. Serum markers of inflammation are increased in those at greatest risk of development of coronary artery disease. STEMI occurs when coronary blood flow decreases abruptly because of acute thrombus formation after a plaque fissures, ruptures, or ulcerates.

a. Plaques with rich lipid cores and thin fibrous caps *[vulnerable plaques]* are most prone to rupture but are rarely large enough to cause coronary obstruction by themselves. Plaque rupture results in a thrombogenic environment; collagen, adenosine diphosphate (ADP), epinephrine, and serotonin stimulate platelet aggregation, vasoconstrictor thromboxane A_2 is released, and activated platelets promote growth and stabilization of thrombus.

b. Flow-restrictive plaques that cause angina pectoris and stimulate growth of collateral circulation are less likely to rupture.

c. Rarely, STEMI is the result of acute coronary spasm or coronary artery embolization.

2. Signs and Symptoms of Acute Myocardial Infarction (Table 1-3)

TABLE 1-3 ■ **Signs and Symptoms of Acute Myocardial Infarction**
Anginal pain that does not resolve with rest
Anxiety
Pallor
Diaphoresis
Sinus tachycardia
Hypotension
Pulmonary rales
New cardiac murmur
Dysrhythmia
Abnormal ECG
Increased cardiac biomarkers (CPK, troponins)

CPK, Creatine phosphokinase; *ECG,* electrocardiogram.

3. **Diagnosis.** Diagnosis of acute MI requires the rise and fall in plasma levels of biochemical markers of myocardial necrosis plus at least one of these three criteria: (1) ischemic symptoms, (2) development of pathologic Q waves on ECG, (3) ECG changes indicative of ischemia (ST-segment elevation or depression), or (4) imaging evidence of a new loss of viable myocardium or new regional wall motion abnormality. Two thirds of patients describe new-onset angina or change in anginal pattern during the 30 days preceding acute MI.
   a. ***Laboratory Studies.*** Cardiac troponins (troponin T or I) increase within 3 hours after myocardial injury and remain elevated for 7 to 10 days. They are more specific than creatine kinase–MB for determining myocardial injury (Table 1-4).
   b. ***Imaging Studies.*** Echocardiography to look for regional wall motion abnormalities is useful in patients with left bundle branch block or an abnormal ECG (but without ST-segment elevation) in whom the diagnosis of acute MI is uncertain.
4. **Acute Treatment** (Table 1-5)
5. **Adjunctive Medical Therapy for Acute Myocardial Infarction** (Table 1-6)

B. **Unstable Angina/Non–ST-Elevation Myocardial Infarction.** UA/NSTEMI results from a reduction in myocardial oxygen supply caused by rupture or erosion of an atherosclerotic coronary plaque with thrombosis, inflammation, and vasoconstriction. Most affected arteries have less than 50% stenosis. Embolization of platelets or clot fragments into the coronary microcirculation leads to microcirculatory ischemia or infarction. Other causes can include dynamic obstruction from vasoconstriction; worsening coronary luminal narrowing from progressive atherosclerosis, in-stent restenosis, or stenosis of bypass grafts; vasculitis; and myocardial ischemia from increased oxygen demand (e.g., thyrotoxicosis).
   1. **Diagnosis.** UA/NSTEMI has three principal presentations: (1) angina at rest lasting for more than 20 minutes, (2) chronic angina pectoris that becomes more frequent and

TABLE 1-4 ■ **Biomarkers for Evaluation of Patients with ST-Elevation Myocardial Infarction**

BIOMARKER	RANGE OF TIME TO INITIAL ELEVATION	MEAN TIME TO PEAK ELEVATION*	TIME TO RETURN TO NORMAL
FREQUENTLY USED IN CLINICAL PRACTICE			
CK-MB†	3-12 hr	24 hr	48-72 hr
Troponin I‡	3-12 hr	24 hr	5-10 days
Troponin T	3-12 hr	12 hr–2 days	5-14 days
INFREQUENTLY USED IN CLINICAL PRACTICE			
Myoglobin	1-4 hr	6-7 hr	24 hr
CK-MB tissue isoform	2-6 hr	18 hr	Unknown
CK-MM tissue isoform	1-6 hr	12 hr	38 hr

Modified from Antman EM, Anbe DT, Armstrong PW, et al. ACC/AHA guidelines for the management of patients with ST-elevation myocardial infarction. A report of the American College of Cardiology/American Heart Association Task Force on Practice Guidelines (Committee to Revise the 1999 Guidelines for the Management of Patients with Acute Myocardial Infarction). *Circulation.* 2004;110:e82-e292.

*Nonreperfused patients.

†Increased sensitivity can be achieved by sampling every 6 or 8 hr.

‡Multiple assays available for clinical use; the clinician should be familiar with the cutoff value used in his or her institution.

CK-MB, Creatine kinase–MB.

TABLE 1-5 ■ Treatment of Acute Myocardial Infarction

Immediate	Evaluate hemodynamic stability Obtain 12-lead ECG Supplemental oxygen Pain relief: nitroglycerin, morphine Aspirin (clopidogrel if aspirin intolerant) β-Blockers for patients not in heart failure or low cardiac output state or with heart block
Within 30-60 minutes of arrival and within 12 hours of symptom onset	Thrombolytic therapy (streptokinase, tissue plasminogen activator, reteplase, tenecteplase) Note: *Not* recommended in patients with UA or NSTEMI
Within 90 minutes of arrival and within 12 hours of symptom onset	Coronary angioplasty Coronary stenting followed by treatment with glycoprotein IIb/IIIa inhibitor
If coronary anatomy precludes a percutaneous intervention or angioplasty fails	CABG (also indicated with acute mitral regurgitation or infarction-related ventricular septal defect)

CABG, Coronary artery bypass grafting; *ECG,* electrocardiogram; *NSTEMI,* non–ST-elevation myocardial infarction; *UA,* unstable angina.

TABLE 1-6 ■ Adjunctive Medical Therapy in Acute Myocardial Infarction

DRUG	INDICATION AND TIMING
Heparin (unfractionated or low molecular weight)	For 24-48 hours after thrombolytic therapy to reduce thrombin regeneration
Bivalirudin, hirudin	For 24-48 hours in patients with heparin-induced thrombocytopenia
β-Blockers	For *all* patients without specific contraindications, starting as early as possible and continued indefinitely
ACEIs	Large anterior MI Clinical evidence of left ventricular failure EF lower than 40% Diabetes mellitus
Angiotensin II receptor blockers	Patients with indications who are intolerant of ACEIs
Calcium channel blockers	Only in patients with persistent ischemia despite aspirin, β-blockers, nitrates, and intravenous heparin
Hypoglycemic agents	Glycemic control in patients with diabetes
Magnesium	Only in torsade de pointes ventricular tachycardia
Statins	Should be started as soon as possible after acute MI

ACEI, Angiotensin-converting enzyme inhibitor; *EF,* ejection fraction; *MI,* myocardial infarction.

more easily provoked, and (3) new-onset angina that is severe, prolonged, or disabling. UA/NSTEMI can also manifest with hemodynamic instability or CHF. ECG findings can include ST-segment depression and T-wave inversions. Elevation of cardiac biomarkers, troponins, and/or CK-MB distinguishes NSTEMI from UA.

2. **Treatment of Unstable Angina/Non–ST-Elevation Myocardial Infarction** (Table 1-7)

TABLE 1-7 ■ **Treatment of Unstable Angina/Non–ST-Elevation Myocardial Infarction**

Decrease oxygen demand and increase oxygen supply	Bed rest Supplemental oxygen Analgesia β-Blockers Sublingual or intravenous nitroglycerin Treatment of severe anemia
Reduce further thrombus formation	Aspirin or clopidogrel Intravenous unfractionated heparin or subcutaneous low-molecular-weight heparin for 48 hours *Note:* Thrombolytic therapy is *not* indicated and has been shown to *increase* mortality.
For high-risk patients	Coronary angiography Revascularization by PCI or CABG
For lower-risk patients	Medical therapy Later stress testing

CABG, Coronary artery bypass grafting; *PCI,* percutaneous coronary intervention.

III. COMPLICATIONS OF ACUTE MYOCARDIAL INFARCTION (TABLE 1-8)

IV. PERIOPERATIVE IMPLICATIONS OF PERCUTANEOUS CORONARY INTERVENTION

PCI includes percutaneous transluminal coronary angioplasty (PTCA) with and without placement of a coronary stent. PTCA alone is associated with restenosis of the coronary vessel in 15% to 60% of patients. Restenosis rates are significantly reduced by placement of a coronary stent at the time of PTCA. Two classes of stents are available: bare metal stents (BMSs) and drug-eluting stents (DESs). Two issues associated with stent placement are thrombosis at the stent site and increased risk of bleeding caused by dual antiplatelet therapy.

A. Thrombosis. Endothelial injury associated with PTCA and stent placement increases risk of thrombosis within the vessel. Risk of thrombosis declines after reendothelialization of the vessel or stent (2 to 3 weeks after PTCA, 12 weeks after BMS, and ≥1 year after DES). During that vulnerable time, dual antiplatelet therapy is indicated.

1. Stent Thrombosis

a. Defined in relation to timing of stent placement as acute (≤24 hours), subacute (2 to 30 days), late (between 30 days and 1 year), and very late (≥1 year).

b. Risk of thrombosis is increased more than fourteenfold and 1-year mortality is increased tenfold if dual antiplatelet therapy (aspirin with clopidogrel) is stopped prematurely (<2 weeks for PTCA, <6 weeks for BMS, <1 year for DES).

2. Surgery and Stent Thrombosis

a. ***Bare Metal Stent.*** Risk of death, MI, stent thrombosis, and need for urgent revascularization is increased 5% to 30% if surgery is performed within 6 weeks of placement. Emergency surgery triples the risk of adverse events compared with elective surgery.

b. ***Drug-Eluting Stent.*** Risk of major adverse cardiac events is very significant if antiplatelet therapy is discontinued and noncardiac surgery performed within 1 year of placement. Emergency surgery is associated with a 3.5-fold increase in adverse events compared with elective surgery.

TABLE 1-8 ■ **Complications of Acute Myocardial Infarction**

COMPLICATION	TREATMENT
Dysrhythmia	Ventricular fibrillation: rapid defibrillation followed by treatment with amiodarone and/or β-blockers, treatment of hypokalemia Ventricular tachycardia: cardioversion if sustained, amiodarone and/or lidocaine; implanted defibrillator in patients with recurrent ventricular tachycardia or fibrillation despite adequate revascularization Atrial fibrillation: cardioversion if hemodynamically unstable, β-blocker or calcium channel blocker to control rate Sinus bradycardia: atropine, temporary cardiac pacing Second- or third-degree heart block: temporary cardiac pacing
Pericarditis—acute and delayed (Dressler's syndrome)	Aspirin or indomethacin, corticosteroids only for refractory symptoms and preferably deferred until 4 weeks after acute MI
Severe mitral regurgitation	Intravenous nitroprusside or other therapies to decrease left ventricular afterload IABP Prompt surgical repair: 24-hr mortality is high in the setting of total papillary muscle rapture.
Ventricular septal rupture	IABP Prompt surgical repair
Congestive heart failure and cardiogenic shock	Treat reversible causes Support blood pressure Decrease left ventricular overload Treat pulmonary edema Restore coronary blood flow via thrombolytic therapy, PCI, or CABG Consider circulatory assist device (VAD) or IABP
Myocardial rupture	Emergency surgery
Right ventricular infarction	Intravascular volume replacement Inotropic support Pulmonary artery vasodilation Atrioventricular sequential pacing if needed
Cerebrovascular accident	Echocardiography and immediate initiation of anticoagulation for left ventricular thrombus if present, followed by 6 months of warfarin therapy

CABG, Coronary artery bypass grafting; *IABP,* intraaortic balloon pump; *MI,* myocardial infarction; *PCI,* percutaneous coronary intervention; *VAD,* ventricular assist device.

B. Risks of Perioperative Bleeding with Antiplatelet Agents

1. **Spontaneous Bleeding.** Aspirin therapy is associated with an increased risk that is about 1.5 times normal, but severity of bleeding episodes is not increased.
2. **Bleeding after Noncardiac Surgery.** Risks of bleeding are increased about 50% in patients taking clopidogrel and aspirin (clopidogrel alone has not been well studied). However, mortality has been seen to increase only with intracranial surgery.

C. Bleeding versus Stent Thrombosis in the Perioperative Period

1. Premature discontinuation of antiplatelet therapy should be avoided when the risk of bleeding is low and the potential bleeding is manageable.

TABLE 1-9 ■ **Recommended Time Intervals for Withholding Antiplatelet Therapy Before and After Neuraxial Puncture or Catheter Removal**

DRUG	TIME *BEFORE* PUNCTURE OR CATHETER MANIPULATION OR REMOVAL	TIME *AFTER* PUNCTURE OR CATHETER MANIPULATION OR REMOVAL
Clopidogrel	7 days	After catheter removal
Ticlopidine	10 days	After catheter removal
Prasugrel	7-10 days	6 hr after catheter removal
Ticagrelor	5 days	6 hr after catheter removal

Data from recommendations of the European Society of Anaesthesiology.

2. For those in whom antiplatelet therapy should be discontinued (e.g., neurosurgery, spinal cord decompression, aortic aneurysm surgery, prostatectomy), clopidogrel should be stopped 5 to 7 days before surgery and resumed as quickly as possible postoperatively.

D. Management of Patients with Stents Undergoing Noncardiac Surgery: Five Factors to Consider

1. **Interval between Percutaneous Coronary Intervention and Surgery.** Patients with a BMS should wait at least 6 weeks, and preferably 90 days, after stent placement to undergo elective surgery. Patients with a DES should wait at least 1 year.
2. **Continuation of Dual Antiplatelet Therapy.** Platelets can be administered for bleeding but may have reduced efficacy if clopidogrel has been recently administered (<4 hours before). Platelet infusions will be most effective at least 14 hours after the last dose. If dual antiplatelet therapy must be stopped prematurely, then aspirin should be continued if possible. Patients who have had antiplatelet therapy prematurely discontinued should be monitored closely.
3. **Perioperative Monitoring.** Urgent cardiac evaluation should be performed if perioperative angina occurs in a patient with a stent.
4. **Anesthetic Technique.** Neuraxial blockade is not prudent in patients undergoing dual antiplatelet therapy. Times for withholding antiplatelet therapy before neuraxial puncture or placement or removal of a neuraxial catheter are summarized in Table 1-9.
5. **Availability of Interventional Cardiology.** Patients should be triaged to an interventional cardiologist within 90 minutes of a diagnosis or suspicion of acute MI or acute stent thrombosis.

V. PERIOPERATIVE MYOCARDIAL INFARCTION

Approximately 500,000 to 900,000 perioperative MIs occur annually worldwide. The incidence of perioperative MI in patients who undergo elective high-risk vascular surgery is 5% to 15%, and mortality of perioperative MIs approaches 20%.

A. Pathophysiology. Most perioperative MIs occur within 24 to 48 hours after surgery. Two mechanisms appear to play a role in perioperative MI: (1) increased myocardial oxygen demand relative to supply and (2) thrombosis associated with vulnerable plaque rupture. These processes are not mutually exclusive. However, one process or the other can predominate in a particular patient.

B. Diagnosis of Perioperative Myocardial Infarction. The diagnosis of acute MI traditionally requires the presence of at least two of the following three elements: (1) ischemic chest pain, (2) evolutionary changes on the ECG, and (3) increase and decrease in cardiac biomarker levels. In the perioperative period, ischemic episodes are often not associated with chest pain, and many postoperative ECGs are nondiagnostic. An acute increase in troponin levels should be considered an MI in the perioperative setting, requiring careful attention and referral to a cardiologist for further evaluation and management.

VI. PREOPERATIVE ASSESSMENT OF PATIENTS WITH KNOWN OR SUSPECTED ISCHEMIC HEART DISEASE

A. History (Table 1-10)

1. **Silent Myocardial Ischemia.** A history of ischemic heart disease or an abnormal ECG suggestive of a previous MI is associated with an increased incidence of silent myocardial ischemia. Treatment of silent myocardial ischemia is the same as that for classic angina pectoris.
2. **Previous Myocardial Infarction.** Acute (1 to 7 days) and recent (8 to 30 days) MI and UA incur the highest risk of perioperative myocardial ischemia, MI, and cardiac death.
   a. Elective surgery should be delayed for more than 30 days after acute MI.
   b. Elective noncardiac surgery should be delayed for 4 to 6 weeks after coronary angioplasty.
   c. Elective noncardiac surgery should be delayed for at least 6 weeks after PCI with BMS placement and as long as 12 months after DES placement. Elective noncardiac surgery should be delayed for 6 weeks after CABG surgery.

TABLE 1-10 ■ **Clinical Predictors of Increased Perioperative Cardiovascular Risk**

MAJOR
Unstable coronary syndromes
Acute or recent myocardial infarction (MI) with evidence of significant ischemic risk by clinical symptoms or noninvasive study
Unstable or severe angina
Decompensated heart failure
Significant dysrhythmias
High-grade atrioventricular block
Symptomatic ventricular dysrhythmias in the presence of underlying heart disease
Supraventricular dysrhythmias with uncontrolled ventricular rate
Severe valvular heart disease
INTERMEDIATE
Mild angina pectoris
Previous MI by history or Q waves on electrocardiogram (ECG)
Compensated or previous heart failure
Diabetes mellitus (particularly insulin dependent)
Renal insufficiency
MINOR
Advanced age (older than 70 years)
Abnormal ECG (left ventricular hypertrophy, left bundle branch block, ST-T abnormalities)
Rhythm other than sinus
Low functional capacity
History of stroke
Uncontrolled systemic hypertension

Adapted from Fleisher LA, Beckman JA, Brown KA, et al. ACC/AHA 2006 guideline update on perioperative cardiovascular evaluation for noncardiac surgery: focused update on perioperative beta-blocker therapy: a report of the American College of Cardiology/American Heart Association Task Force on Practice Guidelines. *Circulation.* 2006;113:2662-2674, with permission.

3. **Co-existing Noncardiac Diseases.** The history should elicit symptoms of relevant co-existing noncardiac diseases (peripheral vascular disease, syncope, cough, dyspnea, orthopnea, paroxysmal nocturnal dyspnea, history of cigarette smoking, renal insufficiency, and diabetes mellitus).
4. **Current Medications.** The presence of effective β-blockade is suggested by a resting heart rate of 50 to 60 beats per minute. Many recommend withholding angiotensin-converting enzyme inhibitors (ACEIs) for 24 hours before surgical procedures involving significant fluid shifts or blood loss. A history of current use of clopidogrel and ticlopidine precludes neuraxial anesthesia. Both can also increase the risk of perioperative bleeding and necessitate platelet transfusion in urgent clinical situations.

B. **Physical Examination.** The physical examination findings of patients with ischemic heart disease are often normal (Table 1-11).

C. **Specialized Preoperative Testing** (Table 1-12)

VII. MANAGEMENT OF ANESTHESIA IN PATIENTS WITH KNOWN OR SUSPECTED ISCHEMIC HEART DISEASE UNDERGOING NONCARDIAC SURGERY

The preoperative assessment of patients with ischemic heart disease or risk factors for ischemic heart disease is geared toward (1) determining the extent of ischemic heart disease and any previous interventions (CABG, PCI), (2) determining the severity and stability of the disease, and (3) reviewing medical therapy and noting drugs that can increase the risk of surgical bleeding or contraindicate a particular anesthetic technique.

A. **Risk Stratification.** For stable patients undergoing elective major noncardiac surgery, six independent predictors of major cardiac complications have been described in Lee's Revised Cardiac Risk Index (Table 1-13). The presence of several risk factors increases the incidence

TABLE 1-11 ■ Possible Physical Examination Findings in Patients with Ischemic Heart Disease

Left ventricular failure (S_3 gallop, rales)
Right ventricular failure (jugular venous distention, peripheral edema)
Cerebrovascular disease (carotid bruit)
Orthostatic hypotension (caused by antihypertensive medication)

TABLE 1-12 ■ Specialized Preoperative Testing in Patients with Ischemic Heart Disease

Preoperative stress test—usually not indicated in patients with stable coronary disease and acceptable exercise tolerance
Echocardiography—can assess left ventricular EF and valve function
Stress echocardiography—wall motion abnormalities during pharmacologic stress testing (atropine, dipyridamole, dobutamine) can indicate presence and extent of ischemic heart disease
Radionuclide ventriculography—can evaluate left ventricular EF
Thallium scintigraphy—"cold spots" show areas of possible ischemia or infarction
Computed tomography—can visualize coronary artery calcifications
Positron emission tomography—demonstrates regional myocardial blood flow and metabolism

EF, Ejection fraction.

TABLE 1-13 ■ Cardiac Risk Factors in Patients Undergoing Elective Major Noncardiac Surgery

1. High-risk surgery
   - Abdominal aortic aneurysm
   - Peripheral vascular operation
   - Thoracotomy
   - Major abdominal operation
2. Ischemic heart disease
   - History of myocardial infarction
   - History of a positive exercise test result
   - Current complaints of angina pectoris
   - Use of nitrate therapy
   - Q waves on electrocardiogram
3. Congestive heart failure
   - History of congestive heart failure
   - History of pulmonary edema
   - History of paroxysmal nocturnal dyspnea
   - Physical examination showing rales or S_3 gallop
   - Chest radiograph showing pulmonary vascular redistribution
4. Cerebrovascular disease
   - History of stroke
   - History of transient ischemic attack
5. Insulin-dependent diabetes mellitus
6. Preoperative serum creatinine concentration >2 mg/dL

Adapted from Lee TH, Marcantonio ER, Mangione CM, et al. Derivation and prospective validation of a simple index for prediction of cardiac risk of major noncardiac surgery. *Circulation.* 1999;100:1043-1049, with permission.

of postoperative cardiac complications. These risk factors have been incorporated into the American College of Cardiology/American Heart Association (ACC/AHA) guidelines for perioperative cardiovascular evaluation for noncardiac surgery. Preoperative intervention is rarely necessary just to lower the risk of surgery. Interventions are indicated or not indicated irrespective of the need for surgery. Preoperative testing should be performed only if it is likely to influence perioperative management. The need for perioperative cardiac evaluation is determined in several steps.

1. Assess the urgency of surgery. The need for emergency surgery takes precedence over the need for additional workup.
2. Assess whether the patient has undergone revascularization and whether and when the patient underwent invasive or noninvasive cardiac evaluation (Figure 1-1).
3. If no prior revascularization was performed, stratify risk according to clinical risk factors (Table 1-14), surgery-specific risk factors (Table 1-15), and functional capacity (≥4 metabolic equivalent tasks [METs]). Patients able to meet a 4-MET demand during normal daily activities without chest pain or dyspnea have good functional capacity. Patients with two of the following three factors—high-risk surgery, low exercise tolerance, and moderate clinical risk factors—could be considered for further cardiac evaluation. Patients who have low functional capacity or in whom it is difficult to assess functional capacity are good candidates for further evaluation (Figure 1-2).

B. Management after Risk Stratification. Three therapeutic options are available before elective noncardiac surgery: (1) revascularization by surgery, (2) revascularization by PCI, and (3) optimal medical management.

1. **Coronary Artery Bypass Grafting.** The indications for preoperative coronary revascularization are the same as those in the nonoperative setting.

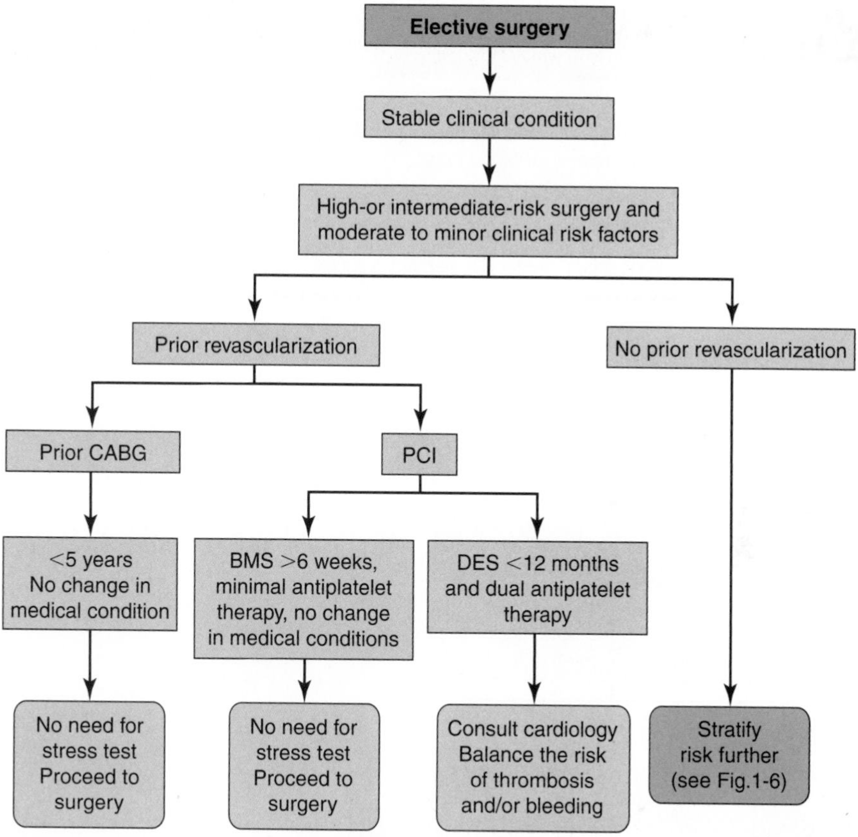

FIGURE 1-1 ■ Algorithm for preoperative assessment of patients with ischemic heart disease scheduled for elective intermediate- to high-risk surgery who are in stable clinical condition with moderate clinical risk factors. Determine whether previous coronary intervention was performed, and assess the stability of the cardiac condition. If no change in cardiac condition has occurred, proceed with surgery with medical management. For patients with intracoronary stents, determine the date of insertion and location of the stent(s), the kind of stent(s), and the status of current antiplatelet therapy. Patients receiving antiplatelet therapy may require consultation with the cardiologist and the surgeon. *BMS,* Bare metal stent; *CABG,* coronary artery bypass grafting; *DES,* drug-eluting stent; *PCI,* percutaneous coronary intervention.

TABLE 1-14 ■ Clinical Risk Factors for Perioperative Cardiac Risk

Major risk factors: may require delay of elective surgery and cardiology evaluation	Unstable coronary syndrome, decompensated heart failure, significant dysrhythmias, severe valvular heart disease
Intermediate risk factors: well-validated markers of increased cardiac risk	Stable angina, previous myocardial infarction, compensated or previous heart failure, insulin-dependent diabetes mellitus, renal insufficiency
Minor risk factors: markers of coronary disease not demonstrated to increase perioperative risk	Hypertension, left bundle branch block, nonspecific ST-T wave changes, history of stroke

TABLE 1-15 ■ Surgery-Specific Risk Factors for Perioperative Cardiac Complications

High-risk surgery	Emergency major surgery, aortic or other major vascular surgery, peripheral vascular surgery, prolonged surgery involving large fluid shifts and/or blood loss
Intermediate-risk surgery	Carotid endarterectomy, head and neck surgery, intraperitoneal and intrathoracic surgery, orthopedic surgery, prostate surgery
Low-risk surgery	Endoscopic surgery, superficial surgery, cataract surgery, breast surgery

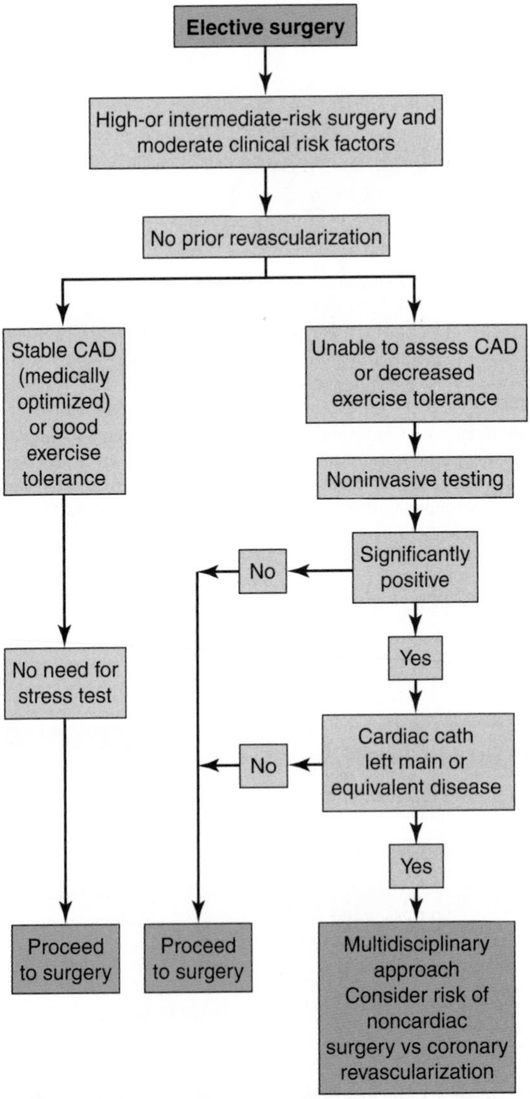

FIGURE 1-2 ■ Algorithm for preoperative assessment of patients scheduled for intermediate- to high-risk surgery who have moderate clinical risk factors and poor exercise tolerance (or in whom exercise tolerance cannot be established). Consider noninvasive stress testing to determine whether significant myocardium is at risk. If significant myocardium is at risk, consider coronary angiography. For patients with one or two clinical risk factors, consider noninvasive stress testing only if it will affect patient management; otherwise proceed to surgery with medical management. *CAD,* Coronary artery disease.

2. **Percutaneous Coronary Intervention.** There is no value in preoperative coronary intervention in patients with stable ischemic heart disease. Angioplasty is now often accompanied by stenting, which requires postprocedure antiplatelet therapy to prevent acute coronary thrombosis and maintain long-term vessel patency. Discontinuation of antiplatelet therapy predisposes to stent thrombosis with significant morbidity and mortality.
3. **Pharmacologic Management**
   a. β-Blockers: Currently, the only class I recommendation is to continue them perioperatively in patients who are already receiving them. Other patients who may benefit from β-blockers include those undergoing vascular surgery who have multiple cardiac risk factors and those who show reversible cardiac ischemia on preoperative testing.
   b. α_2-Agonists have analgesic, sedative, and sympatholytic effects and may be useful in patients in whom β-blockers are contraindicated.
   c. Statin therapy may be beneficial if started 1 to 4 weeks before high-risk surgery. Discontinuation of statins in the perioperative period is not recommended, due to a possible rebound effect.
   d. Perioperative hyperglycemia must be controlled, with a goal of keeping perioperative glucose levels under 180 mg/dL.
   e. Anxiety must be treated.

C. **Intraoperative Management.** Goals are (1) to prevent myocardial ischemia by optimizing myocardial oxygen supply and reducing myocardial oxygen demand and (2) to monitor for and treat ischemia. Factors influencing the balance of myocardial oxygen demand and supply are summarized in Table 1-16. Avoid persistent and excessive changes in heart rate and systemic blood pressure. A common recommendation is to keep the heart rate and blood pressure within 20% of the normal awake value. Increased heart rate increases myocardial oxygen requirements while decreasing supply because of decreased diastolic coronary artery perfusion time. HTN results in increased myocardial oxygen demand that is only partially offset by increased coronary perfusion pressure. Maintenance of the balance between myocardial oxygen supply and demand is more important than the specific anesthetic technique or drugs selected to produce anesthesia and muscle relaxation.

TABLE 1-16 ■ Intraoperative Events that Influence the Balance Between Myocardial Oxygen Delivery and Myocardial Oxygen Requirements

DECREASED OXYGEN DELIVERY
Decreased coronary blood flow
Tachycardia
Diastolic hypotension
Hypocapnia (coronary artery vasoconstriction)
Coronary artery spasm
Decreased oxygen content
Anemia
Arterial hypoxemia
Shift of the oxyhemoglobin dissociation curve to the left
INCREASED OXYGEN REQUIREMENTS
Sympathetic nervous system stimulation
Tachycardia
Hypertension
Increased myocardial contractility
Increased afterload
Increased preload

1. **Induction of Anesthesia.** Many different induction drugs are appropriate. (Ketamine is an unlikely choice because it increases heart rate and systemic blood pressure.) Myocardial ischemia may accompany the sympathetic nervous system stimulation that results from direct laryngoscopy and tracheal intubation. Short-duration direct laryngoscopy (≤15 seconds) and/or administration of drugs to minimize the pressor response, such as laryngotracheal lidocaine, intravenous lidocaine, esmolol, and/or fentanyl, is indicated.
2. **Maintenance of Anesthesia.** Drug selection for maintenance of anesthesia is based in part on the patient's estimated left ventricular function.
   - *a.* In patients with normal left ventricular function, controlled myocardial depression with a volatile anesthetic (with or without nitrous oxide) may minimize sympathetic nervous system activity during intense stimulation. However, volatile agents can be detrimental if drug-induced hypotension leads to decreases in coronary perfusion pressure. Equally acceptable is use of a nitrous oxide–opioid technique with the addition of a volatile anesthetic to treat undesirable increases in blood pressure at critical points.
   - *b.* In patients with severely impaired left ventricular function, opioids may be selected for maintenance of anesthesia. The addition of nitrous oxide, a benzodiazepine, or a low-dose volatile anesthetic should be considered because total amnesia cannot be ensured with an opioid alone.
   - *c.* Regional anesthesia is acceptable in patients with ischemic heart disease, but decreases in blood pressure associated with epidural or spinal anesthesia must be controlled. Hypotension that exceeds 20% of the preblock blood pressure should be treated promptly. Despite presumed benefits of regional anesthesia, the postoperative cardiac morbidity and mortality are not significantly different between general and regional anesthesia.
3. **Choice of Muscle Relaxant.** Muscle relaxants with minimal or no effect on heart rate and systemic blood pressure (vecuronium, rocuronium, cisatracurium) are preferred. Histamine release and the resulting decrease in blood pressure caused by atracurium are less desirable. Glycopyrrolate is preferred to atropine for the anticholinergic component in combination therapy to reverse neuromuscular blockade, because it is associated with less increase in heart rate.
4. **Monitoring.** Intraoperative monitoring should aim for early detection of myocardial ischemia. However, most myocardial ischemia occurs in the absence of hemodynamic alterations, so one should be cautious when endorsing routine use of expensive or complex monitors to detect myocardial ischemia (Table 1-17).
5. **Intraoperative Management of Myocardial Ischemia.** Treatment of myocardial ischemia should be instituted when there are 1-mm or greater ST-segment changes on the ECG. A persistent increase in heart rate can be treated by intravenous administration of a β-blocker (e.g., esmolol). Nitroglycerin is appropriate when myocardial ischemia is associated with a normal to modestly elevated blood pressure. Hypotension is treated with

TABLE 1-17 ■ Intraoperative Monitoring for Myocardial Ischemia

Electrocardiogram (ECG)	Ischemia is characterized by ST-segment elevation or depression of ≥1 mm. The degree of ST change parallels the severity of ischemia. Monitoring of three leads (either II, V_4, and V_5 or V_3, V_4, and V_5) is recommended.
Pulmonary artery catheter (PAC)	Increased pulmonary capillary wedge pressure may indicate ischemia. V waves indicate mitral regurgitation and papillary muscle dysfunction. PAC can guide treatment of myocardial dysfunction.
Transesophageal echocardiography	Development of regional wall motion abnormalities precedes ECG changes.

sympathomimetic drugs to restore coronary perfusion pressure. Fluid infusion can be useful to help restore blood pressure.

D. Postoperative Management

1. Prevent or treat events that increase myocardial oxygen demand, such as pain, shivering, hypercarbia, and sepsis.
2. Avoid or treat conditions that lead to decreased myocardial oxygen supply, such as anemia, hypoxemia, hypovolemia, and hypotension.
3. Continue treatments in the perioperative period, such as β-blockers, that reduce the risks of adverse cardiac events.
4. Manage the timing of weaning and tracheal extubation to avoid detrimental alterations in blood pressure and heart rate.
5. Continuous ECG monitoring is useful for detecting postoperative myocardial ischemia, which is often silent.

VIII. CARDIAC TRANSPLANTATION

Heart transplantation is most often considered in patients with end-stage heart failure caused by dilated cardiomyopathy or ischemic heart disease. Preoperatively, the ejection fraction is often less than 20%. Irreversible pulmonary HTN is a contraindication to cardiac transplantation.

A. Management of Anesthesia

1. Etomidate is a preferred induction agent because it has little effect on hemodynamics. Opioids are often chosen for maintenance of anesthesia. Volatile anesthetics may produce undesirable degrees of myocardial depression and peripheral vasodilation. Nitrous oxide is rarely used because of its additive effects on myocardial depression, detrimental effects on pulmonary artery pressure, and potential to enlarge air emboli.
2. After cardiopulmonary bypass, isoproterenol is commonly administered to support heart rate and lower pulmonary artery pressure. Additional treatments of pulmonary HTN may include a prostaglandin, nitric oxide, or a phosphodiesterase inhibitor.
3. The denervated transplanted heart initially assumes an intrinsic heart rate of about 110 beats per minute, which is not responsive to drugs that normally raise or lower the heart rate. After transplantation, about 25% of patients eventually develop bradycardia that necessitates the use of a permanent cardiac pacemaker. Cardiac transplant patients tolerate hypovolemia poorly because the heart is denervated, that is, it no longer has innervation from sympathetic or parasympathetic nerve fibers because these fibers are cut during the transplant surgery. The transplanted heart does respond to direct-acting catecholamines, but drugs such as ephedrine that act by indirect mechanisms have less effect. Vasopressin may be needed to treat severe hypotension unresponsive to catecholamines.

B. Postoperative Complications

1. Early postoperative morbidity after heart transplantation surgery is usually related to sepsis and rejection. The most common early cause of death after cardiac transplantation is opportunistic infection as a result of immunosuppressive therapy. CHF and development of dysrhythmias can be late signs of rejection. Nephrotoxicity is a potential complication of cyclosporine therapy. Long-term corticosteroid use can result in skeletal demineralization and glucose intolerance.
2. Late complications of cardiac transplantation include development of coronary artery disease in the allograft and an increased incidence of cancer.

C. Anesthetic Considerations in Heart Transplant Recipients

1. Cardiac Innervation

a. The transplanted heart has no sympathetic, parasympathetic, or sensory innervation, and the loss of vagal tone results in a higher-than-normal resting heart rate. Carotid sinus massage and the Valsalva maneuver have no effect on heart rate. There is no sympathetic response to direct laryngoscopy and tracheal intubation, and the denervated heart has a blunted heart rate response to light anesthesia or intense pain. The transplanted heart is unable to increase its heart rate immediately in response to hypovolemia or hypotension but responds instead with an increase in stroke volume (Frank-Starling mechanism).

b. Adrenergic receptors are intact on the transplanted heart, which will eventually respond to circulating catecholamines.

2. Responses to Drugs

a. Responses to direct-acting sympathomimetic drugs are intact. Epinephrine, isoproterenol, and dobutamine have similar effects in normal and denervated hearts.

b. Indirect-acting sympathomimetics such as ephedrine have a blunted effect on denervated hearts.

c. Vagolytic drugs such as atropine do not increase the heart rate. Pancuronium does not increase the heart rate, and neostigmine and other anticholinesterases do not slow the heart rate of transplanted hearts.

3. Preoperative Evaluation

a. Heart transplant recipients may have ongoing rejection manifesting as myocardial dysfunction, accelerated coronary atherosclerosis, or dysrhythmias.

b. All preoperative drug therapy must be continued, and proper functioning of a cardiac pacemaker, if in place, must be confirmed. Cyclosporine-induced HTN may require treatment with calcium channel–blocking drugs or ACEIs. Cyclosporine-induced nephrotoxicity may manifest as an increased creatinine concentration, and anesthetic drugs excreted mainly by renal clearance mechanisms should then be avoided.

c. Proper hydration is important and should be confirmed preoperatively because heart transplant patients are preload dependent.

4. Management of Anesthesia

a. Maintain intravascular volume. These patients are preload dependent, and the denervated heart is unable to respond to sudden shifts in blood volume with an increase in heart rate.

b. General anesthesia is often preferable to spinal or epidural anesthesia because of a potentially impaired response to vasodilation. Avoid significant vasodilation and acute reductions in preload. Volatile agents are usually well tolerated in heart transplant patients who do not have significant heart failure.

c. Pay careful attention to aseptic technique and antibiotic prophylaxis. Patients are immunosuppressed and have increased susceptibility to infection.

CHAPTER 2

Valvular Heart Disease

Management of the patient with valvular heart disease during the perioperative period requires an understanding of the hemodynamic alterations that accompany valvular dysfunction. The most commonly encountered cardiac valve lesions produce *pressure overload* (mitral stenosis [MS], aortic stenosis [AS]) or *volume overload* (mitral regurgitation [MR], aortic regurgitation [AR]) on the left atrium or left ventricle. Anesthetic management during the perioperative period is based on the likely effects of drug-induced changes in cardiac rhythm, heart rate, preload, afterload, myocardial contractility, systemic blood pressure, systemic vascular resistance, and pulmonary vascular resistance relative to the pathophysiology of the heart disease.

I. PREOPERATIVE EVALUATION

Preoperative evaluation of patients with valvular heart disease includes assessment of (1) the severity of the cardiac disease, (2) the degree of impaired myocardial contractility, and (3) the presence of associated major organ system disease. Recognition of compensatory mechanisms for maintaining cardiac output (increased sympathetic nervous system activity, cardiac hypertrophy) and knowledge of current drug therapy are important. The presence of prosthetic heart valves requires special consideration in the preoperative evaluation, especially if noncardiac surgery is planned.

A. **History and Physical Examination.** Defining exercise tolerance is necessary to evaluate cardiac reserve in the presence of valvular heart disease and to provide a functional classification according to the criteria established by the New York Heart Association (Table 2-1). Congestive heart failure (CHF) is a common complication of chronic valvular heart disease. Elective surgery should be deferred until CHF can be treated and myocardial contractility optimized. The character, location, intensity, and direction of radiation of a heart murmur provide clues to the location and severity of the valvular lesion. Cardiac dysrhythmias, especially atrial fibrillation, are common. Valvular heart disease and ischemic heart disease often co-exist.

B. **Drug Therapy.** Modern drug therapy for valvular heart disease may include β-blockers, calcium channel blockers, and digitalis for heart rate control; angiotensin-converting enzyme inhibitors (ACEIs) and vasodilators to control blood pressure and afterload; and diuretics, inotropes, and vasodilators as needed to control heart failure. Antidysrhythmic therapy may also be necessary.

C. **Laboratory Data**

   1. **Electrocardiography.** The electrocardiogram (ECG) often exhibits broad and notched P waves (P mitrale), left and/or right axis deviation, and high voltage. Dysrhythmias, conduction abnormalities, and evidence of ischemia or previous infarction may be present.
   2. **Chest Radiography.** The chest radiograph may show cardiomegaly (heart size exceeds 50% of the internal width of the thoracic cage on a posteroanterior chest radiograph).
   3. **Echocardiography with Doppler Color Flow Imaging.** Doppler echocardiography is essential for noninvasive evaluation of valvular heart disease (Table 2-2).

TABLE 2-1 ■ New York Heart Association Functional Classification of Patients with Heart Disease

CLASS	DESCRIPTION
I	Asymptomatic
II	Symptoms with ordinary activity but comfortable at rest
III	Symptoms with minimal activity but comfortable at rest
IV	Symptoms at rest

TABLE 2-2 ■ Doppler Echocardiography in Evaluation of Valvular Heart Disease

Determine significance of cardiac murmurs.
Identify hemodynamic abnormalities associated with physical findings.
Determine transvalvular pressure gradient.
Determine valve area.
Determine ventricular ejection fraction.
Diagnose valvular regurgitation.
Evaluate prosthetic valve function.

TABLE 2-3 ■ Complications Associated with Prosthetic Heart Valves

Valve thrombosis
Systemic embolization
Structural failure
Hemolysis
Paravalvular leak
Endocarditis

4. **Cardiac Catheterization.** Cardiac catheterization can demonstrate the presence and severity of valvular stenosis and/or regurgitation, coronary artery disease, intracardiac shunting, transvalvular pressure gradients, the presence of pulmonary hypertension, and the presence of right-sided heart failure.

D. **Presence of Prosthetic Heart Valves**

1. **Assessment of Prosthetic Heart Valve Function.** Prosthetic heart valve dysfunction is suggested by the appearance of a new murmur or a change in an existing murmur. Transesophageal echocardiography is indicated for evaluation of the mitral valve. Cardiac catheterization permits measurement of transvalvular pressure gradients.
2. **Complications Associated with Prosthetic Heart Valves** (Table 2-3). Patients with mechanical prosthetic heart valves require long-term anticoagulant therapy, whereas those with bioprosthetic valves may not. Antibiotic prophylaxis is necessary in certain situations to decrease the risk of endocarditis.
3. **Management of Anticoagulation in Patients with Prosthetic Heart Valves**
   a. Anticoagulation can be continued for minor surgery in which blood loss is expected to be minimal.

TABLE 2-4 ■ Cardiac Conditions Associated with the Highest Risk of Adverse Outcomes from Endocarditis
1. Prosthetic cardiac valve or prosthetic material used for cardiac valve repair
2. Previous infective endocarditis
3. Congenital heart disease:
Unrepaired cyanotic congenital heart disease, including palliative shunts and conduits
Completely repaired congenital heart defect with prosthetic material or device, whether placed by surgery or by catheter intervention, during the first 6 months after the procedure*
Repaired congenital heart disease with residual defects at the site or adjacent to the site of a prosthetic patch or prosthetic device (which inhibit endothelialization)
4. Cardiac transplantation recipients who develop cardiac valve pathology

From Wilson W, Taubert KA, Gewitz M, et al. Prevention of infective endocarditis. Guidelines from the American Heart Association. *Circulation*. 2007;116:1736-1754, with permission.

Except for the conditions listed above, antibiotic prophylaxis is no longer recommended for any other form of congenital heart disease.

*Prophylaxis is reasonable because endothelialization of prosthetic material occurs within 6 months after the procedure.

b. Discontinue warfarin 2 to 3 days preoperatively for surgery that may be associated with significant bleeding.

c. Substitute intravenous unfractionated heparin or subcutaneous low-molecular-weight (LMW) heparin for the warfarin. The day before surgery (LMW heparin) or 2 to 4 hours before surgery (intravenous unfractionated heparin) the heparin must be discontinued

d. Warfarin is contraindicated during pregnancy; administer subcutaneous unfractionated or LMW heparin. Low-dose aspirin may also be used in conjunction with heparin therapy.

E. Prevention of Bacterial Endocarditis

1. New American Heart Association (AHA) guidelines focus endocarditis prophylaxis only on patients with conditions listed in Table 2-4.
2. The recommendations regarding which antibiotic to use for endocarditis prophylaxis are not dissimilar from previous recommendations.
3. Antibiotic prophylaxis is recommended for the following procedures:
   a. Dental procedures that involve manipulation of gingival tissues or the periapical regions of teeth or perforation of the oral mucosa. Recommended antibiotics are listed in Table 2-5.
   b. Invasive procedures (i.e., those that involve incision or biopsy) on the respiratory tract or infected skin, skin structures, or musculoskeletal tissue. These infections are often polymicrobial laub only staphylococci and β-hemolytic streptococci are likely to cause infective endocarditis, A Therapeutic regimen consisting of an antistaphylococcal penicillin or a cephalosporin is commonly used. Vancomycin or clindamycin can be given to those allergic to penicillin or who have an infection with a methicillin-resistant strain of staphylococcus (MRSA).
4. Antibiotic prophylaxis *is not* recommended for genitourinary (GU) or gastrointestinal (GI) tract procedures.

II. MITRAL STENOSIS

A. Pathophysiology. The normal mitral orifice is 4 to 6 cm^2. Symptoms usually develop when the valve orifice is less than 1.5 cm^2. MS causes progressive mechanical obstruction to left ventricular diastolic filling, with resulting increase in left atrial volume and pressure. Stroke volume decreases during stress-induced tachycardia or when atrial contraction is lost, as in atrial fibrillation. Pulmonary venous pressure increases with the increase in left atrial pressure.

TABLE 2-5 ■ **Antibiotic Prophylaxis for Dental Procedures**

		REGIMEN: SINGLE DOSE 30 TO 60 MIN BEFORE PROCEDURE	
SITUATION	**AGENT**	**ADULTS**	**CHILDREN**
Oral	Amoxicillin	2 g	50 mg/kg
Unable to take oral medication	Ampicillin OR Cefazolin or ceftriaxone	2 g IM or IV 1 g IM or IV	50 mg/kg IM or IV 50 mg/kg IM or IV
Allergic to penicillins or ampicillin—oral	Cephalexin*† OR Clindamycin*† OR Azithromycin or clarithromycin	2 g 600 mg 500 mg	50 mg/kg 20 mg/kg 15 mg/kg
Allergic to penicillins or ampicillin and unable to take oral medication	Cefazolin or ceftriaxone† OR Clindamycin	1 g IM or IV 600 mg IM or IV	50 mg/kg IM or IV 20 mg/kg IM or IV

From Wilson W, Taubert KA, Gewitz M, et al. Prevention of infective endocarditis. Guidelines from the American Heart Association. *Circulation*. 2007;116:1736-1754, with permission.
*Or other first- or second-generation oral cephalosporin in equivalent adult or pediatric dosage.
†Cephalosporins should not be used in an individual with a history of anaphylaxis, angioedema, or urticaria with penicillins or ampicillin.
IM, Intramuscularly; *IV*, intravenously.

TABLE 2-6 ■ **Treatment of Mitral Stenosis**

1. Diuretics to reduce left atrial pressure
2. Heart rate control (β-blockers, digoxin, calcium channel blockers)
3. Anticoagulation therapy
4. Surgical correction (commissurotomy, valvuloplasty, valve reconstruction, valve replacement) when symptoms increase or evidence of pulmonary hypertension appears

Transudation of fluid into the pulmonary interstitial space results in decreased pulmonary compliance, increased work of breathing, and dyspnea on exertion. Overt pulmonary edema occurs when the pulmonary venous pressure exceeds the oncotic pressure of plasma proteins.

B. Diagnosis. Echocardiography is used to assess the severity of MS and to calculate valve area. Pulmonary hypertension is likely if the left atrial pressure is chronically above 25 mm Hg, which is common when the mitral valve area is less than 1 cm^2. Clinically, MS is recognized by the characteristic opening snap that occurs early in diastole and by a rumbling diastolic heart murmur best heard at the apex or in the axilla. Owing to stasis of blood in the left atrium, patients are at a higher risk of systemic thromboembolism. Decreased activity predisposes them to venous thromboembolism as well.

C. Treatment (Table 2-6)

D. Management of Anesthesia (Table 2-7)

1. Preoperative Medication. Preoperative medication is used to decrease anxiety-induced tachycardia. Drugs used for heart rate control should be continued. Diuretic-induced hypokalemia should be treated preoperatively. Anticoagulation should be discontinued for major surgery with anticipated significant blood loss. Neuraxial anesthesia may be acceptable in the absence of anticoagulation.

TABLE 2-7 ■ **Anesthetic Considerations for Patients with Mitral Stenosis**

PROBLEM	MANAGEMENT
Sinus tachycardia or rapid ventricular response to atrial fibrillation decreases cardiac output and can cause pulmonary edema	Administer intravenous β-blocker, calcium channel blocker, or digoxin. Cardioversion may be helpful if the atrial fibrillation is of new onset.
Congestive heart failure caused by central blood volume changes	Avoid excessive fluid administration, do not place patient in Trendelenburg's position
Sudden decrease in systemic vascular resistance with hypotension and increased heart rate decreases cardiac output	Administer sympathomimetic amines. Ephedrine may increase cardiac output but also increase heart rate; phenylephrine may be preferable because it avoids increases in heart rate.
Pulmonary hypertension and right-sided heart failure	Avoid hypercarbia, hypoxemia, lung hyperinflation. Right-sided heart failure may require inotropic support and pulmonary artery vasodilators.

2. **Induction of Anesthesia.** Avoid drugs likely to increase heart rate (e.g., ketamine) or to precipitate hypotension from histamine release.
3. **Maintenance of Anesthesia.** Anesthesia should be designed to minimize sustained changes in heart rate, myocardial contractility, and systemic and pulmonary vascular resistance. A nitrous-narcotic anesthetic or a balanced anesthetic with low concentrations of a volatile anesthetic usually achieves this goal. Nitrous oxide may cause pulmonary vasoconstriction, particularly if pulmonary hypertension is present.
4. **Monitoring.** Use of invasive monitoring depends on the complexity of the procedure and the severity of MS. Asymptomatic patients without evidence of pulmonary congestion do not generally require special monitoring. In patients with symptomatic MS, transesophageal echocardiography and/or continuous monitoring of intraarterial pressure, pulmonary artery pressure, and left atrial pressure should be considered.
5. **Postoperative Management.** In patients with MS, the risk of pulmonary edema and right-sided heart failure continues into the postoperative period. Pain and hypoventilation can cause increased heart rate and increased pulmonary vascular resistance. Patients may require continued mechanical ventilation, particularly after major thoracic or abdominal surgery. Anticoagulation should be resumed as soon as possible.

III. MITRAL REGURGITATION

A. **Pathophysiology.** MR is characterized by decreases in forward left ventricular stroke volume and cardiac output associated with increased left atrial pressure. Volume and pressure overload of the left atrium are especially increased in patients with combined MS and MR.

B. **Diagnosis.** MR is recognized clinically by the presence of a holosystolic apical murmur with radiation to the axilla. The ECG and chest radiograph may indicate left ventricular hypertrophy. Echocardiography documents the presence, severity, and sometimes the cause of MR. The presence of a V wave in a pulmonary artery occlusion pressure waveform reflects regurgitant flow through the mitral valve.

C. **Treatment.** Surgical repair or replacement is indicated when the ejection fraction is less than 0.6 or before the left ventricle end-systolic dimension is 45 mm or greater. Symptomatic patients should undergo mitral valve surgery even if ejection fraction is normal. Although vasodilators are useful in the treatment of acute MR, there is no apparent benefit to long-term use of vasodilator drugs in *asymptomatic* patients with chronic MR.

TABLE 2-8 ■ Anesthetic Considerations for Patients with Mitral Regurgitation
Prevent bradycardia.
Prevent increases in systemic vascular resistance.
Minimize drug-induced myocardial depression.
Monitor the magnitude of regurgitant flow with a pulmonary artery catheter (size of the V wave) and/or echocardiography.

ACEIs or β-blockers and biventricular pacing have been shown to decrease *functional* MR (usually due to a dilated cardiomyopathy) and improve symptoms and exercise tolerance in symptomatic patients.

D. Management of Anesthesia (Table 2-8). Modest increases in heart rate and reduction in left ventricular afterload (e.g., with nitroprusside) with or without inotropic drugs improve left ventricular output. The decrease in systemic vascular resistance caused by regional anesthesia may be beneficial in some patients.

1. **Induction of Anesthesia.** Avoid increases in systemic vascular resistance or decreases in heart rate. Pancuronium may be a useful muscle relaxant due to a modest increase in heart rate.
2. **Maintenance of Anesthesia.** The increase in heart rate and decrease in systemic vascular resistance plus the minimal negative inotropic effects of isoflurane, desflurane, and sevoflurane make them all acceptable choices for maintenance of anesthesia. When myocardial function is severely compromised, opioid-based anesthesia may be considered, although caution is advised because narcotics can produce significant bradycardia that is very deleterious in severe MR.
3. **Monitoring.** Invasive monitoring is not needed for minor surgery in asymptomatic patients. In patients with severe MR, pulmonary artery occlusion pressure monitoring may be helpful.

IV. MITRAL VALVE PROLAPSE

Mitral valve prolapse (MVP) is defined as the prolapse of one or both mitral leaflets into the left atrium during systole with or without MR. It is usually a benign condition, affecting 1% to 2.5% of the population; however, MVP can have devastating complications, such as cerebral embolic events, infective endocarditis, severe MR requiring surgery, dysrhythmias, and sudden death.

A. Diagnosis. The diagnosis of MVP is based on echocardiographic findings of valve prolapse of 2 mm or more above the mitral annulus. Cardiac dysrhythmias associated with MVP include both supraventricular and ventricular dysrhythmias and respond well to β-blocker therapy. Cardiac conduction abnormalities are not uncommon.

B. Management of Anesthesia. Management of anesthesia in patients with MVP follows the same principles outlined earlier for patients with MR (see Table 2-8). The degree of MVP is adversely affected by increased ventricular emptying, decreased left ventricular filling, and smaller ventricular dimensions, such as occur with increased myocardial contractility, decreased systemic vascular resistance, upright posture, and hypovolemia.

1. **Preoperative Evaluation.** Preoperative evaluation should focus on distinguishing patients with purely functional disease (often women younger than 45 years treated with β-blockers) from patients with significant MR (older men with symptoms of mild to moderate CHF). Patients taking β-blockers should continue taking them perioperatively. Anxiolytic medications should be used to avoid tachycardia. Antithrombotic medications such as aspirin or warfarin may be continued in patients undergoing minor surgery when significant blood loss is not expected.
2. **Selection of Anesthetic Technique.** Most patients with MVP have normal left ventricular function; volatile agents are well tolerated. The decrease in systemic vascular resistance associated with regional anesthesia should be offset by fluid administration to avoid

TABLE 2-9 ■ **Severity of Aortic Stenosis Measured by Echocardiography**

	MILD	MODERATE	SEVERE
Mean transvalvular pressure gradient (mm Hg)	<20	20-50	>50
Peak transvalvular pressure gradient (mm Hg)	<36	>50	>80
Aortic valve area (cm^2)	1.0-1.5	0.8-1.0	<0.8

changes in left ventricular volume that could adversely affect MVP and the degree of mitral regurgitation.

3. **Induction of Anesthesia.** Avoid sudden decreases in systemic vascular resistance. Etomidate is an attractive choice for induction in patients with significant MVP, because it causes minimal myocardial depression or alterations in sympathetic nervous system activity. Ketamine stimulates the sympathetic nervous system and enhances the degree of prolapse and regurgitation.
4. **Maintenance of Anesthesia.** Minimize sympathetic nervous system activation resulting from surgical stimuli (volatile anesthetics with or without nitrous oxide and/or opioids). Unexpected ventricular dysrhythmias can occur, especially during operations performed in the head-up or sitting position, presumably because of increased left ventricular emptying and accentuation of MVP. Generous intravenous fluid therapy and prompt replacement of intraoperative blood loss is indicated. If vasopressors are needed, an α-agonist such as phenylephrine is more desirable than inotropes, which may enhance MVP and MR.
5. **Monitoring.** Routine monitoring is all that is necessary in the majority of patients with MVP. An intraarterial catheter and pulmonary artery catheter are needed only in patients with significant MR and left ventricular dysfunction.

V. AORTIC STENOSIS

A. **Pathophysiology.** The normal aortic valve area is 2.5 to 3.5 cm^2. Obstruction to ejection of blood into the aorta caused by decreases in the aortic valve area necessitates an increase in left ventricular pressure to maintain forward stroke volume. Angina pectoris may occur in patients with AS despite the absence of coronary disease. *Severe AS* is defined as transvalvular pressure gradients greater than 50 mm Hg and/or a valve area of less than 0.8 cm^2.

B. **Diagnosis.** The classic symptoms of *critical* AS are angina pectoris, syncope, and CHF. Physical examination reveals a characteristic systolic murmur heard best in the aortic area, often radiating to the neck. Because many patients with AS are asymptomatic, it is important to listen for the systolic murmur of AS in older patients scheduled for surgery. The ECG may demonstrate left ventricular hypertrophy.

1. *Echocardiography* with Doppler examination of the aortic valve provides a more accurate assessment of the severity of AS (Table 2-9) than does clinical evaluation.
2. *Cardiac catheterization* and coronary angiography may be necessary when the severity of AS cannot be determined by echocardiography.
3. *Exercise stress testing* may be useful in risk-stratifying asymptomatic patients with moderate to severe AS. Patients with exercise-induced symptoms may benefit from aortic valve replacement.

C. **Treatment.** In asymptomatic patients with AS, it appears to be safe to continue medical management and delay valve replacement surgery until symptoms develop. Surgical and procedural interventions include balloon valvotomy and valve replacement by traditional open heart surgery or by transcatheter techniques.

TABLE 2-10 ■ Anesthetic Considerations in Patients with Aortic Stenosis
Maintain normal sinus rhythm.
Avoid bradycardia or tachycardia.
Avoid hypotension.
Optimize intravascular fluid volume to maintain venous return and left ventricular filling.

D. Management of Anesthesia. Management of anesthesia in patients with AS includes the prevention of hypotension and any hemodynamic change that will decrease cardiac output (Table 2-10). Cardiopulmonary resuscitation is unlikely to be effective in patients with AS because it is difficult, if not impossible, to create an adequate stroke volume across a stenotic aortic valve with cardiac compressions.

1. **Induction of Anesthesia.** General anesthesia is usually preferable to epidural or spinal anesthesia, which can decrease systemic vascular resistance and precipitate significant hypotension. Induction of anesthesia can be accomplished with an intravenous induction drug that does not decrease systemic vascular resistance.
2. **Maintenance of Anesthesia.** Management of anesthesia can be accomplished with a combination of nitrous oxide and volatile anesthetic and opioids or by opioids alone. Decreases in systemic vascular resistance are undesirable. Intravascular fluid volume should be maintained at normal levels. The onset of junctional rhythm or bradycardia requires prompt treatment with glycopyrrolate, atropine, or ephedrine. Persistent tachycardia can be treated with β-antagonists such as esmolol. Supraventricular tachycardia should be promptly terminated with electrical cardioversion. Lidocaine and a defibrillator should be kept available, as these patients have a propensity to develop ventricular dysrhythmias.
3. **Monitoring.** The use of invasive monitoring is determined by the complexity of the surgery and severity of AS and may include continuous arterial blood pressure monitoring, a pulmonary artery catheter, and/or transesophageal echocardiography.

VI. AORTIC REGURGITATION

A. Pathophysiology. Regurgitation of some of the ejected stroke volume from the aorta back into the right ventricle during diastole results in a combined pressure and volume overload on the left ventricle. The magnitude of the regurgitant volume depends on (1) the duration of diastole, which is determined by heart rate, and (2) the pressure gradient across the aortic valve, which is dependent on systemic vascular resistance. The magnitude of AR is decreased by tachycardia and peripheral vasodilation. Patients with acute AR experience severe left ventricular volume overload before compensation can occur and therefore may have presenting signs of coronary ischemia, rapid deterioration in left ventricular function, and heart failure.

B. Diagnosis. AR is recognized clinically by a characteristic diastolic murmur heard best along the right sternal border, and peripheral signs of a hyperdynamic circulation (widened pulse pressure, decreased diastolic blood pressure, bounding pulses). Signs of left ventricular hypertrophy may be seen on the chest radiograph and ECG. Echocardiography with Doppler examination identifies the presence and severity of AR.

C. Treatment. Surgical replacement of a diseased aortic valve is recommended before the onset of permanent left ventricular dysfunction, even in asymptomatic patients. Medical therapy of AR is directed at decreasing systolic hypertension and ventricular wall stress and improving left ventricular function.

D. Management of Anesthesia (Table 2-11). Management of anesthesia in patients with AR is directed toward maintaining forward left ventricular stroke volume. The heart rate should be

TABLE 2-11 ■ Anesthetic Considerations in Patients with Aortic Regurgitation

Avoid bradycardia.
Avoid increases in systemic vascular resistance.
Minimize myocardial depression.

kept at greater than 80 beats per minute because bradycardia increases the amount of backward blood flow; leading to left ventricular volume overload. Abrupt increases in systemic vascular resistance can precipitate left ventricular failure, requiring treatment with a vasodilator for afterload reduction and an inotrope to increase contractility. Overall, modest increases in heart rate and modest decreases in systemic vascular resistance are reasonable hemodynamic goals.

1. **Induction of Anesthesia.** Induction of anesthesia in the presence of AR can be achieved with any intravenous induction drug with or without inhalation anesthesia that ideally does not decrease heart rate or increase systemic vascular resistance.
2. **Maintenance of Anesthesia.** Maintenance of anesthesia is often provided with nitrous oxide plus a volatile anesthetic and/or opioid. Intravascular fluid volume should be maintained at normal levels to provide for adequate cardiac preload. Bradycardia and junctional rhythm require prompt treatment.
3. **Monitoring.** Minor surgery in patients with asymptomatic AR does not require invasive monitoring. For severe AR, monitoring with a pulmonary artery catheter or transesophageal echocardiography is helpful to monitor myocardial depression, facilitate intravascular volume replacement, and measure the response to vasodilating drugs.

VII. TRICUSPID REGURGITATION

A. Pathophysiology. Tricuspid regurgitation (TR) is usually functional, caused by tricuspid annular dilations secondary to right ventricular enlargement or pulmonary hypertension. Right atrial volume overload results in only a minimal increase in right atrial pressure even in the presence of a large regurgitant volume, owing to high compliance of the right atrium and vena cavae. Clinical signs include jugular venous distention, hepatomegaly, ascites, and peripheral edema.

B. Management of Anesthesia. Intravascular fluid volume and central venous pressure should be maintained in the high-normal range to facilitate adequate right ventricular preload and left ventricular filling. Events known to increase pulmonary artery pressure (e.g., hypoxemia, hypercarbia) should be avoided. Nitrous oxide can be a weak pulmonary artery vasoconstrictor and could increase the degree of TR, so it is best avoided. Right atrial pressure monitoring may help to guide intravenous fluid replacement and to detect changes in the amount of TR during anesthesia.

VIII. TRICUSPID STENOSIS

Tricuspid stenosis (TS) is rare in the adult population and may be associated with a history of rheumatic fever, carcinoid syndrome, and endomyocardial fibrosis. TS increases right atrial pressure and the pressure gradient between the right atrium and right ventricle.

IX. PULMONIC VALVE REGURGITATION

Pulmonic valve regurgitation results from pulmonary hypertension and annular dilation of the pulmonic valve. Other causes include connective tissue diseases, carcinoid syndrome, infective endocarditis, and rheumatic heart disease. It is rarely symptomatic.

X. PULMONIC STENOSIS

Pulmonic stenosis (PS) is usually congenital and detected and corrected in childhood. An acquired form can be caused by rheumatic fever, carcinoid syndrome, or infective endocarditis. Significant obstruction can cause syncope, angina, right ventricular hypertrophy, and right ventricular failure. Surgical valvotomy can be used to relieve the obstruction.

XI. NEW FRONTIERS IN TREATMENT OF VALVULAR HEART DISEASE

New interventions are being developed to allow for treatment of valvular heart disease without the need for open heart surgery or cardiopulmonary bypass. Transcatheter aortic valve implantation (TAVI) is a relatively new technique that can be performed percutaneously via the femoral artery or via puncture of the apex of the left ventricle. General anesthesia is required in most instances, particularly with the transapical approach. This treatment is associated with a lower 30-day and 1-year mortality, better improvement in symptoms, and reduced number of repeat hospitalizations than medical therapy or balloon valvuloplasty. However, stroke and cognitive impairment are increased compared with aortic valve replacement by open heart surgery. Transcatheter pulmonic valve placement has also been successfully performed.

CHAPTER 3

Congenital Heart Disease

Congenital anomalies of the heart and cardiovascular system occur in 7 to 10 per 1000 live births (Table 3-1). Signs and symptoms of congenital heart disease in infants and children (Table 3-2) are apparent during the first week of life in approximately 50% of affected neonates and before 5 years of age in virtually all remaining patients. Echocardiography is the initial diagnostic step. Certain complications are likely to accompany the presence of congenital heart disease (Table 3-3). Cardiac dysrhythmias are not usually a prominent feature.

I. ACYANOTIC CONGENITAL HEART DISEASE

Acyanotic congenital heart disease is characterized by a left-to-right intracardiac shunt (Table 3-4). Such shunts, regardless of their locations, often result in increased pulmonary blood flow with pulmonary hypertension, right ventricular hypertrophy, and eventually congestive heart failure (CHF). The onset and severity of clinical symptoms vary with the site and magnitude of the vascular shunt.

A. Atrial Septal Defect. Atrial septal defect (ASD) accounts for about one third of the congenital heart disease detected in adults and is two to three times more common in females than in males. The physiologic consequences of ASDs reflect the shunting of blood from one atrium to the other; the direction and magnitude of the shunt are determined by the size of the defect and the relative compliance of the ventricles. When the diameter of the ASD approaches 2 cm, it is likely that left-to-right shunt has led to increased pulmonary blood flow. A systolic ejection murmur audible in the second left intercostal space may be mistaken for an innocent flow murmur. Transesophageal echocardiography and Doppler color flow echocardiography are both useful for detecting and determining the location and size of ASDs.

1. **Signs and Symptoms.** ASDs initially produce no symptoms or signs and may remain undetected for years. Symptoms resulting from large ASDs include dyspnea on exertion, supraventricular dysrhythmias, right-sided heart failure, paradoxical embolism, and recurrent pulmonary infections. When pulmonary blood flow is 1.5 times the systemic blood flow, closure of the ASD is indicated to prevent right ventricular dysfunction and irreversible pulmonary hypertension. Prophylaxis against infective endocarditis is not indicated for ASD.
2. **Management of Anesthesia** (Table 3-5)

B. Ventricular Septal Defect. Ventricular septal defect (VSD) is the most common congenital cardiac abnormality in infants and children, and many close spontaneously by 2 years of age. Echocardiography with Doppler flow ultrasonography confirms the presence and location of the VSD, and color-flow mapping provides information about the magnitude and direction of the intracardiac shunt.

1. **Signs and Symptoms.** The physiologic significance of a VSD depends on the size of the defect and the relative resistance in the systemic and pulmonary circulations. If the defect is large, over time the pulmonary vascular resistance increases; the direction of the shunt may reverse, resulting in cyanosis. Adults with small defects and normal pulmonary

TABLE 3-1 ■ **Classification and Incidence of Congenital Heart Disease**

DISEASE	INCIDENCE (%)
ACYANOTIC DEFECTS	
Ventricular septal defect	35
Atrial septal defect	9
Patent ductus arteriosus	8
Pulmonary stenosis	8
Aortic stenosis	6
Coarctation of the aorta	6
Atrioventricular septal defect	3
CYANOTIC DEFECTS	
Tetralogy of Fallot	5
Transposition of the great vessels	4

TABLE 3-2 ■ **Signs and Symptoms of Congenital Heart Disease**

INFANTS
Tachypnea Failure to gain weight Heart rate >200 beats/min Heart murmur Congestive heart failure Cyanosis
CHILDREN
Dyspnea Slow physical development Decreased exercise tolerance Heart murmur Congestive heart failure Cyanosis Clubbing of digits Squatting Hypertension

arterial pressures are generally asymptomatic, and pulmonary hypertension is unlikely. The murmur of a VSD is holosystolic and loudest at the lower left sternal border. Closure of the defect is recommended in patients with large VSDs in whom the magnitude of the pulmonary hypertension is not prohibitive (pulmonary/systemic vascular resistance ratio <0.7).

2. **Management of Anesthesia.** Management of anesthesia for VSD is similar to management for ASD in most respects (see Table 3-5). Right ventricular infundibular hypertrophy may be present in patients with VSDs and increased myocardial contractility, or hypovolemia may exaggerate right ventricular obstruction. Third-degree atrioventricular heart block may follow surgical closure if the cardiac conduction system is near the VSD.

TABLE 3-3 ■ Common Problems Associated with Congenital Heart Disease

Infective endocarditis
Cardiac dysrhythmias
Complete heart block
Hypertension (systemic or pulmonary)
Erythrocytosis
Thromboembolism
Coagulopathy
Brain abscess
Increased plasma uric acid concentration
Sudden death

TABLE 3-4 ■ Congenital Heart Defects Resulting in a Left-to-Right Intracardiac Shunt or Its Equivalent

Secundum atrial septal defect
Primum atrial septal defect (endocardial cushion defect)
Ventricular septal defect
Aorticopulmonary fenestration

TABLE 3-5 ■ Anesthetic Considerations in Patients with Left-to-Right Intracardiac Shunts

Pharmacology of inhaled anesthetics is not altered as long as systemic blood flow remains normal.
Avoid increases in systemic vascular resistance; this increases left-to-right shunting.
Avoid measures that decrease pulmonary vascular resistance (e.g., high F_{IO_2}, pulmonary vasodilators); this increases left-to-right shunt.
Decreased systemic vascular resistance and increased pulmonary vascular resistance decrease left-to-right shunt.
Positive-pressure ventilation is well tolerated.
Antibiotic prophylaxis is indicated for ASD only when a valvular abnormality is also present. Antibiotic prophylaxis is indicated for VSD and PDA.
Avoid introducing air into the circulation, such as through IV solutions.
Transient supraventricular dysrhythmias and atrioventricular conduction changes are common after closure of the ASD.

ASD, Atrial septal defect; *IV,* intravenous; *PDA,* patent ductus arteriosus; *VSD,* ventricular septal defect.

C. Patent Ductus Arteriosus. Patent ductus arteriosus (PDA) is present when the ductus arteriosus (which arises just distal to the left subclavian artery and connects the descending aorta to the left pulmonary artery) fails to close spontaneously shortly after birth, resulting in continuous flow of blood from the aorta to the pulmonary artery. The PDA can usually be visualized on echocardiography, with Doppler studies confirming the continuous flow into the pulmonary circulation.

1. **Signs and Symptoms.** Most patients are asymptomatic, and most PDAs are recognized by the presence of a characteristic continuous systolic and diastolic murmur. If severe pulmonary hypertension develops, closure of the PDA is contraindicated.
2. **Treatment.** The PDA is treated by either medical management (cyclooxygenase inhibitors such as indomethacin) or surgical closure.

3. **Management of Anesthesia.** Management of anesthesia includes the same considerations as for other patients with left-to-right cardiac shunts (see Table 3-5). Ligation of the PDA is often associated with significant systemic hypertension during the postoperative period, which can be managed with vasodilator drugs such as nitroprusside. Long-acting antihypertensive drugs can be gradually substituted for nitroprusside if systemic hypertension persists. Antibiotic prophylaxis for protection against endocarditis is recommended for patients with PDAs who undergo noncardiac surgery.

D. **Aorticopulmonary Fenestration.** Aorticopulmonary fenestration is characterized by a communication between the ascending aorta and the main pulmonary artery. The physiologic consequences and anesthesia management are similar to those associated with a large PDA.

E. **Aortic Stenosis.** Bicuspid aortic valves occur in 2% to 3% of the U.S. population, and about 20% of these patients have other cardiovascular abnormalities, such as PDA or coarctation of the aorta. Transthoracic echocardiography with Doppler flow studies permits assessment of the severity of the aortic stenosis and of left ventricular function.

1. **Signs and Symptoms.** AS is associated with a systolic murmur that is audible over the aortic area (second right intercostal space) and often radiates into the neck. Most patients are asymptomatic until adulthood. Infants with severe AS may have CHF. The electrocardiogram (ECG) may show left ventricular hypertrophy. Angina in the absence of coronary artery disease reflects the inability of coronary blood flow to meet increased myocardial oxygen requirements of the hypertrophied left ventricle. Syncope can occur when the pressure gradient across the aortic valve exceeds 50 mm Hg. In patients with supravalvular AS, associated findings can include prominent facial bones, rounded forehead, pursed upper lip, strabismus, inguinal hernias, dental abnormalities, and developmental delay. Supravalvular aortic stenosis (SVAS) may be associated with a characteristic appearance of prominent facial bones, rounded forehead, and pursed upper lip. Nonsyndromic SVAS is less common but has been implicated in cases of sudden death in conjunction with anesthesia or sedation.
2. **Treatment.** Treatment of symptomatic congenital AS is valve replacement, and considerations for anesthesia management are similar to those for acquired AS.

F. **Pulmonic Stenosis.** Pulmonic stenosis (PS) producing obstruction to right ventricular outflow is valvular in 90% of patients and supravalvular or subvalvular in the remainder. Supravalvular PS often co-exists with other congenital cardiac abnormalities (e.g., ASD, VSD, PDA, tetralogy of Fallot [TOF]). Valvular PS is typically an isolated abnormality, but it may occur in association with a VSD. Echocardiography and Doppler flow studies can determine the site of the obstruction and the severity of the stenosis. Treatment of PS is with percutaneous balloon valvuloplasty.

1. **Signs and Symptoms.** In asymptomatic patients, the presence of PS is identified by the presence of a loud systolic ejection murmur, best heard at the second left intercostal space. Dyspnea may occur on exertion, and eventually right ventricular failure with peripheral edema and ascites develops.
2. **Treatment.** Treatment is percutaneous balloon valvuloplasty.
3. **Management of Anesthesia.** Management of anesthesia is designed to avoid increases in right ventricular oxygen requirements (tachycardia, increased myocardial contractility). Decreases in systemic blood pressure should be promptly treated with sympathomimetic drugs.

G. **Coarctation of the Aorta.** Coarctation of the aorta is usually a result of a discrete, diaphragm-like ridge extending into the aortic lumen just distal to the left subclavian artery (postductal coarctation).

1. **Signs and Symptoms.** Most adults are asymptomatic, and the diagnosis is made when systemic hypertension is detected in the arms in association with diminished or absent femoral arterial pulses. The ECG shows left ventricular hypertrophy. Clinical symptoms include headache, dizziness, epistaxis, and palpitations.

TABLE 3-6 ■ Anesthetic Considerations for Patients with Coarctation of the Aorta

Maintain adequate perfusion to the lower body during aortic cross-clamping (mean arterial pressure ≥40 mm Hg); consider partial circulatory bypass if pressure cannot be maintained.
Continuously monitor systemic pressure above and below the coarctation (right radial and femoral artery catheterization).
Upper-body systemic hypertension during cross-clamping can cause increased workload to the heart and make surgical repair more difficult (consider nitroprusside).
Consider somatosensory evoked potentials to monitor spinal cord function and adequacy of blood flow to the spinal cord during cross-clamping of the aorta.

TABLE 3-7 ■ Congenital Heart Defects Resulting in a Right-to-Left Intracardiac Shunt

Tetralogy of Fallot
Eisenmenger's syndrome
Ebstein's anomaly (malformation of the tricuspid valve)
Tricuspid atresia
Foramen ovale

2. **Treatment.** Surgical resection of the coarctation of the aorta is indicated for patients with a transcoarctation pressure gradient of more than 30 mm Hg. Balloon dilation is a therapeutic alternative.
3. **Management of Anesthesia** (Table 3-6)
4. **Postoperative Management.** Immediate postoperative complications include paradoxical hypertension, aortic regurgitation, and paraplegia. Administration of intravenous (IV) nitroprusside with or without esmolol usually controls systemic blood pressure during the early postoperative period. Paraplegia may result from ischemic damage to the spinal cord during the aortic cross-clamping. Abdominal pain may occur, presumably because of sudden increases in blood flow to the gastrointestinal tract.

II. CYANOTIC CONGENITAL HEART DISEASE

Cyanotic congenital heart disease is characterized by a right-to-left intracardiac shunt (Table 3-7) with associated decreases in pulmonary blood flow and the development of arterial hypoxemia.

A. **Tetralogy of Fallot.** TOF, the most common cyanotic congenital heart defect, is characterized by a large single VSD, an aorta that overrides the right and left ventricles, obstruction to right ventricular outflow, and right ventricular hypertrophy. The resistance to flow across the right ventricular outflow tract is relatively fixed; changes in systemic vascular resistance may affect the magnitude of the shunt. Decreases in systemic vascular resistance increase right-to-left shunt and arterial hypoxemia, whereas increases in systemic vascular resistance (e.g., by squatting) decrease left-to-right shunt and increase pulmonary blood flow.
   1. **Diagnosis.** Echocardiography is used to establish the diagnosis and assess the presence of associated abnormalities. Cardiac catheterization further confirms the diagnosis and permits confirmation of anatomic and hemodynamic data.
   2. **Signs and Symptoms** (Table 3-8)
   3. **Treatment.** Treatment of TOF is complete surgical correction (closure of the VSD with a Dacron patch and relief of right ventricular outflow obstruction by placing a synthetic

graft) when patients are extremely young. Three palliative operations in infancy include Waterston's operation (side-to-side anastomosis of the ascending aorta to the right pulmonary artery), Pott's operation (side-to-side anastomosis of the descending aorta to the left pulmonary artery), and the Blalock-Taussig operation (end-to-side anastomosis of the subclavian artery to the pulmonary artery).

4. **Management of Anesthesia.** For patients with TOF, management of anesthesia aims to avoid events that acutely increase the magnitude of the right-to-left shunt (Table 3-9).
   a. *Preoperative preparation* includes avoiding dehydration by maintaining oral feedings in extremely young patients or by providing IV fluids before the patient's arrival in the operating room. Crying associated with intramuscular administration of drugs used for preoperative medication can lead to hypercyanotic attacks. Continue β-adrenergic antagonists in patients receiving these drugs for prophylaxis against hypercyanotic attacks.
   b. *Induction of anesthesia* is often with ketamine, which preserves systemic vascular resistance. Induction of anesthesia with a volatile anesthetic such as sevoflurane is acceptable but must be accomplished with caution and careful monitoring of systemic oxygenation.
   c. *Maintenance of anesthesia* is often achieved with nitrous oxide combined with ketamine. The principal disadvantage of using nitrous oxide is the associated decrease in the inspired oxygen concentration. Ventilation of the patient's lungs should be controlled, but excessive positive airway pressure may increase the resistance to blood flow through the lungs. Intravascular fluid volume must be maintained because acute hypovolemia increases right-to-left intracardiac shunt. Meticulous care must be taken to avoid infusion of air

TABLE 3-8 ■ **Signs and Symptoms of Tetralogy of Fallot**
Cyanosis
Systolic ejection murmur along the left sternal border
Squatting (particularly in children; increases systemic vascular resistance)
Right axis deviation and right ventricular hypertrophy on electrocardiogram
Compensatory erythropoiesis
Hypercyanotic attacks (sudden episode of arterial hypoxemia, tachypnea, syncope, seizures, often precipitated by crying or exercise; treatment is esmolol and/or phenylephrine)
Cerebrovascular accident caused by cerebrovascular thrombosis or arterial hypoxemia
Cerebral abscess
Infective endocarditis

TABLE 3-9 ■ **Events that Increase Right-to-Left Intracardiac Shunting**

Decreased systemic vascular resistance	Volatile anesthetic agents Histamine release Ganglionic blockade β-Adrenergic blockade
Increased pulmonary vascular resistance	Intermittent positive airway pressure Positive end-expiratory pressure Negative intrapleural pressure
Increased myocardial contractility (accentuates infundibular obstruction to right ventricular ejection)	Surgical stimulation Inotropic agents

through IV tubing because of the risk of systemic air embolization. α-Adrenergic agonist drugs (phenylephrine) are used to treat decreases in systemic vascular resistance.

5. **Patient Characteristics after Repair of Tetralogy of Fallot.** Ventricular cardiac dysrhythmias and atrial fibrillation or flutter are common. Right bundle branch block is common, but third-degree atrioventricular heart block is uncommon.

B. **Eisenmenger's Syndrome.** Eisenmenger's syndrome is a condition in which a left-to-right intracardiac shunt is reversed when pulmonary vascular resistance increases to a level that equals or exceeds the systemic vascular resistance. It occurs in approximately 50% of patients with an untreated VSD and approximately 10% of patients with an untreated ASD. The murmur associated with these cardiac defects disappears when Eisenmenger's syndrome develops.

1. **Signs and Symptoms** (Table 3-10)
2. **Treatment.** Epoprostenol may help decreased pulmonary vascular resistance. Hyperviscosity can be treated with phlebotomy and isovolemic replacement. Pregnancy is discouraged in women with Eisenmenger's syndrome. Lung transplantation with repair of the cardiac defect or combined heart-lung transplantation may be an option. Surgical correction of the underlying heart defect is contraindicated in the presence of irreversible pulmonary hypertension.
3. **Management of Anesthesia.** Management of anesthesia is based on maintenance of preoperative levels of systemic vascular resistance, recognizing that increases in right-to-left shunt are likely if sudden vasodilation occurs. Continuous IV infusions of norepinephrine may be useful, but β-adrenergic agonists that may decrease systemic vascular resistance should be avoided. Minimizing blood loss and hypovolemia and the prevention of iatrogenic paradoxical embolization are important considerations. If epidural anesthesia is selected, it seems prudent to avoid epinephrine in the local anesthetic solution owing to its peripheral β-agonist effects.

C. **Ebstein's Anomaly.** Ebstein's anomaly is an abnormality of the tricuspid valve in which the valve leaflets are malformed or displaced downward into the right ventricle.

1. **Signs and Symptoms** (Table 3-11). The severity of the hemodynamic derangements depends on the degree of displacement and the functional status of the tricuspid valve leaflets and can vary from CHF in neonates to asymptomatic adults. Echocardiography is used to assess right atrial dilation, distortion of the tricuspid valve leaflets, and the severity of the tricuspid regurgitation or stenosis.
2. **Treatment.** Treatment of Ebstein's anomaly is based on preventing associated complications. It includes antibiotic prophylaxis against infective endocarditis, diuretics and digoxin to manage CHF, pharmacologic treatment of arrhythmias, and catheter ablation if accessory pathways are present. Surgical treatment by systemic-to-pulmonary shunt, Glenn's shunt, or Fontan's procedure may be considered.

TABLE 3-10 ■ **Signs and Symptoms of Eisenmenger's Syndrome**
Arterial hypoxemia
• Cyanosis
• Erythrocytosis
• Increased blood viscosity
Decreased exercise tolerance
Atrial fibrillation
Hemoptysis (pulmonary infarction)
Thrombosis
Cerebrovascular accident
Brain abscess
Syncope
Sudden death

TABLE 3-11 ■ Signs and Symptoms of Ebstein's Anomaly
Cyanosis
Congestive heart failure
Paradoxical embolization
Hepatomegaly (caused by passive hepatic congestion secondary to increased right atrial pressure)
Massive enlargement of the right atrium
First-degree atrioventricular block
Paroxysmal arrhythmias, both supraventricular and ventricular
Brain abscess
Sudden death

3. **Management of Anesthesia.** Hazards during anesthesia in patients with Ebstein's anomaly include accentuation of arterial hypoxemia as a result of increases in the magnitude of the right-to-left intracardiac shunt and the development of supraventricular tachydysrhythmias.

D. **Tricuspid Atresia.** Tricuspid atresia is characterized by arterial hypoxemia, a small right ventricle, a large left ventricle, and marked decreases in pulmonary blood flow.

1. **Treatment.** Treatment is anastomosis of the right atrial appendage to the right pulmonary artery to bypass the right ventricle and provide direct atriopulmonary communication (Fontan's procedure).
2. **Management of Anesthesia.** For patients undergoing Fontan's procedure, management of anesthesia has been successfully achieved with opioids or volatile anesthetics. Immediately after cardiopulmonary bypass and continuing into the early postoperative period, it is important to maintain increased right atrial pressures (16 to 20 mm Hg) to facilitate pulmonary blood flow and avoid increases in pulmonary vascular resistance (acidosis, hypothermia, peak airway pressures higher than 15 cm H_2O, or reactions to the tracheal tube), which may cause right-sided heart failure. Early tracheal extubation and spontaneous ventilation are desirable. Subsequent management of anesthesia in patients who have undergone Fontan's procedure is facilitated by monitoring the central venous pressure (which equals the pulmonary artery pressure in these patients) to assess the intravascular fluid volume and to detect sudden impairment of left ventricular function and increased pulmonary vascular resistance.

E. **Transposition of the Great Arteries.** Transposition of the great arteries results in complete separation of the pulmonary and systemic circulations. Survival is possible only if there is communication between the two circulations (VSD, ASD, or PDA).

1. **Signs and Symptoms.** Persistent cyanosis and tachypnea at birth may be the first clues, and CHF is often present.
2. **Treatment.** Immediate management involves creating intracardiac mixing such as using prostaglandin E to maintain patency of the ductus arteriosus and/or balloon atrial septostomy (Rashkind's procedure). Ultimately, correction involves an "arterial switch" operation in which the pulmonary artery and ascending aorta are reanastomosed with the "correct" ventricles, and coronary arteries are reimplanted, so that the aorta is connected to the left ventricle and the pulmonary artery is connected to the right ventricle.
3. **Management of Anesthesia.** Anesthesia is often managed with ketamine combined with or without opioids or benzodiazepines for maintenance of anesthesia. The use of nitrous oxide is limited, as it is important to administer high inspired oxygen concentrations. Dehydration must be avoided during the perioperative period because these patients may have hematocrits in excess of 70%, predisposing them to cerebral venous thrombosis.

F. **Mixing of Blood between the Pulmonary and Systemic Circulations.** Rare congenital heart defects that result in mixing of blood from the pulmonary and systemic circulations manifest

TABLE 3-12 ■ Congenital Heart Defects Resulting in Mixing of Blood from the Pulmonary and Systemic Circulations

DEFECT	CONSIDERATIONS
Truncus arteriosus (single arterial trunk is the origin of both the aorta and pulmonary artery)	Manifests as cyanosis, arterial hypoxemia, failure to thrive, and CHF. Surgical treatment consists of banding of the right and left pulmonary arteries to decrease pulmonary blood flow. PEEP may decrease pulmonary blood flow and decrease symptoms of CHF.
Partial anomalous pulmonary venous return (pulmonary vein empties into the right atrium instead of the left)	Manifests as fatigue, exertional dyspnea, CHF. Angiography is useful for diagnosis.
Total anomalous pulmonary venous return (all four veins drain into the systemic venous circulation)	Manifests as CHF. PEEP may decrease pulmonary blood flow. IV infusions can increase right atrial pressure and cause pulmonary edema. Surgical manipulation of the right atrium can cause obstruction.
Hypoplastic left-sided heart syndrome	Treatment is initial reconstruction of the ascending aorta using the proximal pulmonary artery, followed by Fontan's procedure. Coronary blood flow is compromised, and ventricular fibrillation is a high risk. Anesthetic management is with high-dose opioids and muscle relaxation. High Pa_{O_2} implies excessive pulmonary blood flow at the expense of systemic blood flow—treatments are maneuvers to increase pulmonary vascular resistance.

CHF, Congestive heart failure; *IV,* intravenous; *PEEP,* positive end-expiratory pressure.

as cyanosis and arterial hypoxemia of varying severity depending on the magnitude of the pulmonary blood flow (Table 3-12).

III. MECHANICAL OBSTRUCTION OF THE TRACHEA

The trachea can be obstructed by circulatory anomalies that produce a vascular ring or by dilation of the pulmonary artery secondary to absence of the pulmonic valve and can present as stridor or other upper airway obstruction (Table 3-13).

IV. THE ADULT PATIENT WITH CONGENITAL HEART DISEASE UNDERGOING NONCARDIAC SURGERY

The prevalence of congenital heart disease in adult patients is increasing as increasing numbers of children with congenital heart disease survive to adulthood. Hospitalization rates in this population are twice that of the general population, and adults with congenital heart disease often have chronic comorbidities, such as chronic heart failure, pulmonary hypertension, dysrhythmias, cardiac conduction system disease, residual shunts, valvular lesions, hypertension, and aneurysms. Noncardiac issues include developmental abnormalities, central nervous system disease, erythrocytosis, nephrolithiasis,

TABLE 3-13 ■ **Mechanical Obstruction of the Trachea**

DEFECT	CONSIDERATIONS
Double aortic arch	Vascular ring presses on the trachea and esophagus. Manifests as inspiratory stridor, difficulty managing secretions, and dysphagia. Treatment is surgical resection. Endotracheal tube should be inserted beyond the level of tracheal compression if possible. Gastric tube can cause occlusion of the trachea if the endotracheal tube is above the level of compression.
Aberrant left pulmonary artery	Manifests as expiratory stridor or wheezing. Esophageal obstruction is rare. Surgical division of the aberrant pulmonary artery is the treatment of choice.
Absent pulmonary valve	Results in dilation of the pulmonary artery, which can compress the trachea and left main bronchus. Tracheal intubation and continuous airway pressure of 4-6 mm Hg can keep the trachea distended. Treatment is surgical insertion of a tubular graft with artificial pulmonic valve.

hearing or visual impairments, and lung disease. The most common lesions seen in adult patients are conotruncal abnormalities after repair (TOF, truncus arteriosus, double outlet right ventricle), coarctation after repair, transposition of the great vessels after arterial switch operation, complex single ventricle after Fontan's procedure, pulmonary valve stenosis, congenital aortic valve stenosis, atrioventricular canal defects, secundum ASDs, and sinus venosus ASDs.

A. Common Issues

1. Premedication must be undertaken cautiously, because hypercapnia can increase pulmonary vascular resistance.
2. Endocarditis prophylaxis is important in some lesions.
3. Dysrhythmias are common, with 20% to 45% of adult patients having atrial dilatation. The most common tachyarrhythmia is intraatrial reentrant tachycardia.
4. Pulmonary hypertension is common.
5. Heart failure is common in both corrected and uncorrected congenital heart disease.
6. Congenital bleeding abnormalities can occur owing to low circulating levels of vitamin K clotting factors.

B. Intraoperative Management. Intraoperative management will depend the combination of residual congenital heart disease and comorbidities present. There are no evidence-based recommendations for anesthetic management strategies. Regional anesthesia may be appropriate but must be considered in the context of potential bleeding disorders and the risks of reduction in systemic vascular resistance in patients with unrestricted intracardiac shunts.

C. Postoperative Management. Postoperative management relies first on stratifying the patient to the appropriate postoperative environment based on the severity of disease, type of procedure and perioperative course.

V. INFECTIVE ENDOCARDITIS ANTIBIOTIC PROPHYLAXIS IN REPAIRED AND UNREPAIRED CONGENITAL HEART DISEASE

Patients for whom antibiotic prophylaxis should be considered include those with prosthetic valves or prosthetic material used in valve repair, palliative shunts and conduits, completely repaired congenital heart disease with prosthetic material or a device placed during surgery or by catheter intervention within 6 months of the placement procedure, and repaired congenital heart disease with residual defects at or adjacent to the site of a prosthetic patch or prosthetic device, patients with previous endocarditis, unrepaired congenital heart disease, cyanotic heart disease, or cardiac transplantation with valvulopathy. Except for patients with the above mentioned conditions, antibiotic prophylaxis is no longer recommended. Patients who have the previously listed conditions who are having gingival tissue manipulation or surgery in the periapical region of the teeth or perforation of the oral mucosa are at particular risk and should receive prophylaxis. However, antibiotic prophylaxis for genitourinary or gastrointestinal tract operations is not recommended for these patients.

CHAPTER 4

Abnormalities of Cardiac Conduction and Cardiac Rhythm

The clinical significance of cardiac dysrhythmias for the anesthesiologist depends on the effect they have on vital signs and the potential for deterioration into a life-threatening rhythm. The electrical impulse in the heart moves along the cardiac conduction system, propagating a wave of depolarization and causing progressive contraction of cardiac muscle cells. The depolarization and repolarization events correspond to electrical waves recorded on an electrocardiogram (ECG) (Figure 4-1).

I. ANATOMY OF INTRINSIC CARDIAC PACEMAKERS AND THE CONDUCTION SYSTEM

A. Sinoatrial Node. The sinoatrial (SA) node is the primary site for impulse initiation. It is located at the junction of the superior vena cava and the right atrium. In 60% of individuals, arterial blood supply is via the right coronary artery. The SA node normally discharges at 60 to 100 beats per minute. Any rhythm resulting from accelerated firing of a pacemaker other than the SA node is called an *ectopic* rhythm.

B. Atrioventricular Node. Located in the septal wall of the right atrium, anterior to the coronary sinus, above the septal leaf of the tricuspid valve, the atrioventricular (AV) node has a long refractory period to prevent overstimulation of the ventricles during abnormally rapid atrial impulses. In 85% to 90% of people, the blood supply is the right coronary artery. In the AV node, atrial conduction is briefly slowed.

C. Bundle of His. The bundle of His divides into two branches in the intraventricular septum. Both branches receive blood supply from the left anterior descending coronary artery (LAD).

1. The right bundle branch (RBB) courses down the right ventricle (RV) and divides near the RV apex. The RBB is more susceptible than the left bundle branch (LBB) to interruption because of its late branching.
2. The LBB divides early into the left anterior fascicle (LAF) and left posterior fascicle (LPF). The LPF receives additional blood supply from the posterior descending coronary artery (PDA) and is less vulnerable to damage by an anterior myocardial infarction.

II. ELECTROPHYSIOLOGY OF THE CONDUCTION SYSTEM

The resting cardiac cell is negative inside relative to the outside (−80 to −90 mV) owing to the active concentration of potassium internally and the extrusion of sodium externally. Electrical impulses cause opening of ion channels, and membrane potential rises, reaching +20 mV to initiate an action potential (AP). After cell depolarization, it is refractory to subsequent APs during phase 4 of the depolarization.

A. Electrocardiography. The normal ECG tracing is made of up three parts: P wave, QRS complex, and T wave.

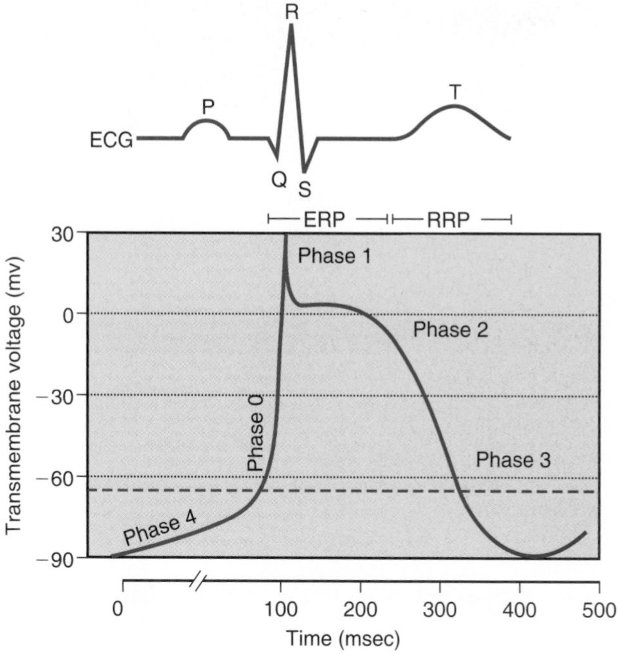

FIGURE 4-1 ■ Transmembrane action potential generated by an automatic cardiac cell and the relationship of this action potential to events depicted on the electrocardiogram.

1. PR interval: from atrial depolarization to ventricular depolarization. Normally 0.12 to 0.20 second.
2. QRS complex: during depolarization of the right and left ventricles. Normally 0.05 to 0.10 second.
3. ST segment: between the S portion of the QRS complex and the T wave. Normally isoelectric. May be elevated up to 1 mm. Is *never* normally depressed.
4. T wave: normally in the same direction as the QRS, and ≤5 mm in amplitude in standard leads or ≤10 mm in precordial leads.
5. QT interval: from the Q wave to the end of the T wave. Varies with heart rate; generally the QT is less than half the R-R interval.

III. MECHANISMS OF TACHYDYSRHYTHMIAS

Tachydysrhythmia is defined as a cardiac rhythm of more than 100 beats per minute.

A. Automaticity. Automaticity is affected by the slope of phase 4 depolarization and/or the resting membrane potential. Sympathetic stimulation increases heart rate by increasing the slope of phase 4 depolarization and decreasing the resting membrane potential. Parasympathetic stimulation decreases heart rate by decreasing the slope of phase 4 depolarization and increasing the resting membrane potential. Dysrhythmias caused by enhanced automaticity can involve almost any cell in the heart and are not limited to secondary pacemakers within the conduction system.

B. Reentry Pathway Dysrhythmias. Reentry pathways account for most premature beats and tachydysrhythmias. Reentry requires two pathways over which electrical impulses can be conducted at different velocities. In a reentry circuit, anterograde conduction occurs over the slower normal conduction pathways, and retrograde conduction occurs over a second, accessory pathway. Pharmacologic or physiologic events (hypoxemia, electrolyte disturbance,

TABLE 4-1 ■ Perioperative Causes of Sinus Tachycardia

PHYSIOLOGIC INCREASE IN SYMPATHETIC TONE
Pain
Anxiety, fear
Light anesthesia
Hypovolemia, anemia
Arterial hypoxemia
Hypotension
Hypoglycemia
Fever, infection
PATHOLOGIC INCREASE IN SYMPATHETIC TONE
Myocardial ischemia, infarction
Congestive heart failure
Pulmonary embolism
Hyperthyroidism
Pericarditis
Pericardial tamponade
Malignant hyperthermia
Ethanol withdrawal
DRUG-INDUCED INCREASE IN HEART RATE
Atropine, glycopyrrolate
Sympathomimetic drugs
Caffeine
Nicotine
Cocaine, amphetamines

acid-base changes, autonomic nervous system changes, myocardial ischemia, drugs) may alter the balance between conduction velocities and refractory periods of the dual pathways, resulting in the initiation or termination of reentrant dysrhythmias.

C. **Afterdepolarizations.** Afterdepolarizations are oscillations in membrane potential that occur during or after repolarization. Under special circumstances these afterdepolarizations can trigger a complete depolarization that can be self-sustaining and result in a triggered dysrhythmia.

IV. SUPRAVENTRICULAR DYSRHYTHMIAS

A. **Sinus Dysrhythmia.** Sinus dysrhythmia is a normal variation in sinus rhythm caused by changes in intrathoracic pressure during inspiration and expiration (Bainbridge reflex).

B. **Sinus Tachycardia** (Table 4-1). Sinus tachycardia is characterized by a gradual change of heart rate to 100 to 160 beats per minute. The ECG shows a normal P wave before each QRS complex and normal PR unless a co-existing conduction block is present. Treatment is correction of the underlying cause (e.g., hypovolemia, pain, anxiety, hypoxemia, hypotension, fever, heart failure). Administration of a β-blocker may lower the heart rate and decrease myocardial oxygen demand. Prognosis is related to the physiologic or pathologic process causing the acceleration of sinus node activity.

C. **Premature Atrial Contractions.** Premature atrial contractions (PACs) are common in patients with and without heart disease. Noncardiac precipitating factors include caffeine, emotional stress, alcohol, nicotine, recreational drugs, and hyperthyroidism. PACs, unlike ventricular premature beats (VPBs), are not followed by a compensatory pause on the ECG. PACs do not require acute therapy unless they are associated with initiation of a tachydysrhythmia. Then treatment is directed at controlling or converting the secondary dysrhythmia.

D. Supraventricular Tachycardia. Supraventricular tachycardia (SVT) is any tachydysrhythmia (average heart rate of 160 to 180 beats/min) initiated and sustained by tissue at or above the AV node. AV nodal reentrant tachycardia (AVNRT) is the most common type of SVT and accounts for 50% of diagnosed SVTs. AVNRT is most commonly a result of a reentry circuit in which there is anterograde conduction over the slower AV nodal pathway and retrograde conduction over a faster accessory pathway. Atrial fibrillation and atrial flutter are SVTs, but their electrophysiology and treatment are distinctly different from those of other forms of SVT and they are discussed separately.

1. **Treatment.** Often, initial treatment involves a vagal maneuver such as carotid sinus massage or a Valsalva maneuver. If this is not effective, pharmacologic treatment directed at blocking AV nodal conduction is indicated. Adenosine, calcium channel blockers, and β-blockers may be used to terminate SVT. Intravenous digoxin is not clinically useful in acute control of SVT because of a delayed peak effect and narrow therapeutic index. Electrical cardioversion is indicated for SVT unresponsive to drug therapy or SVT associated with hemodynamic instability. Radiofrequency catheter ablation may be used to treat recurrent AVNRT.
2. **Anesthetic Management.** For patients with a history of SVT, anesthetic management focuses on avoiding precipitating events, such as increased sympathetic tone, electrolyte imbalances, and acid-base disturbances.

E. Multifocal Atrial Tachycardia. Multifocal atrial tachycardia (MAT) is an irregular rhythm with a rate above 100 beats per minute in which the ECG shows three or more P wave morphologies with variable PR intervals. Treatment consists of treating the underlying abnormality (exacerbation of pulmonary disease, methylxanthine toxicity, congestive heart failure, sepsis, electrolyte abnormalities). Pharmacologic treatment has limited success and is considered secondary, and cardioversion is generally ineffective. Anesthetic management consists of treatment of hypoxemia and avoidance of medications or procedures that worsen pulmonary status.

F. Atrial Flutter. Atrial flutter is an organized atrial rhythm with an atrial rate of 250 to 350 beats per minute and varying degrees of AV block. Flutter waves are usually seen on the ECG, with an associated ventricular rate of 120 to 160 beats per minute. If atrial flutter is hemodynamically significant, the treatment of choice is cardioversion. Patients with atrial flutter lasting longer than 48 hours should be anticoagulated and evaluated by transesophageal echocardiography for the presence of atrial thrombus before any attempt at cardioversion. Pharmacologic control of the ventricular response with intravenous amiodarone, diltiazem, or verapamil may be attempted if vital signs are stable. Elective surgery should be postponed until control of the rhythm has been achieved.

G. Atrial Fibrillation. Atrial fibrillation is the most common sustained cardiac dysrhythmia in the U.S. population (0.4% incidence). Postoperative atrial fibrillation is common in elderly patients undergoing cardiothoracic surgery. Predisposing factors for atrial fibrillation include rheumatic heart disease (especially mitral valve disease), hypertension, thyrotoxicosis, ischemic heart disease, chronic obstructive pulmonary disease, acute alcohol intoxication, pericarditis, pulmonary embolus, and atrial septal defect. The most important clinical consequence of atrial fibrillation is a thromboembolic event causing a stroke due to the presence of atrial thrombi.

1. **Sign and Symptoms.** Signs and symptoms may include palpitations, angina pectoris, CHF, pulmonary edema, hypotension, fatigue, and generalized weakness.
2. **Diagnosis.** The ECG shows chaotic atrial activity and no discernible P waves. Ventricular rate is about 180 beats per minute in patients with a normal AV node.
3. **Treatment.** Treatment goals are control of ventricular rate and conversion to sinus rhythm. Electrical cardioversion is indicated when hemodynamic compromise is present. The preferred drug for chemical conversion of patients with atrial fibrillation is amiodarone. Other choices are propafenone, ibutilide, and sotalol. Control of the ventricular response in patients with atrial fibrillation is typically achieved with drugs that slow AV nodal conduction, such as β-blockers, calcium channel blockers, and digoxin.

4. **Anticoagulation.** Individuals with atrial fibrillation are at increased risk of stroke and are usually treated with anticoagulants. Intravenous heparin is the most commonly used anticoagulant for acute treatment. For chronic anticoagulation, warfarin or dabigatran is most often used, but aspirin therapy may be sufficient for individuals considered to be at low risk of thromboembolic complications.
5. **Anesthetic Management.** If new-onset atrial fibrillation occurs before induction of anesthesia, surgery should be postponed if possible until control of the dysrhythmia has been achieved. Hemodynamically significant atrial fibrillation should be treated with electrical cardioversion. Pharmacologic control may be attempted if vital signs allow. Patients with chronic atrial fibrillation should be maintained on their antidysrhythmic drugs perioperatively, with close attention paid to serum magnesium and potassium levels, particularly if the patient is taking digoxin.

V. VENTRICULAR DYSRHYTHMIAS

A. **Ventricular Ectopy.** Ventricular premature beats (VPBs) arise from single (unifocal) or multiple (multifocal) foci located below the AV node. Characteristic ECG findings include a premature and wide QRS complex, no preceding P wave, ST-segment and T-wave deflection opposite to the QRS deflection, and a compensatory pause before the next sinus beat. A "vulnerable" period occurs in the middle third of the T wave, during which a VPB may initiate repetitive beats, including ventricular tachycardia (VT) or ventricular fibrillation (VF). This is known as the *R-on-T phenomenon.* Symptoms of VPBs include palpitations, near syncope, and syncope.

1. **Treatment.** VPBs should be treated when they are frequent, polymorphic, occurring in runs of three or more, or taking place during the vulnerable period, because these characteristics are associated with an increased incidence of VT and VF. The first step is to eliminate or correct the underlying cause (Table 4-2). Amiodarone, lidocaine, and other antidysrhythmics are not indicated unless VPBs progress to VT or are frequent enough to cause hemodynamic instability. Drug therapy is not at all effective in suppression of ventricular dysrhythmias caused by mechanical irritation of the heart.
2. **Prognosis.** Benign VPBs occur at rest and disappear with exercise. An increased frequency of VPBs with exercise may be an indication of underlying heart disease. In the absence of structural heart disease, asymptomatic ventricular ectopy is not associated with an increased risk of sudden death. The most common pathologic conditions associated with VPBs are myocardial ischemia, valvular heart disease, cardiomyopathy, QT-interval

TABLE 4-2 ■ **Factors Associated with Ventricular Premature Beats**
Normal heart
Arterial hypoxemia
Myocardial ischemia
Myocardial infarction
Myocarditis
Sympathetic nervous system activation
Hypokalemia
Hypomagnesemia
Digitalis toxicity
Caffeine
Cocaine
Alcohol
Mechanical irritation (central venous or pulmonary artery catheter)

prolongation, and the presence of electrolyte abnormalities, especially hypokalemia and hypomagnesemia.

3. **Anesthetic Management.** When receiving an anesthetic, if a patient exhibits six or more VPBs per minute and repetitive or multifocal forms of ventricular ectopy, there is an increased risk of development of a life-threatening dysrhythmia. Treatment should be directed at correcting underlying causes, including repositioning of intracardiac catheters. β-Blockers may be helpful. Amiodarone, lidocaine, and other antidysrhythmics are indicated only if the VPBs progress to VT or are frequent enough to cause hemodynamic instability.

B. **Ventricular Tachycardia.** VT is present when three or more consecutive VPBs occur at a calculated heart rate of greater than 120 beats per minute (usually 150 to 200 beats/min). The rhythm is regular with wide QRS complexes and no discernible P waves. Palpitations, presyncope, and syncope are the three most common symptoms. VT is common after an acute myocardial infarction and in the presence of inflammatory or infectious diseases of the heart. Digitalis toxicity may manifest as VT. Torsade de pointes (TdP) is a distinct form of VT initiated by a VPB in the setting of a prolonged QT interval.

1. **Treatment.** In patients with symptomatic or unstable VT, cardioversion should be performed immediately. If vital signs are stable and the VT is persistent or recurrent after cardioversion, amiodarone is recommended. Alternative drugs include procainamide, sotalol, and lidocaine. Catheter ablation and implantation of a cardioverter-defibrillator are options for drug-refractory VT.

C. **Ventricular Fibrillation.** VF is a rapid, grossly irregular ventricular rhythm with marked variability in QRS cycle length, morphology, and amplitude. A pulse or blood pressure *never* accompanies VF.

1. **Treatment.** Treatment is electrical defibrillation as soon as possible. The best chance for survival is when defibrillation occurs within 3 to 5 minutes of cardiac arrest. For refractory VF, administration of epinephrine or vasopressin may improve response to electrical defibrillation. After three defibrillation attempts, amiodarone, lidocaine, or, in the case of TdP, magnesium is indicated. Contributing factors (hypoxia, hypovolemia, acidosis, hypokalemia, hyperkalemia, hypoglycemia, hypothermia, drug or environmental toxins, cardiac tamponade, tension pneumothorax, coronary ischemia, pulmonary embolus, and hemorrhage) should be sought and treated. Long-term treatment for recurrent VF is placement of an automatic implanted cardioverter-defibrillator (AICD).

2. **Anesthetic Management.** Cardiopulmonary resuscitation (CPR) must be initiated immediately, followed as soon as possible with defibrillation. Underlying causes should be sought and corrected.

VI. VENTRICULAR PREEXCITATION SYNDROMES

Congenital alternate (accessory) pathways can conduct electrical impulses in the heart, with the potential for initiating reentrant tachydysrhythmias.

A. **Wolff-Parkinson-White Syndrome**

1. **Signs and Symptoms** (Table 4-3)

2. **Treatment** (Table 4-4). Although antidysrhythmics can provide therapeutic management of the dysrhythmias associated with WPW syndrome, catheter ablation is considered the best treatment for symptomatic WPW syndrome.

3. **Anesthetic Management.** Patients with known WPW syndrome should continue to receive their antidysrhythmic drugs. The goal of management is to avoid any event (e.g., increased sympathetic nervous system activity resulting from pain, anxiety, or hypovolemia) or drug (e.g., digoxin, verapamil) that could enhance anterograde conduction of cardiac impulses through an accessory pathway. Equipment for electrical cardioversion-defibrillation must be available.

TABLE 4-3 ■ Manifestations of Wolff-Parkinson-White Syndrome

Symptomatic tachydysrhythmia is typically first seen in early adulthood.
Dysrhythmias may first be seen perioperatively.
Symptoms may include palpitations with or without dizziness, syncope, dyspnea, or angina.
Sudden death may be the first sign (presumably due to VF).
ECG findings include delta wave and supraventricular tachycardia that is most commonly orthodromic (narrow QRS) but may be antidromic (wide QRS).
Atrial fibrillation and/or atrial flutter may be present, which can result in very rapid ventricular response rates and/or VF.

ECG, Electrocardiogram; *VF*, ventricular fibrillation.

TABLE 4-4 ■ Treatment of Wolff-Parkinson-White Syndrome

Orthodromic (narrow QRS) tachycardia	Vagal maneuvers Adenosine Verapamil β-Blockers Amiodarone
Antidromic (wide QRS) tachycardia	Procainamide if systolic BP > 90 mm Hg Cardioversion if systolic BP < 90 mm Hg
Atrial fibrillation	Procainamide Cardioversion if hemodynamically unstable

VII. LONG QT SYNDROME

Long QT syndrome (LQTS) can be congenital or acquired. Several genetically determined syndromes usually manifest as syncope in late childhood. Episodes may be precipitated by stress, exercise, or other events that stimulate the sympathetic nervous system. Acquired LQTS may be caused by many prescription medications, such as antibiotics, antidysrhythmics, antidepressants, and antiemetics.

A. Diagnosis. LQTS is associated with prolongation of the QTc to more than 460 to 480 milliseconds. During a syncopal episode, the most common finding on the ECG is polymorphic VT (TdP).

B. Treatment. Treatment of LQTS includes correction of electrolyte abnormalities and discontinuation of drugs associated with QT prolongation. Additional treatment options include β-blocker therapy, cardiac pacing, and AICD implantation.

C. Anesthetic Management (Table 4-5)

VIII. MECHANISMS OF BRADYDYSRHYTHMIAS

Bradydysrhythmias (heart rate less than 60 beats/min) are most commonly caused by SA node dysfunction or a conduction block.

A. Sinus Bradycardia

1. **Diagnosis.** Sinus bradycardia occurs at a heart rate of less than 60 beats per minute. The ECG shows a regular rhythm with a normal-appearing P wave before each QRS complex.
2. **Treatment.** Atropine, epinephrine, or dopamine may be used to treat severely symptomatic patients, but cardiac pacing is the long-term treatment of choice.

TABLE 4-5 ■ Anesthesia Management in Patients with Long QT Syndrome (LQTS)

- Perform preoperative electrocardiography to exclude LQTS in a patient with a family history of sudden death.
- Consider preoperative β-blockade.
- Consider the effects of volatile agents, droperidol, and antiemetic medications on the QT interval.
- Avoid events that lead to sympathetic activation and prolongation of the QT interval.
- Treat hypokalemia and hypomagnesemia.
- Administer esmolol to treat acute dysrhythmias.
- A defibrillator should be immediately available.

3. **Anesthetic Management.** Sinus bradycardia in asymptomatic patients requires no treatment. If patients are severely symptomatic, immediate transcutaneous or transvenous pacing is indicated, with or without pharmacologic support.
4. **Bradycardia Associated with Spinal and Epidural Anesthesia.** Bradycardia or asystole may develop suddenly (within seconds or minutes) in a patient with a previously normal or even increased heart rate, or the heart rate slowing may be progressive. It most often occurs approximately an hour after spinal or epidural anesthetic is initiated. Arterial oxygen saturation is typically normal. Approximately half of patients note shortness of breath, nausea, restlessness, light-headedness, or tingling fingers and manifest a deterioration in mental status before arrest. The risk of bradycardia and asystole may persist into the postoperative period. Proposed mechanisms include reflex-induced bradycardia resulting from decreased venous return and activation of vagal reflex arcs. Another possibility is unopposed parasympathetic nervous system activity resulting from an anesthetic-induced sympathectomy. Bradydysrhythmias associated with spinal or epidural anesthesia should be treated aggressively.
5. **Bradycardia Associated with Sinus Node Dysfunction.** Dysfunction of the SA node, also referred to as *sick sinus syndrome,* is a common cause of bradycardia and accounts for more than 50% of the indications for placement of a permanent cardiac pacemaker.

B. Junctional Rhythm. Junctional (nodal) rhythm is caused by activity of the cardiac pacemaker in the tissues surrounding the AV node. Junctional pacemakers usually have an intrinsic rate of 40 to 60 beats per minute. The ECG can show either no P wave or a P wave preceding the QRS but with a shortened PR interval. Atropine can be used to treat hemodynamically significant junctional rhythms.

IX. CONDUCTION DISTURBANCES

Abnormalities of the conduction system can lead to heart block (Table 4-6).

X. TREATMENT OF CARDIAC DYSRHYTHMIAS

A. Antidysrhythmic Drugs (Table 4-7)

B. Electrical Cardioversion

1. **Synchronized Cardioversion.** Synchronized cardioversion entails delivery of an electrical discharge synchronized to the R wave of the ECG so that the current is delivered during the QRS complex and not during the vulnerable period of the T wave. It is used to treat acute unstable SVTs (such as atrial flutter and atrial fibrillation) and to convert chronic stable rate-controlled atrial flutter or atrial fibrillation to sinus rhythm.

TABLE 4-6 ■ **Conduction Disturbances of the Heart**

CONDUCTION DISTURBANCE	CHARACTERISTICS
First-degree atrioventricular (AV) block	PR interval > 0.2 sec Usually asymptomatic Atropine is usually effective treatment
Second-degree AV block: Mobitz I (Wenckebach)	Progressive prolongation of the PR interval until a beat is dropped Usually transient and asymptomatic
Second-degree AV block: Mobitz II	Complete interruption of cardiac conduction with dropped beats Usually symptomatic with palpitations and near syncope Higher risk to progress to third-degree heart block than Mobitz I Treatment is cardiac pacing (atropine usually not effective)
Right bundle branch block (RBBB)	QRS > 0.12 sec and rSR in V_1 and V_2 Usually benign
Left bundle branch block (LBBB)	QRS > 0.12 sec and absence of Q waves in leads I and V_6 Often associated with ischemic heart disease
Third-degree heart block (complete heart block)	If block is nodal, heart rate 45-55 beats/min If block is infranodal, heart rate 30-40 beats/min Treatment is cardiac pacing—intravenous isoproterenol may temporize until pacing can be initiated

TABLE 4-7 ■ **Antidysrhythmic Drugs**

DRUG/INDICATION	COMMON SIDE EFFECTS
β-Adrenergic blockers: Ventricular rate control in atrial fibrillation, atrial flutter, and narrow-complex tachycardias	Bradycardia AV conduction delay Hypotension
Adenosine: Supraventricular tachydysrhythmias, AVNRT	Peripheral vasodilation, flushing Dyspnea Bronchospasm Angina
Amiodarone: Supraventricular tachydysrhythmias, VT, prevention of recurrent atrial fibrillation, improved response to defibrillation	Slows metabolism of other drugs that undergo hepatic metabolism Bradycardia Hypotension Pulmonary fibrosis Thyroid dysfunction
Atropine: Symptomatic bradycardia	Tachycardia
Calcium channel blockers: SVT, atrial fibrillation, atrial flutter; *contraindicated* in WPW syndrome	Second- or third-degree heart block Myocardial depression Peripheral vasodilation Bradycardia

TABLE 4-7 ■ **Antidysrhythmic Drugs—cont'd**

DRUG/INDICATION	COMMON SIDE EFFECTS
Catecholamines:	
Dopamine: Symptomatic bradycardia unresponsive to atropine	Tachycardia Hypertension Peripheral vasoconstriction
Epinephrine: To support circulation during cardiopulmonary resuscitation, cardiac arrest resulting from β-blocker or calcium channel blocker overdose	Hypertension Tachycardia
Isoproterenol: Symptomatic bradycardia, complete heart block, cardiac transplantation patients	Bronchodilation Tachycardia Peripheral vasodilation
Digoxin: Atrial tachydysrhythmias, atrial fibrillation, atrial flutter	Toxicity, especially with renal failure and/or hypokalemia Enhanced conduction through accessory pathways
Lidocaine: VPBs, ventricular tachydysrhythmias, recurrent ventricular fibrillation	Accumulation and toxicity with decreased hepatic blood flow Central nervous system toxicity
Magnesium: May be useful for torsade de pointes	Muscle weakness
Procainamide: Ventricular tachycardia with pulse, atrial flutter or fibrillation, atrial fibrillation in WPW syndrome, SVT resistant to vagal maneuvers or adenosine	Prolonged QT interval Hypotension Lupus-like syndrome Myocardial depression Accumulation in patients with renal failure
Sotalol: Ventricular tachycardia, atrial fibrillation or flutter in WPW syndrome	Bronchospasm Lethargy Myocardial depression
Vasopressin: To support circulation during cardiopulmonary resuscitation	Vasoconstriction
20% Lipid emulsion: Bupivacaine overdose with ventricular dysrhythmias	None known

AV, Atrioventricular; *SVT,* supraventricular tachycardia; *VPB,* ventricular premature beat; *VT,* ventricular tachycardia; *WPW,* Wolff-Parkinson-White.

Propofol and short-acting benzodiazepines are commonly used for sedation during elective cardioversion.

C. Defibrillation. Defibrillation is the delivery of an electrical discharge that is not synchronized (because there are no R waves) for treatment of VF. Modern defibrillators are classified as either monophasic or biphasic.

D. Radiofrequency Catheter Ablation. Cardiac dysrhythmias amenable to radiofrequency catheter ablation include reentrant supraventricular dysrhythmias and some ventricular dysrhythmias. The procedure is usually performed under conscious sedation.

E. Artificial Cardiac Pacemakers

1. **Transcutaneous Cardiac Pacing.** Patients with symptomatic bradycardia or severe conduction block require immediate pacing. Transcutaneous pacing should be considered a temporizing measure until transvenous cardiac pacing can be instituted.
2. **Permanently Implanted Cardiac Pacemakers.** Cardiac pacing is the only long-term treatment for symptomatic bradycardia regardless of cause. An artificial cardiac pacemaker can be inserted intravenously (endocardial lead) or via a subcostal approach (epicardial or myocardial lead).
3. **Pacing Modes.** A five-letter generic code is used to describe the various characteristics of cardiac pacemakers. (1) the cardiac chamber(s) being paced (*A*, atrial; *V*, ventricular; *D*, dual chamber); (2) the cardiac chamber(s) that detect(s) (sense[s]) electrical signals (*A*, atrial; *V*, ventricular; *D*, dual; 0, none); (3) the response to sensed signals (*I*, inhibition; *T*, triggering; *D*, dual: inhibition and triggering; 0, none); (4) *R*, denotes activation of rate response features; and (5) for multisite pacing, the chamber(s) in which multisite pacing is delivered. The most common pacing modes are AAI, VVI, and DDD (Table 4-8).
   a. ***DDD Pacing.*** The pacemaker responds to increases in sinus node discharge rate, such as during exercise. DDD pacing minimizes the incidence of pacemaker syndrome (syncope, weakness, orthopnea, paroxysmal nocturnal dyspnea, hypotension, pulmonary edema) that is a result of loss of AV synchrony and the consequent decrease in cardiac output.
   b. ***DDI Pacing.*** Sensing occurs in both the atrium and ventricle, but the only response to a sensed event is inhibition. DDI pacing is useful in the presence of atrial tachydysrhythmias.
   c. ***Asynchronous Pacing.*** With A00, V00, and D00 pacing, leads fire at a fixed rate regardless of the patient's underlying rhythm.
   d. ***Rate-Adaptive Pacemakers.*** Rate-adaptive pacemakers are used in patients who lack an appropriate heart rate response to exercise.
   e. ***Single-Chamber Pacing.*** Single-chamber pacing is used often in patients with symptomatic bradycardia resulting from SA or AV node disease. Pacemaker syndrome can result because of loss of AV synchrony in single-chamber pacing.
   f. ***Dual-Chamber Pacing.*** Dual-chamber pacing is also called "physiologic pacing" because it maintains AV synchrony.
4. **Choice of Pacing Mode.** Choice of pacing mode depends on the primary indication for the artificial pacemaker. (Sinus node disease necessitates an atrial pacemaker; AV node disease calls for a dual-chamber pacemaker; the need for a rate response to exercise necessitates a rate-adaptive pacemaker.)
5. **Complications of Permanent Cardiac Pacing.** Early complications related to insertion (e.g., pneumothorax, hemothorax, air embolism) occur in about 5% of patients, and late complications in 2% to 7%. Early pacemaker failure is usually caused by electrode displacement or breakage. Pacemaker failure that occurs more than 6 months after implantation is usually a result of premature battery depletion.

F. Implanted Cardioverter-Defibrillator Therapy. Implanted cardioverter-defibrillators (ICDs) were approved by the U.S. Food and Drug Administration in 1985 for use in patients at risk of VF. The ICD senses VF, the capacitor charges, and, before shock delivery, a confirmatory algorithm is fulfilled by signal analysis. This process prevents inappropriate shocks for self-terminating events or spurious signals. Approximately half of patients with ICDs will have an adverse event related to the device within the first year after implantation, such as failure to sense or pace, inappropriate therapy, or dislodgment. A coding system for ICDs is similar to that for pacemakers. The first letter is the chamber shocked (*0*, none; *A*, atrium; *V*, ventricle; *D*, dual), the second letter is the *antitachycardia* pacing chamber (*0*, *A*, *V*, or *D*), the third indicates the tachycardia detection mechanism (*E*,

TABLE 4-8 ■ **Types of Pacemaker Pulse Generators**

LETTER CODE	DESCRIPTION
SINGLE-CHAMBER PACING MODES	
AOO	Asynchronous (fixed rate) atrial pacing
VOO	Asynchronous ventricular pacing
AAI	"Demand" atrial pacing: pacemaker senses and is inhibited by intrinsic atrial depolarization (P wave)
VVI	"Demand" ventricular pacing: pacemaker senses and is inhibited by intrinsic ventricular depolarization (R wave)
DUAL-CHAMBER PACING MODES	
DDD	Paces and senses both atrium and ventricle
DDI	Senses both the atrium and ventricle and is inhibited if a *P* wave or *R* wave are present
DDDR	Sensors detect changes in movement or minute ventilation as sings of exercise and make rate adjustments

A, Atrium; *V*, ventricle; D, dual; *0*, none—asynchronous; *I*, inhibited; *R*, rate-adaptive.

electrocardiogram; *H*, hemodynamic), and the fourth is the *antibradycardia* pacing chamber (0, A, V, D).

G. Surgery in Patients with Cardiac Devices

1. **Preoperative Evaluation.** Evaluation includes determining the reason for the device and assessment of its current function. A preoperative history of presyncope, or syncope in a patient with a pacemaker or a decrease in heart rate from the initial heart rate setting, could reflect pacemaker dysfunction. The ECG is not a diagnostic aid if the intrinsic heart rate is greater than the preset pacemaker rate. In such cases, proper function of a synchronous or sequential artificial cardiac pacemaker is best confirmed by electronic evaluation. ICDs are often switched off preoperatively and switched back on postoperatively.
2. **Management of Anesthesia.** In patients with artificial cardiac pacemakers, management of anesthesia includes (1) monitoring the ECG to confirm proper functioning of the pulse generator and (2) ensuring the availability of equipment (external defibrillator-pacer magnet) and drugs (atropine, isoproterenol) to maintain an acceptable intrinsic heart rate should the cardiac pacemaker unexpectedly fail. Pulmonary artery catheters may become entangled in, or dislodge, recently placed transvenous (endocardial) electrodes but are unlikely to dislodge electrodes more than 4 weeks after implantation. Improved shielding of cardiac pacemakers has reduced the problems associated with electromagnetic interference from electrocautery, which can either cause a device to revert to asynchronous functioning or be completely inhibited. The grounding pad for electrocautery should be as far as possible from the pulse generator; the electrocautery current should be kept as low as possible and applied in short bursts. The presence of a temporary transvenous cardiac pacemaker presents a special risk of VF resulting from microshock currents conducted by the pacing electrodes. If cardioversion or defibrillation becomes necessary, care should be taken to keep the therapeutic current away from the pulse generator and lead system. Postoperative management includes interrogating the device and restoring appropriate baseline settings if necessary. This should be done as soon as possible after surgery.

3. **Anesthesia for Cardiac Pacemaker Insertion.** Most pacemakers are inserted using conscious sedation and routine monitoring. Drugs such as atropine or isoproterenol should be available in the event that a decrease in heart rate compromises hemodynamics before the new pacemaker is functional.

CHAPTER 5

Systemic and Pulmonary Arterial Hypertension

I. SYSTEMIC HYPERTENSION

Systemic hypertension (HTN) affects approximately 30% of adults in the United States. HTN is defined in adults as a systemic blood pressure (BP) of 140/90 mm Hg or more on at least two occasions measured at least 1 to 2 weeks apart (Table 5-1). Prehypertension is a systemic BP of 120 to 139 mm Hg or a diastolic BP of 80 to 89 mm Hg. HTN is a significant risk factor for the development of ischemic heart disease and a major cause of congestive heart failure (CHF), stroke, arterial aneurysm, and end-stage renal disease. A widened pulse pressure (the difference between systolic and diastolic BP) has been linked with intraoperative hemodynamic instability and adverse perioperative outcomes.

A. Pathophysiology. Systemic HTN is termed *essential* or *primary* when a cause cannot be identified and *secondary* when an identifiable cause is present.

1. *Essential HTN* accounts for more than 95% of all cases of HTN and is characterized by a familial incidence and inherited biochemical abnormalities (Table 5-2).
2. *Secondary HTN* accounts for less than 5% of all cases of systemic HTN and is most commonly a result of renal artery stenosis (Table 5-3).

B. Treatment of Essential Hypertension. The standard goal of therapy is to decrease systemic BP to less than 140/90 mm Hg or, in the presence of diabetes mellitus or renal disease, to less than 130/80 mm Hg. Treatment resulting in normalization of blood pressure lowers the incidence of cerebrovascular accidents and progression to CHF and/or renal failure.

1. **Lifestyle Modification.** Lifestyle modifications of proven value for lowering BP include weight reduction, moderation of alcohol intake, smoking cessation, increased physical activity, maintenance of recommended levels of dietary calcium and potassium, and moderation in dietary salt intake.
2. **Pharmacologic Therapy.** Thiazide diuretics are recommended as initial therapy for uncomplicated HTN. The hypertensive patient may have comorbid conditions that provide indications for antihypertensive therapy with drugs of a particular class (Table 5-4). Angiotensin-converting enzyme inhibitors (ACEIs) or angiotensin receptor blockers (ARBs) are particularly useful for patients with a history of CHF.

C. Treatment of Secondary Hypertension. Treatment of secondary HTN is usually surgical with pharmacologic therapy reserved for patients in whom surgery is not possible. Conditions treated surgically include renovascular HTN, hyperaldosteronism, Cushing's disease, and pheochromocytoma.

D. Hypertensive Crises. A hypertensive crisis typically manifests with a BP higher than 180/120 and is categorized as either a *hypertensive urgency or emergency,* based on the presence or absence of impending or progressive target organ damage.

1. **Hypertensive Emergency.** Patients with evidence of acute or ongoing target organ damage (encephalopathy, intracerebral hemorrhage, acute left ventricular failure, pulmonary

TABLE 5-1 ■ Classification of Systemic Hypertension

CATEGORY	SYSTOLIC BLOOD PRESSURE (mm Hg)	DIASTOLIC BLOOD PRESSURE (mm Hg)
Normal	<120	<80
Prehypertension	120-139	80-89
Stage 1 hypertension	140-159	90-99
Stage 2 hypertension	≥160	≥100

Data from Chobanian AV, Bakris G, Black H, et al. Seventh Report of the Joint National Committee on Prevention, Detection, Evaluation and Treatment of High Blood Pressure. *Hypertension*. 2003;42:1206-1252.

TABLE 5-2 ■ Conditions Associated with Essential Hypertension

- Increased sympathetic nervous system activity
- Sodium and water retention
- Hypercholesterolemia
- Insulin resistance
- Obesity
- Alcohol and tobacco use
- Obstructive sleep apnea
- Glucose intolerance
- Ischemic heart disease and angina pectoris
- Left ventricular hypertrophy
- Congestive heart failure
- Cerebrovascular disease
- Peripheral vascular disease
- Renal insufficiency

edema, unstable angina, dissecting aortic aneurysm, acute myocardial infarction, eclampsia, microangiopathic hemolytic anemia, renal insufficiency) require prompt treatment. The treatment goal is to decrease the diastolic BP by about 20% within the first 60 minutes, and then more gradually. In parturients, a diastolic BP of greater than 109 mm Hg is considered a hypertensive emergency. Placement of an intraarterial catheter for continuous BP monitoring treatment is advised.

2. **Hypertensive Urgency.** Hypertensive urgency is said to be present when BP is severely elevated without evidence of target organ damage. Presenting symptoms and signs can include headache, epistaxis, or anxiety. Some patients benefit from oral antihypertensive therapy because noncompliance with or unavailability of prescribed medications is often responsible for this problem.
3. **Pharmacologic Therapy** (Table 5-5). Pharmacologic therapy depends on the patient's comorbidities and symptoms and signs at presentation.

E. **Management of Anesthesia in Patients with Essential Hypertension** (Table 5-6). There is no evidence that postoperative complications are increased when most hypertensive patients (diastolic BP as high as 110 mm Hg) undergo elective surgery (Table 5-7). However, co-existing HTN may increase the incidence of postoperative myocardial reinfarction in patients with prior myocardial infarction and the incidence of neurologic complications in patients undergoing carotid endarterectomy.

TABLE 5-3 ■ **Common Causes of Secondary Hypertension**

CAUSES	CLINICAL FINDINGS	LABORATORY EVALUATION
Renovascular disease	Epigastric or abdominal bruit Severe hypertension in young patient	MRA Aortography Duplex ultrasonography CT angiography
Hyperaldosteronism	Fatigue Weakness Headache Paresthesias Nocturnal polyuria and polydipsia	Urinary potassium Serum potassium Plasma renin Plasma aldosterone
Aortic coarctation	Elevated blood pressure in upper limbs relative to lower limbs Weak femoral pulses Systolic bruit	Aortography Echocardiography MRI or CT
Pheochromocytoma	Episodic headache, palpitations, and diaphoresis Paroxysmal hypertension	Plasma catecholamines Urinary metanephrines Adrenal CT or MRI scan
Cushing's syndrome	Truncal obesity Proximal muscle weakness Purple striae "Moon facies" Hirsutism	Dexamethasone suppression test Urinary cortisol Adrenal CT scan Glucose tolerance test
Renal parenchymal disease	Nocturia Edema	Urinary glucose, protein, and casts Serum creatinine Renal ultrasonography Renal biopsy
Pregnancy-induced hypertension	Peripheral and pulmonary edema Headache Seizures Right upper quadrant pain	Urinary protein Uric acid Cardiac output Platelet count

CT, Computed tomography; *MRI,* magnetic resonance imaging; *MRA,* magnetic resonance angiography.

1. **Preoperative Evaluation**
   a. Evaluate for the presence of end-organ damage (angina pectoris, left ventricular hypertrophy, CHF, cerebrovascular disease, stroke, peripheral vascular disease, renal insufficiency). Elective surgery should be postponed if end-organ damage can be improved or further evaluation would alter the anesthetic plan.
   b. A diastolic BP of 100 to 115 mm Hg is often used as a criterion for postponing elective surgery, although no universal guidelines exist.
   c. Electrolyte imbalance, such as hypokalemia (<3.5 mEq/L), is a common perioperative finding in patients taking diuretic medication but does not appear to increase the incidence of cardiac dysrhythmias in the perioperative period. Hyperkalemia may be seen in patients taking ACEIs or ARBs who are also receiving potassium supplementation or have renal dysfunction.
   d. Most antihypertensive drugs should be continued throughout the perioperative period to ensure optimal control of BP.

TABLE 5-4 ■ **Common Antihypertensive Drugs**

CLASS	SUBCLASS	GENERIC NAME	TRADE NAME
Diuretics	Thiazides	Chlorothiazide Hydrochlorothiazide Indapamide Metolazone	Diuril HydroDiuril, Microzide Lozol Zaroxolyn, Mykrox
	Loop	Bumetanide Furosemide Torsemide	Bumex Lasix Demadex
	Potassium-sparing	Amiloride Spironolactone Triamterene	Midamor Aldactone Dyrenium
Adrenergic antagonists	β-Blockers	Atenolol Bisoprolol Metoprolol Nadolol Propranolol Timolol	Tenormin Zebeta Lopressor Corgard Inderal Blocadren
	α_1-Blockers	Doxazosin Prazosin Terazosin	Cardura Minipress Hytrin
	Combined α- and β-blockers	Carvedilol Labetalol	Coreg Normodyne, Trandate
Adrenergic agonists	Centrally acting α-agonists	Clonidine Methyldopa	Catapres Aldomet
Vasodilators		Hydralazine	Apresoline
ACEIs		Benazepril Captopril Enalapril Fosinopril Lisinopril Moexipril Quinapril Ramipril Trandolapril	Lotensin Capoten Vasotec Monopril Prinivil, Zestril Univasc Accupril Altace Mavik
Angiotensin receptor blockers		Candesartan Eprosartan Irbesartan Losartan Olmesartan Telmisartan Valsartan	Atacand Teveten Avapro Cozaar Benicar Micardis Diovan
Calcium channel blockers	Dihydropyridine	Amlodipine Clevidipine Felodipine Israpidine Nicardipine Nifedipine Nisoldipine	Norvasc Cleviprex Plendil DynaCirc Cardene Adalat, Procardia Sular
	Nondihydropyridine	Diltiazem Verapamil	Cardizem, Dilacor, Tiazac Calan, Isoptin SR, Covera

ACEI, Angiotensin-converting enzyme inhibitor.

TABLE 5-5 ■ Treatment of Hypertensive Emergencies

CAUSE AND MANIFESTATION	PRIMARY AGENTS	CAUTIONS	COMMENTS
Encephalopathy and intracranial hypertension	Nitroprusside, labetalol, fenoldopam, nicardipine	Cerebral ischemia may result from lowering blood pressure as a result of altered autoregulation. Risk of cyanide toxicity with nitroprusside. Nitroprusside increases intracranial pressure.	Lower blood pressure may lessen bleeding in intracerebral hemorrhage.
Myocardial ischemia	Nitroglycerin	Avoid β-blockers in acute congestive heart failure.	Include morphine and oxygen therapy.
Acute pulmonary edema	Nitroglycerin, nitroprusside, fenoldopam	Avoid β-blockers in acute congestive heart failure.	Include morphine, loop diuretic, and oxygen therapy.
Aortic dissection	Trimethaphan, esmolol, other vasodilators in combination with a β-blocker	Vasodilators may cause reflex tachycardia and increased pulsatile force of left ventricular contraction.	Goal: lessening of pulsatile force of left ventricular contraction.
Renal insufficiency	Fenoldopam, nicardipine	Tachyphylaxis occurs with fenoldopam.	May require emergent hemodialysis. Avoid ACEIs and ARBs.
Preeclampsia and eclampsia	Methyldopa, hydralazine Magnesium sulfate Labetalol, nicardipine	Hydralazine can cause lupuslike syndrome. Patients have risk of flash pulmonary edema. Calcium channel blockers may reduce uterine blood flow and inhibit labor.	Definitive therapy is delivery of fetus. ACEIs and ARBs are contraindicated during pregnancy owing to teratogenicity.
Pheochromocytoma	Phentolamine, phenoxybenzamine, propranolol	Unopposed α-adrenergic stimulation after β-blockade worsens hypertension.	
Cocaine intoxication	Nitroglycerin, nitroprusside, phentolamine	Unopposed α-adrenergic stimulation after β-blockade worsens hypertension.	

ACEIs, Angiotensin-converting enzyme inhibitors; *ARBs,* angiotensin receptor blockers.

TABLE 5-6 ■ Management of Anesthesia for Patients with Hypertension

PREOPERATIVE EVALUATION
Determine adequacy of blood pressure control. Review pharmacology of drugs being administered to control blood pressure. Evaluate for evidence of end-organ damage. Continue drugs used to control blood pressure.
INDUCTION AND MAINTENANCE OF ANESTHESIA
Anticipate exaggerated blood pressure response to anesthetic drugs. Limit duration of direct laryngoscopy. Administer a balanced anesthetic to blunt hypertensive responses. Consider placement of invasive hemodynamic monitors. Monitor for myocardial ischemia.
POSTOPERATIVE MANAGEMENT
Anticipate periods of systemic hypertension. Maintain monitoring of end-organ function.

TABLE 5-7 ■ Risk of General Anesthesia and Elective Surgery in Hypertensive Patients

PREOPERATIVE SYSTEMIC BLOOD PRESSURE STATUS	INCIDENCE OF PERIOPERATIVE HYPERTENSIVE EPISODES (%)	INCIDENCE OF POSTOPERATIVE CARDIAC COMPLICATIONS (%)
Normotensive	8*	11
Treated and rendered normotensive	27	24
Treated but remain hypertensive	25	7
Untreated and hypertensive	20	12

Data from Goldman L, Caldera DL. Risk of general anesthesia and elective operation in the hypertensive patient. *Anesthesiology*. 1979;50:285-292.
*$P < .05$ compared with other groups in the same column.

1. *ACEIs and ARBs*. Surgical procedures involving major fluid shifts in patients treated with ACEIs have been associated with hypotension that is responsive to fluid infusion and administration of sympathomimetic drugs. It may be prudent to discontinue ACEIs 24 to 48 hours preoperatively in patients at high risk of intraoperative hypovolemia and hypotension. The hypotension experienced by patients treated with ARBs can be refractory to conventional vasoconstrictors such as ephedrine and phenylephrine, necessitating use of vasopressin or one of its analogues. ARBs should be discontinued on the day before surgery.

2. **Induction of Anesthesia.** Anesthesia can produce an exaggerated *decrease* in BP owing to peripheral vasodilation in the presence of decreased intravascular fluid volume.
   a. *Direct laryngoscopy* and tracheal intubation can produce significant *increases* in BP patients with essential HTN, even if these patients are normotensive preoperatively. Myocardial ischemia is more likely to occur in association with the HTN and tachycardia that accompany laryngoscopy and intubation. These patients may benefit from

TABLE 5-8 ■ **Calculation of Pulmonary Vascular Resistance (PVR)**

$\frac{(\text{Mean PAP} - \text{PAOP}) \times 80}{\text{CO}}$	PVR is expressed in dynes/sec/cm^{-5}, with normal PVR = 50-150 dynes/sec/cm^{-5}
$\frac{(\text{Mean PAP} - \text{PAOP})}{\text{CO}}$	PVR is expressed in Wood units (mm Hg/L/min), with normal PVR = 1 Wood unit

CO, Cardiac output (L/min); *PAOP,* pulmonary artery occlusion pressure (mm Hg); *PAP,* pulmonary artery pressure (mm Hg).

maneuvers that suppress tracheal reflexes and blunt the autonomic responses to tracheal manipulation (deep inhalation anesthesia; injection of an opioid, lidocaine, β-blocker, or vasodilator before laryngoscopy) and from limiting duration of direct laryngoscopy to 15 seconds or less.

3. **Maintenance of Anesthesia.** Management of intraoperative BP lability is as important as preoperative control of HTN in these patients. Regional anesthesia can be used in hypertensive patients. However, a high sensory level of anesthesia with its associated sympathetic denervation can unmask hypovolemia.
   a. ***Intraoperative Hypertension.*** Hypertension in response to painful stimuli is likely, even in patients whose BP is controlled preoperatively. Volatile anesthetics are useful in attenuating sympathetic nervous system activity responsible for pressor responses. Alternatively, antihypertensive medication can be administered by bolus or by continuous infusion.
   b. ***Intraoperative Hypotension.*** Hypotension may be treated by decreasing the depth of anesthesia, increasing fluid infusion rates, and/or administering sympathomimetic drugs such as ephedrine or phenylephrine. Intraoperative hypotension in patients being treated with ACEIs or ARBs is responsive to administration of intravenous fluids, sympathomimetic drugs, and/or vasopressin.
   c. ***Intraoperative Monitoring.*** Invasive monitoring with an intraarterial catheter and a central venous or pulmonary artery catheter may be useful if extensive surgery is planned and there is evidence of left ventricular dysfunction or other significant end-organ damage. Transesophageal echocardiography can be used to monitor volume status but requires specialized equipment and personnel and is not universally available.
4. **Postoperative Management.** Postoperative HTN is common and requires prompt treatment to decrease the risk of myocardial ischemia, cardiac dysrhythmias, CHF, stroke, and bleeding.

II. PULMONARY ARTERIAL HYPERTENSION

Pulmonary arterial HTN (PAH) is defined as a mean pulmonary artery pressure greater than 25 mm Hg at rest or greater than 30 mm Hg with exercise, and a pulmonary artery occlusion pressure of 15 mm Hg or less, and pulmonary vascular resistance (PVR) greater than 3 Wood units (mm Hg/L/min) (Table 5-8). PAH with no familial context and without evidence of left-sided heart disease, myocardial disease, congenital heart disease, or any clinically significant respiratory, connective tissue, or chronic thromboembolic disease is called idiopathic PAH. For classification of PAH, see Table 5-9. Subsequent discussion will focus on idiopathic PAH. PAH increases perioperative risk of right ventricular (RV) failure, hypoxemia, coronary ischemia, respiratory failure, dysrhythmias, and CHF, as well as perioperative mortality.

A. **Clinical Presentation and Evaluation.** Common symptoms are breathlessness, weakness, fatigue, abdominal distention, syncope, and angina pectoris. Physical findings may include a parasternal lift, murmur of pulmonic insufficiency (Graham-Steell murmur) and/or tricuspid

TABLE 5-9 ■ Clinical Findings in Pulmonary Hypertension

DIAGNOSTIC MODALITY	KEY FINDINGS
Chest radiograph	Prominent pulmonary arteries Right atrial and right ventricular enlargement Parenchymal lung disease
Electrocardiography	P pulmonale Right axis deviation Right ventricular strain or hypertrophy Complete or incomplete right bundle branch block
Two-dimensional echocardiography	Right atrial enlargement Right ventricular hypertrophy, dilation, or volume overload Tricuspid regurgitation Elevated estimated pulmonary artery pressures Congenital heart disease
Pulmonary function tests	Obstructive or restrictive pattern Low diffusing capacity
$\dot{V}/\dot{Q}$ scan	Ventilation/perfusion mismatching
Pulmonary angiography	Vascular filling defects
Chest CT scan	Main pulmonary artery size >30 mm Vascular filling defects Mosaic perfusion defects
Abdominal ultrasound or CT scan	Cirrhosis Portal hypertension
Blood tests	Antinuclear antibody positive Rheumatoid factor positive Platelet dysfunction HIV positive
Sleep study	High respiratory disturbance index

Data from Dincer HE, Presberg KW. Current management of pulmonary hypertension. *Clin Pulm Med.* 2004;11:40-53.

CT, Computed tomography; *HIV,* human immunodeficiency virus; $\dot{V}/\dot{Q}$, ventilation/perfusion.

regurgitation, a pronounced pulmonic component of S_2, an S_3 gallop, jugular venous distention, peripheral edema, hepatomegaly, and ascites. Ortner's syndrome is paralysis of the left recurrent laryngeal nerve caused by compression by the dilated pulmonary artery. Laboratory evaluation and diagnostic studies used in the workup of PAH of any cause are listed in Table 5-9. Right-sided heart catheterization can aid in evaluating disease severity and determining potential response to vasodilator therapy.

B. Physiology and Pathophysiology. PAH develops in response to pulmonary vasoconstriction, vascular wall remodeling, and thrombosis in situ. RV wall stress increases in response to PAH. RV stroke volume and left ventricular filling are reduced, leading to low cardiac output and systemic hypotension. RV dilation results in annular dilation of right-sided heart valves producing tricuspid regurgitation and/or pulmonic insufficiency. RV myocardial perfusion is limited as the RV wall stress increases. Hypoxemia can occur by three mechanisms: (1) right-to-left shunting through a patent foramen ovale; (2) increased oxygen extraction associated with exertion in the face of a fixed cardiac output; and (3) ventilation/perfusion ($\dot{V}/\dot{Q}$) mismatch.

C. Treatment of Pulmonary Arterial Hypertension. A sample treatment algorithm is presented in Figure 5-1.

1. **Oxygen, Anticoagulation, and Diuretics.** Oxygen therapy improves survival and reduces progression of PAH. Anticoagulation may reduce risk of thrombosis and thromboembolism resulting from sluggish pulmonary blood flow, dilation of the right side of the heart, venous stasis, and the limitation in physical activity imposed by this disease. Diuretics can decrease preload in patients with right-sided heart failure.
2. **Calcium Channel Blockers.** Nifedipine, diltiazem, and amlodipine are the most commonly used calcium channel blockers for this purpose and have been shown to improve 5-year survival in patients who are responsive to vasodilators.
3. **Phosphodiesterase Inhibitors.** Phosphodiesterase inhibitors dilate pulmonary blood vessels and improve cardiac output. Sildenafil (Viagra) administration has been associated with improved exercise capacity and reduction in RV mass. Tadalafil (Cialis) is a long-acting phosphodiesterase inhibitor that is well tolerated.
4. **Inhaled Nitric Oxide.** Nitric oxide (NO) improves $\dot{V}/\dot{Q}$ matching and improves oxygenation by relaxing pulmonary vascular smooth muscle. Problems associated with NO administration include rebound PAH, platelet inhibition, methemoglobinemia, formation of toxic nitrate metabolites, and the technical requirements for its application.
5. **Prostacyclins.** Prostacyclins (epoprostenol, treprostinil, iloprost) are systemic and pulmonary vasodilators that also have antiplatelet activity. Prostacyclins reduce PVR and improve cardiac output and exercise tolerance; they can be administered by continuous infusion, by inhalation, and by intermittent subcutaneous injection. All demonstrate short-term improvements in hemodynamics but have not been associated with sustained improvement or decreased mortality.
6. **Endothelin Receptor Antagonists (Bosentan).** Endothelin interacts with two receptors: endothelin A (pulmonary vasoconstriction and smooth muscle proliferation) and endothelin B (vasodilation, enhanced endothelin clearance, increased production of NO and prostacyclin). Endothelin receptor antagonists lower pulmonary arterial pressure and PVR and improve RV function, exercise tolerance, quality of life, and mortality.
7. **Surgical Treatment.** RV assist devices can be used in severe PAH and right-sided heart failure. Balloon atrial septostomy is a procedure that allows right-to-left shunting of blood to decompress the right heart, but it is used only as a treatment of advanced right-sided heart failure and as a bridge to cardiac transplantation. Lung transplantation is the only curative therapy for many types of PAH.

D. Anesthetic Management. Increased RV afterload, hypoxemia, hypotension, and inadequate RV preload contribute to an increased risk of RV failure. Hypoxia, hypercarbia, and acidosis must be aggressively controlled because they cause increased PVR. Reduction in systemic vascular resistance by inhalational anesthetics or sedatives may be dangerous because of the relatively fixed cardiac output. Maintenance of sinus rhythm is crucial because atrial "kick" may be critical for adequate ventricular filling.

1. **Preoperative Preparation and Induction.** In a PAH patient who is not yet on long-term therapy, administration of sildenafil or L-arginine preoperatively may be helpful. Pulmonary vasodilator therapy must be continued in the perioperative period. Ketamine and etomidate may inhibit pulmonary vasorelaxation and should be avoided. NO should be available if possible. Regional anesthesia should be used cautiously because the changes in intravascular volume and systemic vascular resistance may be poorly tolerated.
2. **Monitoring.** Central venous catheterization and intraarterial BP monitoring are recommended.
3. **Maintenance.** Inhalational agents are useful for maintenance of anesthesia. Systemic hypotension can be corrected with fluids, phenylephrine, or more potent vasoconstrictors if needed, because almost all potent systemic vasoconstrictors also increase pulmonary artery pressure. A potent pulmonary vasodilator such as milrinone, nitroglycerin, NO, or prostacyclin should be available to treat PAH should it worsen.

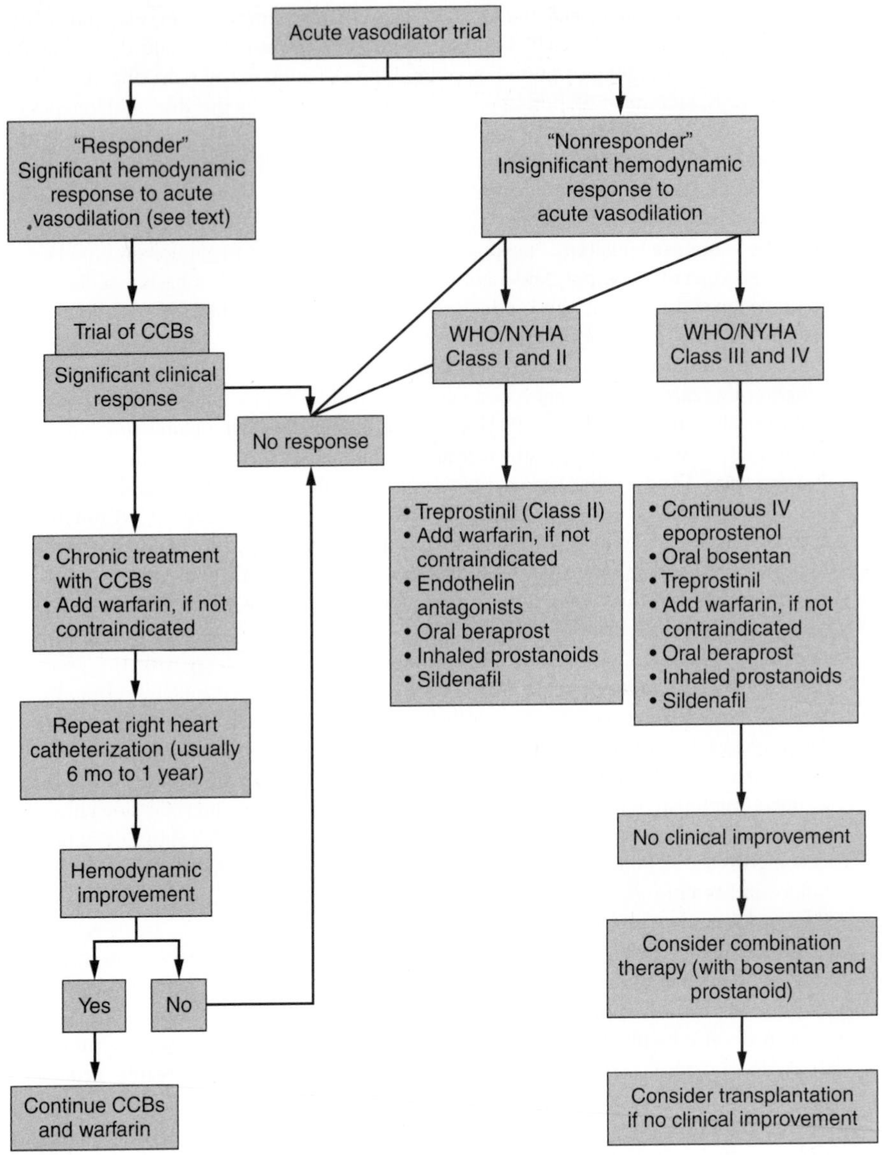

FIGURE 5-1 ■ Outpatient treatment of pulmonary arterial hypertension. *CCBs,* Calcium channel blockers; *IV,* intravenous; *NYHA,* New York Heart Association; *WHO,* World Health Organization. *(Data from Dincer HE, Presberg KW. Current management of pulmonary hypertension.* Clin Pulm Med. *2004;11:40-53.)*

4. **Postoperative Period.** Patients with PAH are at risk of sudden death in the early postoperative period because of worsening PAH, pulmonary thromboembolism, dysrhythmias, and fluid shifts. Intensive monitoring and optimal pain control are essential.
5. **Obstetric Population.** Delivery methods that decrease patient effort are recommended. Nitroglycerin should be immediately available at the time of uterine involution to offset the effects of uterine blood return to the central circulation.

CHAPTER 6

Heart Failure and Cardiomyopathies

I. HEART FAILURE

Heart failure (HF) is defined as the inability of the heart to fill with or eject blood at a rate appropriate to meet tissue requirements. HF affects about 1% of adults over age 65 in the United States. Systolic heart failure (SHF) is more common among middle-aged men, and diastolic heart failure (DHF) is usually seen in elderly women. HF is most often a result of (1) ischemic heart disease or cardiomyopathy; (2) cardiac valve abnormalities; (3) systemic hypertension (HTN); (4) diseases of the pericardium; or (5) pulmonary HTN (cor pulmonale).

A. Forms of Ventricular Dysfunction

1. **Systolic and Diastolic Heart Failure.** Decreased ventricular systolic wall motion reflects systolic dysfunction, whereas diastolic dysfunction is characterized by abnormal ventricular relaxation and reduced compliance.
   a. ***Systolic Heart Failure.*** Causes of SHF include coronary artery disease (CAD), dilated cardiomyopathy (DCM), chronic pressure overload (aortic stenosis and chronic HTN), and chronic volume overload (regurgitant valvular lesions and high-output cardiac failure). Patients with left bundle branch block (LBBB) and SHF are at high risk of sudden death.
   b. ***Diastolic Heart Failure.*** DHF occurs in patients with normal or near-normal left ventricular (LV) systolic function. DHF can be classified into four stages. Class I DHF is characterized by an abnormal LV relaxation pattern with normal left atrial pressure. Classes II, III, and IV include abnormal relaxation and reduced LV compliance resulting in increased left ventricular end-diastolic pressure (LVEDP). Ischemic heart disease, essential HTN, and aortic stenosis are the most common causes of DHF. The major differences between SHF and DHF are presented in Table 6-1.
   c. ***Acute and Chronic Heart Failure.*** *Acute HF* is defined as new-onset HF or a change in the signs and symptoms of chronic HF requiring emergency therapy. Chronic HF occurs in patients with longstanding cardiac disease and is associated with signs and symptoms of venous congestion. In patients with acute HF, systemic hypotension is often present without peripheral edema.
   d. ***Left-Sided and Right-Sided Heart Failure.*** In patients with left-sided HF, high LVEDP leads to pulmonary venous congestion with symptoms of dyspnea, orthopnea, paroxysmal nocturnal dyspnea, and pulmonary edema. Right-sided HF causes systemic venous congestion, with peripheral edema and hepatomegaly. The most common cause of right-sided HF is left-sided HF.
   e. ***Low-Output and High-Output Heart Failure.*** Normal cardiac index (CI) is 2.2 to 3.5 L/min/m^2. Low-output failure may occur in a patient who has a normal CI at rest but has an inadequate response to stress or exercise. The most common causes of low-output HF are CAD, cardiomyopathy, HTN, valvular disease, and pericardial disease. Causes of high output HF include anemia, pregnancy, arteriovenous fistulas, hyperthyroidism, beriberi, and Paget's disease. In high-output HF, ventricular failure is caused by an

TABLE 6-1 ■ **Characteristics of Patients with Diastolic Versus Systolic Heart Failure**

CHARACTERISTIC	DIASTOLIC HEART FAILURE	SYSTOLIC HEART FAILURE
Age	Often elderly	Typically 50-70 yr old
Sex	Often female	More often male
Left ventricular ejection fraction	Preserved, ≥40%	Depressed, ≤40%
Left ventricular cavity size	Usually normal, often with concentric left ventricular hypertrophy	Usually dilated
Chest radiography	Congestion ± cardiomegaly	Congestion and cardiomegaly
Gallop rhythm present	Fourth heart sound	Third heart sound
Hypertension	+++	++
Diabetes mellitus	+++	++
Previous myocardial infarction	+	+++
Obesity	+++	+
Chronic lung disease	++	0
Sleep apnea	++	++
Dialysis	++	0
Atrial fibrillation	+ Usually paroxysmal	+ Usually persistent

+, Occasionally associated; ++, often associated; +++, usually associated; 0, not associated.

increased hemodynamic burden, by myocardial toxicity in thyrotoxicosis and beriberi, and by myocardial anoxia in severe, prolonged anemia.

B. Pathophysiology of Heart Failure. The initiating mechanisms of HF are pressure overload (aortic stenosis, essential HTN), volume overload (mitral or aortic regurgitation), myocardial ischemia or infarction, myocardial inflammatory disease, and restricted diastolic filling (constrictive pericarditis, restrictive cardiomyopathy).

1. **The Frank-Starling Relationship.** *The Frank-Starling relationship* refers to an increase in stroke volume (SV) that accompanies an increase in LV end-diastolic volume. When myocardial contractility is decreased (as in HF), a smaller increase in SV occurs with any given increase in LVEDV. Constriction of venous capacitance vessels shifts blood centrally, increases preload, and helps maintain cardiac output (CO).
2. **Activation of the Sympathetic Nervous System.** Activation of the sympathetic nervous system (SNS) promotes arteriolar and venous constriction that maintains systemic blood pressure and shifts blood to the central circulation. Blood is redistributed from the kidneys, splanchnic organs, skeletal muscles, and skin to the coronary and cerebral circulations, resulting in activation of the renin-angiotensin-aldosterone system (RAAS) and increased renal sodium and water retention. Downregulation of β-adrenergic receptors occurs during HF, and plasma catecholamine concentrations are increased. High norepinephrine levels promote myocyte necrosis and ventricular remodeling. β-Blocker therapy may decrease the deleterious effects of catecholamines on the heart.

TABLE 6-2 ■ Signs and Symptoms of Congestive Heart Failure

SIGNS AND SYMPTOMS OF PULMONARY VASCULAR CONGESTION	
Left ventricular failure	• Dyspnea and/or tachypnea (increased lung stiffness caused by interstitial pulmonary edema) • Orthopnea (inability of the ventricle to tolerate increased venous return when recumbent) • Paroxysmal nocturnal dyspnea (shortness of breath that awakens the patient from sleep) • Nocturia • Rales • S_3 gallop • Acute pulmonary edema • Decreased cerebral blood flow (confusion, insomnia, anxiety, memory deficits) • Systemic hypotension and cool extremities (severe heart failure)
SIGNS AND SYMPTOMS OF SYSTEMIC VENOUS CONGESTION	
Right ventricular failure	• Jugular venous distention • Organomegaly (e.g., hepatic congestion) • Right upper quadrant tenderness • Ascites • Peripheral edema

3. **Alterations in the Inotropic State, Heart Rate, and Afterload.** The maximum velocity of contraction of cardiac muscle is referred to as V_{max}. V_{max} is increased in inotropic states (increased catecholamines) and decreased in HF. Afterload is the tension the ventricular muscle must develop to open the aortic or pulmonic valve and is increased in the presence of systemic HTN. Forward SV can be increased in patients with HF by administering vasodilating drugs and decreasing afterload. In the presence of SHF, the SV is relatively fixed and CO is dependent on heart rate. In SHF, increased heart rate maintains CO. In DHF, tachycardia reduces ventricular filling time and reduces CO. Heart rate control is a target of therapy for DHF.
4. **Humoral-Mediated Responses and Biochemical Pathways.** During HF, vasoconstriction is initiated via increased activity of the SNS and RAAS, parasympathetic withdrawal, high levels of circulating vasopressin, endothelial dysfunction, and release of inflammatory mediators. B-type natriuretic peptide (BNP), which promotes diuresis, natriuresis, vasodilation, antiinflammatory effects, and inhibition of the RAAS and SNS, is secreted by both atrial and ventricular myocardium. In HF the ventricle becomes the principal site for BNP production.
5. **Myocardial Remodeling.** Myocardial remodeling is the process by which mechanical, neurohormonal, and genetic factors change the LV size, shape, and function to maintain CO. Angiotensin-converting enzyme inhibitors (ACEIs) and aldosterone antagonists have been shown to promote a "reverse-remodeling" process and are first-line therapy for HF.

C. **Signs and Symptoms of Heart Failure** (Table 6-2)

D. **Diagnosis of Heart Failure**

1. **Laboratory Diagnosis.** Plasma BNP levels below 100 pg/mL indicate that HF is unlikely (90% negative predictive value), and levels above 500 pg/mL are consistent with the diagnosis of HF (90% positive predictive value). Abnormal renal function test results may indicate decreased renal perfusion due to HF, and abnormal liver function test results may occur if liver congestion occurs. Hyponatremia, hypomagnesemia, and hypokalemia may be present.

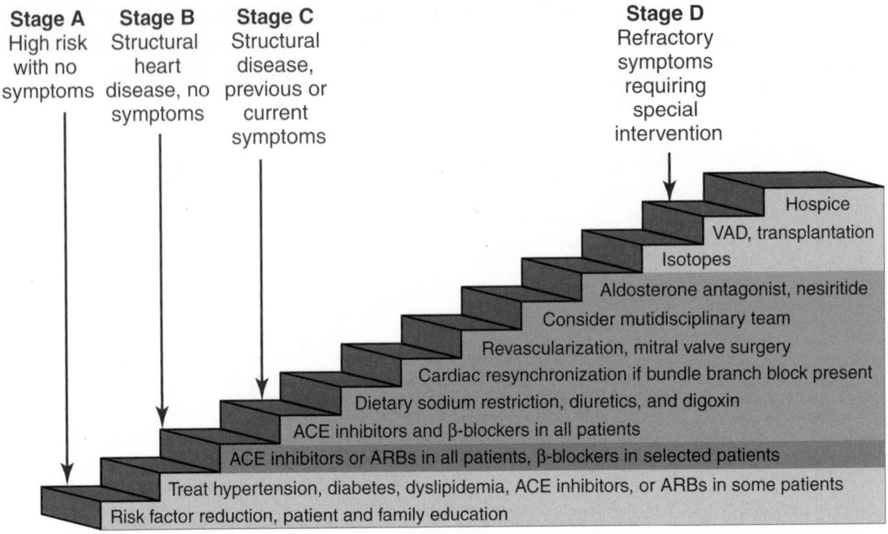

FIGURE 6-1 ■ Stages of heart failure and treatment options for systolic heart failure. Patients with stage A heart failure are at high risk of heart failure but do not yet have structural heart disease or symptoms of heart failure. This group includes patients with hypertension, diabetes, coronary artery disease, previous exposure to cardiotoxic drugs, or a family history of cardiomyopathy. Patients with stage B heart failure have structural heart disease but no symptoms of heart failure. This group includes patients with left ventricular hypertrophy, previous myocardial infarction, left ventricular systolic dysfunction, or valvular heart disease, all of whom would be considered to have New York Heart Association (NYHA) class I symptoms. Patients with stage C heart failure have known structural heart disease and current or previous symptoms of heart failure. Their current symptoms may be classified as NYHA class I, II, III, or IV. Patients with stage D heart failure have refractory symptoms of heart failure at rest despite maximal medical therapy, are hospitalized, and require specialized interventions or hospice care. All such patients would be considered to have NYHA class IV symptoms. *ACE,* Angiotensin-converting enzyme; *ARB,* angiotensin receptor blocker; *VAD,* ventricular assist device. *(Reproduced with permission from Jessup M, Brozena S. Heart failure.* N Engl J Med. *2003;348:2007-2018. Copyright © 2003 Massachusetts Medical Society. All rights reserved.)*

a. The *electrocardiogram* is usually abnormal and has a low predictive value for the diagnosis of HF.
b. *Chest radiography* may reveal cardiomegaly, pulmonary venous congestion, interstitial or alveolar pulmonary edema, Kerley's lines, pleural effusions, or pericardial effusion. Radiographic evidence of pulmonary edema may lag behind the clinical evidence of pulmonary edema by up to 12 hours.
c. *Echocardiography* can assess ejection fraction (EF), LV structure and functionality, the presence of other structural abnormalities such as valvular and pericardial disease, the presence and degree of diastolic dysfunction, and right ventricular (RV) function.

E. Classification of Heart Failure

1. The *New York Heart Association Functional Classification* correlates with survival and quality of life. It groups patients into four classes:
   Class I: Ordinary physical activity does not cause symptoms.
   Class II: Symptoms occur with ordinary exertion.
   Class III: Symptoms occur with less than ordinary exertion.
   Class IV: Inability to carry on any physical activity without discomfort. Symptoms present at rest.
2. The *American College of Cardiology and American Heart Association* classify patients according to disease progression (Figure 6-1):
   Stage A: Patients at high risk of HF but without structural heart disease or symptoms of HF

Stage B: Patients with structural heart disease but without symptoms of HF
Stage C: Patients with structural heart disease with previous or current symptoms of HF
Stage D: Patients with refractory HF requiring specialized interventions

F. Management of Heart Failure

1. **Management of Chronic Heart Failure.** Treatment options include lifestyle modification, patient and family education, medical therapy, corrective surgery, implantable devices, and cardiac transplantation.
2. **Management of Systolic Heart Failure**
    a. ***Inhibitors of the Renin-Angiotensin-Aldosterone System***
        1. *ACEIs* are the first line of treatment for HF. ACEIs have been proven to decrease ventricular remodeling, enhance reverse remodeling, and reduce morbidity and mortality of patients in any stage of HF. These benefits appear to be less in African Americans than in white patients.
        2. *Angiotensin II receptor blockers* have similar but not superior efficacy compared with ACEIs and are recommended for patients who cannot tolerate ACEIs.
        3. *Aldosterone antagonists* may reduce sodium and water retention, hypokalemia, and ventricular remodeling, as well as reduce mortality and hospitalization rates in New York Heart Association class III and IV patients. Eplerenone has been shown to reduce mortality from cardiovascular events and number of hospitalizations related to HF. Aldosterone antagonists are recommended as part of first-line therapy in *all* patients with HF.
        4. *β-Blockers* reduce morbidity and hospitalizations; improve quality of life, survival, and EF; and decrease ventricular remodeling.
        5. *Diuretics* decrease ventricular end-diastolic pressure and decrease diastolic ventricular wall stress, preventing the cardiac distention that interferes with subendocardial perfusion and negatively affects myocardial metabolism and function.
        6. *Vasodilators* in patients with dilated left ventricles increase SV and decrease ventricular filling pressures. African American patients show improved clinical outcomes when treated with a combination of hydralazine and nitrates.
        7. *Statins* decrease morbidity and mortality in patients with SHF, via antiinflammatory and lipid-lowering effects.
        8. *Digitalis* improves cardiac inotropy and decreases activation of the SNS and the RAAS. It is not clear that digitalis treatment improves survival. Digitalis can be added to therapy in patients who are symptomatic despite treatment with diuretics, ACEIs, and β-blockers. Patients with atrial fibrillation (AF) and HF may particularly benefit from digoxin. Elderly patients or those with impaired renal function are at risk for digitalis toxicity, which may be manifested by anorexia, nausea, blurred vision, and cardiac dysrhythmias. Treatment of digitalis toxicity includes reversing hypokalemia, treating cardiac dysrhythmias, administering antidigoxin antibodies, and/or implementing temporary cardiac pacing.
3. **Management of Diastolic Heart Failure** (Table 6-3)
4. **Surgical Management of Heart Failure.** Cardiac resynchronization therapy (CRT), also known as *biventricular pacing,* allows the heart to contract more efficiently and promotes reverse remodeling. Implanted cardioverter-defibrillators (ICDs) prevent sudden death in certain patients with advanced HF (Table 6-4). Treatments that target the cause of HF include coronary revascularization by percutaneous interventions or coronary artery bypass surgery, postinfarction ventricular aneurysmectomy, and heart transplantation. Ventricular assist devices (VADs) may facilitate recovery of heart function in some patients or provide a bridge to transplantation. Total artificial heart implantation as a *bridge* to transplantation or as *destination therapy* in patients who are not candidates for heart transplantation may be recommended for patients with pulmonary HTN requiring biventricular support for extended periods of time.

TABLE 6-3 ■ Management of Diastolic Heart Failure

GOALS	MANAGEMENT STRATEGIES
Prevent development of diastolic heart failure by decreasing risk factors	Treat coronary artery disease Treat hypertension Control weight gain Treat diabetes mellitus
Allow adequate filling time of left ventricle by decreasing heart rate	Administer β-blockers, calcium channel blockers, digoxin
Control volume overload	Treat with diuretics, long-acting nitrates Prescribe low-sodium diet
Restore and maintain sinus rhythm	Treat with cardioversion, amiodarone, digoxin
Decrease ventricular remodeling	Administer ACEIs, statins
Correct precipitating factors	Perform aortic valve replacement, coronary revascularization

ACEIs, Angiotensin-converting enzyme inhibitors.

TABLE 6-4 ■ Indications for Implantable Cardioverter-Defibrillator Devices

CAUSE OF HEART FAILURE	CONDITION
Coronary artery disease	Ejection fraction <30% Ejection fraction <40% if electrophysiologic study demonstrates inducible ventricular dysrhythmias
All other causes	After first episode of syncope or aborted ventricular tachycardia or ventricular fibrillation

5. **Anesthetic Considerations for Patients with Implanted Nonpulsatile Ventricular Assist Devices (e.g., HeartMate).** The system consists of a pump that is implanted extraperitoneally in the left upper abdomen, draining blood from the LV apex and ejecting it into the ascending aorta. A drive line connects the pump to an electrical power source and to an external console.
   a. Although the driveline is the most common infection site, it should not be prepped with povidone-iodine solution, which leads to plastic breakdown. Confirm that the device is plugged into a wall electrical outlet. Avoid chest compressions that might dislodge the cannulas.
   b. General considerations include anticoagulation management, antibiotic prophylaxis, and management of problems related to electromagnetic interferance. Use bipolar cautery and appropriate grounding pad placement to direct electric current away from the VAD generator.
   c. Hemodynamic monitoring is challenging due to lack of pulsatile blood flow. Ultrasound guidance may be needed for arterial catheter placement, and arterial oxygen saturation may be monitored by arterial blood gas sampling. Pulse oximetry cannot be used because there is no "pulse" in these patients. Transesophageal echocardiography is very useful for monitoring volume status, RV function, and cannula function. Maintaining intravascular volume is critical. LV "suck down" occurs when an underfilled LV is continuously drained by the VAD pump; this results in a dramatic decrease in CO. It is treated by decreasing pump speed and initiating volume expansion. RV function is critical to optimal LVAD inflow.
6. **Management of Acute Heart Failure** (Table 6-5). The hemodynamic profile of acute HF is characterized by high ventricular filling pressures, low CO, and HTN or hypotension.

TABLE 6-5 ■ **Management of Acute Heart Failure**

THERAPEUTIC MODALITY	EFFECTS
Diuretics (furosemide, hydrochlorothiazide)	May improve symptoms rapidly, but high doses can adversely affect clinical outcomes.
Vasodilators (nitroglycerin, nitroprusside)	Reduce LV filling pressure and systemic vascular resistance; increase SV.
Inotropes	
Catecholamines (epinephrine, norepinephrine, dopamine, dobutamine)	Catecholamines improve excitation-contraction coupling by direct adrenergic-receptor stimulation.
Phosphodiesterase inhibitors (amrinone, milrinone)	Phosphodiesterase inhibitors block degradation of cyclic adenosine monophosphate.
Calcium sensitizers (levosimendan)	A new class of inotropes that increase contractility without increasing myocardial oxygen consumption, heart rate, or dysrhythmias.
Exogenous B-type natriuretic peptides (nesiritide)	Bind to both A- and B-type natriuretic receptors. Promote arterial, venous, and coronary vasodilation. Decrease LVEDP. Improve dyspnea and induce diuresis and natriuresis.
NO synthase inhibitors	Large amount of inflammation-related NO produced by the heart and endothelium in HF has negative inotropic and profound vasodilatory effect, leading to shock and vascular collapse. NO synthase inhibitors are currently investigational.
Intraaortic balloon pump	Balloon placed via femoral artery into descending aorta inflates during diastole, promoting coronary perfusion, and deflates during systole, creating "suction" that enhances LV ejection.
LV and RV assist devices	Can improve survival in patients with severe cardiogenic shock and allow some myocardial recovery. May be a bridge to transplantation or be destination therapy.

HF, Heart failure; *LV,* left ventricular; *LVEDP,* left ventricular end-diastolic pressure; *NO,* nitric oxide; *RV,* right ventricular; *SV,* stroke volume.

7. **Prognosis.** The mortality rate during the first 4 years after the diagnosis of HF approaches 40%. Factors associated with a poor prognosis include increased blood urea nitrogen and creatinine levels, hyponatremia, hypokalemia, severely depressed EF, high levels of endogenous BNP, very limited exercise tolerance, and the presence of multifocal premature ventricular contractions.

II. MANAGEMENT OF ANESTHESIA IN PATIENTS WITH HEART FAILURE

See Table 6-6.

III. CARDIOMYOPATHIES

According to the American Heart Association, "Cardiomyopathies are a heterogeneous group of diseases of the myocardium associated with mechanical and/or electrical dysfunction that usually (but not invariably) exhibit inappropriate ventricular hypertrophy or dilation and are due to a

TABLE 6-6 ■ Management of Anesthesia in Patients with Heart Failure

Preoperative medications	Continue β-blockers and digoxin. Discontinue ACEIs and ARBs.
Electrolytes	Correct hypokalemia.
Anesthetic induction	All types of general anesthesia have been used successfully. Opioids may be beneficial because they have minimal hymodynamic effects.
Monitoring	Intraarterial pressure, CVP, and PA monitoring according to surgery and patient condition. Transesophageal echocardiography may be helpful.
Regional anesthesia	Decreased systemic vascular resistance may benefit CO but can be difficult to control.
Patients after heart transplant	Patients have high risk of infection due to immunosuppression. Heart rate is not responsive to indirect adrenergic-agonists or to anticholinergic drugs; isoproterenol or epinephrine may be useful to increase the heart rate. Delayed response to β-adrenergic inotropic drugs may occur. Heart is very preload dependent.
Postoperative management	HF during surgery requires postoperative ICU care and monitoring. Treat pain aggressively.

ACEIs, Angiotensin-converting enzyme inhibitors; *ARBs,* angiotensin receptor blockers; *CO,* cardiac output; *CVP,* central venous pressure; *ICU,* intensive care unit; *PA,* pulmonary artery.

TABLE 6-7 ■ Classification of Primary Cardiomyopathies

Genetic	Hypertrophic cardiomyopathy Arrhythmogenic right ventricular cardiomyopathy Left ventricular noncompaction Glycogen storage disease Conduction system disease (Lenègre's disease) Ion channelopathies: long QT syndrome, Brugada's syndrome, short QT syndrome
Mixed	Dilated cardiomyopathy Primary restrictive nonhypertrophic cardiomyopathy
Acquired	Myocarditis (inflammatory cardiomyopathy): viral, bacterial, rickettsial, fungal, parasitic (Chagas disease) Stress cardiomyopathy Peripartum cardiomyopathy

variety of causes that frequently are genetic." Cardiomyopathies are either confined to the heart (primary [Table 6-7]) or are part of systemic disorders (secondary [Table 6-8]). They often lead to cardiovascular death or progressive HF-related disability.

IV. HYPERTROPHIC CARDIOMYOPATHY

Hypertrophic cardiomyopathy (HCM) is the most common genetic cardiovascular disease (1:500), affects people of all ages, and has an autosomal dominant inheritance pattern. HCM is characterized by LV hypertrophy in the absence of other causes (e.g., HTN).

TABLE 6-8 ■ **Classification of Secondary Cardiomyopathies**

Infiltrative	Amyloidosis Gaucher's disease Hunter's syndrome
Storage	Hemochromatosis Glycogen storage disease Niemann-Pick disease
Toxic	Drugs: cocaine, alcohol Chemotherapy drugs: doxorubicin, daunorubicin, cyclophosphamide Heavy metals: lead, mercury Radiation therapy
Inflammatory	Sarcoidosis
Endomyocardial	Hypereosinophilic (Löffler's) syndrome Endomyocardial fibrosis
Endocrine	Diabetes mellitus Hyperthyroidism or hypothyroidism Pheochromocytoma Acromegaly
Neuromuscular	Duchenne-Becker dystrophy Neurofibromatosis Tuberous sclerosis
Autoimmune	Lupus erythematosus Rheumatoid arthritis Scleroderma Dermatomyositis Polyarteritis nodosa

A. **Pathophysiology.** Vigorous contraction of the hypertrophied septum results in accelerated blood flow through a narrow left ventricular outflow tract (LVOT); a Venturi effect on the anterior leaflet of the mitral valve moves the leaflet into the LVOT (systolic anterior movement [SAM]), leading to increased LVOT obstruction and mitral regurgitation. Situations that worsen LVOT obstruction are presented in Table 6-9. Diastolic dysfunction is common. Myocardial ischemia may be present in the absence of CAD. Dysrhythmias result from the disorganized cellular architecture, myocardial scarring, and expanded interstitial matrix and are associated with risk of sudden death.
B. **Signs and Symptoms.** Signs and symptoms vary widely, may include angina pectoris (often relieved by lying down), fatigue or syncope, tachydysrhythmias, and HF. Most patients remain asymptomatic throughout life. Cardiac examination may reveal a double apical impulse, gallop rhythm, and cardiac murmurs (increased by a Valsalva maneuver, nitroglycerin, and standing versus lying down). Sudden death is most likely between the ages of 10 and 30 years.
C. **Diagnosis.** The electrocardiogram (ECG) is abnormal in 75% to 90% of patients (e.g., left ventricular hypertrophy [LVH], ST- and T-wave abnormalities, Q waves, left atrial enlargement) and may be the only sign of the disease in asymptomatic patients. Echocardiography can demonstrate the presence of myocardial hypertrophy and assess EF (usually >80%), systolic anterior motion of the mitral valve, and diastolic dysfunction. Cardiac catheterization allows direct measurement of the increased LVEDP and LVOT pressure gradient. Endomyocardial biopsy and DNA analysis are reserved for patients in whom the diagnosis cannot be otherwise established.
D. **Treatment.** HCM is associated with high risk of sudden death and must be treated aggressively.

TABLE 6-9 ■ Factors Influencing Left Ventricular Outflow Tract Obstruction in Patients with Hypertrophic Cardiomyopathy

EVENTS THAT INCREASE OUTFLOW TRACT OBSTRUCTION
Increased myocardial contractility
β-Adrenergic stimulation (catecholamines)
Digitalis
Decreased preload
Hypovolemia
Vasodilators
Tachycardia
Positive pressure ventilation
Decreased afterload
Hypotension
Vasodilators
EVENTS THAT DECREASE OUTFLOW TRACT OBSTRUCTION
Decreased myocardial contractility
β-Adrenergic blockade
Volatile anesthetics
Calcium entry blockers
Increased preload
Hypervolemia
Bradycardia
Increased afterload
Hypertension
α-Adrenergic stimulation

1. **Medical Therapy.** β-Blockers and calcium channel blockers have been used extensively to treat HCM. Patients at high risk of sudden death may require amiodarone therapy or placement of an internal cardioverter-defibrillator. AF is associated with an increased risk of systemic thromboembolism, congestive HF, and sudden death. Amiodarone is the most effective antidysrhythmic drug for prevention of paroxysms of AF in these patients. β-Blockers and calcium channel blockers can control the heart rate. Long-term anticoagulation is indicated in those with recurrent or chronic AF.
2. **Surgical Therapy.** The small subgroup of patients with HCM who have both large outflow tract gradients (≥50 mm Hg) and severe symptoms despite medical therapy benefit from surgical removal of a small amount of cardiac muscle from the ventricular septum (septal myomectomy). The procedure abolishes or greatly reduces the LVOT gradient in most patients, with subsequent reduction in intraventricular systolic and end-diastolic pressures.

E. **Prognosis.** Annual mortality is approximately 1%. However, the subset of patients at high risk of sudden death (family history of sudden death or history of malignant ventricular dysrhythmias) has a mortality rate of 5% per year.

F. **Management of Anesthesia** (Table 6-10). Management of anesthesia in patients with HCM is directed toward minimizing LVOT obstruction by decreasing myocardial contractility and increasing preload and afterload.

V. DILATED CARDIOMYOPATHY

DCM is characterized by LV or biventricular dilation, systolic dysfunction, and normal LV wall thickness. African American men have an increased risk of developing DCM. DCM is the most

TABLE 6-10 ■ **Anesthetic Considerations in Patients with Hypertrophic Cardiomyopathy**

Preoperative evaluation and management	Obtain ECG and updated echocardiogram. Continue β-blockers and/or calcium channel blockers. Premedicate to reduce anxiety. Correct hypovolemia. Turn off ICD; have external defibrillator immediately available.
Intraoperative management	All induction agents are acceptable if used cautiously. Avoid tachycardia and sudden decreases in SVR. During positive pressure ventilation, use small tidal volumes, avoid PEEP. Maintain preload. Volatile agents may be helpful in decreasing contractility. Treat hypotension with pure α-agonist (phenylephrine). Treat dysrhythmias promptly; perform cardioversion early.
Monitors	Transesophageal echocardiography is very useful. CVP and PA catheters are not accurate in assessing LV filling in patients with HCM.
Parturients	Regional anesthesia may be used safely. Use phenylephrine for hypotension, not ephedrine. Use oxytocin with caution. Avoid diuretics, digoxin, and nitrates in pulmonary edema, because they promote LVOT obstruction.
Postoperative management	Monitor closely throughout recovery. Treat pain, shivering, anxiety aggressively to avoid or reduce SNS activation. Treat hypovolemia promptly.

CVP, Central venous pressure; *ECG*, electrocardiogram; *HCM*, hypertrophic cardiomyopathy; *ICD*, Implanted cardioverter-defibrillator; *LV*, left ventricular; *LVOT*, left ventricular outflow tract; *PA*, pulmonary artery; *PEEP*, positive end-expiratory pressure; *SNS*, sympathetic nervous system; *SVR*, systemic vascular resistance.

common type of cardiomyopathy, the third most common cause of HF, and the most common indication for cardiac transplantation.

A. Signs and Symptoms. Symptoms include those of HF and exertional chest pain that mimics angina pectoris. Ventricular dilation causes functional mitral and/or tricuspid regurgitation. Supraventricular and ventricular dysrhythmias, conduction system abnormalities, and sudden death are common. Systemic embolization is also common.

B. Diagnosis

1. The *ECG* often shows ST-segment and T-wave abnormalities and LBBB. Cardiac dysrhythmias are common.
2. The *chest radiograph* may show LV dilation.
3. *Echocardiography* reveals dilation of all four chambers, especially the left ventricle, and global hypokinesis. Other findings can include regional wall motion abnormalities (in the absence of CAD), mural thrombi, and mitral or tricuspid regurgitation secondary to annular dilation.
4. *Laboratory testing* should eliminate other causes of cardiac dilation such as hyperthyroidism.
5. *Endomyocardial biopsy* is not recommended.

C. Treatment (Table 6-11)

D. Prognosis. The 5-year mortality rate is 50%. Factors that predict a poor prognosis include an EF less than 25%, pulmonary capillary wedge pressure greater than 20 mm Hg, CI less than 2.5 L/min/m^2, systemic hypotension, pulmonary HTN, and increased central venous pressure.

E. Management of Anesthesia. Because DCM is a cause of HF, the anesthetic management of these patients is the same as described in the HF section of this chapter.

TABLE 6-11 ■ Treatment of Dilated Cardiomyopathy

Supportive measures	Weight control, low-sodium diet, fluid restriction, smoking and alcohol cessation
Medical management	Similar to that for chronic heart failure Anticoagulation to prevent systemic embolization Insertion of implantable cardioverter-defibrillator in patients who have had a cardiac arrest
Surgical management	Cardiac transplantation

VI. PERIPARTUM CARDIOMYOPATHY

Peripartum cardiomyopathy (PPCM) is a rare form of DCM of unknown cause that occurs anywhere from the third trimester of pregnancy until 5 months after delivery in women with no history of heart disease (1 per 3000 to 4000 live births). Risk factors include obesity, multiparity, advanced maternal age (>30 years), multifetal pregnancy, preeclampsia, and African American ethnicity.

A. **Signs and Symptoms.** Signs and symptoms are nonspecific and include dyspnea, fatigue, and peripheral edema.

B. **Diagnosis.** Diagnosis is based on the echocardiographic documentation of a new finding of dilated cardiac chambers and LV systolic dysfunction during the period surrounding parturition.

C. **Treatment.** The goal is to alleviate the symptoms of HF. Diuretics, vasodilators (hydralazine, nitrates), and digoxin can be used. ACEIs are teratogenic but can be useful *after* delivery. Anticoagulation is recommended. Heart transplantation is considered in patients whose condition does not improve.

D. **Prognosis.** Mortality ranges from 25% to 50%, with most deaths occurring within 3 months after delivery. Prognosis is correlated with the degree of normalization of left ventricle size and function within 6 months of delivery.

E. **Management of Anesthesia.** Assessment of cardiac status and careful planning of the analgesia and/or anesthesia required for delivery are necessary. Regional anesthesia may provide a desirable decrease in afterload.

VII. SECONDARY CARDIOMYOPATHIES WITH RESTRICTIVE PHYSIOLOGY

Secondary cardiomyopathies with restrictive physiology are caused by systemic diseases that produce myocardial infiltration and severe diastolic dysfunction (e.g., amyloidosis, hemochromatosis, sarcoidosis, and carcinoid). Although diastolic function is impaired and ventricular compliance is reduced, systolic function is usually normal. Cardiomyopathies with restrictive physiology must be differentiated from constrictive pericarditis, which has a similar physiology but is more likely if there is a clinical history of pericarditis.

A. **Signs and Symptoms.** Signs and symptoms of LV and/or RV failure may be present, but cardiomegaly is absent. AF and thromboembolic events are common. Cardiac conduction disturbances are particularly common in amyloidosis and sarcoidosis.

B. **Diagnosis**

1. **General Findings.** The ECG may demonstrate conduction abnormalities. The chest radiograph may show signs of pulmonary congestion and/or pleural effusion, but cardiomegaly is absent. Laboratory tests should be directed toward diagnosis of the systemic disease responsible for the cardiac infiltration.

TABLE 6-12 ■ Treatment of Cor Pulmonale

Reduce right ventricular workload by promoting pulmonary vasodilation. • Maintain Pa_{O_2} >60 mm Hg (Sp_{O_2} >90%) with supplemental oxygen. • Correct P_{CO_2} and pH abnormalities if possible. • Diuretics (use with caution—resulting alkalosis can cause CO_2 retention). • Palmonary vasodilation (e.g., sildenafil and bosentan)
Treat atrial fibrillation with drugs or electrical cardioversion if new onset. Control ventricular response with drugs if atrial fibrillation is chronic.
Lung transplantation (single or double) or heart-lung transplantation may be considered in cases unresponsive to medical therapy.

2. **Echocardiography.** Echocardiography will demonstrate diastolic dysfunction and normal systolic function, enlarged atria, and normal ventricular size. In cardiac amyloidosis, the ventricular mass appears characteristically large.
3. **Endomyocardial Biopsy.** Endomyocardial biopsy can elucidate the exact cause of the infiltrative cardiomyopathy.

C. **Treatment.** Symptomatic treatment is similar to that for DHF. Maintenance of normal sinus rhythm is extremely important. SV is relatively fixed, and the onset of bradycardia may precipitate acute HF. With cardiac sarcoidosis, malignant ventricular dysrhythmias are common and may necessitate insertion of an ICD. Anticoagulation is recommended in patients with AF or low output states. Cardiac transplantation is not a treatment option because myocardial infiltration will recur in the transplanted heart.

D. **Prognosis.** The prognosis is very poor.

E. **Management of Anesthesia.** Management of anesthesia for patients with restrictive cardiomyopathy uses the same principles as for patients with diastolic heart failure.

VIII. COR PULMONALE

Cor pulmonale is RV enlargement (hypertrophy and/or dilation) that may progress to right HF, caused by diseases that induce pulmonary HTN (chronic obstructive pulmonary disease, restrictive lung disease, respiratory insufficiency of central origin, obesity-hypoventilation syndrome, idiopathic pulmonary HTN).

A. **Pathophysiology.** Acute or chronic alveolar hypoxia (Pa_{O_2} < 55 mm Hg) causes pulmonary vasoconstriction. Longstanding chronic hypoxia promotes pulmonary vasculature remodeling and an increase in pulmonary vascular resistance. The right ventricle has an increased workload and undergoes hypertrophy. Eventually, RV dysfunction occurs, leading to RV failure.

B. **Signs and Symptoms.** Signs and symptoms occur late in the course of the disease and include peripheral edema, dyspnea, and effort-related syncope. Accentuation of the pulmonic component of the second heart sound, a diastolic murmur of pulmonic regurgitation, and a systolic murmur caused by tricuspid regurgitation indicate severe pulmonary HTN. Signs of overt RV failure include increased jugular venous pressure, hepatosplenomegaly, and peripheral edema.

C. **Diagnosis.** The ECG may show signs of right atrial and RV hypertrophy (peaked P waves in leads II, III, and aVF—"P pulmonale"), right axis deviation, and a partial or complete right bundle branch block. Echocardiography can assist in estimating pulmonary artery pressure, assessing the size and function of the right atrium and ventricle, and evaluating the presence and severity of tricuspid or pulmonic regurgitation.

D. **Treatment** (Table 6-12)

E. **Prognosis.** The prognosis depends on the underlying cause.

TABLE 6-13 ■ Intraoperative Management of Cor Pulmonale

- Induction of anesthesia can be safely accomplished by any method.
- Use adequate depth of anesthesia for intubation to avoid precipitating bronchospasm.
- Volatile agents can promote bronchodilation.
- Avoid large opioid dosage owing to the potential for respiratory depression and CO_2 retention in the postoperative period.
- Humidification of gases can maintain mucociliary function.
- Intraarterial catheter allows frequent sampling of arterial blood gases.
- Utilize central venous pressure and pulmonary artery monitoring according to the invasiveness of surgery.
- Transesophageal echocardiography may be an alternative method of monitoring right ventricular function.
- Use regional anesthesia with caution: high motor block can interfere with muscles of respiration, and decreased systemic vascular resistance is deleterious in the presence of fixed pulmonary hypertension.

F. Management of Anesthesia

1. **Preoperative Management.** Preoperative preparation is directed toward (1) eliminating and controlling acute and chronic pulmonary infection, (2) reversing bronchospasm, (3) improving clearance of airway secretions, (4) expanding collapsed or poorly ventilated alveoli, (5) hydration, and (6) correcting any electrolyte imbalances.
2. **Intraoperative Management** (Table 6-13)
3. **Postoperative Management.** Avoid factors that exacerbate pulmonary HTN, and maintain oxygen therapy as needed.

CHAPTER 7

Pericardial Diseases and Cardiac Trauma

The three most common responses to pericardial injury are characterized as acute pericarditis, pericardial effusion, and constrictive pericarditis. Cardiac tamponade is a possibility whenever pericardial fluid accumulates under pressure.

I. ACUTE PERICARDITIS (Table 7-1)

A. **Etiology.** Pericarditis may be infective or autoimmune and can follow cardiac surgery, blunt or penetrating trauma, hemopericardium, or epicardial pacemaker implantation.

B. **Diagnosis.** Diagnosis of acute pericarditis is based on the presence of chest pain, pericardial friction rub, and changes on the electrocardiogram (ECG). ECG changes evolve through four stages: stage I, diffuse ST-segment elevation and PR-segment depression; stage II, normalization of the ST and PR segments; stage III, widespread T-wave inversions; and stage IV, normalization of the T waves.

C. **Treatment.** Salicylates or nonsteroidal antiinflammatory drugs may be useful in decreasing pericardial inflammation and chest pain. Corticosteroids can relieve symptoms of acute pericarditis but may be associated with an increased incidence of relapse. They are reserved for patients whose condition does not respond to conventional therapy.

D. **Relapsing Pericarditis.** Relapsing pericarditis may follow acute pericarditis of any cause but is rarely life-threatening. Treatment may include standard treatments for acute pericarditis and/or corticosteroids (prednisone) or immunosuppressive drugs such as azathioprine.

TABLE 7-1 ■ **Causes of Acute Pericarditis and Pericardial Effusion**
Infectious cause
• Viral
• Bacterial
• Fungal
• Tuberculous
Post–myocardial infarction (Dressler's syndrome)
Posttraumatic cause, postcardiotomy
Metastatic disease
Drug use
Mediastinal radiation
Systemic disease
• Rheumatoid arthritis
• Systemic lupus erythematosus
• Scleroderma

TABLE 7-2 ■ Signs and Symptoms of Cardiac Tamponade

- Large effusions—compression of adjacent structures; dyspnea, cough, chest pain, hoarseness, hiccups, dysphagia
- Increase in jugular venous pressure (distention of the jugular vein during inspiration [Kussmaul's sign])
- Pulsus paradoxus (decrease in systolic blood pressure >10 mm Hg during inspiration)—seen in about 75% of patients with acute cardiac tamponade but only 30% of those with chronic pericardial effusions
- Beck's triad: distant heart sounds, increased jugular venous pressure, and hypotension
- Hypotension
- Tachycardia
- Hepatomegaly, ascites, peripheral edema
- Ewart's sign: bronchial breath sounds and dullness to percussion at the inferior angle of the left scapula—a sign of pericardial effusion
- Low voltage on electrocardiogram
- Equalization of right and left atrial pressure and right ventricular pressure
- Activation of the sympathetic nervous system

II. PERICARDIAL EFFUSION AND CARDIAC TAMPONADE

Cardiac tamponade occurs when buildup of the fluid in the pericardial space impairs cardiac filling. In up to 20% of cases, the cause of the pericardial effusion is unknown.

A. ***Signs and Symptoms (Table 7-2).*** Signs and symptoms of a pericardial effusion depend on its size and duration. Acute changes in pericardial volume as small as 100 mL may result in cardiac tamponade. Larger volumes can accumulate if the effusion develops gradually. Right atrial pressure increases as pericardial fluid pressure increases. Cardiac output is maintained as long as central venous pressure exceeds right ventricular end-diastolic pressure. Loculated pericardial effusion may selectively compress one or more cardiac chambers, producing localized cardiac tamponade.

B. ***Diagnosis.*** Echocardiography is the most accurate and practical method for diagnosing pericardial effusion and cardiac tamponade. Computed tomography (CT) and magnetic resonance imaging (MRI) are also useful for detecting both pericardial effusion and pericardial thickening.

C. ***Treatment.*** Removal of fluid is required for definitive treatment.

D. ***Temporizing Measures to Maintain Stroke Volume.*** Temporizing measures to maintain stroke volume until definitive treatment of cardiac tamponade can be instituted include expanding intravascular volume, administering catecholamines to increase myocardial contractility, and correcting metabolic acidosis resulting from low cardiac output.

E. ***Management of Anesthesia.*** General anesthesia and positive-pressure ventilation in the presence of hemodynamically significant cardiac tamponade can result in life-threatening hypotension caused by anesthesia-induced peripheral vasodilation, direct myocardial depression, or decreased venous return from the increased intrathoracic pressure associated with positive-pressure ventilation.

1. Pericardiocentesis performed with local anesthesia is the preferred initial management of hypotensive patients with cardiac tamponade.
2. If it is not possible to relieve cardiac tamponade before induction of anesthesia, the principal goals of anesthetic induction are to maintain adequate cardiac output and blood pressure (Table 7-3).

III. CONSTRICTIVE PERICARDITIS

Chronic constrictive pericarditis is characterized by fibrous scarring and adhesions that obliterate the pericardial space, creating a "rigid shell" around the heart. Subacute constrictive pericarditis is fibroelastic.

TABLE 7-3 ■ Management of Anesthesia in Patients with Cardiac Tamponade

- Avoid or mitigate decreases in myocardial contractility, heart rate, and systemic vascular resistance during induction. Ketamine mat be particularly useful.
- Avoid increases in intrathoracic pressure (coughing, straining).
- Minimize time from initiation of positive-pressure ventilation to incision whenever possible.
- Administer intravenous fluids to maintain preload.
- Administer catecholamines to maintain cardiac output.
- Monitor central venous pressure, intraarterial pressure.
- Anticipate hypertensive response after surgical relief of tamponade.

TABLE 7-4 ■ Signs and Symptoms of Constrictive Pericarditis

- Decreased exercise tolerance and fatigue
- Venous congestion signs that mimic right-sided heart failure: jugular venous distention, hepatic congestion, ascites, peripheral edema
- Equalization of intracardiac pressures
- Atrial dysrhythmias
- Pulsus paradoxus usually *not* seen
- Kussmaul's sign commonly seen
- Early diastolic sound can be heard—"pericardial knock"

A. **Signs and Symptoms** (Table 7-4).

B. **Diagnosis** Diagnosis of constrictive pericarditis depends on the confirmation of an increased central venous pressure without other signs or symptoms of heart disease. Features of constrictive pericarditis may also be present in patients with restrictive cardiomyopathy, but several features help to distinguish these two entities (Table 7-5).

C. **Treatment** Treatment of constrictive pericarditis consists of surgical stripping and removal of the adherent constricting pericardium. This procedure may result in considerable bleeding from the epicardial surface of the heart.

D. **Management of Anesthesia** Anesthetic drugs and techniques should be chosen that minimize changes in heart rate, systemic vascular resistance, venous return, and myocardial contractility. Optimization of intravascular volume is essential. When hemodynamic compromise (hypotension) is present before surgery, management of anesthesia is as described for cardiac tamponade. Invasive monitoring of arterial and central venous pressure is useful because removal of adherent pericardium may result in significant fluid and blood losses. Cardiac dysrhythmias are common.

IV. PERICARDIAL AND CARDIAC TRAUMA

A. Pericardial Trauma

1. **Diagnosis.** Suspicion of pericardial trauma or pericardial rupture should be raised when unexplained alterations in heart rate and blood pressure occur after initial resuscitation, especially if a sternal fracture and/or multiple rib fractures are present. Other indications may be mediastinal air on a chest radiograph or radiographic evidence of cardiac herniation. Cardiac herniation and strangulation can occur with pericardial-pleural tears or with pericardial-diaphragmatic tears.
2. **Treatment.** Severe tears associated with hemodynamic instability and cardiac herniation necessitate emergency thoracotomy.

TABLE 7-5 ■ Differentiation of Constrictive Pericarditis from Restrictive Cardiomyopathy

FEATURE	CONSTRICTIVE PERICARDITIS	RESTRICTIVE CARDIOMYOPATHY
Medical history	Previous pericarditis, cardiac surgery, trauma, radiotherapy, connective tissue disease	No such history
Mitral or tricuspid regurgitation	Usually absent	Often present
Ventricular septal movement with respiration	Movement toward left ventricle on inspiration	Little movement toward left ventricle
Respiratory variation in mitral and tricuspid flow velocity	Greater than 25% in most cases	Less than 15% in most cases
Equilibration of diastolic pressures in all cardiac chambers	Within 5 mm Hg in nearly all cases	In only a small proportion of cases
Respiratory variation in ventricular peak systolic pressures	Right and left ventricular peak systolic pressures are out of phase (discordant)	Right and left ventricular peak systolic pressures are in phase
Magnetic resonance imaging, computed tomography	Show pericardial thickening in most cases	Rarely shows pericardial thickening
Endomyocardial biopsy	Normal or nonspecific	Shows amyloid in some cases

Adapted from Hancock EW. Differential diagnosis of restrictive cardiomyopathy and constrictive pericarditis. *Heart*. 2001;86:343-349.

B. Myocardial Contusion

1. **Signs and Symptoms.** Signs and symptoms typically include chest pain and palpitations in the setting of recent chest trauma. Cardiac failure is uncommon.
2. **Diagnosis.** ECG changes are nonspecific. Serum troponin I and T may be elevated. Echocardiography may demonstrate impaired ventricular wall motion, valvular regurgitation, or pericardial effusion.
3. **Treatment.** Treatment of myocardial contusion is supportive, consisting of hemodynamic support and management of dysrhythmias. When anesthesia and surgery are anticipated in patients with suspected myocardial contusion, invasive hemodynamic monitoring is recommended. Anesthetic drugs that depress myocardial function should be avoided. A cardioverter-defibrillator and drugs for dysrhythmia treatment should be immediately available.

C. Commotio Cordis. Commotio cordis occurs when blunt injury over the heart causes a malignant ventricular dysrhythmia that, untreated, leads to death. This condition is sometimes seen in sports injuries when the athlete sustains a single, focal, high-impact injury to the chest from a ball. Commotio cordis is thought to result from a "mechanical" R-on-T phenomenon caused by mechanical stretching of the cardiac fibers during cardiac repolarization. Treatment is rapid defibrillation.

CHAPTER 8

Vascular Disease

The incidence of perioperative cardiac complications is higher in patients undergoing vascular surgery than in the general population. Vascular surgery patients are at a particularly high risk of perioperative myocardial infarction, but the risk differs based on the type of vascular surgery performed.

I. DISEASES OF THE THORACIC AND ABDOMINAL AORTA

Diseases of the aorta are most often aneurysmal. Occlusive disease is more likely to occur in peripheral arteries. The aorta and its major branches are affected by two entities that may be present simultaneously or may occur at different stages of the same disease process. An *aneurysm* is a dilation of all three layers of the aorta. An *aortic dissection* occurs when a tear in the intima allows blood to create an extraluminal channel called the *false lumen,* potentially compromising blood flow to the aortic branch arteries. Both aneurysms and dissections can rupture, with rapid exsanguination.

II. ANEURYSMS AND DISSECTION OF THE THORACIC AORTA

A. Etiology (Table 8-1)

1. **Marfan's Syndrome.** Marfan's syndrome is the most prevalent hereditary connective tissue disorder (autosomal dominant mutation in fibrillin-1 gene).
2. **Ehlers-Danlos Syndrome.** Ehlers-Danlos syndrome is a group of several disorders associated with skin fragility, easy bruisability, and osteoarthritis. Type IV, a vascular form caused by mutations in the type III procollagen gene, is the only one associated with premature death. The most common presentations of type IV Ehlers-Danlos syndrome are aortic dissection and intestinal rupture.

TABLE 8-1 ■ Etiology of Thoracic Aortic Aneurysm and Dissection

- Systemic hypertension
- Congenital disorders of connective tissue (e.g., Marfan's syndrome, Ehlers-Danlos syndrome, bicuspid aortic valve, nonsyndromic familial aortic dissection)
- Deceleration injury
- Blunt trauma
- Crack cocaine use
- Surgical manipulation of the aorta: aortic cannulation, cross-clamping, or incision (e.g., for aortic valve replacement)
- Pregnancy: implicated in approximately half of aortic dissections in women older than 40 years of age

3. **Bicuspid Aortic Valve.** The most common congenital abnormality associated with aortic dilation and dissection, bicuspid aortic valve occurs in 1% of the population.
4. **Nonsyndromic Familial Aortic Dissection and Aneurysm.** Nonsyndromic familial aortic dissection and aneurysm is found in 20% of patients referred for repair of thoracic aortic aneurysm or dissection. At least three chromosomal regions have been identified.

B. **Classification** (Figure 8-1)

C. **Signs and Symptoms.** See Table 8-2.

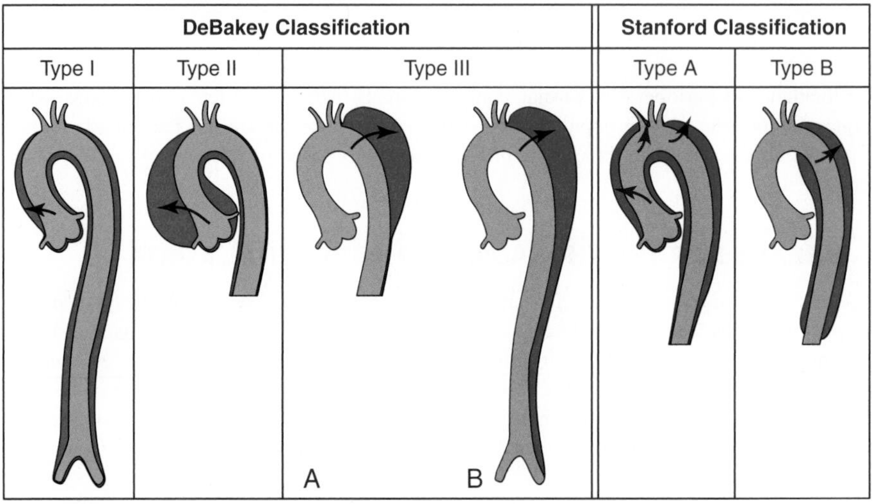

FIGURE 8-1 ■ The two most widely used classifications of aortic dissection. The DeBakey classification includes three types. In type I, the intimal tear usually originates in the proximal ascending aorta and the dissection involves the ascending aorta and variable lengths of the aortic arch and descending thoracic and abdominal aorta. In type II, the dissection is confined to the ascending aorta. In type III, the dissection is confined to the descending thoracic aorta (type IIIa) or extends into the abdominal aorta and iliac arteries (type IIIb). The Stanford classification has two types. Type A includes all cases in which the ascending aorta is involved by the dissection, with or without involvement of the arch or the descending aorta. Type B includes cases in which the ascending aorta is not involved. *(From Kouchoukos NT, Dougenis D. Surgery of the thoracic aorta.* N Engl J Med. *1997;336:1876-1888. Copyright 1997 Massachusetts Medical Society with permission.)*

TABLE 8-2 ■ Signs and Symptoms of Aneurysms and Dissections of the Thoracic Aorta

- Often symptomatic
- Signs and symptoms caused by local compression of adjacent structures; hoarseness, stridor, dysphagia, dyspnea, plethora, and facial edema resulting from superior vena cava obstruction
- Congestive heart failure resulting from aortic regurgitation
- Excruciating tearing chest pain of chest or neck or between the shoulder blades
- Diminished peripheral pulses
- Stroke
- Paraplegia
- Hypertension
- Peripheral vasoconstriction
- Myocardial infarction
- Cardiac tamponade

D. Diagnosis. Widening of the mediastinum on chest radiograph or computed tomography (CT) and magnetic resonance imaging (MRI) may identify thoracic aortic disease. In acute aortic dissection, transesophageal echocardiography (TEE) with color Doppler imaging is both highly sensitive (98%) and specific (95%). Angiography of the aorta may be required for patients undergoing elective surgery on the thoracic aorta to define relevant anatomy.

E. Preoperative Evaluation. Myocardial ischemia or infarction, respiratory failure, renal failure, and stroke are the principal causes of morbidity and mortality associated with thoracic aortic surgery; preoperative assessment of the function of these organ systems is needed. Cigarette smoking and chronic obstructive pulmonary disease (COPD) are important predictors of respiratory failure after thoracic aortic surgery. Patients with severe stenosis of one or both common or internal carotid arteries should be considered for carotid endarterectomy before elective surgery on the thoracic aorta.

F. Indications for Surgery. Thoracic aortic aneurysm repair is indicated when aneurysm size exceeds a diameter of 5 cm. Ascending and aortic arch dissection requires emergent or urgent surgery. Descending thoracic aortic dissection is generally associated with better survival compared with dissection of the ascending aorta and is rarely treated with urgent surgery.

1. **Type A Dissection.** In-hospital mortality is approximately 27% in surgically treated patients and 56% in those treated medically. Long-term survival rates are 90% to 96% versus 69% to 89%, respectively.
2. **Ascending Aorta.** All patients with acute dissection involving the ascending aorta should be considered candidates for surgery.
3. **Aortic Arch.** Resection of the aortic arch requires cardiopulmonary bypass, profound hypothermia, and a period of circulatory arrest. Neurologic deficits are the major complications, occurring in 3% to 18% of patients.
4. **Descending Thoracic Aorta.** Elective resection is advisable if the aneurysm exceeds 5 to 6 cm in diameter or if symptoms are present. Patients with an uncomplicated acute type B aortic dissection can be treated with medical therapy consisting of intraarterial monitoring of systemic blood pressure and urinary output and administration of drugs to control blood pressure and the force of left ventricular contraction (β-blockers, nitroprusside). Surgery is indicated for patients with type B aortic dissection with signs of impending rupture; ischemia of the legs, abdominal viscera, or spinal cord; and/or renal failure.
5. **Endovascular Repair.** Endovascular repair by placement of intraluminal stent grafts to treat patients with aneurysms of the descending thoracic aorta may be particularly useful in the elderly and in those with coexisting medical conditions, such as hypertension, COPD, and renal insufficiency.

G. Unique Risks of Surgery. Surgical resection of thoracic aortic aneurysms can be associated with spinal cord ischemia (anterior spinal artery syndrome), the potential for adverse hemodynamic responses such as myocardial ischemia and heart failure, and renal insufficiency.

1. **Anterior Spinal Artery Syndrome.** Anterior spinal artery syndrome manifests as flaccid paralysis of the lower extremities and bowel and bladder dysfunction. Sensation and proprioception are spared.
   a. ***Spinal Cord Blood Supply.*** The spinal cord is supplied by one anterior spinal artery and two posterior spinal arteries. The anterior spinal artery begins at the fusion of branches of both vertebral arteries and is reinforced by six to eight radicular arteries, the largest of which is the artery of Adamkiewicz. Damage can result from surgical resection of the artery of Adamkiewicz or exclusion of the origin of the artery by the cross-clamp. Anterior spinal artery blood flow is then reduced directly, and collateral blood flow is also reduced because aortic pressure distal to the cross-clamp is very low.
   b. ***Risk Factors.*** A major risk factor for paraplegia is duration of aortic cross-clamping that exceeds 30 minutes. Prolonged cross-clamp (X-clamp) time warrants additional protective techniques for spinal cord protection, such as partial circulatory assistance (left atrium–to–femoral artery shunt); reimplantation of critical intercostal arteries when

possible; cerebrospinal fluid (CSF) drainage; maintenance of proximal hypertension during cross-clamping; reduction of spinal cord metabolism by moderate hypothermia (30° to 32° C); avoidance of hyperglycemia; and the use of mannitol, corticosteroids, and/or calcium channel blockers. The incidence of spinal cord ischemia after endovascular repair is not clear, with some studies showing similar incidence to that of open aortic surgery, and others showing a lower incidence.

2. **Hemodynamic Responses to Aortic Cross-Clamping.** Thoracic aortic clamping and unclamping are associated with severe hemodynamic and homeostatic disturbances in virtually all organ systems owing to decrease in blood flow distal to the X-clamp and substantial increase in blood flow above the level of aortic occlusion. Increased systemic vascular resistance (SVR), decreased cardiac output (CO), and no change in heart rate are common. The level of X-clamp is critical to the nature of hemodynamic change: minimal with infrarenal X-clamp, and dramatic with intrathoracic X-clamp.
   a. ***Vasodilators.*** Vasodilators (nitroprusside, nitroglycerin) may reduce clamp-induced decreases in CO and ejection fraction.
   b. ***Perfusion Pressures Distal to the X-Clamp.*** Perfusion pressures distal to the X-clamp are decreased and may be adversely affected by vasodilator therapy, compromising perfusion of distal organs. Drugs and volume replacement must be adjusted to maintain distal aortic perfusion pressure even if that results in an increase in blood pressure proximal to the clamp. Placement of a temporary shunt, hypothermia, and reimplantation of spinal arteries may be considered and may influence the choice of drug therapy.
   c. ***Increase in Cerebrospinal Fluid Pressure.*** Increase in CSF and decrease in anterior spinal artery pressure occurs with X-clamping the thoracic aorta. CSF drainage might increase spinal cord blood flow and decrease the incidence of neurologic complications.
   d. ***Pulmonary Effects.*** Pulmonary effects such as increased pulmonary vascular resistance and pulmonary edema sometimes occur and may be the effects of increased pulmonary vascular volume and release of vasoactive mediators.
3. **Hemodynamic Responses to Aortic Unclamping.** Hemodynamic responses include substantial decreases in SVR and systemic blood pressure. Gradual release of the aortic clamp is recommended to allow time for volume replacement and to slow the washout of the vasoactive and cardiodepressant mediators from ischemic tissues. Correction of metabolic acidosis does not significantly influence the degree of hypotension after aortic declamping.

H. Management of Anesthesia

1. **Monitoring.** Proper monitoring is more important than the selection of specific anesthetic drugs (Table 8-3).
2. **Temporary Shunts.** Temporary shunts (proximal aorta–to–femoral artery or left atrium–to–femoral artery shunts) or partial cardiopulmonary bypass may be considered when attempting to maintain renal and spinal cord perfusion.

I. Postoperative Management. Amelioration of pain is essential for patient comfort and to facilitate coughing and maneuvers designed to prevent atelectasis. If neuraxial analgesia is used during the immediate postoperative period, opioids are preferred over local anesthetics to prevent masking of anterior spinal artery syndrome. Patients recovering from thoracic aortic aneurysm resection are at risk of developing cardiac, pulmonary, and renal failure during the immediate postoperative period. Systemic hypertension may require treatment with drugs such as nitroglycerin, nitroprusside, hydralazine, and labetalol.

III. ANEURYSMS OF THE ABDOMINAL AORTA

A. Diagnosis. Abdominal aortic aneurysms are usually detected as asymptomatic, pulsatile abdominal masses. Abdominal ultrasonography, CT, and MRI are useful for accurate measurement of aneurysm size and evaluation of relevant vascular anatomy.

TABLE 8-3 ■ **Anesthesia Management: Monitoring During Thoracic Aortic Surgery**

SYSTEM MONITORED	MANAGEMENT CONSIDERATIONS
Systemic blood pressure	Place arterial catheter in right upper extremity and femoral artery. • X-clamp proximal to the left subclavian artery will prevent monitoring of blood pressure if catheter is in the left upper extremity. • Loss of pressure tracing warns of innominate artery occlusion. • Simultaneous blood pressure monitoring allows assessment of cerebral perfusion pressure and distal organ perfusion pressure. • Common recommendation: Maintain upper extremity mean arterial pressure (MAP) ≥100 mm Hg and lower extremity MAP ≥50 mm Hg during X-clamp.
Neurologic function	Somatosensory evoked potentials are not helpful. Motor evoked potentials may reflect anterior spinal cord function but are not useful in the presence of muscle relaxants.
Cardiac function	Perform transesophageal echocardiography. Insert pulmonary artery catheter.
Intravascular volume	Maintain urine flow; consider diuretics, steroids, mannitol.
Induction and maintenance of anesthesia	Selective endobronchial intubation facilitates surgical exposure. Volatile agents and opioids are commonly used.

B. **Treatment.** Surgery is usually recommended for abdominal aortic aneurysms larger than 5.5 cm in diameter. Endovascular aneurysm repair is an alternative to surgical repair.

C. **Preoperative Evaluation.** Coexisting medical conditions, especially coronary artery disease, COPD, and renal dysfunction, are important to identify preoperatively. Myocardial ischemia or infarction is responsible for most postoperative deaths after elective abdominal aortic aneurysm resection. Preoperative evaluation of cardiac function might include stress testing with or without echocardiography or radionuclide imaging. Severe reductions in vital capacity and forced expiratory volume in 1 second and abnormal renal function significantly increase the risk of elective aneurysm repair.

D. **Rupture of an Abdominal Aortic Aneurysm.** The classic triad of hypotension, back pain, and a pulsatile abdominal mass is present in only about half of patients.

1. **Stable Patients.** Exsanguination may be prevented by clotting and the tamponade effect of the retroperitoneum. Euvolemic resuscitation is deferred until the aortic rupture is surgically controlled in the operating room, because euvolemic resuscitation and increase in blood pressure without surgical control of bleeding may lead to loss of retroperitoneal tamponade, further bleeding, hypotension, and death.
2. **Unstable Patients.** Unstable patients with a suspected ruptured abdominal aortic aneurysm require immediate operation and control of the proximal aorta without preoperative confirmatory testing or optimal volume resuscitation.

E. **Management of Anesthesia** (Table 8-4). Management of anesthesia for resection of an abdominal aortic aneurysm requires consideration of commonly associated medical conditions, including ischemic heart disease, hypertension, COPD, diabetes mellitus, and renal dysfunction.

TABLE 8-4 ■ Anesthesia Considerations in Abdominal Aortic Aneurysm Resection

Monitoring	Intraarterial pressure monitoring. PA catheter, particularly in patients with history of LV dysfunction or history of previous MI and when suprarenal X-clamping is anticipated. Consider echocardiography. Urine output monitoring.
Anesthetic maintenance	Volatile agents and opioids. Consider combined GA/epidural anesthesia.
Fluid management	Administration of crystalloid and colloid before unclamping to minimize declamping hypotension.
Cross-clamping	Increased SVR, decreased venous return. With infrarenal clamping, myocardial performance often remains stable.
Unclamping	Hypotension can be anticipated: preemptive volume loading before unclamping should be considered. Gradual opening of the cross-clamp may mitigate effect. Consider occult source of bleeding if hypotension does not resolve promptly with fluid therapy. TEE may be useful in assessing volume status.

GA, General anesthetic; *LV*, left ventricular; *MI*, myocardial infarction; *PA*, pulmonary artery; *SVR*, systemic vascular resistance; *TEE*, transesophageal echocardiography.

F. Postoperative Management

1. **Analgesia.** Adequate analgesia from use of either neuraxial opioids or patient-controlled analgesia is very important in facilitating early tracheal extubation.
2. **Systemic Hypertension.** Systemic hypertension is common during the postoperative period and may be more likely in patients with preoperative hypertension.

G. Endovascular Aortic Aneurysm Repair. Endovascular aortic aneurysm repair involves percutaneous placement of stents via small incisions over the femoral vessels, using general or regional anesthesia. Successful repair is achieved in more than 85% of patients, and perioperative mortality is comparable to that associated with open repair (up to 14%). Monitoring consists of at least intravascular blood pressure and urine output monitoring. The potential for conversion to an open aneurysm repair must be considered.

1. **Complications.** Complications include endograft leaks, vascular injury, inadequate fixation of graft to the vessel wall with graft migration, stent frame fractures, and graft breakdown. Although endovascular grafting does not require aortic cross-clamping, spinal cord ischemia is still a risk owing to exclusion of intercostal arteries.
2. **Anesthesia Management.** General or regional anesthesia is acceptable, with intravascular blood pressure monitoring and urine output monitoring. The possibility of having to convert to an open procedure must be considered, and adequate access for intravenous fluid resuscitation established. Spinal drainage may be considered in thoracic aortic endovascular repair.
3. **Postoperative Management.** Thoracic aortic endovascular repair usually necessitates an intensive care unit stay. Patients who have undergone abdominal aortic endovascular repair should also be followed closely, particularly for the development or worsening of renal dysfunction.

IV. CAROTID ARTERY DISEASE AND STROKE

Cerebrovascular accidents (strokes) are characterized by sudden neurologic deficits resulting from ischemic, hemorrhagic, or thrombotic events. Hemorrhagic stroke is classified as intracerebral or subarachnoid. A transient ischemic attack is a sudden vascular-related focal neurologic deficit that resolves within 24 hours.

A. Cerebrovascular Anatomy. The blood supply to the brain (20% of CO) is transported via two pairs of blood vessels: the internal carotid arteries and the vertebral arteries. These vessels join to form the major intracranial blood vessels (anterior cerebral arteries, middle cerebral arteries, posterior cerebral arteries) and the circle of Willis.

1. **Etiology of Acute Ischemic Stroke.** Acute ischemic stroke is usually caused by cardioembolism, large-vessel atherothromboembolism (such as from disease at the carotid bifurcation), or small-vessel occlusive disease (lacunar infarction).
2. **Risk Factors for Stroke.** Risk factors include age, hypertension, cigarette smoking, hyperlipidemia, diabetes mellitus, excessive alcohol consumption (more than six drinks daily), atrial fibrillation, heart failure, obesity, physical inactivity, African American race, sickle cell disease, male gender, and increased homocysteine levels.
3. **Evaluation of Stroke.** Conventional angiography or CT angiography can be used to identify vascular occlusions, thrombi, aneurysms, or arteriovenous malformations. Echocardiography is very useful in evaluating the source of cardioembolism. Carotid ultrasound can identify carotid stenosis.
4. **Treatment.** Medical management includes administration of recombinant tissue plasminogen activator within 4.5 hours of onset of stroke. Interventional neuroradiology may offer intraarterial thrombolysis or endovascular clot removal. Low-frequency transcranial ultrasound-mediated thrombolysis is under investigation. Additional considerations are management of hypoxia, glycemic derangements, hyperthermia, hypotension, severe hypertension, and arrhythmias.

B. Carotid Endarterectomy. Surgical treatment of symptomatic carotid artery stenosis greatly decreases the risk of stroke, especially in men with severe carotid stenosis. Surgical treatment for asymptomatic disease is still controversial. Carotid angioplasty and stenting may become alternatives to carotid endarterectomy.

1. **Preoperative Evaluation.** Patients should be examined for co-existing cardiovascular and renal disease. Ischemic heart disease is a major cause of morbidity and mortality after carotid endarterectomy. Patients with severe coronary artery disease and severe carotid occlusive disease present a dilemma. No randomized studies have determined the benefit of combined versus staged procedures. It is useful to establish the usual range of blood pressure for each patient preoperatively in order to have a guide for acceptable perfusion pressures during anesthesia and surgery. The effect of a change in head position on cerebral function should also be ascertained, so that positions that further impede cerebral blood flow can be avoided.
2. **Management of Anesthesia.** Anesthesia for carotid endarterectomy must meet two goals: maintenance of hemodynamic stability and prompt emergence allowing immediate assessment of neurologic status in the operating room. Carotid endarterectomy can be performed with the patient under general anesthesia or under regional (cervical plexus) block, allowing the patient to remain awake to facilitate neurologic assessment during carotid artery cross-clamping. Maintenance of an adequate blood pressure and normocarbia is important because cerebral autoregulation may be abnormal in these patients. Monitoring usually includes an intraarterial catheter. Patients with poor left ventricular function and/or severe coronary artery disease might require a central venous or pulmonary artery catheter or TEE. The utility of electroencephalographic monitoring during carotid endarterectomy is limited because electroencephalography may not detect subcortical or small cortical infarcts, false-negative results are not uncommon, and the electroencephalogram (EEG) can be affected by changes in temperature, blood pressure, and depth of anesthesia. Transcranial Doppler ultrasonography allows continuous monitoring of blood flow velocity and the presence of microemboli.
3. **Postoperative Management and Complications.** Complications include hypertension or hypotension, myocardial ischemia or infarction, development of significant soft tissue edema or a hematoma in the neck, and the onset of neurologic signs and symptoms of a new stroke or thrombosis at the endarterectomy site. Hypertension is common, and infusion of nitroprusside or nitroglycerin and the use of longer-acting drugs such as hydralazine or

labetalol are treatment options. Hypotension resulting from carotid sinus hypersensitivity is usually treated with vasopressors such as phenylephrine.

4. **Endovascular Treatment.** Endovascular treatment of carotid disease may become the leading alternative to carotid endarterectomy. The major complication of carotid stenting is microembolization of atherosclerotic material into the cerebral circulation during the procedure.

V. PERIPHERAL VASCULAR DISEASE

Peripheral arterial disease results in compromised blood flow to the extremities. Chronic impairment of blood flow to the extremities is most often a result of atherosclerosis, whereas arterial embolism is most likely to be responsible for acute arterial occlusion. Vasculitis may also be responsible for compromised peripheral blood flow (Table 8-5). An ankle-brachial index (ratio of systolic blood pressure at the ankle to the systolic blood pressure in the brachial artery) of less than 0.90 correlates extremely well with angiogram-positive disease.

A. **Risk Factors.** Risk factors associated with development of peripheral atherosclerosis are similar to those for ischemic heart disease: diabetes mellitus, hypertension, tobacco use, dyslipidemia, hyperhomocysteinemia, and a family history of premature atherosclerosis.

B. **Signs and Symptoms.** Intermittent claudication and pain at rest are the principal symptoms of peripheral arterial disease. Decreased or absent arterial pulses are the most reliable physical findings associated with peripheral arterial disease. Bruits, subcutaneous atrophy, hair loss, coolness, pallor, cyanosis, and dependent rubor in the extremities may be additional findings.

C. **Diagnostic Tests.** Doppler ultrasonography and the resulting pulse volume waveform are used to identify arterial vessels with stenotic lesions. Duplex ultrasonography can identify areas of plaque formation and stenosis. Transcutaneous oximetry may identify severity of skin ischemia. MRI and contrast angiography guide interventional therapy.

D. **Treatment**

1. **Medical Therapy.** Medical therapy includes exercise programs and identification and treatment or modification of risk factors for atherosclerosis, such as smoking cessation, lipid-lowering therapy, and treatment of hypertension and diabetes.

2. **Revascularization.** Revascularization procedures are indicated for patients with disabling claudication, ischemic rest pain, or impending limb loss.

   a. ***Percutaneous Transluminal Angioplasty.*** Percutaneous transluminal angioplasty of iliac arteries has a high initial success rate that may be further improved by stent placement. Femoral and popliteal artery percutaneous transluminal angioplasty has a lower success rate than iliac artery percutaneous transluminal angioplasty.

TABLE 8-5 ■ Peripheral Vascular Diseases

Chronic peripheral arterial occlusive disease (atherosclerosis)
Distal abdominal aorta or iliac arteries
Femoral arteries
Subclavian steal syndrome
Coronary-subclavian steal syndrome
Acute peripheral arterial occlusive disease (embolism)
Systemic vasculitis
Takayasu's arteritis
Thromboangiitis obliterans
Wegener's granulomatosis
Temporal arteritis
Polyarteritis nodosa
Other vascular syndromes
Raynaud's phenomenon
Kawasaki's syndrome

b. ***Surgical Procedures.*** Surgical procedures used for vascular reconstruction include aortobifemoral bypass, axillobifemoral bypass, femoral-femoral bypass, and femoropopliteal and tibioperoneal reconstruction. Amputation is necessary for patients with advanced limb ischemia in whom revascularization is not possible or has failed.

i. Operative risk of reconstructive peripheral arterial surgery is primarily related to the presence of associated atherosclerotic vascular disease, particularly ischemic heart disease and cerebrovascular disease.

ii. Mortality is usually a result of myocardial infarction in patients with preoperative evidence of ischemic heart disease, a history of coronary artery bypass grafting, or congestive heart failure. In patients with severe or unstable ischemic heart disease, percutaneous coronary intervention or coronary artery bypass grafting might be considered before revascularization surgery is performed. In patients with stable coronary artery disease, outcomes are not improved by prior coronary revascularization.

E. Management of Anesthesia. Management of anesthesia for surgical revascularization of the lower extremities incorporates principles similar to those described for the management of patients undergoing abdominal aortic aneurysm repair.

1. **Perioperative β-Blockade.** The American College of Cardiology and the American Heart Association identify the following patients as candidates for perioperative β-blockade: (1) patients undergoing vascular surgery with or without evidence of preoperative ischemia and with or without high or intermediate risk factors, (2) patients receiving long-term β-blocker therapy, and (3) patients undergoing vascular surgery even if they have only low risk factors.
2. **Regional (Epidural or Spinal) Anesthesia.** Regional anesthesia promotes increased graft blood flow, postoperative analgesia, less activation of the coagulation system, and fewer postoperative respiratory complications. Placement of an epidural catheter at least 1 hour before intraoperative heparinization is not associated with an increased incidence of untoward neurologic events.
3. **Infrarenal Aortic Cross-Clamping and Unclamping.** Infrarenal aortic cross-clamping and unclamping are associated with fewer hemodynamic derangements than occur in patients undergoing resection of an abdominal aortic aneurysm.
4. **Monitoring.** A central venous catheter or echocardiography may be useful.

F. Postoperative Management. Postoperative management includes provision of analgesia, treatment of fluid and electrolyte derangements, and control of heart rate and blood pressure to reduce the incidence of myocardial ischemia and infarction. Dexmedetomidine, an α_2-agonist, can attenuate the increase in heart rate and plasma catecholamine concentrations.

G. Subclavian Steal Syndrome. Occlusion of the subclavian or innominate artery proximal to the origin of the vertebral artery results in diversion of blood flow from the ipsilateral vertebral artery to the distal subclavian artery. Central nervous system symptoms (syncope, vertigo, ataxia, hemiplegia) and/or arm ischemia is usually present and accentuated by exercise of the ipsilateral arm. Pulse is absent or diminished in the ipsilateral arm, and systolic blood pressure is likely to be at least 20 mm Hg lower in that arm. Subclavian endarterectomy may be curative.

H. Coronary-Subclavian Steal Syndrome. Coronary-subclavian steal syndrome is a rare complication of using the internal mammary artery (IMA) for coronary revascularization. Proximal stenosis in the left subclavian artery leads to reversal of blood flow through the patent IMA graft. Signs and symptoms include angina pectoris, central nervous system ischemia, and a 20-mm Hg or more decrease in systolic blood pressure in the ipsilateral arm.

VI. ACUTE ARTERIAL OCCLUSION

Acute arterial occlusion differs from the gradual development of arterial occlusion caused by atherosclerosis and is usually a result of cardiogenic embolism.

A. Signs and Symptoms. Signs and symptoms include intense pain, paresthesias, motor weakness distal to the site of arterial occlusion, loss of a palpable peripheral pulse, cool skin, and sharply demarcated skin color changes (pallor or cyanosis) distal to the arterial occlusion.

B. Diagnosis. The diagnosis is confirmed by arteriography.

C. Treatment. Treatment is surgical embolectomy and anticoagulation. Intra-arterial thrombolysis may be effective.

D. Management of Anesthesia. Anesthesia is similar to that for patients with chronic peripheral arterial disease.

VII. RAYNAUD'S PHENOMENON

Raynaud's phenomenon is episodic vasospastic ischemia of the digits. It affects women more often than men.

A. Classification. Raynaud's phenomenon is categorized as primary (Raynaud's disease) or secondary when it is associated with other diseases such as scleroderma or systemic lupus erythematosus.

B. Etiology. Mechanisms postulated to cause Raynaud's phenomenon include increased sympathetic nervous system activity, digital vascular hyperreactivity to vasoconstrictive stimuli, circulating vasoactive hormones, and decreased intravascular pressure.

C. Diagnosis. Noninvasive tests that can be used to evaluate patients with Raynaud's phenomenon include digital pulse volume recording and measurement of digital systolic blood pressure and digital blood flow. Raynaud's phenomenon is the initial complaint in most patients with a limited form of scleroderma called *CREST syndrome*. CREST is an acronym for subcutaneous calcinosis, Raynaud's phenomenon, esophageal dysmotility, sclerodactyly (scleroderma limited to the fingers), and telangiectasia.

D. Treatment. Treatment includes protecting the hands and feet from exposure to cold. Calcium channel blockers such as nifedipine and sympathetic nervous system antagonists such as prazosin can be used to treat Raynaud's phenomenon. In rare instances, surgical sympathectomy might be considered for treatment of persistent, severe digital ischemia.

E. Management of Anesthesia. Increasing the ambient temperature of the operating room and maintaining normothermia are basic considerations. Systemic blood pressure is usually monitored via a noninvasive technique. Regional anesthesia is acceptable for peripheral operations in patients with Raynaud's phenomenon, but it may be prudent not to include epinephrine in the anesthetic solution because the catecholamine could provoke undesirable vasoconstriction.

VIII. PERIPHERAL VENOUS DISEASE

Superficial thrombophlebitis occurs in up to 50% of patients undergoing total hip replacement. It can be associated with localized pain and inflammation but is rarely associated with pulmonary embolism. Deep vein thrombosis (DVT; usually involving a leg vein) with subsequent pulmonary embolism is a leading cause of postoperative morbidity and mortality. Factors that predispose to thromboembolism are multiple and include events associated with anesthesia and surgery (Table 8-6).

A. Deep Vein Thrombosis

1. **Diagnosis.** Diagnosis of DVT by clinical signs is unreliable. Compression ultrasonography, venography, and impedance plethysmography are all used (Figure 8-2). Inherited abnormalities associated with initial and recurrent venous thrombosis and embolism include congenital deficiency of antithrombin III, protein C, protein S, or plasminogen.
2. **Prevention of Venous Thromboembolism**
3. **Clinical Risk Factors and Recommended Prophylaxis.** See Table 8-7.
4. **Regional Anesthesia.** Regional anesthesia is associated with reduced risk (20% to 40%) of deep venous thromboembolism and pulmonary embolism after total knee or total hip arthroplasty.

TABLE 8-6 ■ Factors Predisposing to Thromboembolism

Venous stasis
- Recent surgery
- Trauma
- Lack of ambulation
- Pregnancy
- Low cardiac output (congestive heart failure, myocardial infarction)
- Stroke

Abnormality of the venous wall
- Varicose veins
- Drug-induced irritation

Hypercoagulable state
- Surgery
- Estrogen therapy (oral contraceptives)
- Cancer
- Deficiencies of endogenous anticoagulants (antithrombin III, protein C, protein S)
- Stress response associated with surgery
- Inflammatory bowel disease

History of previous thromboembolism
- Morbid obesity
- Advanced age

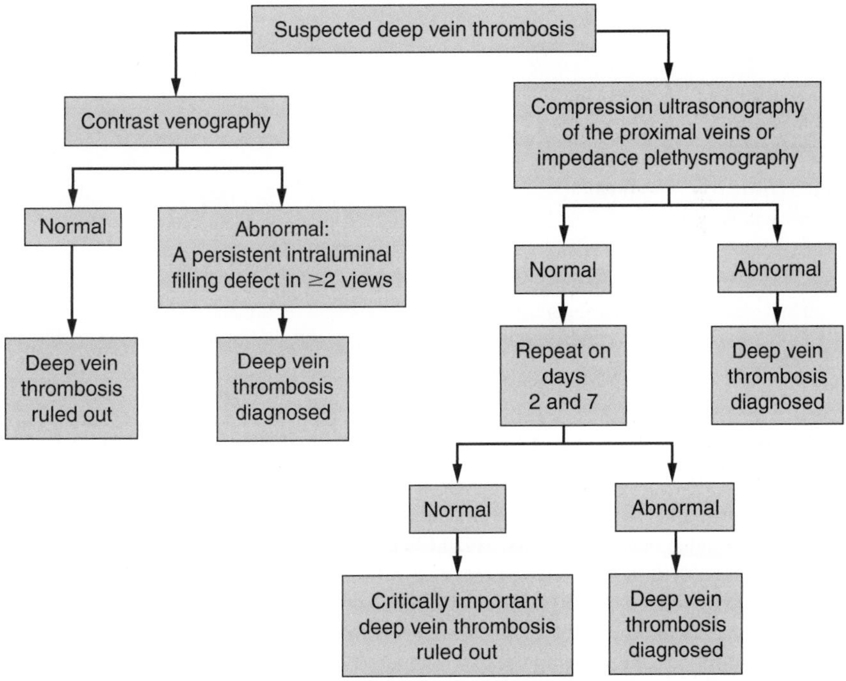

FIGURE 8-2 ■ Steps in the diagnosis of deep vein thrombosis. *(Adapted from Ginsberg JS. Management of venous thromboembolism.* N Engl J Med. *1996;335:1816-1828. Copyright 1996 Massachusetts Medical Society.)*

TABLE 8-7 ■ **Risk and Predisposing Factors for Development of Deep Venous Thrombosis After Surgery or Trauma**

ASSOCIATED CONDITIONS	LOW RISK	MODERATE RISK	HIGH RISK
General surgery	<40 yr old Operation <60 min	>40 yr old Operation >60 min	>40 yr old Operation >60 min Previous deep vein thrombosis Previous pulmonary embolism Extensive trauma Major fractures
Orthopedic surgery			Knee or hip replacement
Trauma			Extensive soft tissue injury Major fractures Multiple trauma sites
Medical conditions	Pregnancy	Postpartum period Myocardial infarction Congestive heart failure	Stroke
Incidence of deep vein thrombosis without prophylaxis	2%	10%-40%	40%-80%
Symptomatic pulmonary embolism	0.2%	1%-8%	5%-10%
Fatal pulmonary embolism	0.002%	0.1%-0.4%	1%-5%
Recommended steps to minimize deep vein thrombosis	Graduated compression stockings Early ambulation	External pneumatic compression Subcutaneous heparin Intravenous dextran	External pneumatic compression Subcutaneous heparin Intravenous dextran Vena caval filter Warfarin

Adapted from Weinmann EE, Salzman EW. Deep-vein thrombosis. *N Engl J Med.* 1994;331:1630-1642.

5. **Treatment.** Anticoagulation is the first-line treatment. Therapy is initiated with heparin (unfractionated or low-molecular-weight heparin) followed by an oral vitamin K antagonist (warfarin), dose-adjusted to achieve a prothrombin time with an international normalized ratio between 2.0 and 3.0. Oral anticoagulants are continued for 3 to 6 months. Inferior vena cava filters may be used in patients with recurrent pulmonary embolism despite adequate anticoagulant therapy or in whom anticoagulation is contraindicated.
6. **Complications of Anticoagulation.** Complications include bleeding and thrombocytopenia associated with heparin administration. Heparin-induced thrombocytopenia (HIT) can be divided into two types:
   a. Type 1 is mild thrombocytopenia (platelet count usually remains higher than 100,000) seen within the first few days of initiation of heparin therapy. It resolves spontaneously and does not preclude future treatment with heparin.

TABLE 8-8 ■ Signs and Symptoms of Takayasu's Arteritis

CENTRAL NERVOUS SYSTEM
Vertigo Visual disturbances Syncope Seizures Cerebral ischemia or infarction
CARDIOVASCULAR SYSTEM
Multiple occlusions of peripheral arteries Ischemic heart disease Cardiac valve dysfunction Cardiac conduction defects
LUNGS
Pulmonary hypertension Ventilation-perfusion mismatch
KIDNEYS
Renal artery stenosis
MUSCULOSKELETAL SYSTEM
Ankylosing spondylitis Rheumatoid arthritis

b. Type 2 occurs in 1% to 3% of patients receiving unfractionated heparin and is caused by antibodies to heparin-platelet factor 4 complex. It results in severe thrombocytopenia and platelet activation that causes microvascular thrombosis. Diagnosis is made on the basis of heparin antibodies together with a positive result of platelet serotonin release assay. Treatment with a direct thrombin inhibitor such as argatroban or lepirudin is required to prevent further thrombosis. All future heparin exposure must be avoided.

IX. SYSTEMIC VASCULITIS

Peripheral vascular disease may manifest as part of a systemic vasculitis caused by a connective tissue disease, sepsis, or malignancy.

A. Takayasu's Arteritis. Takayasu's arteritis is an idiopathic, progressive occlusive vasculitis that causes narrowing, thrombosis, or aneurysms of systemic and pulmonary arteries. It is diagnosed definitively based on contrast angiography.

1. **Signs and Symptoms.** See Table 8-8.
2. **Treatment is Corticosteroids.** Anticoagulation may be indicated in some patients.
3. **Management of Anesthesia.** See Table 8-9.

B. Temporal (Giant Cell) Arteritis. Temporal arteritis is inflammation of the arteries of the head and neck, manifesting as headache, scalp tenderness, or jaw claudication. Prompt initiation of treatment with corticosteroids is indicated in patients with visual symptoms to prevent blindness. Evidence of arteritis on a biopsy specimen of the temporal artery is present in approximately 90% of patients.

C. Kawasaki's Syndrome. Kawasaki's syndrome (mucocutaneous lymph node syndrome) occurs primarily in children and manifests as fever, conjunctivitis, inflammation of the mucous membranes, swollen erythematous hands and feet, truncal rash, and cervical lymphadenopathy and vasculitis.

TABLE 8-9 ■ **Anesthesia Considerations in Takayasu's Arteritis**

Preoperative considerations	Monitor for adrenal suppression caused by chronic corticosteroid use. In laryngoscopy and intubation, consider that neck hyperextension can compromise blood flow through the carotid arteries.
Choice of anesthetic technique	Regional may not be possible owing to anticoagulation. Hypotension can compromise perfusion to vital organs. Adequate arterial pressure must be maintained.
Monitoring	Noninvasive blood pressure measurement may be difficult owing to subclavian and brachial artery stenosis. Electroencephalographic monitoring may be helpful for detecting cerebral ischemia.

1. **Treatment.** Treatment consists of γ-globulin and aspirin.
2. **Management of Anesthesia.** With regard to anesthesia, the possibility of intraoperative myocardial ischemia must be considered.

D. **Thromboangiitis Obliterans (Buerger's Disease).** Thromboangiitis obliterans is an inflammatory vasculitis leading to occlusion of small- and medium-sized arteries and veins in the extremities. The diagnosis is confirmed by biopsy of active vascular lesions.
1. **Signs and Symptoms.** Signs and symptoms include claudication of the upper or lower extremities. Raynaud's phenomenon is common.
2. **Treatment.** Treatment is smoking cessation. Surgical revascularization is not usually feasible because of the involvement of small distal blood vessels.
3. **Management of Anesthesia.** With regard to anesthesia, it is necessary to avoid events that might damage already ischemic extremities. Positioning and padding of pressure areas and maintenance of normothermia are critical. Systemic blood pressure should be measured noninvasively. If regional anesthetic techniques are selected, epinephrine should be omitted from the local anesthetic solution to avoid the possibility of accentuating vasospasm.

E. **Wegener's Granulomatosis.** Wegener's granulomatosis is characterized by formation of necrotizing granulomas in inflamed blood vessels in multiple organ systems (Table 8-10).
1. **Treatment.** Treatment with cyclophosphamide can produce remissions in approximately 90% of patients.
2. **Management of Anesthesia.** In patients with Wegener's granulomatosis, management of anesthesia requires an appreciation of the widespread organ system involvement of this disease. Immunosuppression results from cyclophosphamide treatment. Avoidance of trauma during laryngoscopy is important because bleeding from granulomas and dislodgment of friable ulcerated tissue can occur. A smaller than expected endotracheal tube may be required if the glottic opening is narrowed by granulomatous changes. Arteritis involving peripheral vessels may interfere with placement of an indwelling arterial catheter to monitor blood pressure or may limit the frequency of arterial punctures to obtain samples for blood gas analysis.

F. **Churg-Strauss Syndrome.** Churg-Strauss syndrome is a vasculitis of medium to small vessels, associated with inflammation of the respiratory tract with symptoms of rhinitis and asthma, as well as eosinophilia. Cardiac, renal, neurologic, and gastrointestinal manifestations can occur. Treatment is with glucocorticoids and maintenance immunosuppressive therapy.

G. **Polyarteritis Nodosa.** Polyarteritis nodosa most often occurs in women, often in association with hepatitis B antigenemia and allergic reactions to drugs. Renal failure is the most common cause of death.

TABLE 8-10 ■ Signs and Symptoms of Wegener's Granulomatosis

CENTRAL NERVOUS SYSTEM
Cerebral aneurysms
Peripheral neuropathy
RESPIRATORY TRACT AND LUNGS
Sinusitis
Laryngeal stenosis
Epiglottic destruction
Ventilation-perfusion mismatch
Pneumonia
Hemoptysis
Bronchial destruction
CARDIOVASCULAR SYSTEM
Cardiac valve destruction
Disturbances of cardiac conduction
Myocardial ischemia
KIDNEYS
Hematuria
Azotemia
Renal failure

1. **Diagnosis.** The diagnosis depends on histologic evidence of vasculitis on biopsy and demonstration of characteristic aneurysms on arteriography.
2. **Treatment.** Treatment usually includes corticosteroids and cyclophosphamide, removal of offending drugs, and treatment of underlying diseases such as cancer.
3. **Management of Anesthesia.** In patients with polyarteritis nodosa, management of anesthesia should take into consideration the likelihood of co-existing renal disease, cardiac disease, and systemic hypertension. Supplemental corticosteroids may be indicated.

CHAPTER 9

Respiratory Diseases

Pulmonary complications play an important part in determining morbidity, hospital length of stay, and long-term mortality after surgery. Preoperative modification of disease severity and patient optimization decrease the incidence of these complications. Respiratory diseases and conditions can be divided into the following categories: acute upper respiratory tract infection (URI), asthma, chronic obstructive pulmonary disease (COPD), acute respiratory failure, restrictive lung disease, pulmonary embolism (PE), and lung transplantation.

I. ACUTE UPPER RESPIRATORY TRACT INFECTION

Infectious (viral or bacterial) nasopharyngitis accounts for approximately 95% of all URIs. Noninfectious nasopharyngitis is allergic and vasomotor in origin.

A. **Signs and Symptoms.** Signs of acute URI include sneezing and runny nose. A history of allergies may indicate an allergic cause rather than infection. With infectious causes, there is usually fever, purulent nasal discharge, productive cough, fever, and malaise. The patient may be tachypneic or wheezing or may have an appearance that suggests toxicity.

B. **Diagnosis.** Diagnosis is usually based on clinical signs and symptoms. Viral cultures and laboratory tests lack sensitivity and are impractical in a busy clinical setting.

C. **Management of Anesthesia**

1. **Preoperative Considerations.** Most studies regarding URIs and postoperative complications have been done in pediatric patients. Patients with systemic signs of infection (fever, purulent rhinitis, productive cough, rhonchi) undergoing elective surgery, particularly airway surgery, are at risk of adverse events, and delaying surgery should be considered. More respiratory complications are also reported in pediatric patients with prematurity and those with a history of parental smoking. Patients who have had a URI for days or weeks and are stable to improving can be safely managed without postponing surgery. Delaying surgery does not reduce the incidence of adverse respiratory events if anesthesia is administered within 4 weeks of the URI. Airway hyperreactivity may require 6 weeks or more to resolve.
2. **Intraoperative Management.** Intraoperatively, management of patients with a URI includes adequate hydration, reducing secretions, and limiting manipulation of a potentially sensitive airway. The laryngeal mask airway (LMA) (versus endotracheal intubation) may reduce the risk of bronchospasm. It has not been proven that prophylactic bronchodilators reduce the incidence of perioperative bronchospasm.
3. **Postoperative Adverse Respiratory Events.** Postoperative events include bronchospasm, laryngospasm, airway obstruction, postintubation croup, desaturation, and atelectasis. Intraoperative and immediate postoperative hypoxemia is common and amenable to treatment with supplemental oxygen. Long-term complications have not been demonstrated.

II. ASTHMA

Asthma is characterized by chronic airway inflammation, reversible expiratory airflow obstruction in response to various stimuli, and bronchial hyperreactivity. It is estimated that asthma affects 300 million people worldwide, and the prevalence is increasing. The prevalence of asthma is significantly greater in women than in men.

A. Signs and Symptoms. Asthma is an episodic disease characterized by acute exacerbations interspersed with symptom-free periods. Symptoms and signs include wheezing, productive or nonproductive cough, dyspnea, chest discomfort or tightness that may lead to "air hunger," and eosinophilia. Particular attention should be paid to factors associated with increased risk, such as previous intubation or intensive care unit (ICU) admission for exacerbations, two or more hospitalizations in the last year, and the presence of co-existing diseases. *Status asthmaticus* is defined as life-threatening bronchospasm that persists despite treatment.

B. Pathogenesis: Allergen-Induced versus Abnormal Autonomic Regulation

1. **Evidence for Allergen-Induced Immunologic Model.**
   a. Atopy is the single greatest risk factor for the development of asthma.
   b. A personal and/or family history of allergic diseases is often present.
   c. There is usually a positive wheal-and-flare skin reaction to intradermal injection of extracts of airborne antigens.
   d. Serum immunoglobulin E (IgE) levels are increased, and/or there is a positive response to provocative tests involving the inhalation of specific antigens.
   e. Evidence of genetic linkage of high total serum IgE levels and atopy has been observed.
2. **Model of Abnormal Autonomic Nervous System Regulation of Neural Function.** Chemical mediators released from mast cells probably interact with the autonomic nervous system. Some chemical mediators can stimulate airway receptors and trigger bronchoconstriction, whereas other mediators sensitize bronchial smooth muscle to the effects of acetylcholine. Stimulation of muscarinic receptors can facilitate mediator release from mast cells, providing a positive feedback loop for sustained inflammation and bronchoconstriction.

C. Diagnosis

1. **Forced Expiratory Volume in 1 Second.** Forced expiratory volume in 1 second (FEV_1) and maximum mid-expiratory flow rate (MMEF) are direct measures of the severity of expiratory airflow obstruction (Figure 9-1 and Table 9-1).
2. **Flow-Volume Loops.** Flow-volume loops show characteristic downward scooping of the expiratory limb of the loop (Figure 9-2).
3. **Mild Asthma Is Usually Accompanied by a Normal Pa_{O_2} and Pa_{CO_2}.** Hypocarbia and respiratory alkalosis are the most common arterial blood gas findings in the presence of asthma. Hypercarbia may indicate failure of the skeletal muscles necessary for breathing.
4. **Chest X-Ray Examination and Electrocardiography.** The chest radiograph may show hyperinflation of the lungs or reveal superimposed pulmonary pathology, such as pneumonia or congestive heart failure. The electrocardiogram (ECG) may show evidence of right heart strain and cardiac irritability.
5. **Differential Diagnosis.** The differential diagnosis includes viral tracheobronchitis, sarcoidosis, rheumatoid arthritis with bronchiolitis, extrinsic compression (thoracic aneurysm, mediastinal neoplasm) or intrinsic compression (epiglottitis, croup) of the upper airway, congestive heart failure, PE, and pulmonary edema.

D. Treatment (Table 9-2). Asthma treatment has two components: (1) "controller" treatments, which modify the airway environment such that acute airway narrowing occurs less frequently (e.g., inhaled and systemic corticosteroids, theophylline, and antileukotrienes), and (2) "reliever" or rescue agents for acute bronchospasm (e.g., β-adrenergic agonists and anticholinergic drugs). Treatment of *status asthmaticus* is summarized in Table 9-3.

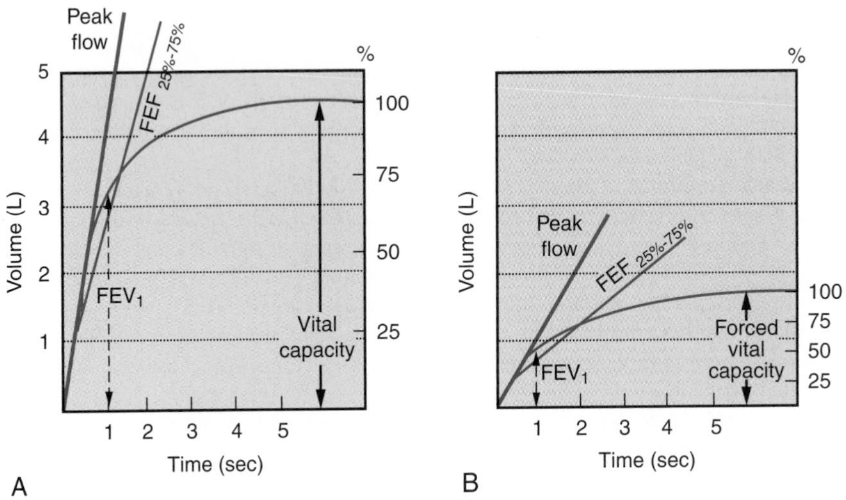

FIGURE 9-1 ■ Spirographic changes of a normal subject **(A)** and a patient in bronchospasm **(B).** The FEV_1 is typically less than 80% of the vital capacity in the presence of obstructive airway disease. Peak flow and maximum mid-expiratory flow rate ($FEF_{25\%-75\%}$) are also decreased in these patients **(B).** *(Adapted from Kingston HGG, Hirshman CA. Perioperative management of the patient with asthma.* Anesth Analg. *1984;63:844-855.)*

TABLE 9-1 ■ Classification of Asthma Based on Severity of Expiratory Airflow Obstruction

SEVERITY	FEV_1 (% PREDICTED)	$FEF_{25\%-75\%}$ (% PREDICTED)	Pa_{O_2} (mm Hg)	Pa_{CO_2} (mm Hg)
Mild (asymptomatic)	65-80	60-75	>60	<40
Moderate	50-64	45-59	>60	<45
Marked	35-49	30-44	<60	>50
Severe (status asthmaticus)	<35	<30	<60	>50

Adapted from Kingston HGG, Hirschman CA. Perioperative management of the patient with asthma. *Anesth Analg.* 1984;63:844-855.

$FEF_{25\%-75\%}$, Forced expiratory flow at 25% to 75% of forced vital capacity.

E. Management of Anesthesia

1. **Preoperative Evaluation.** Disease severity, effectiveness of current therapy, and the potential need for additional therapy should be assessed before surgery. Preoperative evaluation begins with a clinical history to elicit the severity and characteristics of the patient's asthma (Table 9-4). Auscultation of the chest to detect wheezing or crepitations is important. Pulmonary function tests (especially FEV_1) before and after bronchodilator therapy may be indicated in patients scheduled for major elective surgery. Measurement of arterial blood gases is indicated if there is any question about the adequacy of ventilation or oxygenation.
   a. ***Preoperative Medication.*** Use of anticholinergic drugs should be individualized. Anti-inflammatory and bronchodilator therapy should be continued until the time of anesthesia induction. Supplementation with "stress dose" corticosteroids may be indicated before major surgery. Patients should be free of wheezing and have a peak expiratory

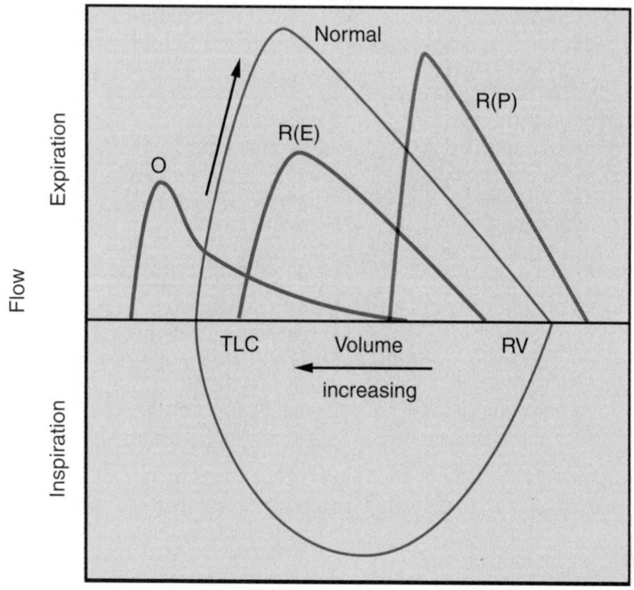

FIGURE 9-2 ■ Flow-volume curves in different conditions: *O,* obstructive disease; *R(E),* extraparenchymal restrictive disease with limitation in inspiration and expiration; *R(P),* parenchymal restrictive disease. Forced expiration is plotted in all conditions; forced inspiration is shown only for the normal curve. *RV,* Residual volume; *TLC,* total lung capacity. By convention, lung volume increases to the left on the abscissa. The arrow alongside the normal curve indicates the direction of expiration from TLC to RV. *(Adapted from Weinberger SE. Disturbances of respiratory function. In: Fauci B, Braunwald E, Isselbacher KJ, et al, eds.* Harrison's Principles of Internal Medicine. *14th ed. New York, NY: McGraw-Hill; 1998.)*

flow greater than 80% of predicted or at the level of the patient's personal best value before surgery.

2. **Induction and Maintenance of Anesthesia.** A goal of induction and maintenance of anesthesia in the asthmatic patient is to suppress airway reflexes to avoid bronchoconstriction in response to mechanical stimulation of the airways.
   a. ***Regional Anesthesia.*** The use of regional anesthesia when the operative site is suitable for this may avoid instrumentation of the airway and tracheal intubation.
   b. ***General Anesthesia.*** Induction of anesthesia with propofol is preferable to induction with thiopental, which is associated with a higher incidence of wheezing. Ketamine may produce smooth muscle relaxation and contribute to decreased airway resistance.
      i. After unconsciousness is produced, the lungs are ventilated with a volatile anesthetic agent to establish a depth of anesthesia sufficient to permit tracheal intubation without precipitating bronchospasm. Intravenous or intratracheal injection of lidocaine 1 to 1.5 mg/kg 1 to 3 minutes before tracheal intubation can be helpful. Opioids may suppress the cough reflex and deepen anesthesia. It may be preferable to use short-acting opioids that have limited risk of causing postoperative respiratory depression, such as remifentanil (continuous infusion of 0.05 to 0.1 mcg/kg/min).
      ii. LMA insertion is less likely than endotracheal intubation to result in bronchoconstriction and may be a better method of airway management in asthmatic patients in whom it is appropriate. After endotracheal intubation, it may be difficult to differentiate light anesthesia from bronchospasm as the cause of a decrease in pulmonary compliance. Administration of neuromuscular blocking drugs relieves the difficulty of ventilation resulting from light anesthesia but has no effect on bronchospasm.

TABLE 9-2 ■ **Pharmacologic Agents Used in the Treatment of Asthma**

CLASS	DRUG	ACTIONS	ADVERSE EFFECTS
Antiinflammatory drugs	Corticosteroids: beclomethasone, triamcinolone, flunisolide, fluticasone, budesonide	Decrease airway inflammation, reduce airway hyperresponsiveness	Dysphonia, myopathy of laryngeal muscles, oropharyngeal candidiasis
	Cromolyn	Inhibit mediator release from mast cells, membrane stabilization	
	Leukotriene modifiers: zafirlukast, pranlukast, montelukast, zileuton	Reduce synthesis of leukotrienes by inhibiting 5-lipoxygenase enzyme	Minimal
Bronchodilators	β-adrenergic agonists: albuterol, metaproterenol, salmeterol	Stimulate β_2-receptors of tracheobronchial tree	Tachycardia, tremors, dysrhythmias, hypokalemia
	Anticholinergics: ipratropium, atropine, glycopyrrolate	Decrease vagal tone by blocking muscarinic receptors in airway smooth muscle	Dry mouth, cough, blurred vision
Methylxanthines	Theophylline	Increase cAMP by inhibiting phosphodiesterase, block adenosine receptors, release endogenous catecholamines	Disrupted sleep cycle, nervousness, nausea, vomiting, anorexia, headache, dysrhythmias

cAMP, Cyclic adenosine monophosphate.

TABLE 9-3 ■ **Treatment of Status Asthmaticus**

β_2-Agonists by metered-dose inhaler every 15-20 min or by continuous nebulizer administration
Intravenous corticosteroids (cortisol 2 mg/kg followed by 0.5 mg/kg/hr or methylprednisolone 60-125 mg every 6 hr)
Supplemental oxygen to maintain $Sa_{O_2} > 90\%$
IV magnesium sulfate may improve lung function
Oral leukotriene inhibitors
Tracheal intubation and mechanical ventilation (when $Pa_{CO_2} > 50$ mm Hg)

- High gas flows permit short inspiration times and longer expiration times.
- Expiration time must be prolonged to avoid air-trapping and "auto PEEP."
- Permissive hypercarbia to avoid barotrauma.

Empirical broad-spectrum antibiotics
General anesthesia with volatile agents to produce bronchodilation

TABLE 9-4 ■ Characteristics of Asthma to Evaluate Preoperatively

Age at onset
Triggering events
Hospitalization for asthma
Frequency of emergency department visits
Need for intubation and mechanical ventilation
Allergies
Cough
Sputum characteristics
Current medications
Anesthetic history

TABLE 9-5 ■ Differential Diagnosis of Intraoperative Bronchospasm and Wheezing

Mechanical obstruction of endotracheal tube
Kinking
Secretions
Overinflation of the tracheal tube cuff
Inadequate depth of anesthesia
Active expiratory efforts
Decreased functional residual capacity
Endobronchial intubation
Pulmonary aspiration
Pulmonary edema
Pulmonary embolus
Pneumothorax
Acute asthmatic attack

iii. Drugs with limited ability to evoke the release of histamine should be selected. Although all opioids have some histamine-releasing effects, fentanyl and analogous agents have been used safely in asthma patients.

iv. Theoretically, antagonism of neuromuscular blockade with anticholinesterase drugs could precipitate bronchospasm secondary to stimulation of postganglionic cholinergic receptors in airway smooth muscle. Bronchospasm does not predictably occur after administration of anticholinesterase drugs, probably because of the protective bronchodilating effects provided by the simultaneous administration of anticholinergic drugs.

v. During mechanical ventilation in asthmatic patients, a slow inspiratory flow rate provides optimal distribution of ventilation relative to perfusion. Sufficient time for exhalation is necessary to prevent air trapping. Humidification and warming of inspired gases may be especially helpful.

vi. Maintenance of adequate hydration ensures less viscous secretions in the airway.

vii. If possible, extubation should be performed while anesthesia is still sufficient to suppress hyperreactive airway reflexes. When it is unwise to extubate the trachea before the patient is fully awake, suppressing airway reflexes and/or the risk of bronchospasm by administration of intravenous lidocaine or pretreatment with inhaled bronchodilators should be considered.

3. **Intraoperative Bronchospasm.** Intraoperative bronchospasm is often a result of factors other than asthma (Table 9-5).

TABLE 9-6 ■ **Comparative Features of Chronic Obstructive Pulmonary Disease**

FEATURE	CHRONIC BRONCHITIS	EMPHYSEMA
Mechanism of airway obstruction	Decreased airway lumen resulting from mucus and inflammation	Loss of elastic recoil
Dyspnea	Moderate	Severe
FEV_1	Decreased	Decreased
Pao_2	Marked decrease ("blue bloater")	Modest decrease ("pink puffer")
$Paco_2$	Increased	Normal to decreased
Diffusing capacity	Normal	Decreased
Hematocrit	Increased	Normal
Cor pulmonale	Marked	Mild
Prognosis	Poor	Good

FEV_1, Forced expiratory volume in 1 second.

III. CHRONIC OBSTRUCTIVE PULMONARY DISEASE

COPD is characterized by the progressive development of airflow limitation that is not fully reversible. It includes chronic bronchitis with obstruction of small airways and emphysema with enlargement of air sacs, destruction of lung parenchyma, loss of elasticity, and closure of small airways. Risk factors for COPD are (1) cigarette smoking; (2) respiratory infection; (3) occupational exposure to dust, especially in coal mining, gold mining, and the textile industry; and (4) genetic factors such as α_1-antitrypsin deficiency.

A. Signs and Symptoms. Physical findings vary with severity of COPD. As expiratory airflow obstruction increases in severity, tachypnea and a prolonged expiratory phase are evident. Breath sounds are decreased, and expiratory wheezes are common.

B. Diagnosis. A chronic productive cough and progressive exercise limitation are the hallmarks of the persistent expiratory airflow obstruction characteristic of COPD (Tables 9-6 and 9-7). Patients with predominant chronic bronchitis have a chronic productive cough, whereas patients with predominant emphysema report dyspnea. Wheezing is common with mucus accumulation in the airways and may mimic asthma.

1. **Pulmonary Function Tests.** Decreases in the FEV_1/forced vital capacity (FVC) ratio and even greater decreases in the forced expiratory flow between 25% and 75% of vital capacity ($FEF_{25\%-75\%}$) are found on pulmonary function testing. Lung volumes show an increased residual volume and normal to increased functional residual capacity (FRC) and total lung capacity (TLC) (see Figure 9-2).
2. **Chest Radiography.** Abnormalities may be minimal, even with severe COPD. Hyperlucency and hyperinflation (flattening of the diaphragm with loss of its normal domed appearance and a very vertical cardiac silhouette) suggest the diagnosis of emphysema.

C. Treatment (Table 9-8)

1. **Smoking Cessation and Long-Term Oxygen Therapy.** Smoking cessation reduces or eliminates the symptoms of chronic bronchitis. Long-term oxygen therapy is recommended if Pao_2 is less than 55 mm Hg on room air, the hematocrit greater than 55%, or there is evidence of cor pulmonale. The goal of oxygen therapy is to achieve a Pao_2 of 60 to 80 mm Hg, which can usually be accomplished with oxygen delivered by nasal cannula at 2 L/min.
2. **Drug Therapy** (see Table 9-8)

TABLE 9-7 ■ Spirometric Classification of the Severity of Chronic Obstructive Pulmonary Disease Based on Postbronchodilator FEV_1 Measurements

STAGE	CHARACTERISTICS
0: At risk	Normal spirometry Chronic symptoms (cough, sputum production)
I: Mild COPD	$FEV_1/FVC < 70\%$ $FEV_1 \geq 80\%$ predicted, with or without chronic symptoms (cough, sputum production)
II: Moderate COPD	$FEV_1/FVC < 70\%$ $50\% \leq FEV_1 < 80\%$ predicted, with or without chronic symptoms (cough, sputum production)
III: Severe COPD	$FEV_1/FVC < 70\%$ $30\% \leq FEV_1 < 50\%$ predicted, with or without chronic symptoms (cough, sputum production)
IV: Very severe COPD	$FEV_1/FVC < 70\%$ $FEV_1 < 30\%$ predicted or $FEV_1 < 50\%$ predicted plus chronic respiratory failure (i.e., $Pa_{O_2} < 60$ mm Hg and/or $P_{CO_2} > 50$ mm Hg)

Adapted from the Global Initiative for Chronic Obstructive Lung Disease. Global strategy for the diagnosis, management and prevention of COPD: update 2010. www.goldcopd.com.

COPD, Chronic obstructive pulmonary disease; *FEV_1*, forced expiratory volume in 1 sec; *FVC,* forced vital capacity.

TABLE 9-8 ■ Treatment of Patients with Chronic Obstructive Pulmonary Disease

Cessation of cigarette smoking
β_2-Agonists (even small improvements in airway resistance decrease symptoms and may decrease infective exacerbations)
Anticholinergic drugs (most effective in patients with COPD)
Inhaled corticosteroids
Intermittent broad-spectrum antibiotics
Annual vaccination against influenza and pneumococci
Supplemental oxygen if $Pa_{O_2} < 55$ mm Hg, hematocrit > 55%, or evidence of cor pulmonale is present
Diuretics in patients with cor pulmonale and right-sided heart failure with peripheral edema

COPD, Chronic obstructive pulmonary disease.

3. **Lung Volume Reduction Surgery.** In selected patients with emphysema who have regions of overdistended, poorly functioning lung tissue, lung volume reduction surgery may be considered. Surgical removal of the overdistended areas allows more normal areas of the lung to expand and improves not only lung function but quality of life.
   a. ***Management of Anesthesia.*** For lung volume reduction surgery, management of anesthesia includes use of a double-lumen endobronchial tube to permit lung separation, avoidance of nitrous oxide, and avoidance of excessive positive airway pressure.

D. Management of Anesthesia

1. **Preoperative Management**
   a. ***Pulmonary Function Testing.*** Preoperative pulmonary function testing is controversial and does not reliably predict the likelihood of postoperative pulmonary complications after nonthoracic surgery. Pulmonary function tests and arterial blood gases may be

TABLE 9-9 ■ Anesthesia Management Strategies to Reduce Risks of Postoperative Pulmonary Complications in Patients with Chronic Obstructive Pulmonary Disease

PREOPERATIVE
Encourage cessation of smoking for at least 6 weeks.
Treat expiratory airflow obstruction, if evidence suggests its presence.
Treat respiratory infection with antibiotics.
Initiate patient education regarding lung volume expansion maneuvers.
INTRAOPERATIVE
Use minimally invasive surgery (endoscopic) techniques when possible.
Consider use of regional anesthesia.
Avoid surgical procedures likely to require more than 3 hours.
POSTOPERATIVE
Institute lung volume expansion maneuvers (voluntary deep breathing, incentive spirometry, continuous positive airway pressure).
Maximize analgesia (neuraxial opioids, intercostal nerve blocks, patient-controlled analgesia).

Adapted from Smetana GW. Preoperative pulmonary evaluation. *N Engl J Med.* 1999;340:937-944, copyright 1999 Massachusetts Medical Society.

useful for predicting pulmonary function after lung resection. Indications for a preoperative pulmonary evaluation include (1) hypoxemia on room air or the need for home oxygen therapy without a known cause, (2) bicarbonate greater than 33 mEq/L or Pco_2 greater than 50 mm Hg in a patient whose pulmonary disease has not been previously evaluated, (3) a history of respiratory failure resulting from a problem that still exists, (4) severe shortness of breath attributed to respiratory disease, (5) planned pneumonectomy, (6) difficulty assessing pulmonary function by clinical signs, (7) the need to distinguish among potential causes of significant respiratory compromise, (8) determination of the response to bronchodilators, and (9) suspected pulmonary hypertension. Right ventricular function should be carefully assessed by clinical examination and echocardiography in patients with advanced pulmonary disease.

i. ***Flow Volume Loops.*** Patients with COPD experience a decrease in the expiratory flow rate at any given lung volume. The expiratory curve is concave upward, and the residual volume is increased. Patients with restrictive lung disease will show a decrease in all lung volumes (see Figure 9-2).

b. ***Risk Reduction Strategies*** *(Table 9-9)*

i. ***Smoking Cessation.*** Within 12 hours after cessation of smoking, the Pao_2 at which hemoglobin is 50% saturated with oxygen (P_{50}) increases from 22.9 to 26.4 mm Hg and plasma levels of carboxyhemoglobin decrease from 6.5% to approximately 1%. The effects of nicotine on the heart are transient, lasting only 20 to 30 minutes. It likely takes 6 weeks for hepatic enzyme activity to return to normal after cessation of smoking. Aids to smoking cessation include nicotine replacement therapy, which is well tolerated, and administration of bupropion, typically started 1 to 2 weeks before smoking is stopped.

2. **Intraoperative Management**

a. ***Regional Anesthesia.*** Peripheral nerve block carries a lower risk of pulmonary complications than either spinal or general anesthesia. Regional anesthesia is a useful choice in patients with COPD only if large doses of sedative and anxiolytic drugs will not be needed. Small doses of a benzodiazepine (e.g., midazolam, in increments of 1 to 2 mg

TABLE 9-10 ■ **Major Risk Factors Associated with Postoperative Pulmonary Complications**

PATIENT RELATED
1. Age > 60 years
2. ASA class higher than II
3. Congestive heart failure
4. Preexisting pulmonary disease (COPD)
5. Functionally dependent
6. Cigarette smoking
PROCEDURE RELATED
1. Emergency surgery
2. Abdominal or thoracic surgery; head and neck surgery; neurosurgery; vascular/aortic aneurysm surgery
3. Prolonged duration of anesthesia (>2.5 hr)
4. General anesthesia
TEST PREDICTORS
1. Albumin level <3.5 g/dL

Adapted from Smetana GW, Lawrence VA, Cornell JE. Preoperative pulmonary risk stratification for noncardiothoracic surgery. A systematic review for the American College of Physicians. *Ann Intern Med.* 2006;144:581-595.
ASA, American Society of Anesthesiologists; *COPD,* chronic obstructive pulmonary disease.

intravenously) can be administered without producing significant ventilatory depression. Regional anesthetic techniques that produce sensory anesthesia above T6 can impair ventilatory function.

b. *General Anesthesia.* Volatile anesthetics are rapidly eliminated through the lungs and cause bronchodilation. Desflurane, however, may cause bronchial irritation and increased airway resistance and may not be an ideal choice. Nitrous oxide should be used with caution due to the possibility of enlargement or rupture of bullae resulting in development of a tension pneumothorax. Inhaled anesthetics may attenuate regional hypoxic pulmonary vasoconstriction and cause more intrapulmonary shunting, and an increased FIO_2 may be necessary. Humidification of inspired gases and low gas flows can help to keep airway secretions moist. Mechanical ventilation with tidal volumes (TVs) of 6 to 8 mL/kg combined with slow inspiratory flow rates minimizes the likelihood of turbulent airflow and helps maintain optimal ventilation/perfusion matching. Slow respiratory rates (6 to 10 breaths/min) provide sufficient time for complete exhalation to occur and for venous return and are less likely to be associated with undesirable degrees of hyperventilation. Air trapping can be detected by the following: (1) capnography showing that the CO_2 level does not plateau but is up-sloping at the time of the next breath, (2) expiratory flow rate that does not reach zero before initiation of the next breath, (3) positive end-expiratory pressure (PEEP), which may develop or increase, and (4) blood pressure that falls as PEEP increases.

3. Postoperative Management. Prevention of pulmonary complications is based on maintaining adequate lung volumes, especially FRC, and facilitating an effective cough. Risk factors for postoperative complications are summarized in Table 9-10.

a. *Lung Expansion Maneuvers.* Deep breathing exercises, incentive spirometry, chest physiotherapy, and positive-pressure breathing techniques are of proven benefit for preventing postoperative pulmonary complications in high-risk patients.

b. *Postoperative Neuraxial Analgesia.* Postoperative neuraxial analgesia with opioids may permit early tracheal extubation and early ambulation with increased FRC and improved oxygenation. Neuraxial opioids may be especially useful after intrathoracic and upper abdominal surgery. Sedation and delayed respiratory depression can be seen, especially when poorly lipid-soluble opioids such as morphine are used. Neuraxial analgesia has not been proven to decrease the incidence of clinically significant postoperative pulmonary complications nor to be superior to parenteral opioids. Postoperative neuraxial analgesia is recommended after high-risk thoracic, abdominal, and major vascular surgery.

c. ***Mechanical Ventilation.*** During the immediate postoperative period, mechanical ventilation may be necessary in patients with severe COPD (FEV_1/FVC ratio < 0.5 or with a preoperative $Paco_2$ > 50 mm Hg). Fio_2 and ventilator settings should be adjusted to keep the Pao_2 between 60 and 100 mm Hg and the $Paco_2$ in a range that maintains the arterial pH at 7.35 to 7.45.

d. ***Chest Physiotherapy.*** Chest physiotherapy may decrease the incidence of postoperative pulmonary complications.

IV. LESS COMMON CAUSES OF EXPIRATORY AIRFLOW OBSTRUCTION

A. **Bronchiectasis.** A chronic suppurative disease of the airways, bronchiectasis may cause expiratory airflow obstruction similar to that seen with COPD.

1. **Pathophysiology.** Bacterial or mycobacterial infections are presumed responsible for most cases of bronchiectasis.
2. **Diagnosis.** The history of a chronic cough productive of large amounts of purulent sputum is highly suggestive of bronchiectasis. Digital clubbing occurs in most patients with significant bronchiectasis and is a valuable clue, especially because this change is not characteristic of COPD. Computed tomography (CT) provides excellent images of bronchiectatic airways.
3. **Treatment.** Bronchiectasis is treated with antibiotics and postural drainage. Massive hemoptysis (>200 mL over a 24-hour period) may require surgical resection of the involved lung or selective bronchial arterial embolization.
4. **Management of Anesthesia.** A double-lumen endobronchial tube may be used to prevent spillage of purulent sputum into normal areas of the lungs. Nasal intubation should be avoided due to high rates of chronic sinusitis.

B. **Cystic Fibrosis**

1. **Pathophysiology.** Cystic fibrosis (CF) is caused by a mutation in a single gene on chromosome 7 that encodes the CF transmembrane conductance regulator. The result is defective chloride ion transport in epithelial cells causing damage to the lungs (bronchiectasis, COPD, sinusitis), pancreas (diabetes mellitus), liver (cirrhosis), gastrointestinal tract (meconium ileus), and reproductive organs (azoospermia).
2. **Diagnosis.** Sweat chloride concentration higher than 80 mEq/L plus the characteristic clinical manifestations (cough, chronic purulent sputum production, exertional dyspnea) or a family history of the disease confirm the diagnosis of CF.
3. **Treatment.** Treatment is similar to treatment of bronchiectasis and is directed toward symptomatic relief (mobilization and clearance of lower airway secretions and treatment of pulmonary infection) and correction of organ dysfunction (pancreatic enzyme replacement).
4. **Management of Anesthesia.** The same principles as outlined for management of anesthesia in patients with COPD and bronchiectasis are used in CF. Elective surgical procedures should be delayed until optimal pulmonary function can be ensured by controlling bronchial infection and facilitating removal of airway secretions. Vitamin K treatment may be necessary if hepatic function is poor or if absorption of fat-soluble vitamins is impaired. Volatile anesthetics permit the use of high inspired concentrations of oxygen, decrease airway resistance, and decrease the responsiveness of hyperreactive airways. Humidification of inspired gases, hydration, and avoidance of anticholinergic drugs are important for maintaining secretions in a less viscous state. Frequent tracheal suctioning is often necessary.

C. Primary Ciliary Dyskinesia. Primary ciliary dyskinesia is characterized by congenital impairment of ciliary activity in respiratory and reproductive tract ciliated cells and sperm tails (spermatozoa are alive but immobile). As a result of impaired ciliary activity in the respiratory tract, chronic sinusitis, recurrent respiratory infections, and bronchiectasis develop. Fertility in both men and women is impaired. The triad of chronic sinusitis, bronchiectasis, and situs inversus is known as *Kartagener's syndrome.* Preoperative preparation is directed at treating active pulmonary infection and determining the presence of any significant organ involvement. In view of the high incidence of sinusitis, nasopharyngeal airways should be avoided.

D. Bronchiolitis Obliterans. A disease of childhood, bronchiolitis obliterans is most often the result of infection with respiratory syncytial virus. It may accompany viral pneumonia, collagen vascular disease (especially rheumatoid arthritis), and inhalation of nitrogen dioxide (silo filler's disease), or it may be a sequela of graft-versus-host disease after bone marrow transplantation.

E. Tracheal Stenosis. Tracheal stenosis may develop after prolonged endotracheal intubation.

1. **Diagnosis.** Tracheal stenosis becomes symptomatic when the lumen of the adult trachea is decreased to less than 5 mm. Dyspnea is prominent even at rest. Peak expiratory flow rates are decreased. Stridor is usually audible. Flow-volume loops display flattened inspiratory and expiratory curves.
2. **Management of Anesthesia.** Surgical resection of the stenotic tracheal segment with primary anastomosis is often required. Translaryngeal endotracheal intubation is initially established, and after surgical exposure the distal normal trachea is opened and a sterile cuffed tube inserted and attached to the anesthetic circuit. Maintenance of anesthesia with volatile anesthetics is useful for ensuring maximum inspired concentrations of oxygen. High-frequency ventilation is useful in selected patients. Addition of helium to the inspired gases may improve gas flow through the area of tracheal narrowing.

V. RESTRICTIVE LUNG DISEASE

Restrictive lung disease is characterized by decreases in all lung volumes, decreased lung compliance, and preservation of expiratory flow rates (Figure 9-3). Causes are summarized in Table 9-11.

A. Acute Intrinsic Restrictive Lung Disease: Pulmonary Edema. Pulmonary edema is usually caused by leakage of intravascular fluid into the interstitium of the lungs and into the alveoli.

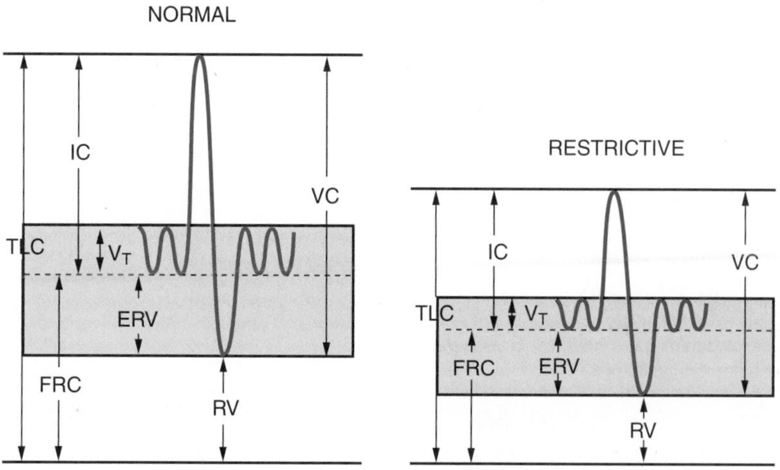

FIGURE 9-3 ■ Lung volumes in restrictive lung disease compared with normal values. *ERV,* Expiratory reserve volume; *IC,* inspiratory capacity; *RV,* residual volume; *TLC,* total lung capacity; *VC,* vital capacity; V_T, tidal volume.

Acute pulmonary edema can be caused by increased capillary pressure (hydrostatic or cardiogenic pulmonary edema) or by increased capillary permeability. Diffuse alveolar damage is typically present with the increased permeability pulmonary edema associated with acute respiratory distress syndrome (ARDS).

1. **Aspiration Pneumonitis.** Aspirated acidic gastric fluid is rapidly distributed throughout the lung, destroying surfactant-producing cells and damaging the pulmonary capillary endothelium with resulting atelectasis and leakage of intravascular fluid into the lungs. The clinical picture is similar to that of ARDS, with arterial hypoxemia, tachypnea, bronchospasm, and acute pulmonary hypertension. Chest radiographs may not demonstrate evidence of aspiration pneumonitis for 6 to 12 hours after the event.
   a. ***Treatment.*** Treatment includes endotracheal intubation, delivery of supplemental oxygen and PEEP, and administration of bronchodilators. There is no evidence that prophylactic

TABLE 9-11 ■ **Causes of Restrictive Lung Disease**

ACUTE INTRINSIC RESTRICTIVE LUNG DISEASE (PULMONARY EDEMA)
Acute respiratory distress syndrome
Aspiration
Neurogenic problems
Opioid overdose
High altitude
Reexpansion of collapsed lung
Upper airway obstruction (negative pressure)
Congestive heart failure
CHRONIC INTRINSIC RESTRICTIVE LUNG DISEASE
Sarcoidosis
Hypersensitivity pneumonitis
Eosinophilic granuloma
Alveolar proteinosis
Lymphangioleiomyomatosis
Drug-induced pulmonary fibrosis
DISORDERS OF THE CHEST WALL, PLEURA, AND MEDIASTINUM
Deformities of the costovertebral skeletal structures
Kyphoscoliosis
Ankylosing spondylitis
Deformities of the sternum
Flail chest
Pleural effusion
Pneumothorax
Mediastinal mass
Pneumomediastinum
Neuromuscular disorders
Spinal cord transection
Guillain-Barré syndrome
Neuromuscular transmission diseases
Muscular dystrophies
OTHER
Obesity
Ascites
Pregnancy

antibiotics decrease the incidence of pulmonary infection or alter outcome, and corticosteroid treatment is controversial.

2. **Neurogenic Pulmonary Edema.** In a small proportion of patients experiencing acute brain injury, neurogenic pulmonary edema develops owing to massive outpouring of sympathetic impulses from the injured central nervous system that results in generalized vasoconstriction and a shift of blood volume into the pulmonary circulation.
   a. ***Diagnosis.*** The association of pulmonary edema with a recent central nervous system injury suggests neurogenic pulmonary edema. The principal entity in the differential diagnosis is aspiration pneumonitis.
   b. ***Treatment.*** Treatment is directed at decreasing intracranial pressure and supporting oxygenation and ventilation.
3. **Drug-Induced Pulmonary Edema.** After administration of a number of drugs, especially heroin and cocaine, drug-induced pulmonary edema can occur. High-permeability pulmonary edema is suggested by high protein concentrations in the pulmonary edema fluid. Treatment is supportive and may include tracheal intubation for airway protection and mechanical ventilation.
4. **High-Altitude Pulmonary Edema.** High-altitude pulmonary edema is presumed to be due to hypoxic pulmonary vasoconstriction, which increases pulmonary vascular pressures. Onset typically occurs within 48 to 72 hours at high altitude (2500 to 5000 m). Treatment includes administration of oxygen and prompt descent from the high altitude. Inhalation of nitric oxide may improve oxygenation.
5. **Reexpansion of Collapsed Lung.** Reexpansion of a collapsed lung may lead to pulmonary edema in that lung. Treatment is supportive.
6. **Negative-Pressure Pulmonary Edema.** Relief of acute upper airway obstruction caused by postextubation laryngospasm, epiglottitis, tumors, obesity, hiccups, or obstructive sleep apnea in spontaneously breathing patients may be followed by negative-pressure pulmonary edema. The time of onset after relief of airway obstruction ranges from a few minutes to as long as 2 to 3 hours. Tachypnea, cough, and failure to maintain oxygen saturation above 95% are common presenting signs and may be confused with pulmonary aspiration or PE.
   a. ***Pathogenesis.*** The pathogenesis involves the development of high negative intrapleural pressure caused by vigorous inspiratory efforts against an obstructed upper airway. This decreases interstitial hydrostatic pressure, increases venous return, and increases left ventricular afterload. In addition, such negative pressure leads to intense sympathetic nervous system activation, hypertension, and central displacement of blood volume. Together these factors produce acute pulmonary edema by increasing the transcapillary pressure gradient.
   b. ***Treatment.*** Treatment involves maintenance of a patent upper airway and administration of supplemental oxygen. This form of pulmonary edema is typically transient and self-limited.
7. **Management of Anesthesia in Patients with Acute Restrictive Lung Disease**
   a. ***Preoperative.*** Elective surgery should be delayed in patients with acute restrictive pulmonary disease to optimize cardiorespiratory function. Large pleural effusions may need to be drained. Persistent hypoxemia may require mechanical ventilation and PEEP.
   b. ***Intraoperative.*** These patients are critically ill. It is reasonable to ventilate with low TVs (e.g., 6 mL/kg) with a compensatory increase in ventilatory rate (14 to 18 breaths/min) to keep the end-inspiratory plateau pressure under 30 cm H_2O.

B. **Chronic Restrictive Lung Diseases: Interstitial Lung Disease.** Interstitial lung disease is characterized by pulmonary fibrosis and loss of pulmonary vasculature, with pulmonary hypertension, cor pulmonale, dyspnea, and tachypnea.
   1. **Sarcoidosis.** Sarcoidosis is a systemic granulomatous disorder involving many tissues (liver, spleen, heart) but with a predilection for intrathoracic lymph nodes and the lungs. Laryngeal sarcoidosis occurs in up to 5% of patients and may interfere with tracheal intubation. Hypercalcemia is an uncommon but classic manifestation of this disease.

a. ***Lymph Node Biopsy.*** Mediastinoscopy may be necessary to provide lymph node tissue for the diagnosis of sarcoidosis but usually peripheral lymph nodes are accessible for this purpose.

b. ***Corticosteroids.*** Corticosteroids are administered to suppress the manifestation of sarcoidosis and to treat hypercalcemia.

2. **Hypersensitivity Pneumonitis.** Hypersensitivity pneumonitis is characterized by diffuse interstitial granulomatous reactions in the lungs after inhalation of dust containing fungi, spores, or animal or plant material. Repeated episodes can lead to pulmonary fibrosis.
3. **Eosinophilic Granuloma (Histiocytosis X).** Eosinophilic granuloma is associated with pulmonary fibrosis. No known treatment exists.
4. **Pulmonary Alveolar Proteinosis.** Pulmonary alveolar proteinosis is characterized by the deposition of lipid-rich proteinaceous material in the alveoli, resulting in dyspnea and hypoxemia. Treatment of severe cases requires whole-lung lavage, which is facilitated by using a double-lumen endobronchial tube.
5. **Lymphangioleiomyomatosis.** A proliferation of smooth muscle in airways, lymphatics, and blood vessels, lymphangioleiomyomatosis occurs in women of reproductive age. Clinical presentation is progressive dyspnea, hemoptysis, recurrent pneumothorax, and pleural effusions. Most patients die within 10 years of the onset of symptoms.
6. **Management of Anesthesia with Chronic Intrinsic Restrictive Lung Disease**

a. ***Preoperative.*** Presenting signs include dyspnea and cough. Cor pulmonale may be present. A vital capacity of less than 15 mL/kg indicates severe pulmonary dysfunction. Infection should be treated, secretions cleared, and smoking stopped preoperatively.

b. ***Intraoperative.*** Patients tolerate apneic periods poorly because of their small FRC. Uptake of inhaled anesthetics is faster in these patients because of the small FRC. Peak airway pressures should be kept as low as possible to minimize the risk of barotrauma.

C. **Chronic Extrinsic Restrictive Lung Disease: Disorders of the Chest Wall, Pleura and Mediastinum.** Chronic extrinsic restrictive lung disease includes disorders that interfere with lung expansion or compress the lungs, and reduce lung volumes.

1. **Deformities of the Costovertebral Skeletal Structures.** Deformities include scoliosis (lateral curvature with rotation of the vertebral column) and kyphosis (anterior flexion of the vertebral column). Severe deformities (scoliotic angle greater than 100 degrees) may lead to chronic alveolar hypoventilation, hypoxemia, secondary erythrocytosis, pulmonary hypertension, and cor pulmonale. Patients with severe kyphoscoliosis are at increased risk for pneumonia and hypoventilation after administration of central nervous system depressant drugs.
2. **Deformities of the Sternum and Costochondral Articulations.** Deformities include pectus excavatum (inward concavity of the lower sternum) and pectus carinatum (outward protuberance of the upper, middle, or lower sternum). Surgical correction is indicated when the sternal deformity is accompanied by evidence of pulmonary restriction or cardiovascular dysfunction.
3. **Flail Chest.** Multiple rib fractures, especially when they occur in a parallel vertical orientation, can produce a flail chest, with paradoxical inward movement of the unstable portion of the thoracic cage during inspiration, as the remainder of the thoracic cage moves outward. The result is progressive hypoxemia and alveolar hypoventilation. Treatment is positive-pressure ventilation until definitive stabilization procedures can be accomplished or the rib fractures stabilize.
4. **Disorders of the Pleura and Mediastinum.** Disorders of the pleura and mediastinum may contribute to mechanical changes that interfere with optimal lung expansion (Table 9-12).

a. ***Tension Pneumothorax.*** Gas enters the pleural space during inhalation and is prevented from escaping during exhalation, causing progressive trapping of more air and increasing pressure in the pleural space. Dyspnea, hypoxemia and hypotension can be severe. Tachycardia is the most common finding. Treatment is immediate evacuation of air by small-bore needle or plastic catheter, oxygen supplementation, and, in some cases, placement of a chest tube.

TABLE 9-12 ■ Disorders of the Pleura and Mediastinum that Cause a Restrictive Pattern of Pulmonary Dysfunction and Their Treatments

Pleural fibrosis—after hemothorax, empyema, surgical pleurodesis
Pleural effusion—treatment is via thoracentesis; analysis of fluid may point to further treatment
Pneumothorax—treatment indicated in larger (>15%) pneumothoraces or if symptomatic
Mediastinal tumors—can be accompanied by superior vena cava compression
Mediastinitis—treated with broad-spectrum antibiotics and surgical drainage
Pneumomediastinum—often resolves spontaneously, may need surgical drainage and repair
Bronchogenic cysts—caution must be exercised regarding use of nitrous oxide or mechanical ventilation due to the potential to expand the cyst

5. **Neuromuscular Disorders.** Disorders that interfere with the transfer of central nervous system input to respiratory muscles can result in restrictive lung disease. Vital capacity is an important indicator of the total impact of a neuromuscular disorder on ventilation.
   a. ***Spinal Cord Transection.*** Breathing is maintained solely or predominantly by the diaphragm in quadriplegic patients (transection must be at or below C5 or the diaphragm is paralyzed). Because the diaphragm is active only during inspiration, cough—which requires activity by expiratory muscles, including those of the abdominal wall—is almost totally absent. Respiratory failure almost never occurs in quadriplegic patients in the absence of complications such as pneumonia.
   b. ***Guillain-Barré Syndrome.*** Guillain-Barré syndrome may result in respiratory insufficiency that requires mechanical ventilation in 20% to 25% of patients.
   c. ***Disorders of Neuromuscular Transmission.*** Myasthenia gravis is the most common of the disorders affecting neuromuscular transmission that may result in respiratory failure. The myasthenic syndrome (Eaton-Lambert syndrome) may be confused with myasthenia gravis. Prolonged skeletal muscle paralysis or weakness may occur after administration of nondepolarizing neuromuscular blocking drugs.
   d. ***Muscular Dystrophy.*** Muscular dystrophy predisposes patients to pulmonary complications and respiratory failure. Chronic alveolar hypoventilation caused by inspiratory muscle weakness may develop. Expiratory muscle weakness impairs cough, and accompanying weakness of the swallowing muscles may lead to pulmonary aspiration.
6. **Diaphragmatic Paralysis.** In the absence of respiratory disease, most adult patients with unilateral diaphragmatic paralysis are asymptomatic. Transient diaphragmatic dysfunction may occur after abdominal surgery. Atelectasis and arterial hypoxemia may then occur. Incentive spirometry may alleviate these abnormalities.
7. **Management of Anesthesia**
   a. ***Preoperative.*** In the presence of mediastinal tumors, severity of preoperative pulmonary symptoms bears no relationship to the degree of respiratory compromise that can be encountered during anesthesia. CT scan and/or flexible fiberoptic bronchoscopy using topical anesthesia may be useful for evaluating airway obstruction. Preoperative radiation therapy should be considered whenever possible. Under anesthesia, tumor compression of the airway, vena cava, pulmonary artery, or atria can cause life-threatening hypoxemia, hypotension, or even cardiac arrest.
   b. ***Intraoperative.*** Restrictive lung disease does not influence the choice of drugs used for induction or maintenance of anesthesia. The method of induction of anesthesia and tracheal intubation in the presence of mediastinal tumors depends on the preoperative assessment of the airway. Symptomatic patients may need to undergo induction of anesthesia while sitting. Superior vena cava syndrome can cause upper airway edema. Invasive blood pressure monitoring should be considered. Spontaneous ventilation

TABLE 9-13 ■ Diagnosis of Acute Respiratory Failure
Pao_2 < 60 mm Hg despite supplemental oxygen and absence of right-to-left cardiac shunt
$Paco_2$ > 50 mm Hg in the absence of respiratory compensation for metabolic alkalosis
Decreased pH (distinguishes acute from chronic respiratory failure, in which pH is usually 7.35-7.45)
Decreased FRC and lung compliance
Increased pulmonary vascular resistance and pulmonary artery hypertension often present

FRC, Functional residual capacity.

throughout surgery is recommended whenever possible. Surgical bleeding is often increased due to increased central venous pressure.

c. ***Postoperative.*** Tumor swelling as a result of partial resection or biopsy may increase airway obstruction and necessitate reintubation of the trachea.

VI. DIAGNOSTIC PROCEDURES IN PATIENTS WITH LUNG DISEASE

A. **Fiberoptic Bronchoscopy.** Generally, fiberoptic bronchoscopy has replaced rigid bronchoscopy for visualizing the airways and obtaining tissue samples from the lung. The principal contraindication to pleural biopsy is a coagulopathy.

B. **Mediastinoscopy.** With the patient under general anesthesia, mediastinoscopy is performed through a small transverse incision just above the suprasternal notch. Complications include pneumothorax, mediastinal hemorrhage, venous air embolism, and injury to the recurrent laryngeal nerve leading to hoarseness and vocal cord paralysis. The mediastinoscope can also press against the right innominate artery, causing loss of the pulse in the right arm and compromise of right carotid artery blood flow.

VII. ACUTE RESPIRATORY FAILURE (Table 9-13)

Acute deterioration in lung function is most often triggered by events such as pneumonia, congestive heart failure, and increased metabolic production of carbon dioxide as produced by febrile states. Acute respiratory failure is present when the Pao_2 is below 60 mm Hg despite oxygen supplementation and in the absence of a right-to-left cardiac shunt. It is distinguished from chronic respiratory failure based on the presence of abrupt increases in $Paco_2$ and a corresponding decrease in pH. (In chronic respiratory failure, pH is often normal or nearly normal despite an increase in $Paco_2$).

A. **Treatment**

1. **Supplemental Oxygen.** Oxygen is administered to maintain the Pao_2 at more than 60 mm Hg.
2. **Bronchopulmonary Drainage.** Bronchopulmonary drainage is achieved by encouragement to cough, administration of inhaled bronchodilators and systemic corticosteroids, and treatment of underlying infection with antibiotics.
3. **Mechanical Support of Ventilation.** Mechanical ventilation is necessary when hypercarbia is severe enough to decrease the pH below 7.2, when patients show signs of mental status deterioration or respiratory muscle fatigue, when there is hemodynamic instability, or when secretions cannot be cleared.

B. **Risk Factors for Postoperative Pulmonary Complications** (see Table 9-10)

VIII. ACUTE OR ADULT RESPIRATORY DISTRESS SYNDROME (ARDS)

ARDS is characterized by acute inflammatory lung injury (aspiration, sepsis, trauma, multiple blood transfusions) and arterial hypoxemia. There is an influx of protein-rich edema fluid into the

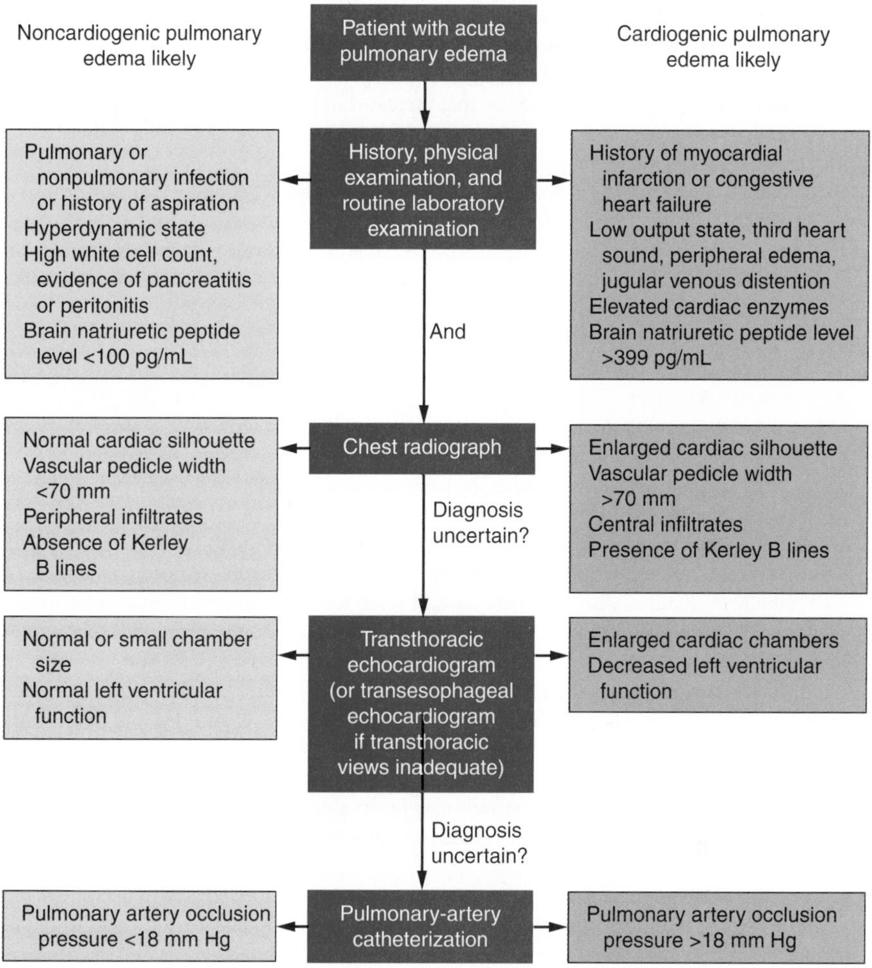

FIGURE 9-4 ■ Differentiation of cardiogenic from noncardiogenic pulmonary edema. *(Adapted from Ware LB, Matthay MA. Acute pulmonary edema.* N Engl J Med. *2005;353:2788-2796. Copyright Massachusetts Medical Society, 2005.)*

alveoli as a result of neutrophil-mediated lung injury and increased alveolar capillary membrane permeability.

A. Signs and Symptoms. Arterial hypoxemia resistant to treatment with supplemental oxygen is often the first sign. Radiographic signs are indistinguishable from cardiogenic pulmonary edema. Pulmonary hypertension can cause right heart failure.

B. Diagnosis. Diagnosis of ARDS is dependent on the presentation of acute, refractory hypoxemia, diffuse infiltrates on chest radiography consistent with pulmonary edema, and a pulmonary capillary wedge pressure of less than 18 mm Hg. The PaO_2/FIO_2 ratio is typically less than 200 mm Hg. Cardiogenic pulmonary edema must be distinguished from noncardiogenic pulmonary edema (Figure 9-4).

C. Treatment. Treatment of acute respiratory failure is directed at initiating specific therapies that support oxygenation and ventilation. The three principal goals in the management of acute respiratory failure are (1) correction of hypoxemia, (2) removal of excess carbon dioxide, and (3) provision of a patent upper airway. Additional measures include provision of adequate nutrition and prevention of gastrointestinal bleeding and thromboembolic events.

1. **Tracheal Intubation and Mechanical Ventilation**
   a. ***Inspired Oxygen Concentrations.*** Inspired oxygen concentrations are adjusted to maintain the $Pa{O_2}$ between 60 and 80 mm Hg.
   b. ***Tidal Volumes.*** TVs are adjusted so that increases in peak airway pressure do not exceed 35 to 40 cm H_2O. Ideal TV is determined by assessing lung mechanics rather than by measuring arterial blood gases.
   c. ***Positive End-Expiratory Pressure.*** PEEP is indicated when high concentrations of inspired oxygen ($F{IO_2} > 0.5$) are needed for prolonged periods and risk of oxygen toxicity increases. PEEP helps prevent alveolar collapse at end-expiration and thereby increases lung volumes (especially FRC), improves ventilation/perfusion matching, and decreases the magnitude of right-to-left intrapulmonary shunting. A pulmonary artery catheter is useful for monitoring the adequacy of intravascular fluid replacement, myocardial contractility, and tissue oxygenation in patients being treated with PEEP.
   b. ***Inverse-Ratio Ventilation.*** Inverse-ratio ventilation is characterized by an inspiratory time that exceeds the expiratory time owing to an end-inspiratory pause to maintain the alveolar pressure briefly at the plateau level. Prospective studies have not confirmed a specific benefit in most patients.
2. **Fluid and Hemodynamic Management.** A reasonable goal is to maintain the intravascular fluid volume at the lowest level consistent with adequate organ perfusion as assessed by metabolic evaluation, acid-base balance and renal function. If organ perfusion cannot be maintained after restoration of intravascular fluid volume, as in patients with septic shock, treatment with vasopressors may be necessary to improve organ perfusion pressures and normalize tissue oxygen delivery. Indicators of possible intravascular volume depletion include pulmonary artery occlusion pressure (PAOP) below 15 mm Hg and urine output below 0.5 to 1.0 mL/kg/hr.
3. **Corticosteroids.** The value of corticosteroid administration early in the course of the disease remains unproven. Corticosteroids may have value in the treatment of the later fibrosing-alveolitis phase of ARDS or as rescue therapy in patients with severe ARDS that is not resolving.
4. **Removal of Secretions.** Tracheal suctioning, chest physiotherapy, and postural drainage are used for removal of secretions. Fiberoptic bronchoscopy may be indicated to remove thicker accumulated secretions that are contributing to atelectasis.
5. **Control of Infection.** Specific antibiotic therapy based on sputum culture and sensitivity is important, but the use of prophylactic antibiotics is not recommended.
6. **Nutritional Support.** Nutritional support is important to prevent skeletal muscle weakness.
7. **Mechanical Support of Ventilation** (Figure 9-5)
   a. ***Volume-Cycled Ventilation.*** TV is fixed, and inflation pressure varies. TV is maintained despite changes in peak airway pressure, in contrast to pressure-cycled ventilators.
      i. ***Assist-Control Ventilation (ACV).*** In the control mode the patient receives a predetermined number of mechanically delivered breaths even if there are no inspiratory efforts. In the assist mode, if the patient can create a small negative airway pressure, a breath at the preset TV will be delivered (assisted).
      ii. ***Synchronized Intermittent Mandatory Ventilation (SIMV).*** SIMV allows patients to breathe spontaneously at any rate and TV while a preset minute ventilation is provided by the ventilator. Theoretic advantages of SIMV compared with ACV include continued use of respiratory muscles, lower mean airway and mean intrathoracic pressure, prevention of respiratory alkalosis, and improved patient-ventilator coordination.
   b. ***Pressure-Cycled Ventilation.*** Pressure-cycled ventilation provides gas flow into the lungs until a preset airway pressure is reached. TV is variable and changes with alterations in lung compliance and airway resistance.

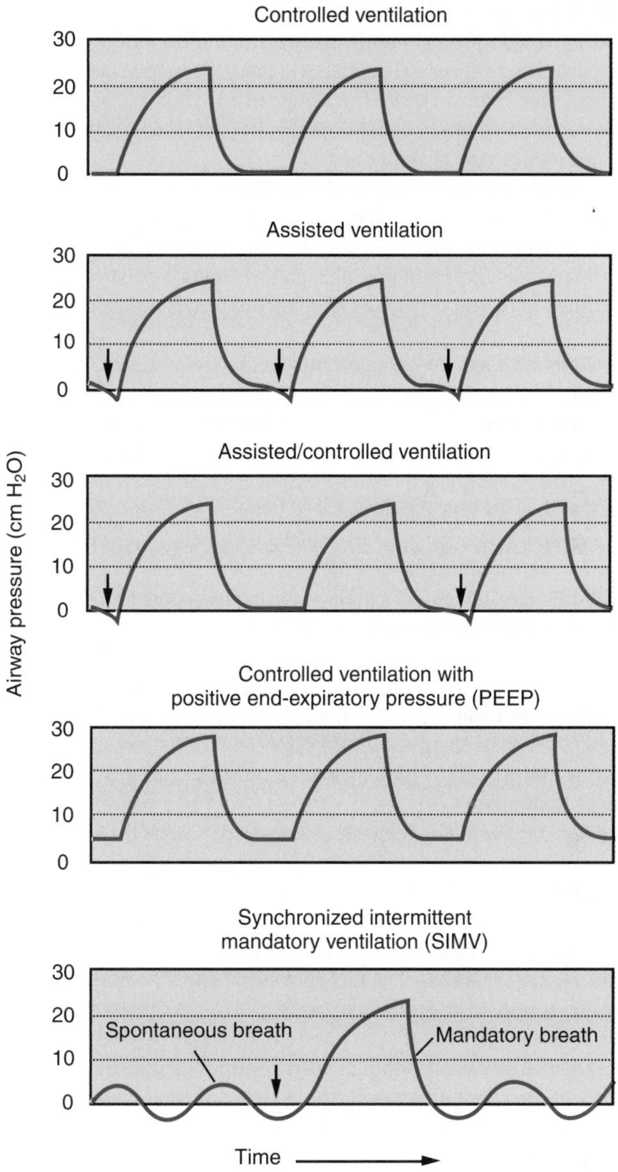

FIGURE 9-5 ■ Tidal volume and airway pressures produced by various modes of ventilation delivered through an endotracheal tube. Arrows indicate initiation of a spontaneous breath by the patient who triggers the ventilator to deliver a mechanically assisted breath.

8. **Management of Patients Receiving Mechanical Support of Ventilation.** Critically ill patients who require mechanical ventilation may benefit from continuous infusion of sedative drugs to treat anxiety and agitation and to facilitate coordination with ventilator-delivered breaths.
   a. ***Sedation.*** Benzodiazepines, propofol, and narcotics are the drugs most commonly administered to decrease anxiety, produce amnesia, increase patient comfort, and provide analgesia during mechanical ventilation. Continuous infusion of drugs rather than intermittent injection provides a more consistent level of drug effect.

b. ***Paralysis.*** When sedation is inadequate or hypotension accompanies the administration of drugs used for sedation, the administration of nondepolarizing neuromuscular blocking drugs to produce skeletal muscle relaxation may be necessary to permit optimal mechanical ventilation. A risk of prolonged drug-induced skeletal muscle paralysis is accentuation of the diffuse polyneuropathy that may accompany critical illness.

9. **Complications of Mechanical Ventilation**

a. ***Infection.*** In mechanically ventilated patients with acute respiratory failure, tracheal intubation is the single most important predisposing factor for developing nosocomial pneumonia (ventilator-associated pneumonia). Nosocomial sinusitis is strongly related to the presence of a nasotracheal tube, and treatment includes antibiotics, replacement of nasal tubes with oral tubes, and decongestants and head elevation to facilitate sinus drainage.

b. ***Alveolar Overdistention.*** Alveolar overdistention from large TVs (10 to 12 mL/kg) and high airway pressures (greater than 50 cm H_2O) may cause alveolar rupture and intrapulmonary hemorrhage. TVs of 5 to 8 mL/kg and airway pressures 30 cm H_2O or less may be indicated for treating acute respiratory failure and ARDS. This form of ventilation may require acceptance of some hypercarbia and respiratory acidosis as well as a PaO_2 of less than 60 mm Hg. Permissive hypercapnia is not recommended in patients with increased intracranial pressure, cardiac dysrhythmias, or pulmonary hypertension.

c. ***Barotrauma.*** Barotrauma may manifest as subcutaneous emphysema, pneumomediastinum, pulmonary interstitial emphysema, pneumoperitoneum, pneumopericardium, arterial gas embolism, or tension pneumothorax.

d. ***Atelectasis.*** A common cause of hypoxemia that develops during mechanical ventilation, atelectasis is not responsive to an increase in FIO_2.

e. ***Critical Illness Myopathy.*** Patients who undergo mechanical ventilation are at risk of neuromuscular weakness that persists after the cause of the respiratory failure has resolved and may be exacerbated by prolonged use of muscle relaxants.

10. **Monitoring of Treatment**

a. ***Weaning from the Ventilator.*** Some guidelines that indicate the feasibility of discontinuing mechanical ventilation include (1) vital capacity greater than 15 mL/kg; (2) $PAO_2 - PaO_2$ less than 350 cm H_2O while breathing 100% oxygen; (3) PaO_2 more than 60 mm Hg with FIO_2 less than 0.5; (4) negative inspiratory pressure greater than −20 cm H_2O; (5) normal pHa; (6) respiratory rate less than 20 breaths per minute; and (7) dead-space ventilation/TV ratio (V_D/V_T) less than 0.6. Tachypnea and low TVs usually signify an inability to tolerate extubation.

b. ***Tracheal Extubation.*** Tracheal extubation should be considered when patients tolerate 30 minutes of spontaneous breathing with a continuous positive airway pressure of 5 cm H_2O without deterioration of arterial blood gases, mental status, or cardiac function. The PaO_2 should remain higher than 50 mm Hg while the patient is breathing less than 50% oxygen. $PaCO_2$ should remain less than 50 mm Hg, and the pHa should remain higher than 7.30.

c. ***Supplemental Oxygen.*** Often patients require supplemental oxygen after tracheal extubation. SpO_2 monitoring facilitates weaning from supplemental oxygen.

d. ***Oxygen Exchange and Arterial Oxygenation.*** Oxygen exchange and arterial oxygenation are reflected by the PaO_2. Calculation of $PAO_2 - PaO_2$ is useful for distinguishing among various mechanisms of arterial hypoxemia (Table 9-14).

e. ***Carbon Dioxide Elimination.*** The adequacy of alveolar ventilation relative to the metabolic production of carbon dioxide is reflected by the $PaCO_2$ (Table 9-15). The efficacy of carbon dioxide transfer across alveolar-capillary membranes is detected by the V_D/V_T. This ratio reflects areas in the lungs that receive adequate ventilation but inadequate blood flow. Hypercarbia is defined as $PaCO_2$ greater than 45 mm Hg. Acute increases in $PaCO_2$ are associated with increased cerebral blood flow and increased intracranial pressure.

TABLE 9-14 ■ **Mechanisms of Arterial Hypoxemia**

MECHANISM	$Pa{O_2}$	$Pa{CO_2}$	$P{A}{O_2}-Pa{O_2}$	RESPONSE TO SUPPLEMENTAL OXYGEN
Low inspired oxygen concentration (altitude)	Decreased	Normal to decreased	Normal	Improved
Hypoventilation (drug overdose)	Decreased	Increased	Normal	Improved
Ventilation-to-perfusion mismatching (COPD, pneumonia)	Decreased	Normal to decreased	Increased	Improved
Right-to-left intrapulmonary shunt (pulmonary edema)	Decreased	Normal to decreased	Increased	Poor to none
Diffusion impairment (pulmonary fibrosis)	Decreased	Normal to decreased	Increased	Improved

COPD, Chronic obstructive pulmonary disease; *PaO_2 − PaO_2*, alveolar-arterial difference in partial pressure of oxygen.

TABLE 9-15 ■ **Mechanisms of Hypercarbia**

MECHANISM	$Pa{CO_2}$	V_D/V_T	$P{A}{O_2}-Pa{O_2}$
Drug overdose	Increased	Normal	Normal
Restrictive lung disease (kyphoscoliosis)	Increased	Normal to increased	Normal to increased
Chronic obstructive pulmonary disease	Increased	Increased	Increased
Neuromuscular disease	Increased	Normal to increased	Normal to increased

PaO_2 − PaO_2, Alveolar-arterial difference in partial pressure of oxygen; *V_D/V_T*, dead space ventilation/tidal volume ratio.

Extreme increases in the $PaCO_2$ to more than 80 mm Hg may result in central nervous system depression and seizures.

f. ***Mixed Venous Partial Pressure of Oxygen (PvO_2).*** PvO_2 and the arterial-to-venous oxygen difference ($CaO_2 - CvO_2$) reflect the overall adequacy of the oxygen delivery system relative to tissue oxygen extraction. A PvO_2 less than 35 mm Hg or a $CaO_2 - CvO_2$ greater than 6 mL/dL indicates the need to increase the cardiac output or to increase the blood oxygen content to facilitate tissue oxygenation.

g. ***Arterial pH.*** Measurements of arterial pH show acidemia or alkalemia. Metabolic acidosis predictably accompanies arterial hypoxemia and inadequate delivery of oxygen to tissues. Acidemia caused by respiratory or metabolic derangements is associated with dysrhythmias and pulmonary hypertension.

h. ***Intrapulmonary Shunt.*** Right-to-left intrapulmonary shunting occurs when there is perfusion of alveoli that are not ventilated. The net effect is a decrease in PaO_2, reflecting dilution of oxygen in blood exposed to ventilated alveoli with blood containing less oxygen coming from unventilated alveoli. Physiologic shunt normally makes up 2% to 5% of the cardiac output.

IX. PULMONARY THROMBOEMBOLISM

A. **Diagnosis.** The differential diagnosis of PE is extensive (Table 9-16), and clinical signs are often nonspecific (Table 9-17).

1. **Transthoracic Echocardiography.** Transthoracic echocardiography can help identify right ventricular pressure overload as well as myocardial infarction, dissection of the aorta, and pericardial tamponade, which may mimic PE. Echocardiography may show acute dilation of the right atrium and right ventricle, pulmonary arterial hypertension, and occasionally even thrombi in the main pulmonary arteries.
2. **Laboratory Tests.** A positive D-dimer test result means that a PE is possible. A negative D-dimer test result strongly suggests that thromboembolism is absent (negative predictive value >99%). Troponin levels may also be elevated and may represent right ventricular myocyte damage caused by acute right ventricular strain.
3. **Imaging.** Spiral CT scanning with contrast can assist in diagnosis of both acute and chronic PE and has replaced ventilation-perfusion scanning in many centers. Pulmonary arteriography, the gold standard for the diagnosis of PE, is used when results of other testing are inconclusive. Ventilation-perfusion lung scanning and ultrasonography of leg veins are other noninvasive tests that can aid in the diagnosis of deep vein thrombosis and/or PE.

TABLE 9-16 ■ **Differential Diagnosis of Pulmonary Embolism**

Myocardial infarction
Pericarditis
Congestive heart failure
Chronic obstructive pulmonary disease
Pneumonia
Pneumothorax
Pleuritis
Thoracic herpes zoster
Anxiety-hyperventilation syndrome
Thoracic aorta dissection
Rib fractures

TABLE 9-17 ■ **Signs and Symptoms of Pulmonary Embolism**

SIGN OR SYMPTOM	INCIDENCE (%)
Acute dyspnea	75
Tachypnea (>20 breaths/min)	70
Pleuritic chest pain	65
Rales	50
Nonproductive cough	40
Tachycardia (>100 beats/min)	30
Accentuation of pulmonic component of second heart sound	25
Hemoptysis	15
Fever (38°-39° C)	10
Homans's sign	5

B. Treatment of Acute Pulmonary Embolism

1. **Anticoagulation.** An intravenous bolus of unfractionated heparin (5000 to 10,000 units) followed by a continuous intravenous infusion should be administered immediately to any patient considered to have a high clinical likelihood of PE. An alternative is low-molecular-weight heparin given subcutaneously. Extended anticoagulation is usually accomplished with warfarin to maintain an international normalized ratio of 2.0 to 3.0.
2. **Inferior Vena Caval Filter.** Placement of an inferior vena caval filter can be considered for patients who cannot be anticoagulated, have significant bleeding while being anticoagulated, or have recurrent PE despite being anticoagulated.
3. **Thrombolytic Therapy.** If there is hemodynamic instability or severe hypoxemia, thrombolytic therapy may be considered. Inotropic support, pulmonary vasodilators, tracheal intubation and mechanical ventilation, and analgesics may also be warranted.
4. **Hemodynamic Support.** Hypotension may require treatment with inotropes or vasoconstrictors. A pulmonary vasodilator may be needed to control pulmonary hypertension.
5. **Surgical Embolectomy.** Surgical embolectomy is reserved for patients with a massive PE who are unresponsive to medical therapy and cannot receive thrombolytic therapy.

C. Management of Anesthesia. For the surgical treatment of life-threatening PE, the anesthetic chosen must support vital organ function and minimize myocardial depression. Monitoring of intraarterial pressure and cardiac filling pressures is necessary. Cardiac inotropic support may be needed. The phosphodiesterase inhibitors amrinone and milrinone increase myocardial contractility and are also excellent pulmonary artery vasodilators. Induction and maintenance of anesthesia must avoid any accentuation of arterial hypoxemia, systemic hypotension, and pulmonary hypertension. Removal of embolic fragments from the distal pulmonary artery may be facilitated by the application of positive pressure while the surgeon applies suction through the arteriotomy in the main pulmonary artery.

X. FAT EMBOLISM

The syndrome of fat embolism typically appears 12 to 72 hours (lucid interval) after long-bone fractures, especially of the femur or tibia. The triad of hypoxemia, mental confusion, and petechiae, especially over the neck, shoulders, and chest, in patients with tibia or femur fractures should arouse suspicion of fat embolism. Treatment includes management of ARDS and immobilization of long-bone fractures. Prophylactic administration of corticosteroids for patients at risk may be useful, but the efficacy of corticosteroids has not been proven.

XI. LUNG TRANSPLANTATION

A. Indications (Table 9-18). Lung transplantation approaches include single-lung transplant, double-lung transplant, heart-lung transplant, and transplantation of lobes from living donors.

TABLE 9-18 ■ **Indications for Lung Transplantation**

1. Chronic obstructive pulmonary disease
2. Cystic fibrosis
3. Idiopathic pulmonary fibrosis
4. Primary pulmonary hypertension
5. Bronchiectasis
6. Eisenmenger's syndrome

Adapted from Singh H, Bossard RF. Perioperative anaesthetic considerations for patients undergoing lung transplantation. *Can J Anaesth.* 1997;44:284-299.

B. Management of Anesthesia for Lung Transplantation

1. **Preoperative Evaluation.** Smokers should have quit smoking at least 6 to 12 months before transplantation. The ability of the right ventricle to maintain an adequate stroke volume in the presence of the acute increase in pulmonary vascular resistance produced by clamping the pulmonary artery before pneumonectomy must be evaluated. Evaluation of oxygen dependence, steroid use, hematologic and biochemical analyses, and tests of lung and other major organ system function are also required.
2. **Intraoperative and Postoperative Management** (Table 9-19)
3. **Physiologic Effects of Lung Transplantation** (Table 9-20)
4. **Complications of Lung Transplantation** (Table 9-21)

TABLE 9-19 ■ **Intraoperative and Postoperative Management of Lung Transplantation Patients**
Practice strict aseptic technique.
Insert pulmonary artery catheter.
Avoid drugs causing histamine release.
Insert double-lumen endobronchial tube.
Arterial hypoxemia may accompany one-lung ventilation (trial of PEEP if it occurs).
Pulmonary artery hypertension may occur with clamping of the pulmonary artery (prostacyclin infusion, cardiopulmonary bypass).
Bronchospasm may occur.
Maintain postoperative ventilatory support—loss of cough reflex predisposes to pneumonia.
Principal causes of mortality are bronchial dehiscence, and respiratory failure secondary to infection or rejection.

PEEP, Positive end-expiratory pressure.

TABLE 9-20 ■ **Physiologic Effects of Lung Transplantation**
Peak improvement in lung function in 3-6 months
Normalization of arterial oxygenation
Normalization of pulmonary vascular resistance and pulmonary artery pressures
Increased cardiac output
Improved exercise tolerance
Lung denervation
• Loss of cough reflex
• Mucociliary clearance is impaired
• Blunted ventilatory response to carbon dioxide

TABLE 9-21 ■ **Complications of Lung Transplantation**
Pulmonary edema
Dehiscence of the bronchial anastomosis
Anastomotic stenosis
Infection
Acute rejection (most likely in the first 100 days)
Chronic rejection (bronchiolitis obliterans)

C. Management of Anesthesia for Lung Transplantation Recipients. In lung transplant recipients, anesthetic considerations should focus on (1) the function of the transplanted lung, (2) the possibility of rejection or infection in the transplanted lung, (3) the effect of immunosuppressive therapy on other organ systems and the effect of other organ system dysfunction on the transplanted lung, (4) the disease in the native lung, and (5) the planned surgical procedure and its likely effects on the lungs.

1. **Preoperative Evaluation.** If rejection or infection is suspected, elective surgery should be postponed. The side effects of immunosuppressive drugs should be noted. Hypertension and renal dysfunction related to cyclosporine are present in many patients.
   a. ***Chronic Rejection.*** The FEV_1, vital capacity, and TLC decrease, and arterial blood gases show an increased alveolar-to-arterial oxygen gradient, but carbon dioxide retention is rare.
   b. ***Premedication.*** Premedication is acceptable if pulmonary function is adequate. Hypercarbia is common during the early posttransplantation period and can exacerbated by opioid administration. Antisialagogues are useful because secretions can be excessive. Supplemental "stress dose" corticosteroids may be needed. Prophylactic antibiotics are indicated, and strict aseptic technique is required for placement of intravascular catheters. Bronchial hyperreactivity and bronchoconstriction are common. Response to carbon dioxide rebreathing is normal.
2. **Intraoperative Management.** Because of the diminished cough reflex, the potential for bronchoconstriction, and the increased risk of pulmonary infection, it is recommended that regional anesthesia be selected whenever possible. The importance of sterile technique in this high-risk population cannot be overemphasized. Fluid preloading before regional block may be risky in patients with a transplanted lung because disruption of the lymphatic drainage in the transplanted lung can cause interstitial fluid accumulation.
   a. ***Transesophageal Echocardiography.*** Transesophageal echocardiography is useful for monitoring volume status and cardiac function in patients under general anesthesia.
   b. ***Anesthetic Drug Selection.*** An important goal is prompt recovery of adequate respiratory function and early extubation. Volatile anesthetics are well tolerated. Immunosuppressive drugs may interact with neuromuscular-blocking drugs, and the impaired renal function caused by immunosuppressive drugs may prolong the effects of certain muscle relaxants. The effects of nondepolarizing neuromuscular blockers are routinely antagonized pharmacologically because even minimal residual weakness can compromise ventilation in these patients.
   c. ***Positioning an Endotracheal Tube.*** It is best to place the cuff just beyond the vocal cords to minimize the risk of traumatizing the tracheal anastomosis. If the surgical procedure requires a double-lumen endobronchial tube, it is preferable to place the endobronchial portion of the tube into the native bronchus, thus avoiding contact with the tracheal anastomosis.

CHAPTER 10

Diseases Affecting the Brain

Co-existing nervous system diseases often have important implications for selection of anesthetic drugs, techniques, and monitors. Concepts of cerebral protection and resuscitation may assume unique importance in these patients.

I. CEREBRAL BLOOD FLOW, BLOOD VOLUME, AND METABOLISM

Cerebral blood flow (CBF) is governed by cerebral metabolic rate (CMR), cerebral perfusion pressure (CPP) (i.e., cerebral mean arterial pressure [CMAP] minus intracranial pressure [ICP]), arterial carbon dioxide ($Paco_2$) and oxygen (Pao_2) tensions, the influence of various drugs, and intracranial pathology. CBF is normally autoregulated, that is, constant over a given range of perfusion pressure. CBF is normally 50 mL/100 g brain tissue per minute over a CPP range of 50 to 150 mm Hg.

A. Cerebral Metabolic Rate. The rate of oxygen consumption by the brain ($CMRO_2$), or CMR, is 3.0 to 3.8 mL of oxygen per 100 g of brain tissue per minute. $CMRO_2$ decreases with decreased temperature and some anesthetic agents, and increases with temperature and seizures.

B. Cerebral Blood Volume. Intracranial volume and pressure are influenced by cerebral blood volume (CBV) but not directly by CBF. Vasodilatory anesthetics and hypercapnia may produce parallel increases in CBF and CBV. Moderate systemic hypotension may reduce CBF but, because of vessel dilation, increase CBV. Partial cerebral arterial occlusion may reduce regional CBF but increase CBV distal to the occlusion owing to compensatory vasodilation.

C. Arterial Carbon Dioxide Partial Pressure. Variations in $Paco_2$ produce corresponding changes in CBF (Figure 10-1) via vasodilation and constriction. CBF increases 1 mL/100 g/min for every 1 mm Hg increase in the $Paco_2$. CBF is decreased approximately 50% when the $Paco_2$ is acutely lowered to 20 mm Hg. Vasoconstricting anesthetics attenuate the effects of $Paco_2$ on CBV.

D. Arterial Oxygen Partial Pressure. Decreased Pao_2 does not affect CBF until a threshold value of approximately 50 mm Hg has been reached (see Figure 10-1). Below this value, there is abrupt cerebral vasodilation and increased CBF. Arterial hypoxemia plus hypercarbia exerts a synergistic effect (increases in CBF exceed the increase that would be produced by either factor alone).

E. Cerebral Perfusion Pressure and Cerebral Autoregulation. The ability of the brain to maintain constant CBF despite changes in CPP is known as *autoregulation* (see Figure 10-1). This is an active vascular response (arterial constriction with increased blood pressure and arterial dilation during decreased blood pressure). In normotensive patients, the lower limit of CPP associated with autoregulation is about 50 mm Hg. Below that pressure, cerebral blood vessels are maximally vasodilated; and as the pressure drops further, CBF decreases (flow becomes pressure dependent). The upper limit of autoregulation in normotensive patients is believed to be a mean arterial pressure of approximately 150 mm Hg. Above this blood pressure, the cerebral blood vessels are maximally constricted and CBF increases with increased pressure

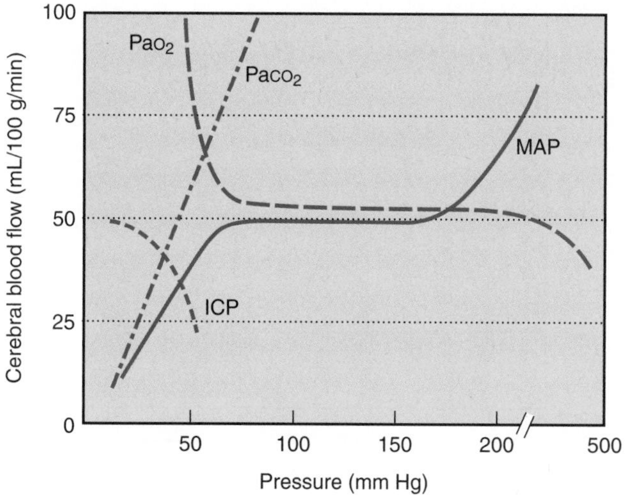

FIGURE 10-1 ■ Impact of intracranial pressure *(ICP)*, Pa_{O_2}, Pa_{CO_2}, and mean arterial pressure *(MAP)* on cerebral blood flow.

(pressure dependent flow). Autoregulation of CBF is shifted to the right (i.e., pressure dependence occurs at higher mean blood pressures at both the upper and lower limits of autoregulation) in chronic, but not acute, hypertension. Decreases in systemic blood pressure are not as well tolerated in patients with chronic hypertension (i.e., stroke and cerebral ischemia can occur at higher pressures than in normal subjects). Autoregulation improves with antihypertensive therapy. Other conditions that may cause loss or impairment of autoregulation include intracranial tumors, head trauma, and volatile anesthetic agent administration.

F. **Venous Blood Pressure.** Venous blood pressure has little effect on CPP or CBF but may profoundly affect CBV. In order for blood to continue to flow out of the cranial vault, ICP must be greater than central venous pressure (CVP). Increases in CVP at a steady ICP lead to increases in CBV. Other causes of increased intracranial venous pressure include venous sinus thrombosis, jugular compression (extreme neck flexion or rotation), and superior vena cava syndrome.

G. **Anesthetic Drugs**

1. **Anesthetic Gases.** Changes in $CMRO_2$ usually cause parallel changes in CBF (CBF/$CMRO_2$ coupling). But volatile anesthetics administered in concentrations greater than 0.6 to 1.0 minimum alveolar concentration (MAC) are potent cerebral vasodilators that produce dose-dependent *increases* in CBF despite concomitant *decreases* in $CMRO_2$. This can cause increases in CBF, CBV, and ICP. With all volatile anesthetics, arterial hypocapnia or supplemental vasoconstricting agents (thiopental, propofol) minimize increases in CBV. Nitrous oxide has less effect on CBF and does not interfere with CBF autoregulation. The initiation of nitrous oxide after closure of the dura may cause a tension pneumocephalus (diffusion into and expansion of the gas bubble left in the intracranial vault), which may manifest as delayed emergence from anesthesia after craniotomy.
2. **Intravenous Anesthetic Agents.** Ketamine is probably a cerebral vasodilator. Barbiturates, etomidate, propofol, and opioids are cerebral vasoconstrictors in the absence of hypercapnia and predictably decrease CBV and ICP. Nondepolarizing neuromuscular blocking drugs do not meaningfully alter ICP but may prevent acute increases in ICP resulting from movement or coughing. Succinylcholine may further raise ICP in the setting of elevated ICP through increases in muscle afferent activity and cerebral arousal, independent of visible muscle fasciculations.

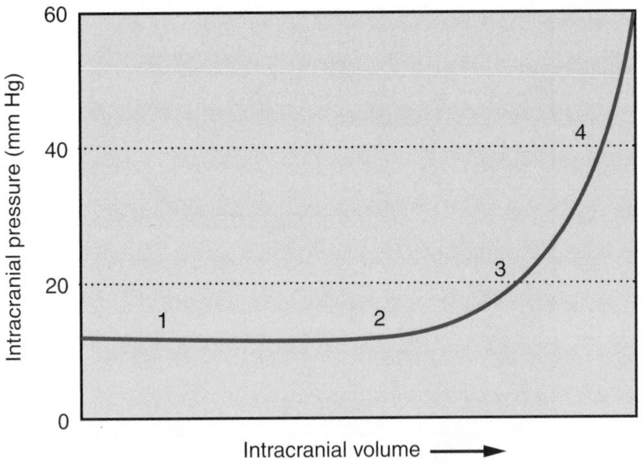

FIGURE 10-2 ■ The intracranial elastance curve depicts the impact of increasing intracranial volume on intracranial pressure (ICP). As intracranial volume increases from point 1 to 2, ICP does not increase because cerebrospinal fluid is shifted from the cranium into the spinal subarachnoid space. Patients on the rising portion of the curve (point 3) can no longer compensate for increases in intracranial volume; the ICP begins to increase, and the increase is likely to be associated with clinical symptoms. Additional increases in intracranial volume at this point (point 3), as produced by anesthetic drug-induced increases in cerebral blood volume, can precipitate abrupt increases in ICP (point 4).

II. INCREASED INTRACRANIAL PRESSURE

The pressure within the dura and cranium is referred to as the *intracranial pressure.* Normal combined volume of the intracranial contents is approximately 1200 to 1500 mL, and normal ICP is usually 5 to 15 mm Hg. An increase in one component of the intracranial volume (brain tissue, cerebrospinal fluid [CSF], blood) must be offset by a decrease in another to prevent an increase in ICP. Normally, these changes are well compensated for, but at some point even a small change in intracranial contents results in a large change in ICP (Figure 10-2). Homeostatic mechanisms increase mean arterial pressure (MAP) to overcome an increase in ICP; when this mechanism eventually fails, CPP falls and cerebral ischemia results.

A. **Cerebrospinal Fluid.** CSF is produced by ultrafiltration and secretion by the cells of the choroid plexus and via the passage of water, electrolytes, and other substances across the blood-brain barrier at a constant rate of 500 to 600 mL/day in adults. CSF is absorbed by arachnoid and granulations within the dura mater bordering venous sinusoids and sinuses. The intracranial vault is compartmentalized by meningeal barriers, and increases in the contents of one region of brain may cause regional increases in ICP and potential herniation of the contents of that compartment into a different compartment. Such herniations may lead to compromise of regional brain function.
B. **Signs and Symptoms.** Signs and symptoms of increased ICP include headache, nausea, vomiting, and papilledema; decreased levels of consciousness and coma can be observed. Acute increases in ICP are not tolerated as well as chronically elevated ICP.
C. **Diagnosis.** Increased ICP is diagnosed based on the symptoms and signs and radiographic evidence (mass, hematoma, midline shift) and by directly measuring ICP.
D. **Monitoring Intracranial Pressure.** A pressure transducer can be placed into the subdural space (known as a *subdural bolt*), brain parenchyma, or ventricle (ventriculostomy). Ventriculostomy also allows the withdrawal of CSF in order to analyze CSF and regulate ICP. A lumbar CSF drain will also allow this, but there is a risk of tonsillar herniation in certain clinical settings (i.e., tumor) with lumbar CSF drainage.
E. **Methods to Decrease Intracranial Pressure** (Table 10-1)
F. **Specific Causes of Increased Intracranial Pressure** (Table 10-2)

TABLE 10-1 ■ Measures to Lower Intracranial Pressure (ICP)

Head position	Elevate 30 degrees above the heart Avoid extreme flexion or rotation Avoid head-down position
Hyperventilation	Goal is Pa_{CO_2} 30-35 mm Hg Effect wanes after 6-12 hr
CSF drainage	Ventriculostomy Lumbar drain (risk of cerebral herniation) Ventriculoperitoneal, ventriculoatrial, and ventriculopleural shunts
Administration of hyperosmolar drugs	Mannitol (0.25-0.5 g/kg over 15-30 min; maximum effect 1-2 hr, duration 6 hr); osmotic diuresis Risk of cerebral edema if blood-brain barrier broken
Loop diuretics	Furosemide; useful in patients with increased vascular volume, such as those with congestive heart failure
Corticosteroids	Not effective in closed head injury; may increase blood glucose concentration, which is detrimental in cerebral ischemia
Barbiturates and propofol	Very useful in acute head injury

CSF, Cerebrospinal fluid.

TABLE 10-2 ■ Causes of Increased Intracranial Pressure (ICP)

Intracranial tumors	Mass effect, related to size Associated edema Obstruction of CSF flow (third ventricle tumors)
Intracranial hematomas	Similar to mass lesions Blood interferes with CSF reabsorption
Infection (meningitis, encephalitis)	Edema Obstruction of CSF reabsorption
Aqueductal stenosis (aqueduct connects third and fourth ventricles)	Common cause of obstructive hydrocephalus Treated with ventricular shunting
Benign intracranial hypertension (pseudotumor cerebri)	No identifiable cause; ICP ≤ 20 mm Hg, normal CSF composition, normal sensorium Symptoms are headaches and bilateral visual disturbances Treatment is removal of 20-40 mL of CSF, administration of acetazolamide to decrease CSF formation, and (rarely) surgical shunt
Normal pressure hydrocephalus	Triad of dementia, gait changes, and urinary incontinence Impaired CSF reabsorption Lumbar puncture shows normal or low CSF pressure; CT or MRI shows large ventricles Treatment is drainage of CSF via shunt

CSF, Cerebrospinal fluid; *CT,* computed tomography; *MRI,* magnetic resonance imaging.

III. INTRACRANIAL TUMORS

Intracranial tumors may be classified as primary (those arising from the brain and its coverings) or metastatic. Supratentorial tumors are more common in adults and often manifest with headache, seizures, or new neurologic deficits. Infratentorial tumors are more common in children and often manifest with obstructive hydrocephalus and ataxia.

A. Tumor Types

1. Astrocytoma

a. *Well-differentiated (low-grade) gliomas* often manifest in young adults with new-onset seizures. Surgical or radiation treatment of low-grade gliomas usually results in symptom-free long-term survival.

b. *Pilocytic astrocytomas* affect children and young adults. They arise in the cerebellum, cerebral hemispheres, hypothalamus, or optic pathways (optic glioma) and appear as a contrast-enhancing, well-demarcated lesion with minimal to no surrounding edema. If the location permits surgical resection, prognosis is very good.

c. *Anaplastic astrocytomas* are poorly differentiated, contrast-enhancing lesions on imaging (as a result of disruption of the blood-brain barrier) that usually evolve into glioblastoma multiforme. Treatment is resection, radiation, or chemotherapy. Prognosis is intermediate between low-grade gliomas and glioblastoma multiforme.

d. *Glioblastoma multiforme* (grade IV glioma) lesions often appear as ring-enhancing lesions as a result of central necrosis and surrounding edema. Treatment typically involves surgical debulking combined with radiation and chemotherapy and is aimed at palliation, not cure. Life expectancy is usually on the order of weeks.

2. **Oligodendrogliomas.** Oligodendrogliomas arise from myelin-producing cells in the central nervous system. Seizures predate the appearance of tumor often by many years. Initial treatment involves resection.

3. **Ependymomas.** Ependymomas arise from cells lining the ventricles and central canal of the spinal cord. Signs and symptoms include obstructive hydrocephalus, headache, nausea, vomiting, and ataxia. Treatment is resection and radiation.

4. **Primitive Neuroectodermal Tumor.** A diverse class of tumors, primitive neuroectodermal tumors include retinoblastoma, medulloblastoma, pineoblastoma, and neuroblastoma. Presentation of medulloblastoma (the most common pediatric primary malignant brain tumor) is similar to that of ependymoma. Treatment is a combination of resection and radiation. Prognosis is very good in children if there is disappearance of both tumor on magnetic resonance imaging (MRI) and tumor cells within the CSF.

5. **Meningiomas.** Usually slow-growing, well-circumscribed, benign tumors, meningiomas arise from arachnoid cap cells, not the dura mater. Surgical resection is the mainstay of treatment. Prognosis is usually excellent. Malignant meningiomas are rare.

6. **Pituitary Tumors.** Pituitary tumors usually arise from cells of the anterior pituitary gland and may occur with tumors of the parathyroids and pancreatic islet cells as part of multiple endocrine neoplasia (MEN) type I. Panhypopituitarism can be caused by either functional or nonfunctional tumors. Tumors can invade the cavernous sinus or internal carotid artery or compress various cranial nerves, causing an array of symptoms.

a. *Functional tumors* (i.e., hormone-secreting tumors) usually occur as a result of an endocrinologic disturbance related to the hormone secreted by the tumor and are usually smaller (<1 cm in diameter) at the time of diagnosis *(microadenomas).*

b. *Nonfunctional tumors* are usually more than 1 cm in diameter when diagnosed *(macroadenomas)* and cause symptoms related to their mass (headache, visual changes resulting from compression of the optic chiasm).

c. *Pituitary apoplexy* is a symptom complex (abrupt onset of headache, visual changes, ophthalmoplegia, altered mental status) secondary to hemorrhage, necrosis, or infarction within the tumor.

d. Treatment depends on tumor type. *Prolactinomas* are often initially treated medically with bromocriptine. Surgical resection via the transsphenoidal or open craniotomy approach is often curative.

7. **Acoustic Neuroma.** Acoustic neuroma is usually a benign schwannoma involving the vestibular component of cranial nerve VIII within the internal auditory canal. Bilateral tumors may occur as part of neurofibromatosis type 2.
   a. Symptoms include hearing loss, tinnitus, and disequilibrium. Larger tumors may cause symptoms related to compression of cranial nerves, most commonly the facial nerve (cranial nerve VII), as well as the brainstem.
   b. Treatment is surgical resection with or without radiation therapy. Surgery usually involves intraoperative cranial nerve monitoring with electromyography or brainstem auditory evoked potentials.
   c. Prognosis is usually very good; however, recurrence of tumor is not uncommon.
8. **Central Nervous System Lymphoma.** Central nervous system lymphoma is a rare tumor that can arise as a primary brain tumor, also known as a *microglioma,* or via metastatic spread from a systemic lymphoma. It may be associated with systemic lupus erythematosus, Sjögren's syndrome, rheumatoid arthritis, immunosuppressed states, and infection with Epstein-Barr virus.
   a. Symptoms depend on the location of the tumor.
   b. Diagnosis is via imaging and biopsy. Steroid treatment should be withheld until pathologic findings are obtained, because steroid-associated tumor lysis before biopsy may result in inadequate sample size for diagnosis.
   c. Treatment is chemotherapy (including intraventricularly delivered drugs) and whole-brain radiation.
   d. Prognosis is poor.
9. **Metastatic Brain Tumors.** Most often, metastatic brain tumors originate from the lung or breast. Malignant melanoma, hypernephroma, and carcinoma of the colon may also spread to the brain. Metastatic brain tumor is likely if more than one intracranial lesion is present.

B. Management of Anesthesia for Tumor Resection (Table 10-3). Goals are maintenance of adequate CPP and oxygenation of normal brain, optimization of operative conditions to facilitate resection, assurance of a rapid emergence from anesthesia to facilitate neurologic assessment, and accommodation of intraoperative electrophysiologic monitoring.

1. **Sitting Position and Venous Air Embolism.** The sitting position is often used for exploration of the posterior cranial fossa because of excellent surgical exposure and enhanced cerebral venous and CSF drainage. These advantages are offset by decreases in systemic blood pressure and cardiac output and the potential hazard of venous air embolism. The cut edge of cranial bone is a common site for the entry of air into veins. Death from massive venous air embolism due to an air lock causing right-sided cardiac output to plummet. The air lock prevents right ventricular outflow of blood to the pulmonary arteries. *Paradoxical air embolism* (embolism into the systemic circulation through a patent foramen ovale or other cardiopulmonary shunt) can occur. For that reason, known right-to-left intracardiac shunts are relative contraindications to use of the sitting position. When the likelihood of venous air embolism is increased, it is useful, but not mandatory, to place a right atrial catheter (for air aspiration) before beginning surgery.
   a. ***Detection of Air Embolism*** *(Table 10-4)*
   b. ***Treatment of Air Embolism*** *(Table 10-5)*

IV. DISORDERS RELATED TO VEGETATIVE BRAIN FUNCTION

A. Coma. Coma is a state of profound unconsciousness produced by drugs, disease, or injury affecting the central nervous system. The causes of coma include structural lesions (tumor, stroke,

TABLE 10-3 ■ **Anesthetic Considerations for Brain Tumor Resection**

Preoperative	Identify the presence or absence of increased ICP (nausea, vomiting, altered consciousness, mydriasis, decreased pupil reactivity, papilledema, bradycardia, systemic hypertension, breathing disturbances, midline shifts on CT or MRI) Sedation may mask neurologic deficits or cause hypoventilation and hypercarbia and further elevate ICP
Induction	Thiopental, etomidate propofol (rapid unconsciousness without increases in ICP) Nondepolarizing muscle relaxants (succinylcholine may transiently increase ICP) Mechanical hyperventilation (avoid hypercapnia)
Laryngoscopy, placement of skull pinions, skin incision	Adequate anesthetic depth for laryngoscopy (avoid increased CBF, CBV, ICP) Intravenous lidocaine (1.5 mg/kg), potent short-acting opioids to blunt response
Maintenance anesthesia	Maintain Pa_{CO_2} around 35 mm Hg Use PEEP with caution Use of nitrous oxide is controversial; may enlarge air embolism, cause tension pneumocephalus after closure Vasodilators can increase CBV, ICP—best used after dura is open Prevent spontaneous movement of the patient; use of muscle relaxants is common
Fluid therapy	Avoid hypo-osmolar solutions Aim for euvolemia Correct blood loss with packed red cells or colloid Use glucose-containing solutions with caution (hyperglycemia exacerbates neuronal injury)
Monitoring	Arterial catheter for blood pressure monitoring, blood gas, and other blood sampling Capnography to monitor ET_{CO_2}, air embolism Continuous ICP monitoring not routine but can be useful Urinary catheter Central venous catheter for sitting craniotomy (aspiration of air) Transesophageal echocardiography may help detect air embolism PA catheter for cardiac indications Peripheral nerve stimulator—place on limb without paresis or paralysis ECG monitoring: changes can reflect increases in ICP or surgical retraction of the brainstem
Postoperative	Limit reaction to endotracheal tube on emergence (narcotics, lidocaine 0.5-1.5 mg/kg IV) Delayed awakening can be caused by anesthetic drugs, hypothermia, residual neuromuscular block, cerebral ischemia, hematoma, or tension pneumocephalus

CBF, Cerebral blood flow; *CBV,* cerebral blood volume; *CT,* computed tomography; *ECG,* electrocardiogram; *ICP,* intracranial pressure; *IV,* intravenously; *MRI,* magnetic resonance imaging; *PA,* pulmonary artery; *PEEP,* positive end-expiratory pressure.

TABLE 10-4 ■ **Detection of Venous Air Embolism**

Doppler transducer over right heart structures	Very sensitive May detect clinically unimportant emboli Does not quantify amount of air entrained
Transesophageal echocardiography	Detects and quantifies air emboli Evaluates cardiac function
$ETco_2$	Sudden decrease can mean increase in alveolar dead space or cardiac impairment caused by air emboli
Decreased end-expired nitrogen concentration	Precedes changes in $ETco_2$ or increased pulmonary artery pressures
Clinical findings	Hypotension, tachycardia, cardiac dysrhythmias, cyanosis (late signs) Gasp reflex (early sign) Millwheel murmur

TABLE 10-5 ■ **Treatment of Air Embolism**

SURGEON

1. Flood the operative site with fluid.
2. Apply occlusive material to bone edges.
3. Identify other sources of air entry.

ANESTHESIOLOGIST

1. Aspirate right atrial catheter to evacuate air (multiorifice catheters are better than single-orifice catheters).
2. Discontinue nitrous oxide, ventilate with 100% oxygen.
3. PEEP or jugular venous compression may be helpful (increases venous back pressure at the surgical site).
4. Provide hemodynamic support (sympathomimetic drugs).
5. Left lateral decubitus position is rarely possible and should not be pursued first.
6. Hyperbaric therapy may be useful for severe venous air embolism or paradoxical air embolism (must be done within 8 hr to be helpful).

PEEP, Positive end-expiratory pressure.

abscess, intracranial bleeding) or diffuse disorders (hypothermia, hypoglycemia, hepatic or uremic encephalopathy, postictal state, encephalitis, drug effects). The most common means used to classify the overall severity of coma is the Glasgow Coma Scale (Table 10-6).

1. **Initial Management.** Initial management includes establishing a patent airway and ensuring the adequacy of oxygenation, ventilation, and circulation.
2. **Determining Cause of Coma**
   a. ***Vital Signs.*** Vital signs may suggest a cause such as hypothermia.
   b. ***Respiratory Patterns.*** Respiratory patterns can also aid in diagnosis. Irregular breathing patterns may reflect an abnormality at a specific site in the central nervous system (Table 10-7).
   c. ***Neurologic Examination***
      i. ***Pupillary Responses.*** Compression of the diencephalon or thalamic structures leads to small (2 mm) but reactive pupils; unresponsive midsize pupils (5 mm) may indicate midbrain compression, and a fixed and dilated pupil (>7 mm) usually indicates

TABLE 10-6 ■ Glasgow Coma Scale

RESPONSE	SCORE
EYE OPENING	
Spontaneous	4
To speech	3
To pain	2
Nil	1
BEST MOTOR RESPONSE	
Obeys	6
Localizes	5
Withdraws (flexion)	4
Abnormal flexion	3
Extensor response	2
Nil	1
VERBAL RESPONSES	
Oriented	5
Confused conversation	4
Inappropriate words	3
Incomprehensible sounds	2
Nil	1

TABLE 10-7 ■ Abnormal Patterns of Breathing

Ataxic (Biot's breathing)	Unpredictable sequence of breaths varying in rate and tidal volume	Medulla
Apneustic breathing	Gasps and prolonged pauses at full inspiration	Pons
Cheyne-Stokes breathing	Cyclic crescendo-decrescendo tidal volume pattern interrupted by apnea	Cerebral hemispheres Congestive heart failure
Central neurogenic hyperventilation	Marked hyperventilation	Cerebral thrombosis or embolism
Posthyperventilation apnea	Awake apnea following moderate decreases in $Paco_2$	Frontal lobes

oculomotor nerve compression (herniation) due to an anticholinergic or sympathomimetic drug intoxication. Pinpoint pupils (1 mm) may indicate opioid or organophosphate intoxication, focal pontine lesions, or neurosyphilis.

ii. ***Extraocular Muscle Function.*** Brainstem function is tested via assessment of the function of the oculomotor, trochlear, and abducens nerves (cranial nerves III, IV, and VI).

(a) ***Passive Head Rotation.*** Passive head rotation (oculocephalic reflex or doll's eyes maneuver) in comatose patients with normal brainstem function will result in full conjugate horizontal eye movements.

(b) ***Cold Water Irrigation.*** Irrigation of the tympanic membrane with cold water (oculovestibular reflex or cold caloric testing) will result in tonic conjugate eye movement toward the side of cold water irrigation if the brainstem is intact. Unilateral oculomotor nerve or midbrain lesions result in failed adduction but intact contralateral abduction. Complete absence of responses can indicate pontine lesions or diffuse disorders.

iii. ***Motor Responses to Painful Stimuli.*** Evaluation of motor responses to painful stimuli may help localize the cause of coma. Patients with mild to moderate diffuse brain dysfunction above the level of the diencephalon will react with purposeful or semipurposeful movements toward the painful stimulus. Unilateral reactions may indicate unilateral lesions such as stroke or tumor.

(a) Decorticate responses (flexion of the elbow, adduction of the shoulder, extension of the knee and ankle) are usually indicative of diencephalic dysfunction.

(b) Decerebrate responses (extension of the elbow, internal rotation of the forearm, leg extension) imply more severe brain dysfunction. Patients with pontine or medullary lesions often exhibit no response to painful stimuli.

iv. ***Laboratory Evaluation and Other Tests.*** Laboratory evaluation should include blood electrolytes and glucose to assess for disorders of sodium and glucose. Liver and renal function tests help evaluate hepatic or uremic encephalopathy. Drug and toxicology screens may help to identify exogenous intoxicants. A complete blood cell count and coagulation studies may suggest intracranial bleeding (i.e., thrombocytopenia or coagulopathy). Computed tomography (CT) or MRI may indicate a structural cause such as tumor or stroke. A lumbar puncture can be performed if meningitis or subarachnoid hemorrhage (SAH) is suspected.

v. ***Management of Anesthesia.*** Comatose patients may be brought to the operating suite either for treatment of the cause of their coma (e.g., burr hole drainage of an intracranial hematoma) or for treatment of injuries that are associated with their comatose state. Goals are establishment of an airway, provision of adequate cerebral perfusion and oxygenation, and optimization of operating conditions. Monitoring of ICP and arterial catheterization for blood pressure monitoring and blood sampling may be indicated. Anesthetic agents that increase ICP (halothane, ketamine) should be avoided, but other potent volatile agents used at low doses (<1 MAC) and intravenous cerebral vasoconstrictive anesthetics are acceptable. Succinylcholine is best avoided because it may transiently increase ICP.

B. Brain Death

1. **Criteria** (Table 10-8)
2. **Management of Anesthesia for Organ Donation** (Table 10-9)

V. CEREBROVASCULAR DISEASE

Stroke is characterized by sudden neurologic deficits resulting from ischemia (88%) or hemorrhage (12%) (Table 10-10). Ischemic stroke is described by the area of the brain affected and the etiologic mechanisms. Hemorrhagic strokes are classified as intracerebral (15%) or subarachnoid (85%).

A. Cerebrovascular Anatomy. Blood supply to the brain is via the internal carotid arteries and the vertebral arteries (Figure 10-3), which join to form the circle of Willis. The vessels arising from the carotid arteries make up the anterior circulation and supply the frontal, parietal, and lateral temporal lobes; the basal ganglia; and most of the internal capsule. Vessels that receive their blood supply from the vertebral-basilar system make up the posterior circulation and typically supply the brainstem, occipital lobes, cerebellum, medial portions of the temporal lobes, and most of the thalamus. Occlusion of specific arteries distal to the circle of Willis results in predictable clinical neurologic deficits (Table 10-11).

B. Acute Stroke

1. **Presentation.** Patients with sudden onset of neurologic dysfunction with signs and symptoms evolving over minutes to hours are more likely having a stroke. Transient ischemic

TABLE 10-8 ■ Criteria for Brain Death

All reversible causes of coma ruled out.
Lack of spontaneous movement (spinal cord reflexes may be intact).
Lack of all cranial nerve reflexes and function.
Failure of heart rate to increase more than 5 beats/min in response to intravenous atropine 0.04 mg/kg (loss of vagal nuclear function).
Apnea test result (loss of ventilatory control nuclei). Test is initiated at $Pa{CO_2}$ 40 ± 5 mm Hg, arterial pH 7.35-7.4, after patient is ventilated with 100% oxygen for ≥10 minutes. Ventilation is discontinued for 10 minutes, with continued tracheal insufflation with 100% oxygen. Arterial blood gases are checked at 5 and 10 min (to ensure $Pa{CO_2}$ ≥ 60 mm Hg). If no respirations, test result is considered confirmatory.
Isoelectric EEG.
Demonstration of absence of cerebral blood flow.

EEG, Electroencephalogram.

TABLE 10-9 ■ Anesthetic Management of the Brain Dead Organ Donor

Hypotension (may be caused by drugs, third-space losses, diabetes insipidus)	Provide aggressive fluid resuscitation. Avoid hypervolemia (pulmonary edema, cardiac failure, hepatic congestion). Avoid vasoconstrictors if possible. Inotropic agents (dobutamine, dopamine) are first-line pharmacologic therapy.
ECG changes	Monitor for electrolyte abnormalities. Monitor for increased ICP. Assess for cardiac contusion (if death is a result of trauma). Consider antiarrhythmic drugs and pacing if needed.
Hypoxemia	Aim for normoxia and normocarbia. Avoid excessive PEEP. Treat anemia and coagulopathy.
Diabetes insipidus	Provide volume replacement with hypotonic solutions. Administer vasopressin (0.4-0.1 units/hr IV) or desmopressin (0.3 mcg/kg IV) if severe. Vasopressin can cause organ ischemia due to its vasoconstrictor effects, so use sparingly.
Temperature regulation	Poikilothermia is common.
Rule of 100s	Systolic BP ≥ 100, urine output ≥ 100 mL/hr, $Pa{O_2}$ ≥ 100 mm Hg, hemoglobin ≥ 100 g/L.

BP, Blood pressure; *ECG,* electrocardiogram; *ICP,* intracranial pressure; *IV,* intravenously; *PEEP,* positive end-expiratory pressure.

attack (TIA) is a sudden vascular-related focal neurologic deficit that resolves within 24 hours and may represent an impending ischemic stroke. Stroke is a medical emergency. Prognosis depends on the amount of time from the onset of symptoms to thrombolytic intervention if thrombosis is the cause.

2. **Risk Factors.** Risk factors include systemic hypertension, cigarette smoking, hyperlipidemia, diabetes mellitus, excessive alcohol consumption, and increased serum homocysteine concentrations.

TABLE 10-10 ■ **Characteristics of Stroke Subtypes**

PARAMETER	SYSTEMIC HYPOPERFUSION	EMBOLISM	THROMBOSIS	SUBARACHNOID HEMORRHAGE	INTRACEREBRAL HEMORRHAGE
Risk factors	Hypotension Hemorrhage Cardiac arrest	Smoking Ischemic heart disease Peripheral vascular disease Diabetes mellitus White men	Smoking Ischemic heart disease Peripheral vascular disease Diabetes mellitus White men	Often absent Hypertension Coagulopathy Drugs Trauma	Hypertension Coagulopathy Drugs Trauma
Onset	Parallels risk factors	Sudden	Often preceded by a TIA	Sudden, often during exertion	Gradually progressive
Signs and symptoms	Pallor Diaphoresis Hypotension	Headache	Headache	Headache Vomiting Transient loss of consciousness	Headache Vomiting Decreased level of consciousness Seizures
Imaging	CT (hypodensity), MRI	CT (hypodensity), MRI	CT (hypodensity), MRI	CT (hyperdensity), MRI	CT (hyperdensity), MRI

Adapted from Caplan LR. Diagnosis and treatment of ischemic stroke. *JAMA*. 1991;266:2413-2418.
CT, Computed tomography; *MRI,* magnetic resonance imaging; *TIA,* transient ischemic attack.

3. **Diagnosis.** Imaging with noncontrast CT reliably distinguishes acute intracerebral hemorrhage from ischemia, which have very different treatments. Conventional angiography is useful in demonstrating arterial occlusion. Other tests include magnetic resonance angiography and transcranial Doppler sonography.
   a. ***Acute Ischemic Strokes.*** Acute ischemic strokes are caused by embolism occurring from a cardiac source, large-vessel atherothromboembolism (often from the carotid bifurcation), or small-vessel occlusive disease (lacunar infarction). Echocardiography is useful for evaluating the patient's cardiac status and looking for cardiac or aortic sources of embolism.
      i. ***Management of Acute Ischemic Stroke.*** Management includes aspirin. *Intravenous* recombinant tissue plasminogen activator (tPA) is used in patients who meet specific eligibility requirements if treatment can be initiated within 3 hours of the onset of symptoms. *Direct infusion of* thrombolytic drugs (prourokinase or tPA) into the occluded artery is another option in the very early phase of a stroke. Supportive therapy includes airway management, oxygenation, ventilation, and control of systemic blood pressure, blood glucose concentrations, and body temperature.
         (a) ***Blood Pressure Control.*** Systemic hypertension is common. Rapid lowering of systemic blood pressure can impair CBF and worsen ischemic injury. Antihypertensive drug therapy (small intravenous doses of labetalol) may be used when necessary to maintain the systemic blood pressure at less than 185/110 mm Hg to lessen myocardial work and irritability. Hypervolemic hemodilution may be considered in attempts to increase CBF while decreasing blood viscosity without significant decreases in oxygen delivery.
         (b) ***Hyperglycemia.*** Normalization of blood glucose concentrations is recommended, using insulin when appropriate. Administration of parenteral glucose should be minimized.

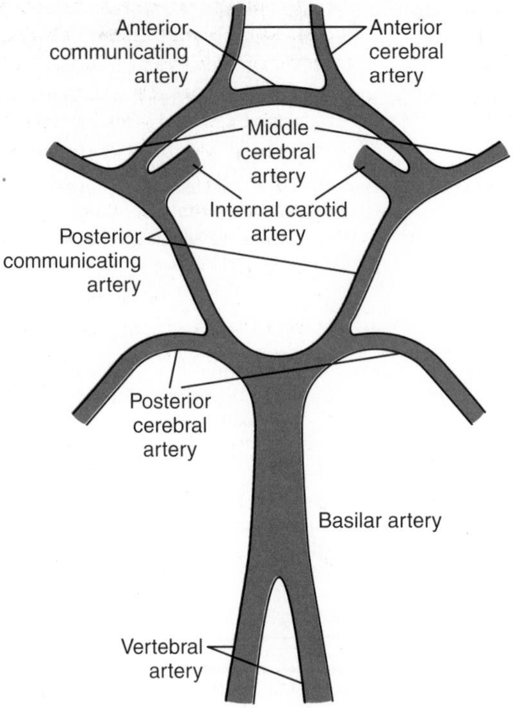

FIGURE 10-3 ■ Cerebral circulation and circle of Willis. The cerebral blood supply is from the vertebral arteries (arising from the subclavian arteries) and the internal carotid arteries (arising from the common carotid arteries).

TABLE 10-11 ■ **Clinical Features of Cerebrovascular Occlusive Syndromes**

OCCLUDED ARTERY	CLINICAL FEATURES
Anterior cerebral artery	Contralateral leg weakness
Middle cerebral artery	Contralateral hemiparesis and hemisensory deficit (face and arm more than leg) Aphasia (dominant hemisphere) Contralateral visual field defect
Posterior cerebral artery	Contralateral visual field defect Contralateral hemiparesis
Penetrating arteries	Contralateral hemiparesis Contralateral hemisensory deficits
Basilar artery	Oculomotor deficits and/or ataxia with "crossed" sensory and motor deficits
Vertebral artery	Lower cranial nerve deficits and/or ataxia with crossed sensory deficits

Adapted from Morgenstern LB, Kasner SE. Cerebrovascular disorders. *Sci Am Med*. 2000:1-15.

(c) ***Temperature Control.*** Benefits of hypothermia are not proven in humans. Fever should be avoided.

(d) ***Deep Vein Thrombosis Prophylaxis.*** Prophylaxis should be initiated early. Administration of 5000 units of heparin subcutaneously every 12 hours is the most common treatment. Patients who cannot be anticoagulated should receive pneumatic compression stockings.

b. *Acute Hemorrhagic Strokes.* Acute hemorrhagic strokes result from either intracerebral or subarachnoid hemorrhage.

i. ***Intracerebral Hemorrhage.*** Intracerebral hemorrhage is four times more likely than ischemic stroke to cause death and cannot be reliably distinguished from ischemic stroke by clinical criteria. A noncontrast CT evaluation is needed. Intravenous administration of recombinant activated factor VII within 4 hours of onset has been shown to decrease hematoma volume and improve clinical outcome. Intraventricular hemorrhage may occlude CSF drainage. Prompt ventricular drainage is performed for signs of hydrocephalus. An ICP monitor is often recommended for patients who are obtunded. Systemic blood pressure management is controversial, as there is concern about decreasing CPP in those with increased ICP. In patients with co-existing essential hypertension, a goal may be to keep the MAP less than 130 mm Hg.

ii. ***Subarachnoid Hemorrhage.*** Spontaneous SAH most commonly results from rupture of intracranial aneurysms. Risk factors for aneurysm rupture are aneurysm size (>25 mm), systemic hypertension, cigarette smoking, cocaine abuse, female sex, and use of oral contraceptives.

(a) ***Diagnosis.*** Diagnosis of SAH is based on clinical symptoms (e.g., "worst headache of my life") and CT demonstration of subarachnoid blood. Rapid onset of photophobia, stiff neck, decreased level of consciousness, and focal neurologic changes also suggest SAH. Establishing the diagnosis promptly followed by treatment of the aneurysm can decrease morbidity and mortality. Two common methods used to grade the severity of SAH are the Hunt and Hess classification and the World Federation of Neurologic Surgeons grading system (Table 10-12). These systems help predict severity and outcome and help to evaluate the efficacy of various therapies.

(b) ***Treatment.*** Treatment involves localizing the aneurysm with conventional or magnetic resonance angiography and excluding the aneurysmal sac from the intracranial circulation while preserving the parent artery, either by surgical or endovascular techniques. Outcomes are optimal when treatment is performed within 72 hours of bleeding. Supportive treatment includes anticonvulsants, control of systemic blood pressure, and ventricular drainage.

(c) ***Vasospasm.*** The incidence and severity of vasospasm correlate with the amount of subarachnoid blood seen on CT. Vasospasm typically occurs 3 to 15 days after SAH. Triple H therapy (Hypertension, Hypervolemia, passive Hemodilution) is initiated if vasospasm occurs. Nimodipine, a calcium channel blocker, has been shown to improve outcome when initiated on the first day and continued for 21 days after SAH.

(d) ***Management of Anesthesia.*** The goals of anesthesia are to limit the risks of aneurysm rupture, prevent cerebral ischemia, and facilitate surgical exposure (Table 10-13).

VI. VASCULAR MALFORMATIONS

A. Arteriovenous Malformations. Arteriovenous malformations (AVMs) are abnormal blood vessels with multiple direct arterial-to-venous connections without intervening capillaries. Rupture is not clinically associated with acute or chronic hypertensive episodes. Although often congenital, they commonly manifest in adulthood as either hemorrhage or new-onset seizures (stealing of blood away from normal brain toward the low-resistance AVM, gliosis caused by previous hemorrhage).

TABLE 10-12 ■ Common Grading Systems for Subarachnoid Hemorrhage

HUNT AND HESS CLASSIFICATION		
SCORE	**NEUROLOGIC FINDING**	**MORTALITY**
0	Unruptured aneurysm	0%-2%
1	Ruptured aneurysm with minimal headache and no neurologic deficits	2%-5%
2	Moderate to severe headache, no deficit other than cranial nerve palsy	5%-10%
3	Drowsiness, confusion, or mild focal motor deficit	5%-10%
4	Stupor, significant hemiparesis, early decerebration	25%-30%
5	Deep coma, decerebrate rigidity	40%-50%

WORLD FEDERATION OF NEUROLOGIC SURGEONS GRADING SYSTEM		
SCORE	**GCS**	**PRESENCE OF MAJOR FOCAL DEFICIT**
0		Intact, unruptured aneurysm
1	15	No
2	13-14	No
3	13-14	Yes
4	7-12	Yes or no
5	3-6	Yes or no

Adapted from Lam AM: Cerebral aneurysms: anesthetic considerations. In: Cottrell JE, Smith DS, eds. *Anesthesia and Neurosurgery*. 4th ed. St Louis: Mosby; 2001.
GCS, Glasgow Coma Scale.

1. *Diagnosis* is made by either MRI or angiography.
2. *Treatment* can involve surgical resection, highly focused (Gamma Knife) radiation, angiographically guided embolization, or a combination of these.
3. *Prognosis* can be estimated using the Spetzler-Martin AVM grading system (Table 10-14).

B. Venous Angiomas. Venous angiomas are tufts of veins that may cause hemorrhage or new-onset seizures.

C. Cavernous Angiomas. Cavernous angiomas are benign lesions that consist of vascular channels without large feeding arteries or large veins that may manifest as new-onset seizures or occasionally as hemorrhage. Treatment usually involves surgical resection for symptomatic lesions.

D. Capillary Telangiectasias. Capillary telangiectasias are low-flow, enlarged capillaries and are probably one of the least understood vascular lesions of the central nervous system. The risk of hemorrhage is low, except for lesions occurring in the brainstem. These lesions are usually not treatable.

E. Arteriovenous Fistulas. Arteriovenous fistulas (AVFs) are direct communications between an artery and a vein that may arise spontaneously or as a result of trauma. They commonly occur between meningeal vessels or between the carotid artery and venous sinuses within the cavernous sinus. They commonly manifest with tinnitus. Treatment is angiographic embolization, or surgical ligation. Diagnosis is made by magnetic resonance or conventional angiography.

TABLE 10-13 ■ **Anesthesia Considerations for Cerebral Aneurysm Surgery**

Induction	Avoid increases in systemic blood pressure. Avoid excessive decreases in ICP before dural opening so that the tamponading force on the external surface of the aneurysm is not decreased. Avoid hyperventilation. Avoid decreases in systemic blood pressure if patient has high ICP or vasospasm (decreased CPP).
Monitoring	Arterial catheter for blood pressure monitoring and frequent blood sampling. CVP for monitoring central volume. PA catheter and/or transesophageal echocardiogram in patients with cardiac indications. EEG and somatosensory and motor evoked potentials are not used routinely.
Induction	Administer intravenous thiopental, propofol, or etomidate. Administer nondepolarizing muscle relaxant.
Intubation	Intravenous short-acting β-blockers, lidocaine, propofol, barbiturates, or short-acting opioids may blunt response.
Intravenous access	Prepare for possible large-volume fluid and blood resuscitation (aneurysm rupture).
Management in case of rupture	Perform aggressive volume resuscitation. Create controlled hypotension (e.g., nitroprusside) until clipped, then return blood pressure to normal or slightly elevated values.
Maintenance	Volatile anesthetic agents with narcotic supplementation. Muscle paralysis during clipping. For elevated ICP: hyperventilation, CSF drainage, diuretics, patient positioning to maximize exposure. Avoid glucose-containing intravenous solutions (hyperglycemia exacerbates cerebral neural injury). Barbiturates may be protective if the parent vessel must be clamped for >10 min.
Emergence	Administer labetalol or esmolol to control BP. Use lidocaine during airway manipulation. Extubate early if possible. Delayed emergence may indicate vasospasm, surgical complication.

BP, Blood pressure; *CPP,* cerebral perfusion pressure; *CSF,* cerebrospinal fluid; *CVP,* central venous pressure; *EEG,* electroencephalogram; *ICP,* intracranial pressure; *PA,* pulmonary artery.

F. **Management of Anesthesia.** Surgical resection of low-flow vascular malformations (i.e., venous angiomas and cavernous angiomas) is generally not associated with the same degree of intraoperative and postoperative complications as of high-flow vascular lesions (i.e., AVMs and AVFs). Considerations include management of high ICP and meticulous blood pressure control (hypotension may result in ischemia in hypoperfused areas, and hypertension may increase the risk of rupture) of an associated aneurysm, exacerbate intraoperative bleeding or worsen intracrania hypertension. Owing to risk of severe intraoperative bleeding, establishment of adequate intravenous access is critical. A smooth, hemodynamically stable induction of general anesthesia is paramount. Muscle relaxation should be accomplished with nondepolarizing neuromuscular blocking. Techniques to blunt the hemodynamic responses to stimulating events

TABLE 10-14 ■ **Spetzler-Martin Arteriovenous Malformation Grading System**

GRADED FEATURE	POINTS ASSIGNED
NIDUS SIZE	
Small (<3 cm)	1
Medium (3-6 cm)	2
Large (>6 cm)	3
ELOQUENCE OF ADJACENT BRAIN*	
Noneloquent	0
Eloquent	1
PATTERN OF VENOUS DRAINAGE	
Superficial only	0
Deep only or deep and superficial	1

SURGICAL OUTCOME BASED ON SPETZLER-MARTIN AVM GRADING SYSTEM

GRADE	PERCENT OF PATIENTS WITH NO POSTOPERATIVE NEUROLOGIC DEFICIT
1	100
2	95
3	84
4	73
5	69

Adapted from Spetzler RF, Martin NA. A proposed grading system for arteriovenous malformations. *J Neurosurg*. 65:476;1986.
Points are assigned and added together to form a grade.
**Eloquent brain* refers to sensory, motor, language, or visual areas as well as hypothalamus, thalamus, internal capsule, brainstem cerebellar peduncles, and deep nuclei.
AVM, Arteriovenous malformation.

such as laryngoscopy, pinion placement, and incision should be used. Hypotonic and glucose-containing solutions should be avoided; mild hyperventilation ($Paco_2$ of 30 to 35 mm Hg) will help facilitate surgical exposure. Lumbar CSF drainage may also help to decrease intracranial volume and improve exposure. Diuretics such as mannitol and furosemide, or, in extreme cases, high-dose barbiturate or propofol anesthesia, may be used to treat cerebral edema.

VII. MOYAMOYA DISEASE

Progressive stenosis of intracranial vessels with the secondary development of an anastomotic capillary network is the hallmark of moyamoya disease. It may be seen after head trauma or in association with other disorders such as neurofibromatosis, tuberous sclerosis, and fibromuscular dysplasia. Intracranial aneurysms occur with increased frequency. Symptoms can be ischemic or hemorrhagic in nature.

A. Diagnosis. The diagnosis is typically made by conventional or magnetic resonance angiography.

B. Medical Treatment. Usually, medical treatment consists of a combination of vasodilators and anticoagulants.

C. Surgical Treatment. Surgical treatment includes direct anastomosis of the superficial temporal artery to the middle cerebral artery (also known as an *extracranial-intracranial bypass*).

D. Prognosis. Even with treatment, the prognosis is not good; only 58% of patients ever attain normal neurologic function.

E. Management of Anesthesia. Preoperative assessment should document preexisting neurologic deficits. Anticoagulants or antiplatelet drugs should be discontinued, if possible, to avoid bleeding complications intraoperatively. The goals of induction and maintenance of anesthesia include hemodynamic stability (hypotension could lead to ischemia in the distribution of the abnormal vessels, and hypertension may cause hemorrhagic complications); avoidance of factors that lead to cerebral or peripheral vasoconstriction (hypocapnia and phenylephrine), which can compromise blood flow in the feeding or recipient vessels; and provision of a rapid emergence from anesthesia so that neurologic function can be assessed. Excessive hyperventilation should be avoided owing to its cerebral vasoconstrictive effect. Hypovolemia should be treated with colloids or nonhypotonic crystalloids. Dopamine and ephedrine are reasonable options for the pharmacologic treatment of hypotension. Anemia should be treated to prevent ischemia in already compromised brain regions. Postoperative complications include stroke, seizure, and hemorrhage.

VIII. TRAUMATIC BRAIN INJURY

Traumatic brain injury is the leading cause of disability and death in young adults in the United States.

A. Diagnosis. Usually diagnosis is by CT scan. The Glasgow Coma Scale provides a reproducible method for assessing the seriousness of brain injury (scores below 8 points indicate severe injury) and for following the patient's neurologic status (see Table 10-6). Head injury patients with scores below 8 are by definition in coma, and approximately 50% of these patients die or remain in vegetative states.

B. Perioperative Management. Perioperative management of patients with acute head trauma must take into consideration the risks of secondary injury from cerebral ischemia as well as injuries affecting organ systems other than the brain. CBF is usually initially decreased and then gradually increases with time. Factors contributing to poor outcome in head injury patients are increased ICP and systolic blood pressures less than 70 mm Hg. Hyperventilation, although effective in controlling ICP, may contribute to cerebral ischemia in head injury patients, and avoidance of hyperventilation is a common recommendation. Barbiturate coma may be useful in some patients as a means to control intracranial hypertension. Associated lung injuries may impair oxygenation and ventilation in these patients and necessitate mechanical ventilation. Neurogenic pulmonary edema may also contribute to acute pulmonary dysfunction. Disseminated intravascular coagulation can occur after severe head injury, possibly due to release of brain thromboplastin into the systemic circulation.

C. Management of Anesthesia. Anesthesia management includes efforts to optimize CPP, minimize the occurrence of cerebral ischemia, and avoid drugs and techniques that could increase ICP. CPP is maintained above 70 mm Hg if possible, and hyperventilation is not used unless it is needed as a temporizing measure to control ICP. Glucose-containing solutions should be avoided unless specifically indicated. In moribund patients, the establishment of a safe and effective airway takes priority over concerns for anesthetic selection, as drugs may not be needed. One should also be aware of the possible presence of hidden extracranial injuries (i.e., bone fractures, pneumothorax), as they may cause problems such as excessive blood loss and perturbations in ventilation and circulation. Nitrous oxide should be avoided because of the risk of pneumocephalus and concern for nonneurologic injuries such as pneumothorax. If acute brain swelling develops, correctable causes such as hypercapnia, arterial hypoxemia, systemic hypertension, and venous obstruction must be considered and corrected if present. Intraarterial monitoring of systemic blood pressure is helpful, whereas time constraints may limit the use of CVP or pulmonary artery catheter monitoring. During the postoperative period, it is common to maintain skeletal muscle paralysis to facilitate mechanical ventilation.

D. Hematomas. Four major types of intracranial hematoma are described based on their location: epidural, subarachnoid, subdural, and intraparenchymal.

1. *Epidural hematoma* results from arterial bleeding into the space between the skull and dura. The cause is usually a tear in a meningeal artery (may be associated with skull fracture). Often, patients experience loss of consciousness in association with the injury, followed by a return of consciousness. Hemiparesis, mydriasis, and bradycardia then suddenly develop a few hours after the head injury, reflecting uncal herniation and brainstem compression. Treatment is prompt drainage.
2. *Traumatic subarachnoid hematoma,* like SAH associated with aneurysmal rupture, is also associated with the development of cerebral vasospasm.
3. *Subdural hematoma* results from lacerated or torn bridging veins that bleed into the space between the dura and arachnoid. Examination of the CSF reveals clear fluid, as subdural blood does not typically have access to the subarachnoid CSF. Diagnosis of a subdural hematoma is confirmed by CT. Head trauma is the most common cause. Patients may view the causative head trauma as trivial, and it may have been forgotten.
   a. ***Signs and Symptoms.*** Signs and symptoms evolve gradually over several days (in contrast to epidural hematomas). Headache is a universal complaint. Drowsiness and obtundation are characteristic findings. Lateralizing neurologic signs eventually occur, manifesting as hemiparesis, hemianopsia, and language disturbances. Elderly patients may have unexplained progressive dementia.
   b. ***Treatment.*** Conservative medical management of subdural hematomas may be acceptable for patients whose condition stabilizes. Most often treatment consists of surgical evacuation of the clot, as the prognosis is poor if coma develops. Because venous bleeding is usually the cause of a subdural hematoma, an attempt to tamponade any sites of venous bleeding is desirable after evacuation of the hematoma. Typically this involves a return to normocapnia to increase brain volume.
4. **Intraparenchymal Hematoma.** Intraparenchymal hematoma is an abnormal collection of blood within the brain tissue proper. Treatment can be difficult.

IX. CONGENITAL ANOMALIES OF THE BRAIN

A. **Chiari Malformations.** Chiari malformations are a group of disorders consisting of congenital displacement of the cerebellum. A Chiari I malformation is downward displacement of the cerebellar tonsils over the cervical spinal cord; Chiari II malformations consist of downward displacement of the cerebellar vermis and are often associated with a meningomyelocele. Chiari III malformations are extremely rare and represent displacement of the cerebellum into an occipital encephalocele.
   1. **Signs and Symptoms.** Chiari I malformation causes an occipital headache that is made worse by coughing or moving the head, often extends into the shoulders and arms, and may have corresponding cutaneous dysesthesia. Visual disturbances, intermittent vertigo, ataxia, and signs of syringomyelia can occur. Chiari II malformations usually manifest in infancy with obstructive hydrocephalus plus lower brainstem and cranial nerve dysfunction.
   2. **Treatment.** Treatment consists of surgical decompression by freeing adhesions and enlarging the foramen magnum. Management of anesthesia must consider the possibility of associated increases in ICP as well as significant intraoperative blood loss, especially in the case of Chiari II malformations.

B. **Tuberous Sclerosis (Bourneville's Disease).** Tuberous sclerosis is characterized by mental retardation, seizures, and facial angiofibromas. Pathologically, tuberous sclerosis can be viewed as a condition in which a constellation of benign hamartomatous proliferative lesions and malformations occurs in virtually every organ of the body (cortical brain tubers, giant cell astrocytomas, cardiac rhabdomyomas, angiomyolipomas, renal cysts, oral lesions [nodular tumors, fibromas, papillomas]). Prognosis depends on the organ systems involved, ranging from no symptoms to life-threatening complications.

TABLE 10-15 ■ Manifestations of Neurofibromatosis

Café au lait spots (present at birth, range from 1 mm to >15 mm in size)
Neurofibromas (cutaneous, neural, vascular)
Intracranial tumor (presence of bilateral acoustic neuromas and café au lait spots establishes diagnosis)
Spinal cord tumor
Pseudarthrosis
Kyphoscoliosis
Short stature
Cancer (neurofibrosarcoma, malignant schwannoma, Wilms's tumor, rhabdomyosarcoma, leukemia)
Endocrine abnormalities (rare pheochromocytoma)
Learning disability
Seizures
Congenital heart disease (pulmonic stenosis)

1. **Anesthesia Management.** The likely presence of mental retardation and treatment of seizures with antiepileptic drugs must be considered. Upper airway abnormalities are determined preoperatively. Cardiac involvement may be associated with intraoperative cardiac dysrhythmias. Impaired renal function may have implications in selection of drugs that depend on renal clearance mechanisms.

C. **von Hippel-Lindau Disease.** von Hippel-Lindau disease is characterized by retinal angiomas, hemangioblastomas, and central nervous system (typically cerebellar) and visceral tumors. Management of anesthesia in patients with von Hippel-Lindau disease must take into consideration the increased risk of pheochromocytomas. The possibility of spinal cord hemangioblastomas may limit the use of spinal anesthesia, although epidural anesthesia has been described for cesarean section. Exaggerated systemic hypertension during direct laryngoscopy or with surgical stimulation may require intervention with esmolol, labetalol, or sodium nitroprusside.

D. **Neurofibromatosis.** Neurofibromatosis is caused by an autosomal dominant mutation that is not limited to racial or ethnic origin and has a diversity of clinical features (Table 10-15). A feature common to all patients is progression of the disease with time.

1. **Treatment.** Treatment consists of symptomatic drug therapy, such as antiepileptic drugs, and appropriately timed surgery. Surgical removal of cutaneous neurofibromas is reserved for those that are particularly disfiguring or functionally compromising. Progressive kyphoscoliosis is best treated with surgical stabilization.
2. **Management of Anesthesia.** Although rare, the possible presence of pheochromocytomas should be considered during the preoperative evaluation. Signs of increased ICP may reflect expanding intracranial tumors. Airway patency may be jeopardized by expanding laryngeal neurofibromas. Selection of regional anesthesia must recognize the possible future development of neurofibromas involving the spinal cord. Nevertheless, epidural analgesia is an effective method of producing analgesia during labor and delivery.

X. DEGENERATIVE DISEASES OF THE BRAIN

A. **Alzheimer's Disease.** A chronic neurodegenerative disorder, Alzheimer's disease is the most common cause of dementia in patients older than 65 years of age. Diffuse amyloid-rich senile plaques and neurofibrillary tangles are the hallmark pathologic findings. Early-onset Alzheimer's disease usually manifests before age 60 and has an autosomal dominant mode of transmission. Late-onset Alzheimer's disease usually develops after age 60, and genetic transmission plays a relatively minor role. With both forms of the disease, patients develop progressive cognitive impairment (problems with memory, apraxia, aphasia, agnosia). Premortem diagnosis is one of exclusion. Treatment focuses on control of symptoms. Pharmacologic options include cholinesterase inhibitors, such as tacrine, donepezil, rivastigmine, and galantamine. Prognosis is poor.

1. **Anesthesia Management.** Shorter-acting sedative-hypnotic drugs, anesthetic agents, and narcotics are preferred because they may allow a more rapid return to baseline mental status. Prolongation of the effect of succinylcholine and relative resistance to nondepolarizing muscle relaxants may occur as a result of the use of cholinesterase inhibitors.

B. **Parkinson's Disease.** Parkinson's disease is a neurodegenerative disorder of unknown cause marked by a characteristic loss of dopaminergic fibers in the basal ganglia; regional dopamine concentrations are also depleted. Depletion of dopamine results in diminished inhibition of neurons controlling the extrapyramidal motor system and unopposed stimulation by acetylcholine.

1. **Signs and Symptoms.** The classic triad of major signs of Parkinson's disease consists of skeletal muscle tremor, rigidity, and akinesia. The earliest manifestations may be loss of associated arm swings when walking and absence of head rotation when turning the body. Facial immobility and tremors occur. Dementia and depression are often present.
2. **Medical Treatment.** Medical treatment is to increase dopamine in the basal ganglia or decrease the neuronal effects of acetylcholine.
   a. *Levodopa* combined with a decarboxylase inhibitor (prevents peripheral conversion of levodopa to dopamine and optimizes the amount of levodopa available to the central nervous system) is the standard medical treatment. Side effects of levodopa include dyskinesias (the most serious side effect, developing in 80% of patients after 1 year of treatment) and psychiatric disturbances (including agitation, hallucinations, mania, and paranoia). Orthostatic hypotension may be prominent in treated patients.
   b. *Amantadine,* an antiviral agent, is reported to help control the symptoms of Parkinson's disease.
   c. *Selegiline* (a type B monoamine oxidase inhibitor) can help control the symptoms of Parkinson's disease by inhibiting the catabolism of dopamine in the central nervous system. Selegiline is not associated with tyramine-associated hypertensive crises.
3. **Surgical Treatment.** Surgery is reserved for disabling and medically refractory symptoms. Stimulation of the subthalamic nuclei via an implanted deep brain stimulator (DBS) device may relieve or help to control tremor. Pallidotomy is associated with significant improvement in levodopa-induced dyskinesias.
4. **Management of Anesthesia.** Levodopa therapy, including the usual morning dose on the day of surgery, should be continued during the perioperative period. (Note: these medications may need to be withheld during placement of a DBS.) Oral levodopa can be administered approximately 20 minutes before inducing anesthesia and may be repeated intraoperatively and postoperatively via an orogastric or nasogastric tube to minimize the likelihood of disease exacerbation (e.g., muscle rigidity interfering with ventilation). Butyrophenones (e.g., droperidol, haloperidol) antagonize the effects of dopamine in the basal ganglia. An acute dystonic reaction after administration of alfentanil has been speculated to reflect opioid-induced decreases in central dopaminergic transmission. Use of ketamine is questionable because of the possible provocation of exaggerated sympathetic nervous system responses.
5. **Anesthesia for Deep Brain Stimulator Placement.** Patients may be told to hold levodopa therapy. DBS placement is usually performed with the patient under sedation, not general anesthesia, to facilitate clinical assessment. Propofol and benzodiazepines can alter microelectrode monitoring and should be avoided. Opioids and dexmedetomidine are acceptable alternatives. Because the patient will be in sitting position, air embolism is a risk and consideration should be given to precordial Doppler monitoring.

C. Hallervorden-Spatz Disease. A rare progressive disorder of the basal ganglia, Hallervorden-Spatz disease starts in childhood and ends in death in approximately 10 years. Dementia and dystonia with torticollis, as well as scoliosis, are commonly present. Skeletal muscle contractures and bony changes may lead to immobility of the temporomandibular joint and cervical spine, even in the presence of deep general anesthesia or drug-induced skeletal muscle paralysis. Noxious stimulation, as produced by attempted awake tracheal intubation, can intensify dystonia. Administration of succinylcholine is questionable. Emergence from anesthesia is predictably accompanied by return of dystonic posturing.

D. Huntington's Disease. Huntington's disease is a degenerative disease of the central nervous system characterized by marked atrophy of the caudate nucleus and, to a lesser degree, the putamen and globus pallidus. Manifestations include progressive dementia combined with choreoathetosis. Involvement of the pharyngeal muscles makes these patients susceptible to pulmonary aspiration. The duration of Huntington's disease, from clinical onset to death, averages 17 years; death is often the result of suicide.

1. **Treatment.** Treatment is symptomatic. Haloperidol and other butyrophenones may be administered to control the chorea and emotional lability associated with the disease.
2. **Anesthesia Management.** The risk of pulmonary aspiration must be taken into consideration. Preoperative sedation using butyrophenones such as droperidol or haloperidol may be helpful in controlling choreiform movements. Decreased plasma cholinesterase activity, with prolonged responses to succinylcholine, has been observed.

E. Torticollis. Torticollis manifests as spasmodic contraction of nuchal muscles, which may progress to involvement of limb and girdle muscles. Hypertrophy of the sternocleidomastoid muscles may be present. There are no known problems relative to the selection of anesthetic drugs, but spasm of nuchal muscles can interfere with maintenance of a patent upper airway before institution of skeletal muscle paralysis. Sudden appearance of torticollis after administration of anesthetic drugs has been reported and responds dramatically to administration of diphenhydramine, 25 to 50 mg intravenously.

F. Transmissible Spongiform Encephalopathies. Transmissible spongiform encephalopathies (Creutzfeldt-Jakob disease [CJD], kuru, Gerstmann-Sträussler-Scheinker syndrome) are noninflammatory diseases of the central nervous system caused by transmissible slow infectious protein pathogens known as *prions.* Prions differ from viruses in that they lack RNA and DNA and fail to produce a detectable immune reaction. Transmissible spongiform encephalopathies are diagnosed on the basis of clinical and neuropathologic findings (diffuse or focally clustered small, round vacuoles that may become confluent). Bovine spongiform encephalopathy (mad cow disease) is a transmissible spongiform encephalopathy that occurs in animals.

1. **Creutzfeldt-Jakob Disease.** CJD is the most common transmissible spongiform encephalopathy. The time interval between infection and development of symptoms is months to years. The disease develops by accumulation of an abnormal protein thought to act as a neurotransmitter in the central nervous system. Rapidly progressive dementia with ataxia and myoclonus suggests the diagnosis, although confirmation may require a brain biopsy. No vaccines or treatments are effective.
   a. *Universal infection* precautions are recommended when caring for patients with CJD, but other precautions are not necessary. Handling CSF calls for special precautions (double gloves, protective glasses, specimen labeled "infectious"), as this has been the only body fluid shown to result in transmission to primates. Surgical instruments should be disposable or should be decontaminated by soaking in sodium hypochlorite or autoclaving. Human-to-human transmission has occurred inadvertently in association with surgical procedures (corneal transplantation, stereotactic procedures with previously used electrodes, contaminated neurosurgical instruments, and human cadaveric dura mater transplantation).
   b. *Management of anesthesia* includes the use of universal infection precautions, disposable equipment, and sterilization of any reusable equipment (laryngoscope blades) using

sodium hypochlorite. Personnel participating in anesthesia are kept to a minimum, and they should wear protective gowns, gloves, and face masks with transparent protective visors to protect the eyes.

G. **Multiple Sclerosis.** Multiple sclerosis is an autoimmune disease affecting the central nervous system; it seems to occur in genetically susceptible persons. It is characterized by diverse combinations of inflammation, demyelination, and axonal damage in the central nervous system. The loss of myelin covering the axons is followed by formation of demyelinative plaques. Peripheral nerves are not affected.

1. **Clinical Manifestations.** Sites of demyelination are present in the central nervous system and spinal cord; clinical manifestations include gait disturbances, limb paresthesias and weakness, urinary incontinence, sexual impotence, optic neuritis (diminished visual acuity, defective pupillary reaction to light), ascending spastic paresis of the skeletal muscles, and Lhermitte's sign (an electrical sensation that runs down the back into the legs in response to flexion of the neck). Increases in body temperature can cause exacerbation of symptoms due to further alterations in nerve conduction in regions of demyelination. There is an increased incidence of seizure disorders. The course of multiple sclerosis is characterized by exacerbations and remissions of symptoms at unpredictable intervals over a period of years.
2. **Diagnosis.** Diagnosis is based on clinical features alone or in combination with oligoclonal abnormalities of immunoglobulins in the CSF, prolonged latency of evoked potentials reflecting slowing of nerve conduction resulting from demyelination, and signal changes in white matter seen on cranial MRI.
3. **Treatment.** Treatment is directed at both symptom control and methods to slow the progression of disease and includes corticosteroids, interferon-β, glatiramer acetate (a mixture of random synthetic polypeptides synthesized to mimic myelin basic protein), mitoxantrone (an immunosuppressive agent), azathioprine, and low-dose methotrexate.
4. **Management of Anesthesia.** The impact of surgical stress on the natural progression of the disease must be taken into consideration (symptoms of multiple sclerosis will likely be exacerbated postoperatively). Any increase in body temperature (e.g., as little as 1° C) that follows surgery may be more likely than drugs to be responsible for exacerbations of multiple sclerosis. Spinal anesthesia has been implicated in postoperative an exacerbation of multiple sclerosis, but exacerbations of the disease after epidural anesthesia or peripheral nerve blocks have not been described. Exaggerated release of muscle potassium and hyperkalemia can follow administration of succinylcholine. Corticosteroid supplementation during the perioperative period may be indicated in patients undergoing long-term treatment with these drugs.

H. **Postpolio Sequelae.** Sequelae of polio include fatigue, skeletal muscle weakness, joint pain, cold intolerance, dysphagia, and sleep and breathing problems (i.e., obstructive sleep apnea) that presumably reflect neurologic damage from the original poliovirus infection. Anesthesia considerations include exquisite sensitivity to sedative effects of anesthetics and delayed awakening from anesthesia, sensitivity to nondepolarizing muscle relaxants, exaggerated postoperative shivering, and increased postoperative pain. Outpatient surgery may not be appropriate for many postpolio patients because they are at increased risk of complications related to respiratory muscle weakness and dysphagia.

XI. SEIZURE DISORDERS

Seizures are caused by transient, paroxysmal, and synchronous discharge of groups of neurons in the brain. *Epilepsy* is defined as recurrent seizures resulting from congenital or acquired (e.g., cerebral scarring) factors. Simple seizures involve no loss of consciousness, whereas altered levels of consciousness are seen in complex seizures. Partial seizures appear to originate from a limited population of neurons in a single hemisphere, whereas generalized seizures appear to involve diffuse activation of neurons in both cerebral hemispheres. A partial seizure that is initially evident in one region of the body (e.g., the right arm) may subsequently become generalized, involving both hemispheres, a process known as the *jacksonian march.*

A. Pharmacologic Treatment. Seizures are treated initially with antiepileptic drugs, starting with a single drug and achieving seizure control by increasing the dose as necessary. Drugs effective for the treatment of partial seizures include carbamazepine, phenytoin, and valproate. Generalized seizure disorders can be managed with carbamazepine, phenytoin, valproate, barbiturates, gabapentin, or lamotrigine. Except for gabapentin, all the useful antiepileptic drugs are metabolized in the liver before undergoing renal excretion. Gabapentin is excreted unchanged by the kidneys. Carbamazepine, phenytoin, and barbiturates cause enzyme induction, and long-term treatment with these drugs can alter the rate of their own metabolism and that of other drugs.

B. Surgical Treatment. Surgery is considered in patients who do not respond to antiepileptic drugs. Such surgery resection of a single pathologic region of the brain, corpus callosotomy, and hemispherectomy. A more conservative surgical approach to medically intractable seizures involves the implantation of a left vagal nerve stimulator. The left side is chosen because the right vagal nerve usually has significant cardiac innervation, which could lead to severe bradydysrhythmias. The mechanism by which vagal nerve stimulation produces its effects is unclear.

C. Status Epilepticus. Status epilepticus is a life-threatening condition that manifests as continuous seizure activity or two or more seizures occurring in sequence without recovery of consciousness between them. The goal of treatment of status epilepticus is prompt establishment of venous access and subsequent pharmacologic suppression of seizure activity combined with support of the airway, ventilation, and circulation and correction of hypoglycemia if present.

D. Management of Anesthesia. In patients with seizure disorders, management of anesthesia includes considering the impact of antiepileptic drugs on organ function, the effect of anesthetic drugs on seizures, and alterations in pharmacokinetics of drugs caused by antiepileptic drug–induced enzyme induction. Methohexital, alfentanil, ketamine, enflurane, isoflurane, and sevoflurane may stimulate epileptiform brainwave activity. Various antiepileptic drugs (phenytoin, carbamazepine) shorten the duration of action of nondepolarizing muscle relaxants. Topiramate may cause unexplained metabolic acidosis. Most inhaled anesthetics, including nitrous oxide, have been reported to produce seizure activity. Thiobarbiturates, opioids, and benzodiazepines are preferred drugs. It is important to maintain treatment with the existing antiepileptic drugs throughout the perioperative period.

XII. NEURO-OCULAR DISORDERS

A. Leber's Optic Atrophy. Characterized by degeneration of the retina and atrophy of the optic nerves, Leber's optic atrophy culminates in blindness. This rare disorder exhibits mitochondrial inheritance and usually manifests as loss of central vision in adolescence or early adulthood, often associated with other neuropathologic conditions, including multiple sclerosis and dystonia.

B. Retinitis Pigmentosa. Retinitis pigmentosa is a genetically and clinically heterogeneous group of inherited retinopathies characterized by degeneration of the retina.

C. Kearns-Sayre Syndrome. Kearns-Sayre syndrome is characterized by retinitis pigmentosa associated with progressive external ophthalmoplegia, typically manifesting before 20 years of age. Cardiac conduction abnormalities (from bundle branch block to complete atrioventricular heart block) are common. Management of anesthesia requires a high index of suspicion for, and preparation to treat, new-onset third-degree atrioventricular heart block.

D. Ischemic Optic Neuropathy. Ischemic optic neuropathy should be suspected in patients who report visual loss during the first week after any type of surgery. If ischemic optic neuropathy is suspected, urgent ophthalmologic consultation should be obtained. Ischemic injury to the optic nerve can result in loss of both central and peripheral vision. The optic nerve can be functionally divided into an anterior and a posterior segment based on difference in blood supply.

1. **Anterior Ischemic Optic Neuropathy.** The visual loss associated with anterior ischemic optic neuropathy is a result of infarction within the watershed perfusion zones between the small branches of the short posterior ciliary arteries. The usual presentation involves sudden, painless, monocular visual deficits varying in severity from slight decreases in visual acuity to blindness. Prognosis is poor for recovery of visual function. Nonarteritic anterior ischemic optic neuropathy is usually attributed to decreased oxygen delivery to the optic disk in association with hypotension and/or anemia. Arteritic anterior ischemic optic neuropathy, which is less common, is associated with inflammation and thrombosis of the short posterior ciliary arteries and may respond to high-dose corticosteroid therapy.
2. **Posterior Ischemic Optic Neuropathy.** Posterior ischemic optic neuropathy is more common than anterior ischemic optic neuropathy as a cause of visual loss in the perioperative period. It manifests as acute loss of vision and visual field defects similar to anterior ischemic optic neuropathy. The cause of postoperative ischemic optic neuropathy appears to be multifactorial (hypotension, anemia, congenital absence of the central retinal artery, altered optic disk anatomy, air embolism, venous obstruction, infection). It has occurred after prolonged spine surgery performed with the patient in the prone position, cardiac surgery, radical neck dissection, and hip arthroplasty. Associated nonsurgical but potentially contributory factors include cardiac arrest, acute treatment of malignant hypertension, blunt trauma, and severe anemia.

E. **Cortical Blindness.** Cortical blindness may follow profound hypotension or circulatory arrest as a result of hypoperfusion and infarction of watershed areas in the parietal or occipital lobes and may also result from air or particulate emboli during cardiopulmonary bypass. Cortical blindness is characterized by loss of vision but retention of pupillary reactions to light and normal funduscopic examination findings. CT or MRI abnormalities in the parietal or occipital lobes confirm the diagnosis.

F. **Retinal Artery Occlusion.** Retinal artery occlusion manifests as painless monocular blindness and occlusion of a branch of the retinal artery that results in limited visual field defects or blurred vision. Visual field defects are often severe initially but improve with time. Central retinal artery occlusion is often caused by emboli from an ulcerated atherosclerotic plaque in the ipsilateral carotid artery.

G. **Ophthalmic Venous Obstruction.** Ophthalmic venous obstruction may occur intraoperatively when patient positioning results in external pressure on the orbits. The prone position and use of headrests during neurosurgical procedures require careful attention to ensure that the orbits are free from external compression.

CHAPTER 11

Spinal Cord Disorders

I. ACUTE TRAUMATIC SPINAL CORD INJURY

A. Spinal Cord Transection. Acute spinal cord transection initially produces flaccid paralysis, with total absence of sensation below the level of the spinal cord injury. The extent of injury is commonly described by the American Spinal Injury Association classification system (Table 11-1). The cord is not usually anatomically transected, but complete or nearly complete neuronal dysfunction occurs below a sentinel dermatomal level. The physiologic effects depend on the level of injury. Severe physiologic derangements occur with injury to the cervical cord, and fewer perturbations occur with more caudal cord injuries. The effects of spinal cord injury collectively known as *spinal shock* include loss of temperature regulation below the level of the injury, hypotension, and bradycardia. Spinal shock typically lasts 1 to 3 weeks.

1. Acute Cervical Spinal Cord Injury

a. Diagnosis. Cervical spine radiographs are obtained in a large fraction of patients with various forms of trauma for fear of missing occult cervical spine injuries. The probability of cervical spine injury is minimal in patients who meet the following criteria: (1) no midline cervical spine tenderness, (2) no focal neurologic deficits, (3) normal sensorium, (4) no intoxication, and (5) no painful distracting injury. Routine imaging studies are not needed in these patients. The sensitivity of plain radiographs is less than 100%, and therefore the likelihood of cervical spine injury must be interpreted in conjunction with other clinical signs and symptoms and risk factors.

b. Treatment. Immediate immobilization is performed to limit neck flexion and extension (halo-thoracic devices are most effective).

c. Management of Anesthesia

i. Direct Laryngoscopy and Tracheal Intubation. Cervical spine movement during direct laryngoscopy is likely to be concentrated at the occipito-atlanto-axial area.

(a) The key principle when performing direct laryngoscopy is to minimize neck movements during the procedure. Extensive clinical experience supports the use of direct laryngoscopy for orotracheal intubation, provided that (1) maneuvers are taken to stabilize the head during the procedure (avoiding hyperextension of the neck) and (2) evaluation of the airway did not suggest the likelihood of any associated technical difficulty.

(b) There is perhaps an even greater risk of compromise of the blood supply to the spinal cord produced by neck motion that elongates the cord, with resultant narrowing of the longitudinal blood vessels. Maintenance of perfusion pressure may be more important than positioning for preventing spinal cord injury in the presence of cervical spine injury.

(c) Topical anesthesia and awake fiberoptic laryngoscopy are alternatives to direct laryngoscopy if patients are cooperative and if airway trauma—with ensuing

TABLE 11-1 ■ **American Spinal Injury Association Impairment Scale**

CATEGORY	DESCRIPTION	DEFINITION
A	Complete	No motor function below level of lesion or in sacral segments S4 and S5
B	Incomplete	Sensory but not motor function is preserved below neurologic level and includes S4-S5 segments
C	Incomplete	Motor function is preserved below level of injury, and more than half of key muscles below neurologic level have a grade less than 3
D	Incomplete	Motor function is preserved below level of injury, and more than half of key muscles below neurologic level have a grade of 3 or more
E	Normal	Sensory and motor function are intact

blood, secretions, and anatomic deformities—does not preclude visualization with the fiberscope.

(d) Awake tracheostomy is reserved for the most challenging airway conditions, in which neck injury, combined with facial fractures or other severe anomalies of airway anatomy, make safely securing the airway by nonsurgical means difficult or unsafe.

ii. ***Cardiopulmonary Support.*** Patients with cervical or high thoracic spinal cord injury are vulnerable to dramatic decreases in systemic blood pressure after acute changes in body posture, blood loss, or positive pressure ventilation. Goals of anesthetic management are optimization of intravascular volume (fluids, blood) to minimize blood pressure changes, ventilatory support, and maintenance of body temperature. Succinylcholine is unlikely to provoke excessive release of potassium during the first few hours after spinal cord transection.

II. CHRONIC SPINAL CORD INJURY

A. Pathophysiology. Early and late sequelae of spinal cord injury are summarized in Table 11-2. Several weeks after acute spinal cord transection, the spinal cord reflexes gradually return. The chronic stage is characterized by overactivity of the sympathetic nervous system and involuntary skeletal muscle spasms.

1. **Treatment.** Baclofen is useful for treating spasticity. Alternative therapies include diazepam and other benzodiazepines, surgical treatment via dorsal rhizotomy or myelotomy, or implantation of a spinal cord stimulator or subarachnoid baclofen pump. Spinal cord injury above C5 may result in apnea owing to denervation of the diaphragm. If diaphragm function is intact, tidal volumes will generally be adequate, but cough and secretion clearance are impaired. Arterial hypoxemia is a frequent early finding after cervical spinal cord injury.
2. **Management of Anesthesia.** Management of anesthesia focuses on preventing autonomic hyperreflexia. Nondepolarizing muscle relaxants are used because succinylcholine is likely to provoke hyperkalemia, particularly during the initial 6 months after spinal cord transection.

B. Autonomic Hyperreflexia. Autonomic hyperreflexia appears after spinal shock and is triggered by cutaneous stimulation (surgical incision) or visceral stimulation (bladder distention) below the level of spinal cord transection. Approximately 85% of patients

TABLE 11-2 ■ **Early and Late Complications in Patients with Spinal Cord Injury**

COMPLICATION	INCIDENCE (%)
2 YEARS AFTER INJURY	
Urinary tract infection	59
Skeletal muscle spasticity	38
Chills and fever	19
Decubitus ulcer	16
Autonomic hyperreflexia	8
Skeletal muscle contractures	6
Heterotopic ossification	3
Pneumonia	3
Renal dysfunction	2
Postoperative wound infection	2
30 YEARS AFTER INJURY	
Decubitus ulcers	17
Skeletal muscle or joint pain	16
Gastrointestinal dysfunction	14
Cardiovascular dysfunction	14
Urinary tract infection	14
Infectious disease or cancer	11
Visual or hearing disorders	10
Urinary retention	8
Male genitourinary dysfunction	7
Renal calculi	6

with lesions above T6 exhibit autonomic hyperreflexia, and it is unlikely to occur in injuries below T10.

1. **Mechanism.** Stimulation below the level of spinal cord transection initiates afferent impulses that enter the spinal cord (Figure 11-1).
2. **Signs and Symptoms.** Signs include systemic hypertension and reflex bradycardia, with cutaneous vasodilation above the level of the spinal cord transection. Patients may report headache, blurred vision, and nasal stuffiness. Cerebral, retinal, or subarachnoid hemorrhage can occur, as well as increased operative blood loss. Other effects may be loss of consciousness, seizures, cardiac dysrhythmias, and pulmonary edema caused by acute left ventricular failure.
3. **Anesthetic Management.** The focus of anesthetic management is on prevention of autonomic hyperreflexia. Although epidural or spinal anesthesia may reduce the risk, epidural anesthesia may be less effective than spinal anesthesia because of its relative sparing of the sacral segments. Regardless of the technique selected for anesthesia, vasodilator drugs with a short half-life (e.g., sodium nitroprusside) should be readily available to treat sudden-onset systemic hypertension. Autonomic hyperreflexia may first manifest postoperatively when the effects of the anesthetic drugs begin to wane.

III. SPINAL CORD TUMORS

Spinal cord tumors can be intramedullary (gliomas, ependymomas), extramedullary intradural (neurofibromas, meningiomas), or extramedullary extradural (metastatic lung, breast, or prostate tumors in location). Other mass lesions of the spinal cord, including abscesses and hematomas, share many of the clinical signs and symptoms seen with tumors.

A. *Symptoms* include pain (often aggravated by coughing or straining), motor symptoms, sphincter dysfunction, and spinal tenderness.

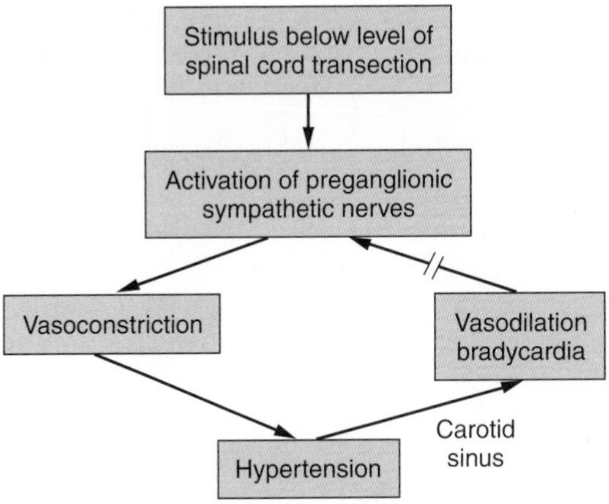

FIGURE 11-1 ■ Sequence of events associated with clinical manifestations of autonomic hyperreflexia. Because the efferent impulses from the brain that produce compensatory vasodilation (in response to increased baroreceptor activity) cannot reach the neurologically isolated portion of the spinal cord, unmodulated vasoconstriction develops below the level of the spinal cord injury, resulting in systemic hypertension.

B. *Diagnosis* involves spinal cord imaging (magnetic resonance imaging [MRI], computed tomography [CT]).

C. *Management of anesthesia* involves ensuring adequate spinal cord oxygenation and perfusion, avoiding hypotension, anemia, and hypoxemia. Tumors involving the cervical spinal cord may influence the approach used to secure the airway. Airway management is similar to that discussed in the management of acute spinal cord injury. Safe resection of a tumor may require the use of intraoperative electrophysiologic monitoring of neurologic function (electromyography, somatosensory evoked potentials, motor evoked potentials). Succinylcholine should be used with caution in patients with spinal cord tumors, given the risk of associated hyperkalemia.

IV. INTERVERTEBRAL DISK DISEASE

Among chronic conditions, low back pain is the most common cause of limitation of activity in patients younger than 45 years of age. Disk disease is the result of trauma or degenerative changes in the intervertebral disk, with nerve root or spinal cord compression from a protruding nucleus pulposus. Pain associated with nerve root compression is usually in a single dermatomal distribution. Spinal cord compression can lead to complex sensory, motor, and autonomic symptoms at and below the level of the insult. CT or MRI confirms the diagnosis and the location.

A. Cervical Disk Disease. Cervical disk disease usually occurs at the C5-C6 or C6-C7 intervertebral spaces. Initial treatment is usually conservative, involving rest, pain control, and possible epidural steroids. Surgical decompression is necessary if symptoms do not abate with conservative treatment.

   1. Anesthesia Management. Airway management is a primary concern and should be based on clinical history, physical examination findings, review of radiographs, and discussion with the surgeon. Retraction of the airway structures during anterior cervical spine approaches may result in injury to the ipsilateral recurrent laryngeal nerve, manifesting as hoarseness, stridor, or even postoperative airway compromise.

B. Lumbar Disk Disease. The most common sites are the L4-L5 and L5-S1 intervertebral spaces. Both sites produce low back pain, which radiates down the posterior and lateral aspects of the thighs and calves (sciatica) and is aggravated by coughing or stretching the sciatic nerve (straight-leg raising).

   1. Treatment. Continuing ordinary activities within the limits permitted by the pain leads to more rapid recovery than bed rest or back-mobilizing exercises. When neurologic symptoms persist despite conservative management, surgical laminectomy or microdiskectomy can be considered. An alternative therapy is epidural steroid injection (e.g., triamcinolone, methylprednisolone), although this treatment offers no significant functional benefit, nor does it decrease the need for surgery.

V. CONGENITAL ANOMALIES AND DEGENERATIVE DISEASES OF THE VERTEBRAL COLUMN

A. Spina Bifida Occulta. Incomplete formation of a single lamina in the lumbosacral spine without other abnormalities (spina bifida occulta) is a congenital defect that is present in an estimated 20% of individuals. It is often an incidental finding during evaluation of another disease process. A variant of spina bifida occulta known as *occult spinal dysraphism* includes a tethered spinal cord (cord ending below the L2-L3 interspace). Up to 50% of individuals with a tethered spinal cord have cutaneous manifestations overlying the anomaly (tufts of hair, hyperpigmented areas, cutaneous lipomas, skin dimples). Performance of spinal anesthesia in patients with a tethered spinal cord may increase the risk of cord injury.

B. Spondylosis. Spondylosis is a noncongenital disorder with osteophyte formation and degenerative disk disease. Narrowing of the spinal canal (spinal stenosis) and compression of the spinal cord by transverse osteophytes or nerve root compression by bony spurs in the intervertebral foramina are seen.

1. **Symptoms.** Symptoms of cervical spondylosis include neck pain and radicular pain in the arms and shoulders that are accompanied by sensory loss and skeletal muscle wasting. Lumbar spondylosis leads to radicular pain and wasting in the lower extremities. Sphincter disturbances are uncommon regardless of the location of spondylosis.

C. Spondylolisthesis. Spondylolisthesis is anterior subluxation of one vertebral body on another, most commonly at the lumbosacral junction. Radicular symptoms usually involve the nerve root inferior to the pedicle of the anteriorly subluxed vertebra. Treatment is initially analgesics, anti-inflammatory medications, and physical therapy if low back pain is the only symptom. Surgery is usually reserved for patients with myelopathy, radiculopathy, or neurogenic claudication.

VI. CONGENITAL ANOMALIES AND DEGENERATIVE DISEASES OF THE SPINAL CORD

A. Syringomyelia. Also known as *syrinx*, syringomyelia is a disorder in which there is cystic cavitation of the spinal cord. The condition may be congenital, may be secondary to spinal cord trauma, or may occur in association with various neoplastic conditions (e.g., gliomas). Rostral extension into the brainstem is called *syringobulbia*. Cysts may have connections to cerebrospinal fluid spaces (communicating) or may be isolated from the cerebrospinal fluid spaces (noncommunicating).

1. **Signs and Symptoms.** Symptoms include sensory impairment of pain and temperature in the upper extremities. Progressive cavitation of the spinal cord leads to destruction of lower motor neurons. Syringobulbia is characterized by paralysis of the palate, tongue, and vocal cords and loss of sensation over the face. MRI is the preferred diagnostic procedure. No known treatment is effective.
2. **Management of Anesthesia.** Lower motor neuron disease with skeletal muscle wasting raises the possibility that hyperkalemia could develop after administration of succinylcholine. Thermal regulation may be impaired. With syringobulbia, any decreased or absent protective airway reflexes may influence the timing of tracheal tube removal postoperatively.

B. Amyotrophic Lateral Sclerosis. Amyotrophic lateral sclerosis (ALS) is a degenerative disease involving (1) the lower motor neurons in the anterior horn gray matter of the spinal cord and (2) the corticospinal tracts (i.e., the primary descending upper motor neurons).

1. **Signs and Symptoms.** Initial signs include skeletal muscle atrophy, weakness, and fasciculations, often beginning in the intrinsic muscles of the hands. Progressive signs eventually

include atrophy and weakness of most of the skeletal muscles, including the tongue, pharynx, larynx, and chest. Other problems include autonomic nervous system dysfunction (orthostatic hypotension, resting tachycardia). ALS has no known treatment, and death is likely within 6 years after the onset of clinical symptoms, usually as a result of respiratory failure.

2. **Anesthesia Considerations.** The possibility of exaggerated ventilatory depression, risk of hyperkalemia after succinylcholine, prolonged responses to nondepolarizing muscle relaxants, and predisposition to pulmonary aspiration resulting from bulbar palsy are considerations with regard to anesthesia.

C. **Friedreich's Ataxia.** Friedreich's ataxia is an autosomal recessive inherited condition characterized by degeneration of the spinocerebellar and pyramidal tracts. Manifestations include cardiomyopathy, kyphoscoliosis with impaired pulmonary function, ataxia, dysarthria, nystagmus, skeletal muscle weakness and spasticity, and diabetes mellitus. Friedreich's ataxia is usually fatal by early adulthood, often as a result of cardiac failure.

1. *Management of anesthesia* is similar to that described for ALS. Response to muscle relaxants seems normal.

CHAPTER 12

Diseases of the Autonomic and Peripheral Nervous Systems

I. AUTONOMIC DISORDERS

A. Shy-Drager Syndrome. Shy-Drager syndrome belongs to a group of three heterogeneous disorders known as *multiple-system atrophy* (striatonigral degeneration, olivopontocerebellar atrophy, Shy-Drager syndrome).

1. **Signs and Symptoms.** Signs are related to autonomic nervous system dysfunction (orthostatic hypotension, syncope, urinary retention, bowel dysfunction, sexual impotence, failure of baroreceptor reflexes to produce increases in heart rate or vasoconstriction in response to hypotension, sluggish pupillary responses).
2. **Treatment.** Treatment is symptomatic and includes elastic stockings, a high-sodium diet to expand the intravascular fluid volume, and administration of α-adrenergic agonists (midodrine). Prognosis is ominous, with death usually occurring within 8 years of diagnosis and as a result of cerebral ischemia.
3. **Management of Anesthesia.** Most patients tolerate general and regional anesthesia without undue risk. Principles of management are prompt correction of hypovolemia and hypotension, the use of direct-acting vasopressor when needed (patients have exaggerated responses to indirect-acting agents), atropine or glycopyrrolate for bradycardia, and adjustment of doses of anesthetic agents to accommodate the patient's diminished compensatory responses.

B. Orthostatic Intolerance Syndrome. A chronic idiopathic disorder of primary autonomic system failure, orthostatic intolerance syndrome is characterized by episodic or postural tachycardia occurring independent of alterations in systemic blood pressure. Symptoms often include palpitations, tremulousness, light-headedness, fatigue, and syncope. Treatment includes maintenance of circulating volume, and possibly long-term administration of α_1-adrenergic agonists, such as midodrine. Anesthetic management involves perioperative volume expansion, low-dose phenylephrine to support blood pressure, and occasionally administration of β-blockers to control tachycardia.

C. Glomus Tumors of the Head and Neck. Glomus tumors of the head and neck are paragangliomas that arise embryologically from neural crest cells and lie along the carotid artery, aorta, glossopharyngeal nerve, and middle ear. Symptoms such as unilateral pulsatile tinnitus, conductive hearing loss, aural fullness, and a bluish red mass behind the tympanic membrane are characteristic of middle ear involvement, and facial paralysis, dysphonia, hearing loss, and pain are indications of cranial nerve invasion.

1. **Glomus Jugulare Tumors.** Glomus jugulare tumors can secrete a variety of hormonal substances such as norepinephrine, cholecystokinin, serotonin, kallikrein, histamine, or bradykinin, thus mimicking pheochromocytoma or carcinoid syndrome.
2. **Treatment.** Most often, treatment is radiation or embolization. Surgery is recommended if bony destruction is present.

3. **Anesthetic Management.** Preoperative determination of serum norepinephrine and catecholamine metabolite (i.e., metanephrine, vanillylmandelic acid) concentrations may detect patients likely to respond as if a pheochromocytoma were present. Administration of phenoxybenzamine or prazosin may be used preoperatively to lower blood pressure and facilitate volume expansion in patients with increased serum norepinephrine concentrations. Invasive hemodynamic monitoring may be warranted. Patients with increased serum 5-hydroxyindoleacetic acid (5-HIAA) concentration, especially those with symptoms similar to those of carcinoid syndrome, should receive preoperative octreotide, often administered subcutaneously. Invasive arterial and central venous pressure monitoring may be warranted, and venous air embolism risks should be appreciated, particularly if the jugular vein is opened to remove tumor.

D. **Carotid Sinus Syndrome.** Carotid sinus syndrome is an exaggeration of normal activity of the carotid baroreceptors in response to mechanical stimulation (profound bradycardia and/or hypotension). Treatment includes drugs, a demand-type artificial cardiac pacemaker, ablation of the carotid sinus, or ablation of the glossopharyngeal nerve with ethanol injection.

1. **Management of Anesthesia.** Management of anesthesia is complicated by hypotension, bradycardia, and cardiac dysrrhythmias. Infiltration of a local anesthetic-containing solution around the carotid sinus before dissection usually improves hemodynamic stability but may also interfere with determining the completeness of the ablation. Drugs such as atropine, isoproterenol, and epinephrine or electrical cardiac pacing may be more effective options.

E. **Hyperhidrosis.** Hyperhidrosis is a rare disorder in which individuals produce excessive sweat. The disorder can be primary, or secondary to such conditions as hyperthyroidism, pheochromocytoma, hypothalamic disorders, spinal cord injury, parkinsonism, or menopause. Conservative treatment consists of topical astringents (potassium permanganate, tannic acid, antiperspirants). Severe cases may require surgical sympathectomy. Anesthetic management is standard for video-assisted thoracoscopy but includes temperature monitoring on a finger or palm to demonstrate vasodilation with sympathectomy.

II. DISEASES OF THE PERIPHERAL NERVOUS SYSTEM

A. **Idiopathic Facial Paralysis (Bell's Palsy).** Bell's palsy is characterized by the rapid onset of motor weakness or paralysis of all the muscles innervated by the facial nerve. A viral inflammatory mechanism (perhaps herpes simplex virus) may be the cause. Spontaneous recovery usually occurs over approximately 12 weeks.

1. **Treatment.** Prednisone (1 mg/kg orally each day for 5 to 10 days) dramatically relieves pain and decreases the number of patients experiencing complete denervation of the facial nerve. If blinking is not possible, the affected eye should be covered to protect the cornea from dehydration. Surgical decompression of the facial nerve may be needed for persistent or severe cases of idiopathic facial paralysis or for facial paralysis secondary to trauma.

B. **Trigeminal Neuralgia (Tic Douloureux).** Tic douloureux is characterized by the sudden onset of brief but intense unilateral facial pain triggered by local sensory stimuli to the affected side of the face. It is diagnosed based on purely clinical signs and symptoms.

1. **Treatment.** Antiepileptic drugs are useful. The anticonvulsant carbamazepine is the drug treatment of choice, but baclofen and lamotrigine are also effective. Surgical therapy (selective radiofrequency destruction of trigeminal nerve fibers, transection of the sensory root of the trigeminal nerve, microsurgical decompression of the trigeminal nerve root) is recommended for individuals who develop pain refractory to drug therapy. Anesthetic management may include intraoperative monitoring of brainstem evoked potentials to asses the integrity of cranial nerve VIII and attention to the possibility of bradycardia caused by the trigeminocardiac reflex.

C. Glossopharyngeal Neuralgia. Glossopharyngeal neuralgia is characterized by intense pain in the throat, neck, tongue, and ear triggered by swallowing, chewing, coughing, or talking. Cardiac symptoms (profound bradycardia, hypotension) associated with glossopharyngeal neuralgia may be confused with sick sinus syndrome or carotid sinus syndrome.

1. *Treatment* of cardiovascular symptoms includes atropine, isoproterenol, an artificial external cardiac pacemaker, or a combination of these modalities. Pain associated with this syndrome is managed by chronic administration of anticonvulsant drugs such as carbamazepine and phenytoin. Permanent pain relief is possible after repeated glossopharyngeal nerve blocks, but this neuralgia is sufficiently life-threatening to justify intracranial transection of the nerve in patients not responsive to medical therapy. Glossopharyngeal neuralgia associated with cardiac symptoms (bradycardia) should be treated promptly due to a risk of sudden death.
2. *Management of anesthesia* is directed at maximizing volume status preoperatively and preparing for intraoperative cardiac pacing if necessary. Topical anesthesia of the oropharynx with lidocaine may prevent bradycardia and hypotension, which can occur in response to stimulation from direct laryngoscopy. Anticholinergic drugs should be promptly available to treat vagus nerve–mediated responses. Systemic hypertension, tachycardia, and ventricular premature beats may occur after surgical transection of the glossopharyngeal nerve and the upper two roots of the vagus nerve.

D. Charcot-Marie-Tooth Disease. The most common inherited cause of chronic motor and sensory peripheral neuropathy, Charcot-Marie-Tooth disease, is characterized by distal skeletal muscle weakness, wasting, and loss of tendon reflexes. Classically this neuropathy is described as being restricted to the lower one third of the legs, producing foot deformities (high pedal arches and talipes) and peroneal muscle atrophy ("stork leg" appearance).

1. *Treatment* is limited to supportive measures, including splints, tendon transfers, and various arthrodeses.
2. *Management of anesthesia* is influenced by concerns about the responses to neuromuscular blocking drugs and the possibility of postoperative respiratory failure resulting from weakness of the muscles responsible for respiration. It appears reasonable to avoid succinylcholine based on theoretic concerns about exaggerated potassium release after administration of this drug to individuals with neuromuscular diseases.

E. Brachial Plexus Neuropathy. Brachial plexus neuropathy (idiopathic brachial neuritis, Parsonage-Turner syndrome, shoulder-girdle syndrome) is characterized by the acute onset of severe pain in the upper arm and patchy paresis or paralysis of the skeletal muscles innervated by branches of the brachial plexus. Skeletal muscle wasting, particularly involving the shoulder girdle and arm, is common. Diagnosis of brachial plexus neuropathy is best accomplished by electrodiagnostic studies. Recovery, though prolonged, is nearly always complete.

F. Guillain-Barré Syndrome. Acute idiopathic polyneuritis, or Guillain-Barré syndrome, is characterized by sudden onset of skeletal muscle weakness or paralysis that typically manifests initially in the legs and spreads cephalad over the ensuing days to involve skeletal muscles of the arms, trunk, and face. Difficulty swallowing as a result of pharyngeal muscle weakness and impaired ventilation as a result of intercostal muscle paralysis are the most serious symptoms of this process. Autonomic nervous system dysfunction is manifested by wide fluctuations in systemic blood pressure, sudden profuse diaphoresis, peripheral vasoconstriction, resting tachycardia, and cardiac conduction abnormalities. Complete recovery can occur within a few weeks, or recovery may take months with some permanent paralysis remaining.

1. **Diagnosis** (Table 12-1)
2. **Treatment.** Treatment is mainly symptomatic and supportive. Corticosteroids are not considered useful therapy for this syndrome. Plasma exchange or infusion of gamma globulin may benefit some patients.
3. **Management of Anesthesia.** Compensatory cardiovascular responses may be absent, resulting in profound hypotension in response to changes in posture, blood loss, or positive

TABLE 12-1 ■ Diagnostic Criteria for Guillain-Barré Syndrome

FEATURES REQUIRED FOR DIAGNOSIS
Progressive bilateral weakness in legs and arms
Areflexia
FEATURES STRONGLY SUPPORTING THE DIAGNOSIS
Progression of symptoms over 2-4 weeks
Symmetry of symptoms
Mild sensory symptoms or signs (definitive sensory level makes diagnosis doubtful)
Cranial nerve involvement (especially bilateral facial weakness)
Spontaneous recovery beginning 2-4 weeks after progression ceases
Autonomic nervous system dysfunction
Absence of fever at onset
Increased concentrations of protein in the cerebrospinal fluid

airway pressure. Noxious stimulation (direct laryngoscopy) could manifest as an exaggerated increase in systemic blood pressure. Patients may exhibit exaggerated responses to indirect-acting vasopressors. Succinylcholine should be avoided. Continued ventilatory support may be needed in the postoperative period.

G. **Neuropathies.** Entrapment neuropathies occur at anatomic sites where peripheral nerves pass through narrow passages (median nerve and carpal tunnel at the wrist, ulnar nerve and cubital tunnel at the elbow), making compression a possibility. Focal demyelination of nerve fibers causes slowing or blocking of nerve impulse conduction through the damaged area. Electromyography studies are adjuncts to nerve conduction studies, showing the presence of denervation impulses and ultimately reinnervation of muscle fibers by surviving axons.

1. **Carpal Tunnel Syndrome.** Carpal tunnel syndrome is the most common entrapment neuropathy, resulting from compression of the median nerve between the transverse carpal ligament forming the roof of the carpal tunnel and the carpal bones at the wrist.
   a. Treatment is immobilizing the wrist with a splint initially. Injection of corticosteroids into the carpal tunnel may relieve symptoms but is seldom curative. Definitive treatment is decompression of the median nerve by surgical division of the transverse carpal ligament.
2. **Cubital Tunnel Entrapment Syndrome.** Cubital tunnel entrapment syndrome results from compression of the ulnar nerve after it passes through the condylar groove and enters the cubital tunnel. Surgical treatment of cubital tunnel entrapment syndrome (by tunnel decompression and transposition of the nerve) may be helpful for relieving symptoms but may also make symptoms worse, perhaps by interfering with the nerve's blood supply.
3. **Meralgia Paresthetica.** Meralgia paresthetica is entrapment of the lateral femoral cutaneous nerve (a purely sensory nerve) as it crosses under the inguinal ligament near the anterior superior iliac spine. It is characterized by burning pain down the lateral thigh as well as possible sensory loss. Risk factors are obesity, abdominal surgery, iliac crest bone graft harvesting, pregnancy, and conditions involving fluid overload. Treatment is conservative, and the condition generally resolves spontaneously. Refractory cases may require local anesthetic and steroid injections at the site of entrapment, or possible surgical decompression.
4. **Diseases Associated with Peripheral Neuropathies**
   a. ***Diabetes Mellitus.*** Up to 7.5% of patients with non–insulin-dependent diabetes mellitus have clinical neuropathy at the time of diagnosis. The principal manifestations are unpleasant tingling, numbness, burning, and aching in the lower extremities; skeletal muscle weakness; and distal sensory loss. The peripheral nerves of patients with diabetes mellitus are more vulnerable to ischemia resulting from compression or stretch injury

(as may occur during intraoperative and postoperative positioning), despite appropriate padding and positioning during these periods.

b. ***Alcohol Abuse.*** Polyneuropathy of chronic alcoholism is nearly always associated with nutritional and vitamin deficiencies. Symptoms characteristically begin in the lower extremities, with pain and numbness in the feet. Restoration of a proper diet, abstinence from alcohol, and multivitamin therapy promote slow but predictable resolution of the neuropathy.

c. ***Vitamin B_{12} Deficiency.*** Neuropathy caused by vitamin B_{12} deficiency resembles the neuropathy typically seen in patients who abuse alcohol. Nitrous oxide is known to inactivate certain vitamin B_{12}–dependent enzymes, which could lead to symptoms of altered nerve function.

d. ***Uremia.*** Distal polyneuropathy with sensory and motor components often occurs in the extremities of patients with chronic renal failure. Symptoms tend to be more prominent in the legs than in the arms. Improved nerve conduction velocity often occurs within a few days after renal transplantation. Hemodialysis does not appear to be equally effective for reversing the polyneuropathy.

e. ***Cancer.*** Peripheral sensory and motor neuropathies occur in patients with a variety of malignancies, especially those involving the lung, ovary, and breast. Myasthenic (Eaton-Lambert) syndrome may be observed in patients with carcinoma of the lung. Invasion of the lower trunks of the brachial plexus by tumors in the apex of the lungs (Pancoast's syndrome) produces arm pain, paresthesias, and weakness of the hands and arms.

f. ***Collagen Vascular Diseases.*** Collagen vascular diseases (systemic lupus erythematosus, polyarteritis nodosa, rheumatoid arthritis, scleroderma) are commonly associated with peripheral neuropathies.

g. ***Sarcoidosis.*** Sarcoidosis is a disorder of unknown cause wherein noncaseating granulomas occur in multiple organ systems, most commonly the lung, lymphatics, bone, liver, and nervous system. Polyneuropathy, resulting from the presence of granulomatous lesions in peripheral nerves, is a common finding in patients with sarcoidosis.

h. ***Refsum's Disease.*** Refsum's disease is a multisystem disorder that manifests as polyneuropathies, ichthyosis, deafness, retinitis pigmentosa, cardiomyopathy, and cerebellar ataxia. Metabolic defects responsible for this disease reflect a failure to oxidize phytanic acid, a fatty acid that subsequently accumulates in excessive concentrations.

i. ***Acquired Immunodeficiency Syndrome (AIDS)–Associated Neuropathy.*** AIDS-associated peripheral neuropathy occurs in patients with AIDS but not in human immunodeficiency virus (HIV)–infected patients without AIDS. The neuropathy is typically distal numbness, tingling, and pain, often in the feet.

5. **Perioperative Peripheral Neuropathies.** Postoperative neuropathies involving many different peripheral nerves have been described that have traditionally been thought to be caused by errors in patient positioning during surgery. Now, however, they are thought to derive from preexisting aberrations of patient anatomy and physiology, although patient positioning may still play a role. Ulnar neuropathy is the most common. The neuropathy typically manifests about 48 hours after surgery. Lower-extremity neuropathies are common after procedures performed in lithotomy position.

   a. ***Management.*** (1) Document a thorough history and physical examination, (2) determine if the deficit is sensory, motor, or mixed, and (3) document the extent and distribution of the deficit. Neurology consultation may be warranted.

CHAPTER 13

Diseases of the Liver and Biliary Tract

Diseases of the liver and biliary tract can be categorized as parenchymal liver disease (hepatitis and cirrhosis) and cholestasis with or without obstruction of the extrahepatic biliary pathway.

I. ASSESSMENT OF LIVER FUNCTION

A. **Bilirubin.** Bilirubin is the degradation product of hemoglobin and myoglobin. Unconjugated bilirubin formed in the periphery is conjugated in the liver by glucuronosyltransferase. *Unconjugated hyperbilirubinemia* occurs with increased bilirubin production, decreased hepatic uptake, or decreased hepatic conjugation. *Conjugated hyperbilirubinemia* occurs with decreased transport of conjugated bilirubin from the liver, acute or chronic hepatocellular dysfunction, or bile duct obstruction (Table 13-1). Scleral icterus can be seen with a serum bilirubin of 3 mg/dL, and overt jaundice at greater than 4 mg/dL.

B. **Aminotransferases.** Alanine aminotransferase (ALT) and aspartate aminotransferase (AST) are involved in hepatic gluconeogenesis. ALT is highly specific to the liver, whereas AST is found in other tissues. Both are released with hepatic injury. An AST/ALT ratio below 1 is characteristic of nonalcoholic steatohepatitis. A ratio of 2 to 4 is typical of alcoholic liver disease. A ratio greater than 4 is typical of Wilson's disease.

C. **Alkaline Phosphatase.** Alkaline phosphatase is elevated in cholestatic disorders and may remain elevated for several days after resolution of biliary obstruction.

D. **International Normalized Ratio.** Elevation may indicate impairment of hepatic synthetic function.

E. **Albumin.** Albumin is synthesized exclusively by hepatocytes. A decreased level may indicate malnutrition, a protein-losing disease, or severe reduction in hepatic synthetic function.

F. **Serologic and Genetic Testing.** Antigen and antibody levels help distinguish viral from autoimmune or other hepatitis. Abnormal protein markers may be diagnostic of α_1-antitrypsin deficiency, Wilson's disease, and hepatocellular carcinoma (HCC). Genetic testing can confirm certain heritable hepatic diseases.

II. HYPERBILIRUBINEMIA

A. **Gilbert's Syndrome.** The most common hereditary hyperbilirubinemia, Gilbert's syndrome is autosomal dominant with variable penetrance. Approximately one third of the normal amount of glucuronosyltransferase is present. Serum bilirubin is typically <3mg/dL but increases with fasting, illness, stress, and fatigue.

B. **Crigler-Najjar Syndrome.** Crigler-Najjar syndrome is a rare hereditary severe unconjugated hyperbilirubinemia caused by mutation of glucuronosyltransferase, which is reduced to less than 10% of normal. Perinatal jaundice and kernicterus can develop. Treatment is exchange transfusion in the neonatal period, phototherapy throughout childhood, and early liver transplantation. Phenobarbital therapy may decrease jaundice. Anesthesia management of children should include bilirubin phototherapy and minimized fasting. Morphine, barbiturates, inhaled anesthetics, and muscle relaxants are all acceptable.

TABLE 13-1 ■ **Causes of Hepatic Dysfunction Based on Liver Function Test Results**

HEPATIC DYSFUNCTION	BILIRUBIN	AMINOTRANSFERASE ENZYMES	ALKALINE PHOSPHATASE	CAUSES
Prehepatic	Increased unconjugated fraction	Normal	Normal	Hemolysis Hematoma resorption Bilirubin overload from blood transfusion
Intrahepatic (hepatocellular)	Increased conjugated fraction	Markedly increased	Normal to slightly increased	Viral infection Drugs Alcohol Sepsis Hypoxemia Cirrhosis
Posthepatic (cholestatic)	Increased conjugated fraction	Normal to slightly increased	Markedly increased	Biliary tract stones or tumors Sepsis

C. **Dubin-Johnson Syndrome.** Conjugated hyperbilirubinemia caused by decreased transport of organic ions from hepatocytes into the biliary system is called Dubin-Johnson syndrome. The disorder is autosomal recessive and benign.

D. **Benign Postoperative Intrahepatic Cholestasis.** Benign postoperative intrahepatic cholestasis may occur after prolonged surgery, especially if complicated by hypotension, hypoxemia, and blood transfusion. Jaundice is usually apparent within 24 to 48 hours. Results of liver function tests (other than bilirubin and alkaline phosphatase) are normal or mildly abnormal. The condition resolves spontaneously.

E. **Progressive Familial Intrahepatic Cholestasis.** A rare hereditary metabolic disease, progressive familial intrahepatic cholestasis causes cholestasis in infancy and end-stage cirrhosis before adulthood. Liver transplantation is the only curative treatment. Anesthesia management is as for all patients with end-stage liver disease.

III. DISEASES OF THE BILIARY TRACT

Cholelithiasis and inflammatory biliary tract disease constitute major health problems in the United States, affecting more than 30 million Americans.

A. **Cholelithiasis and Cholecystitis.** Patients who have gallbladder or biliary tract stones can exhibit no symptoms (silent disease), display acute symptomatic disease, or have chronic intermittently symptomatic disease.

1. **Acute Cholecystitis.** Obstruction of the cystic duct, which is nearly always caused by a gallstone, produces acute inflammation of the gallbladder. Cholelithiasis is present in 95% of patients with acute cholecystitis.

   a. ***Signs and Symptoms.*** Signs and symptoms of acute cholecystitis include nausea, vomiting, fever, abdominal pain, and right upper quadrant tenderness. Patients may notice dark urine and scleral icterus.

b. ***Diagnosis.*** Ultrasonography is the principal diagnostic procedure used in patients with suspected gallstones and acute cholecystitis.

c. ***Differential Diagnosis*** *(see Table 13-1)*

d. ***Treatment.*** Patients with a clinical diagnosis of acute cholecystitis are treated with intravenous fluids and opioids. Febrile patients with leukocytosis are given antibiotics. Laparoscopic cholecystectomy has almost completely replaced open cholecystectomy due to less postoperative pain, fewer pulmonary complications, and more rapid convalescence. Common duct stones can be removed concurrently or subsequently by endoscopic retrograde cholangiopancreatography (ERCP). Operative common bile duct exploration and stone removal may occasionally be needed.

e. ***Complications.*** Localized perforation and abscess formation are likely if symptoms persist for several days. Gallstone ileus results from obstruction of the small bowel, often at the ileocecal valve, by a large gallstone.

f. ***Management of Anesthesia.*** Anesthetic considerations for laparoscopic cholecystectomy are similar to those for other laparoscopic procedures. Insufflation of the abdominal cavity (pneumoperitoneum) may impede ventilation and venous return. The reverse Trendelenburg position favors movement of abdominal contents away from the operative site and may improve ventilation. Mechanical ventilation is recommended to prevent atelectasis, ensure adequate ventilation in the presence of increased intraabdominal pressure, and offset the effects of systemic absorption of carbon dioxide. Endotracheal intubation with a cuffed tube minimizes the risk of pulmonary aspiration. Intraoperative decompression of the stomach with a nasogastric or orogastric tube may decrease the risk of visceral puncture during needle insertion to produce the pneumoperitoneum. Capnography is important for recognizing carbon dioxide embolism. There is no evidence that nitrous oxide significantly expands bowel gas or interferes with surgical working conditions during laparoscopic cholecystectomy. The use of opioids during anesthesia for this operation is controversial because these drugs can cause spasm of the sphincter of Oddi. It is possible to reverse this spasm by administering glucagon, naloxone or nitroglycerin.

2. **Chronic Cholecystitis.** Chronic cholecystitis is usually accompanied by evidence of chronic cholelithiasis. Ultrasonography is a mainstay of diagnosis. Treatment is usually elective cholecystectomy.

   a. *Alternative therapies* include oral dissolution therapy with ursodeoxycholic acid and extracorporeal shockwave lithotripsy.

3. **Choledocholithiasis.** When gallstones are present in the common bile duct, choledocholithiasis occurs. Stones typically lodge at the point of insertion of the duct into the ampulla of Vater.

   a. ***Signs and Symptoms.*** Signs and symptoms may include signs of cholangitis (fever, shaking chills, jaundice, right upper quadrant pain) or jaundice alone and a history of pain suggestive of cholecystitis.

   b. ***Diagnosis.*** Ultrasonography may reveal a dilated common bile duct.

   c. ***Differential Diagnosis.*** Acute obstruction of the common bile duct by a stone may mimic ureterolithiasis, pancreatitis, acute myocardial infarction, or viral hepatitis.

   d. ***Treatment.*** Endoscopic sphincterotomy is the initial treatment for the patient with choledocholithiasis. ERCP can be used to identify the cause of common bile duct obstruction and to remove a stone or place a stent.

IV. ACUTE HEPATITIS

Acute hepatitis is most often caused by a virus but can also be caused by autoimmune processes, drugs, and toxins. Viral hepatitis is typically caused by one of five viruses: hepatitis A virus (HAV), hepatitis B virus (HBV), hepatitis C virus (HCV), hepatitis D virus (HDV), or hepatitis E virus (HEV). Other viruses can include herpes simplex virus (HSV), cytomegalovirus (CMV) and Epstein-Barr virus (EBV).

TABLE 13-2 ■ **Characteristic Features of Viral Hepatitis**

PARAMETER	TYPE A	TYPE B	TYPE C	TYPE D
Mode of transmission	Fecal-oral Sewage-contaminated shellfish	Percutaneous Sexual	Percutaneous	Percutaneous
Incubation period	20-37 days	60-110 days	35-70 days	60-110 days
Results of serum antigen and antibody tests	IgM early and IgG appears during convalescence	HBsAg and anti-HBcAg early and persists in carriers	Anti-HCV in 6 wk to 9 mo	Anti-HDV late and may be short-lived
Immunity	Antibodies in 45%	Antibodies in 5%-15%	Unknown	Protected if immune to type B
Course	Does not progress to chronic liver disease	Chronic liver disease develops in 1%-5% of adults and 80%-90% of children	Chronic liver disease develops in up to 75%	Co-infection with type B
Prevention after exposure	Pooled γ-globulin Hepatitis A vaccine	Hepatitis B immunoglobulin Hepatitis B vaccine	Interferon plus ribavirin	Unknown
Mortality	<0.2%	0.3%-1.5%	Unknown	Acute icteric hepatitis: 2%-20%

Adapted from Keefe EB. Acute hepatitis. *Sci Am Med*. 1999;1-9.
HBcAg, Hepatitis B core antigen; *HBsAg*, hepatitis B surface antigen; *HCV*, hepatitis C virus; *HDV*, hepatitis D virus; *IgG*, immunoglobulin G; *IgM*, immunoglobulin M.

A. Viral Hepatitis. All types of viral hepatitis are similar and cannot be distinguished reliably by clinical features or routine laboratory tests.

1. Diagnosis. Diagnosis of viral hepatitis is dependent on clinical signs and symptoms, laboratory findings, serologic assays, and occasionally liver biopsy (Table 13-2).

a. Signs and Symptoms. The onset of viral hepatitis may be gradual or sudden; the condition most often manifests with dark urine, fatigue, anorexia, and nausea. Other signs may include low-grade fever, upper quadrant pain or generalized abdominal pain, and myalgias or arthralgias. Many of the initial symptoms abate when jaundice develops. Hepatomegaly and splenomegaly may be present. If viral hepatitis is severe, there may be evidence of acute liver failure including confusion, asterixis, peripheral edema, and ascites.

b. Laboratory Tests

i. General. Serum aminotransferase concentrations (AST, ALT) increase 7 to 14 days before the appearance of jaundice and begin to decrease shortly after jaundice develops. The degree of aminotransferase increase does not necessarily parallel the severity of the hepatitis. Anemia and lymphocytosis are typically present. Serum bilirubin concentration rarely exceeds 20 mg/dL. Alkaline phosphatase is not increased unless cholestasis is present. Severe acute hepatitis may result in hypoalbuminemia and/or a prolonged prothrombin time.

ii. ***Serologic Markers*** *(see Table 13-2)*

iii. ***Liver Biopsy.*** Typically biopsy shows spotty necrosis of hepatocytes and widespread parenchymal inflammation.

2. **Treatment.** Treatment of acute viral hepatitis is symptomatic, with restriction of physical activity, sensible nutrition, and intravenous fluids if needed. Abstinence from alcohol is recommended. Liver transplantation is a consideration for fulminant hepatic failure.

3. **Prevention.** Prevention of viral hepatitis includes avoidance of exposure to the virus, passive immunization with γ-globulin, and active immunization with a specific vaccine. Pooled γ-globulin administered intramuscularly as soon as possible after known exposure dramatically decreases the incidence of hepatitis A. Individuals exposed to HBV by percutaneous or mucous membrane routes should receive hepatitis B immunoglobulin and hepatitis B vaccine within 24 hours.

   a. *Hepatitis A vaccine* provides protection for 10 years or longer. Travelers to endemic regions, neonatal intensive care unit staff, food handlers, children in day-care centers, and military personnel should receive this vaccine.

   b. *Hepatitis B vaccine* is recommended for individuals at increased risk of HBV infection, including health care workers with frequent exposure to blood products, homosexual men, intravenous drug users, recipients of certain blood products, and infants born to hepatitis B surface antigen (HBsAg)–positive mothers.

B. **Drug-Induced Hepatitis.** Many drugs (analgesics, volatile anesthetics, antibiotics, antihypertensives, anticonvulsants, tranquilizers) can cause hepatitis indistinguishable histologically from acute viral hepatitis. Most of these drug reactions are idiosyncratic, rare, unpredictable, and not dose dependent.

1. **Acetaminophen Overdose.** Acetaminophen overdose produces profound hepatocellular necrosis in most persons. Oral *N*-acetylcysteine given within 8 hours of an acetaminophen overdose can dramatically decrease the risk of hepatotoxicity.

2. **Volatile Anesthetics.** Volatile anesthetics may produce mild, self-limited postoperative liver dysfunction that likely reflects anesthetic-induced alterations in hepatic oxygen supply relative to demand. Any anesthetic that decreases hepatic blood flow could interfere with adequate hepatocyte oxygenation. Indeed, α-glutathione *S*-transferase concentration (a sensitive marker of hepatocellular damage) increases transiently after administration of isoflurane, desflurane, and sevoflurane.

   a. ***Immune-Mediated Hepatotoxicity ("Halothane Hepatitis").*** A rare but life-threatening form of hepatic dysfunction after administration of volatile anesthetics (most often halothane) likely involves an immune-mediated hepatotoxicity in genetically susceptible individuals. Immunoglobulin G (IgG) antibodies are directed against microsomal proteins on the surface of hepatocytes that have been covalently modified by the reactive oxidative trifluoroacetyl halide metabolite of halothane to form neoantigens. The incidence of halothane-induced hepatitis is estimated at 1 in 20,000 administrations.

   b. ***Enflurane, Isoflurane, and Desflurane.*** These agents may form trifluoroacetyl metabolites, resulting in cross-sensitivity with halothane, but the incidence of hepatitis after these anesthetics is much lower than after halothane because the degree of anesthetic metabolism is substantially less.

   c. ***Sevoflurane.*** Sevoflurane does not undergo metabolism to trifluoroacetylated metabolites and would not be expected to produce immune-mediated hepatotoxicity.

   d. ***Differential Diagnosis of Postoperative Hepatic Dysfunction.*** When postoperative hepatic dysfunction (jaundice) occurs, an analysis of historical data, clinical signs and symptoms, serial liver function tests, and a search for extrahepatic causes of hepatic dysfunction facilitate development of a differential diagnosis. The causes of hepatic dysfunction can be categorized as prehepatic, intrahepatic (hepatocellular), or posthepatic (cholestatic) based on measurement of serum bilirubin, aminotransferases, and alkaline phosphatase (see Table 13-1). Postoperative hepatic dysfunction is often multifactorial.

i. Review all drugs administered.
ii. Check for sources of sepsis.
iii. Evaluate the possibility of an increased exogenous bilirubin load.
iv. Rule out occult hematomas.
v Rule out hemolysis.
vi. Review perioperative records for evidence of hypotension, arterial hypoxemia, hypoventilation, and hypovolemia.
vii. Consider extrahepatic abnormalities (congestive heart failure, respiratory failure, pulmonary embolism, renal insufficiency).
viii. Consider the possibility of benign postoperative intrahepatic cholestasis.
ix. Consider the possibility of immune-mediated hepatotoxicity.

C. **Autoimmune Hepatitis.** Autoimmune hepatitis is an inflammatory liver process caused by a cellular immune response against self-antigens in the liver. Prevalence is 10 to 20 per 100,000, and it is more common in women (70%) and patients with a concurrent autoimmune disease. Treatment with corticosteroids or other immunosuppressive agents is aimed at inducing remission. Liver transplantation may be considered for end-stage liver disease.

V. CHRONIC HEPATITIS

Chronic hepatitis encompasses a diverse group of diseases characterized by long-term (longer than 6 months) elevation of liver chemistries and evidence of inflammation on liver biopsy.

A. **Signs and Symptoms.** Signs of chronic hepatitis vary and range from asymptomatic disease to fulminant hepatic failure. The most common symptoms of chronic hepatitis are fatigue, malaise, and abdominal pain.

B. **Laboratory Tests.** Tests include elevated serum liver enzyme concentrations, and/or bilirubin, and histologic evidence of ongoing inflammation.

C. **Autoimmune Hepatitis.** Autoimmune hepatitis is characterized by hypergammaglobulinemia, increased serum aminotransferase concentrations, and the presence of antinuclear antibodies.

D. **Chronic Hepatitis B.** Chronic hepatitis B is present in 5% of the world's population, and an estimated 0.5% of the U.S. population are carriers of HBsAg. The goal of treatment of chronic hepatitis B is to eradicate HBV infection and prevent the development of cirrhosis or hepatocellular cancer. Currently available therapies, such as lamivudine and adefovir, can suppress HBV replication and lead to improvement in the clinical, biochemical, and histologic features of chronic hepatitis B. Liver transplantation can be performed for liver failure, but HBV will infect the allograft in nearly all recipients. Posttransplantation prophylaxis with lamivudine and hepatitis B immunoglobulin reduces the reinfection rate to approximately 10%.

E. **Chronic Hepatitis C.** Chronic hepatitis C follows acute HCV infection in up to 75% of patients, and an estimated 1.8% of the U.S. population are carriers of HCV.

1. **Diagnosis.** Diagnosis is based on persistently or intermittently increased serum aminotransferase concentrations in association with the presence of anti-HCV antibody. The natural history of chronic hepatitis C may span several decades, progressing insidiously with the ultimate development of cirrhosis or hepatocellular cancer after 10 to 20 years.
2. **Treatment.** Interferon reduces or normalizes serum ALT concentration and decreases inflammation as indicated by liver biopsy in approximately 40% of patients with chronic hepatitis C. It is combined with ribavirin for a better response. Chronic hepatitis C with liver failure is one of the most common indications for liver transplantation.

VI. CIRRHOSIS

Cirrhosis can result from a variety of chronic, progressive liver diseases that are most often the result of excessive chronic alcohol ingestion or chronic viral hepatitis caused by HBV or HCV infection.

A. Diagnosis. Percutaneous liver biopsy establishes the diagnosis of cirrhosis. Computed tomography, magnetic resonance imaging, and hepatic ultrasonography with Doppler flow studies may reveal findings consistent with cirrhosis (splenomegaly, ascites, irregular liver surface). Upper gastrointestinal (GI) endoscopy can establish the presence of esophagogastric varices.

B. Signs and Symptoms (Table 13-3)

C. Portal Hypertension. Caused by increased resistance to hepatic blood flow, portal hypertension results in ascites, hepatomegaly, splenomegaly, and peripheral edema.

D. Ascites and Spontaneous Bacterial Peritonitis. Risk factors include portal hypertension, hypoalbuminemia, and sodium and water retention. Medical therapy includes correction of hypoalbuminemia, adherence to a low-sodium diet, and administration of an aldosterone antagonist. Resistant ascites may require paracentesis or placement of a transjugular intrahepatic portosystemic shunt (TIPS) or LeVeen shunt. Clinical deterioration should raise suspicion of bacterial peritonitis, which has high morbidity and mortality.

E. Gastroesophageal Varices. Resulting from increased splanchnic venous pressure, gastroesophageal varices can lead to significant GI bleeding. Treatment is via endoscopic sclerotherapy and/or banding. A TIPS may be considered. β-Blockers such as nadolol or propranolol reduce portal hypertension and reduce the risk of rebleeding.

F. Hepatic Encephalopathy. Neuropsychiatric changes associated with systemic accumulation of ammonia and other metabolic byproducts can include changes in cognition, motor function, personality, and consciousness. Treatment includes protein restriction, enteral administration of nonabsorbable disaccharides (lactulose) and antibiotics (neomycin), correction of electrolyte imbalance, and avoidance of drugs such as opioids and sedative-hypnotics.

G. Hyperdynamic Circulation. Hyperdynamic circulation is caused by decreased systemic vascular resistance (SVR) and increased cardiac output. Accumulation of vasodilatory compounds such as prostaglandins or interleukins may play a causative role, as may reduced blood viscosity resulting from hypoalbuminemia and anemia.

H. Hepatopulmonary Syndrome. Intrapulmonary shunting occurs in up to 25% of patients. Indicators are dyspnea and hypoxemia. Echocardiography may be needed to rule out intracardiac shunting. Supplemental oxygen therapy is supportive, but definitive treatment is liver transplantation.

TABLE 13-3 ■ **Signs and Symptoms of Cirrhosis of the Liver**

Fatigue and malaise
Hepatomegaly
Splenomegaly
Ascites
Palmar erythema
Spider nevi
Gynecomastia
Testicular atrophy
Decreased serum albumin concentration
Increased INR
Increased serum aminotransferases and alkaline phosphatase

INR, International normalized ratio.

I. Portopulmonary Syndrome Portopulmonary syndrome is the coexistence of portal vein and pulmonary artery hypertension. The condition occurs in less than 4% of patients and typically manifests years after diagnosis of cirrhosis.

1. **Symptoms.** Signs and symptoms include dyspnea, fatigue, and syncope. Signs of right-sided heart failure may be present.
2. **Prognosis.** One-year mortality is higher than 80% with or without liver transplantation. Liver transplantation is the only known curative treatment. However, patients with mean pulmonary artery pressure greater than 45 mm Hg are poor candidates for transplantation.

J. Hepatorenal Syndrome. Hepatorenal syndrome is *functional* renal failure associated with severe liver disease. There is no intrinsic renal abnormality. Prognosis is poor. Renal replacement therapy is the mainstay of treatment.

K. Coagulopathy. Coagulopathy is common in cirrhosis owing to decreased synthesis of coagulation factors. The liver is also responsible for production of many anticoagulant proteins (proteins S, C, Z, and antithrombin III) as well as plasminogen activator inhibitor. Disturbances in coagulation function can be complex.

VII. ACUTE LIVER FAILURE

Acute hepatic failure is characterized by rapid development of jaundice, hypoalbuminemia, coagulopathy, malnutrition, susceptibility to infection, and renal dysfunction in the clinical setting of acute hepatic disease. *Fulminant hepatic failure* refers to acute liver failure with superimposed hepatic encephalopathy that develops within 8 days of the onset of illness in a patient without preexisting liver disease.

A. Signs and Symptoms. Typically, nonspecific symptoms such as malaise or nausea develop in a previously healthy individual and are followed by jaundice, altered mental status, and even coma. The progression of symptoms is rapid. Altered mentation and a prolonged prothrombin time are hallmarks of acute liver failure.

1. *Acute fatty liver of pregnancy* is characterized by accumulation of fat in hepatocytes. Approximately one half of patients have evidence of pregnancy-induced hypertension and/or laboratory evidence of HELLP syndrome (**H**emolysis, **E**levated **L**iver enzymes, and **L**ow **P**latelet count occurring in association with preeclampsia).

B. Treatment. Treatment is primarily supportive; no specific treatments exist for managing acute liver failure. Antidotes must be administered early for acetaminophen or mushroom poisoning. Glucose administration may be indicated. Cerebral edema requires aggressive intervention in the hope of preventing brain herniation. Mortality is 80%, and when survival seems unlikely, the only curative treatment is liver transplantation.

C. Anesthesia Considerations in Acute Liver Failure (Table 13-4)

TABLE 13-4 ■ **Anesthetic Considerations for Patients with Acute Liver Failure**

Only life-saving surgery should be undertaken.
Coagulopathy should be corrected preoperatively.
Low doses of volatile agents, or nitrous oxide alone, may be sufficient for anesthesia.
Consider metabolism and clearance when selecting muscle relaxants.
Glucose may be indicated for hypoglycemia.
Transfuse blood slowly to avoid citrate intoxication.
Judicious fluid management may be needed to maintain urine output (mannitol if necessary).
Use invasive monitoring as needed based on cardiovascular status.
Practice strict aseptic techniques.

VIII. ANESTHESIA FOR PATIENTS WITH DECREASED LIVER FUNCTION

A. **Child-Pugh Score** (Tables 13-5 and 13-6). The Child-Pugh score is based on total bilirubin, serum albumin, international normalized ratio (INR), ascites, and hepatic encephalopathy combined into a single score to categorize patients (class A, B, or C) according to disease severity. The mortality of intraabdominal surgery is 10%, 30% and 80%, respectively for classes A, B, and C.

B. **Preoperative Care.** Care includes optimizing nutrition, to improve hypoalbuminemia and correct vitamin deficiencies which can alter pharmacokinetics. Hypoglycemia and hyponatremia are common.

C. **Encephalopathy.** Encephalopathy can be worsened by infection, GI bleeding, and the presence of a TIPS shunt and is associated with greatly increased perioperative mortality.

D. **Airway Management.** Consideration should be given to rapid sequence induction, because gastric emptying is delayed and gastric volumes are increased.

E. **Renal Function.** Renal function can be adversely affected by GI bleeding, hypotension, hypoperfusion, large-volume paracentesis, and medications. An increasing serum creatinine and decreased glomerular filtration rate in the presence of marginal liver function are ominous signs.

F. **Circulation.** Circulation is hyperdynamic owing to decreased SVR and lower plasma oncotic pressure. Invasive monitoring (arterial line, cardiac output measurement) is advisable. Vasopressors may be useful.

G. **Coagulopathy.** Coagulopathy is often present due to decrease in both coagulation factors and changes in anticoagulant modulators. Vitamin K, fresh frozen plasma, cryoprecipitate, and platelet therapy may be indicated. Diminished capacity to metabolize citrate in the diseased liver leads to calcium ion abnormalities in the face of transfusion, and intravenous calcium administration is often needed.

H. **Pharmacokinetics.** Pharmacokinetics are altered by impaired hepatic function, increased volume of distribution, decreased plasma protein binding and decreased drug clearance. A larger

TABLE 13-5 ■ **Child-Pugh Scoring System to Assess Severity of Liver Disease**

SIGN OF HEPATIC DYSFUNCTION	1 POINT	2 POINTS	3 POINTS
Encephalopathy (grade)	None	Grade I-II	Grade III-IV
Ascites	Absent	Mild	Severe
Bilirubin (mg/dL)	<2	2-3	>3
Albumin (g/dL)	>3.5	2.8-3.5	<2.8
International normalized ratio	<1.7	1.7-2.2	>2.2

TABLE 13-6 ■ **Survival Statistics According to Child-Pugh Class**

POINTS	CLASS	ONE-YEAR SURVIVAL	TWO-YEAR SURVIVAL
5-6	A	100%	85%
7-9	B	81%	57%
10-15	C	45%	35%

initial dose of medication may be needed to achieve desired effects, but subsequent doses may need to be reduced to reflect impaired clearance. Cisatracurium may be a useful muscle relaxant because clearance is independent of hepatic function.

I. Postsurgical Recovery. Liver failure is the most common cause of postoperative death in these patients. Intensive care unit care is usually needed. Early enteral feeding improves outcomes.

IX. LIVER TRANSPLANTATION

Liver transplantation is the only curative therapy for patients with severe acute liver failure or end-stage liver disease with cirrhosis. At present, the typical 1-year survival rate for liver transplant recipients is approximately 85%, and the 5-year survival rate is approximately 70%.

A. Organ Allocation. The Model for End-Stage Liver Disease (MELD) scoring system is used to predict 90-day mortality *without* liver transplantation. Patients with the highest MELD scores are given the highest priority. The MELD score is calculated as follows:

$$3.8 \times \log_e(\text{bilirubin in mg/dL}) + 11.2 \times \log_e(\text{INR}) + 9.6 \times \log_e(\text{creatinine in mg/dL}) + 0.643$$

In the case of hepatocellular carcinoma, liver transplantation is generally considered if there is only a single lesion of 5 cm or less or a total of no more than three tumors, none of which is greater than 3 cm.

B. Surgical Procedure.

1. Management of Anesthesia. Candidates for liver transplantation may have severe multiorgan dysfunction. Many of the physiologic derangements are not correctable until after successful liver transplantation. The likely presence of HBV or HBC in the transplant recipient must be considered by the health care providers.

a. Induction of Anesthesia. As with any patient with end-stage liver disease, anesthesia can be affected by the presence of ascites compromising lung volumes and delaying gastric emptying. Anesthesia can be maintained with opioids and/or inhaled anesthetics combined with muscle relaxants that are not dependent on hepatic clearance mechanisms (atracurium, cisatracurium). Nitrous oxide is usually avoided because of concerns regarding bowel distention that can compromise surgical exposure.

b. Fluid Warming Devices and Rapid Infusion Systems. Devices designed to deliver warmed fluids or blood products at rates exceeding 1 L/min are routinely employed.

c. Invasive Monitoring. Invasive monitoring of systemic blood pressure and cardiac filling pressures and placement of several large-bore intravenous catheters to optimize fluid replacement are important parts of anesthetic management.

d. Surgical Stages During Liver Transplantation

i. Prehepatic or dissection phase involves mobilizing the vascular structures around the liver (hepatic artery, portal vein, suprahepatic and infrahepatic vena cava), isolating the common bile duct, and removing the native liver. Cardiovascular instability resulting from hemorrhage, venous pooling, and impaired venous return is common.

ii. Anhepatic phase begins when the blood supply to the native liver is interrupted by clamping of the hepatic artery and portal vein. To support cardiac output and aid venous return to the heart, a venovenous bypass system is often used. Metabolic acidosis, decreased drug metabolism, and citrate intoxication are likely.

iii. *Reperfusion or neohepatic phase* begins after reanastomosis of the major vascular structures. Unclamping can cause significant hemodynamic instability, dysrhythmias, severe bradycardia, hypotension, and hyperkalemic cardiac arrest. Once the allograft begins to function, hemodynamic and metabolic stability are gradually restored and urine output increases.

iv. Early postoperative extubation may be considered in some patients when the duration of surgery is shorter and the intra operative course has been uneventful.

e. ***Posttransplant Liver Function Tests.*** Test results return to normal and hyperdynamic circulation resolves. Oxygenation usually improves, although intrapulmonary shunting can persist.

CHAPTER 14

Diseases of the Gastrointestinal System

I. ESOPHAGEAL DISEASES

Dysphagia is the classic symptom of all disorders of the esophagus (evaluate by barium contrast study and upper gastrointestinal [GI] endoscopy).

A. **Diffuse Esophageal Spasm.** Most often occurring in elderly patients, diffuse esophageal spasm may mimic angina pectoris and may respond to treatment with nitroglycerin. Nifedipine and isosorbide, which decrease lower esophageal sphincter (LES) pressure, may also relieve pain produced by esophageal spasm.

B. **Achalasia.** Achalasia is a neuromuscular disorder of the esophagus that causes dysfunction of both the esophageal muscles and the LES. It is characterized by hypertension of the LES, failure of the LES to relax when swallowing, reduced esophageal peristalsis, and esophageal dilation.

1. **Symptoms.** Signs and symptoms include the triad of dysphagia, weight loss, and regurgitation.
2. **Comorbidities.** Associated with achalasia are increased risk of esophageal cancer and risk of pulmonary aspiration.
3. **Diagnosis.** Definitive diagnosis is by manometry, but esophagram may show classic "bird's beak" appearance,
4. **Treatment.** All treatments are palliative only, because esophageal motility cannot be restored. Medications include nitrates, nitroglycerin, and calcium channel blockers to relax the LES. Endoscopic injection of botulinum toxin in the LES and endoscopic dilation of the LES are also options. Surgical esophagomyotomy (e.g., laparoscopic Heller's myotomy) offers better results than endoscopic dilation. Esophagectomy may be considered in advanced cases.
5. **Anesthetic Considerations.** Anesthetic considerations include increased risk of aspiration. Full stomach precautions must be taken.

C. **Esophagectomy.** In malignant or obstructive esophageal disease, esophagectomy is considered and can be accomplished via a transthoracic, transhiatal, as minimally invasive (thoracoscopic or laparoscopic) approach.

1. Morbidity and mortality rates are high (10% to 15%). Most postoperative complications are respiratory, and mortality approaches 50% if acute respiratory distress syndrome (ARDS) occurs. Postoperative ARDS occurs in up to 20% of cases and may be related to release of inflammatory mediators and gut-related endotoxins and the use of prolonged one-lung ventilation. Risks for poor outcomes include smoking history, low body mass index, long surgical duration, cardiopulmonary instability, and the occurrence of postoperative anastomotic leak.
2. Anesthesia may be complicated by poor nutritional status of the patient and the effects of recent chemotherapy or radiation therapy.

D. **Gastroesophageal Reflux Disease**

1. **Pathophysiology.** The underlying pathology of esophageal reflux is a decrease in the resting tone of the LES (average 13 mm Hg versus 29 mm Hg in normal patients). Reflux occurs only when the gradient of pressure between the LES and the stomach is lost. Reflux can result in

TABLE 14-1 ■ Effect of Agents on Lower Esophageal Sphincter Tone

INCREASE	DECREASE	NO CHANGE
Metoclopramide	Atropine	Propranolol
Domperidone	Glycopyrrolate	Oxprenolol
Prochlorperazine	Dopamine	Cimetidine
Cyclizine	Sodium nitroprusside	Ranitidine
Edrophonium	Ganglion blockers	Atracurium
Neostigmine	Thiopental	? Nitrous oxide
Succinylcholine	Tricyclic antidepressants	
Pancuronium	β-Adrenergic stimulants	
Metoprolol	Halothane	
α-Adrenergic stimulants	Enflurane	
Antacids	? Nitrous oxide Propofol Opioids	

TABLE 14-2 ■ Some Anesthesia Considerations in Patients with Esophageal Reflux

Anticholinergic medications	Can decreased LES tone and may increase the risk of silent aspiration
Succinylcholine	Increases LES pressure, and intragastric pressure; barrier pressure is uncharged
Prophylactic premedications—histamine blockers	Cimetidine, ranitidine, famotidine, nizatidine all decrease gastric acid secretion and increase gastric pH
Preoperative proton pump inhibitors	Omeprazole (given the night before surgery), rabeprazole, and lansoprazole (both given the morning of surgery) May decrease the antiplatelet effects of clopidogrel or aspirin
Sodium citrate	Oral nonparticulate antacid
Metoclopramide	Gastrokinetic agent to facilitate gastric emptying
Cricoid pressure	Should be applied during induction to prevent aspiration
Tracheal intubation	To protect the airway from aspiration

LES, Lower esophageal sphincter.

chronic cough, bronchoconstriction, pharyngitis, laryngitis, morning hoarseness, bronchitis, or pneumonia. Persistent dysphagia suggests development of a peptic stricture.

2. **Drug Effects on the Lower Esophageal Sphincter** (Table 14-1)
3. **Incidence of Reflux.** More than one third of healthy adults experience symptoms of heartburn at least once every 30 days. The incidence of aspiration during anesthesia is 0.7 to 4.7 per 10,000 general anesthetic procedures.
4. **Anesthesia Considerations** (Table 14-2)

E. **Hiatal Hernia.** Hiatal hernia is a herniation of part of the stomach into the thoracic cavity through the esophageal hiatus in the diaphragm. A sliding hernia is found in approximately 30%

of patients undergoing upper GI radiographic examination. Most patients with hiatal hernia do not have symptoms of reflux esophagitis, emphasizing the importance of the integrity of the LES.

F. **Esophageal Diverticula.** Outpouchings of the wall of the esophagus are called *esophageal diverticula.* Zenker's diverticulum appears in the posterior hypopharyngeal wall (Killian's triangle). Regurgitation of previously ingested food from a Zenker diverticulum can predispose a patient to pulmonary aspiration, even without recent food intake. Treatment is surgical cricopharyngeal myotomy with or without diverticulectomy. A mid-esophageal diverticulum can result from traction from old adhesions or from propulsion associated with esophageal motor abnormalities. An epiphrenic diverticulum may be associated with achalasia.

G. **Mucosal Tear (Mallory-Weiss Syndrome).** Mucosal tears are usually caused by vomiting, retching, or vigorous coughing. Patients have upper GI bleeding, which usually resolves spontaneously. Vasopressin therapy or angiographic embolization may be necessary if bleeding persists.

II. PEPTIC ULCER DISEASE

Burning epigastric pain exacerbated by fasting and improved with meals is the symptom complex associated with peptic ulcer disease (PUD). Benign gastric ulcers are a form of PUD that occurs with one third the frequency of benign duodenal ulceration.

A. **Pathophysiology.** The mucus-bicarbonate layer serves as a physicochemical barrier to multiple agents including hydrogen ions. Surface epithelial cells provide the next line of defense through several factors, including mucus production, epithelial cell ionic transporters that maintain intracellular pH and bicarbonate production, and intracellular tight junctions. Prostaglandins play a central role in gastric epithelial defense and repair.

B. **Causes of Injury**

1. **Hydrochloric Acid and Pepsinogen.** The two principal gastric secretory products capable of inducing mucosal injury are hydrochloric acid and pepsinogen.
2. ***Helicobacter pylori.*** *H. pylori* is a major factor in the pathogenesis of duodenal ulcerations, although early *H. pylori* infection is associated with a decrease in gastric acid secretion. *H. pylori* might induce increased acid secretion through both direct and indirect actions of *H. pylori* and proinflammatory cytokines (interleukin [IL]-8, tumor necrosis factor, and IL-1) on G, D, and parietal cells. *H. pylori* also decreases duodenal mucosal bicarbonate production.

C. **Complications of Peptic Ulcer Disease**

1. **Bleeding.** The leading cause of death associated with PUD is bleeding, and the incidence of this complication has not changed since the introduction of histamine H_2-receptor antagonists. The risk of mortality from bleeding is 10% to 20%.
2. **Perforation.** This complication occurs in about 10% of patients. Mortality of emergent ulcer operations is correlated with preoperative shock, co-existing medical illness, and perforation for more than 48 hours.
3. **Gastric Outlet Obstruction.** Obstruction can occur acutely or chronically in patients with duodenal ulcer disease; hence they should be treated as having a full stomach when they are presented for surgery. Pyloric obstruction is suggested by recurrent vomiting, dehydration, and hypochloremia. Treatment usually consists of nasogastric suction, rehydration, and intravenous administration of antisecretory agents, but surgery may be necessary.

E. **Stress Gastritis.** Major trauma accompanied by shock, sepsis, respiratory failure, hemorrhage, transfusion requirement of more than 6 units, or multiorgan injury is often accompanied by the development of acute stress gastritis. The major complication of stress gastritis is hemorrhage.

D. **Treatment of Peptic Ulcer Disease**

1. **Medical Treatment** (Table 14-3)

TABLE 14-3 ■ Treatment of Peptic Ulcer Disease

ANTACIDS	FOR SYMPTOMATIC RELIEF
H_2-receptor antagonists	Cimetidine, ranitidine, famotidine, nizatidine; bind to cytochrome P-450; can affect metabolism of other medications, and, rarely, affect bone marrow function
Proton-pump inhibitors (PPIs)	Omeprazole, esomeprazole, lansoprazole, rabeprazole, pantoprazole; rapid onset and long duration
Prostaglandin analogues	Misoprostol; enhance mucosal bicarbonate secretion, stimulate mucosal blood flow, and decrease mucosal cell turnover
Cytoprotective agents	Sucralfate provides physicochemical barrier to acid and pepsin; bismuth-containing preparations may exert positive effects through ulcer coating, prevention of further damage, stimulation of prostaglandins
Miscellaneous drugs	Anticholinergics (weak acid-inhibiting effect)
Helicobacter pylori treatment	Combination therapy with amoxicillin, metronidazole, tetracycline, clarithromycin, and bismuth compounds for 14 days; typical triple therapy includes a PPI and two antibiotics

2. **Surgical Treatment.** Surgery is reserved for the treatment of the most complicated ulcer disease. Three procedures—truncal vagotomy and drainage, truncal vagotomy and antrectomy, and proximal gastric vagotomy—have been most widely used for the operative treatment of PUD.

III. ZOLLINGER-ELLISON SYNDROME

Zollinger-Ellison syndrome includes gastroduodenal and intestinal ulceration, with gastric hypersecretion and non-beta islet cell tumors of the pancreas gastrinomas. The incidence of Zollinger-Ellison syndrome varies from 0.1% to 1% of individuals with PUD.

A. **Pathophysiology.** Excess gastrin stimulates acid secretion and exerts a trophic action on gastric epithelial cells. Gastric acid secretion is markedly increased through both parietal cell stimulation and increased parietal cell mass. This increased gastric acid output leads to the PUD, erosive esophagitis, and diarrhea.

B. **Clinical Manifestations.** Abdominal pain and peptic ulceration are seen in up to 90% of patients. Diarrhea and gastroesophageal reflux is seen in up to half of patients. Gastrinomas can develop in the presence of multiple endocrine neoplasia type I (MEN I) syndrome, a disorder involving primarily three organ sites: the parathyroid glands (80% to 90%), pancreas (40% to 80%), and pituitary gland (30% to 60%). An additional distinguishing feature in Zollinger-Ellison syndrome patients with MEN I is the higher incidence of gastric carcinoid tumor development compared with patients with sporadic gastrinomas.

C. **Diagnosis.** Diagnosis is established by clinical presentation and elevated fasting gastrin level. Multiple processes can lead to an elevated fasting gastrin level (Table 14-4).

D. **Treatment.** Initially treatment is with proton pump inhibitors. Curative surgical resection of the gastrinoma is indicated in the absence of evidence of MEN I syndrome and metastatic disease. Anesthetic considerations for gastrinoma resection include the presence of gastric hypersecretion and reflux and depletion of intravascular fluid volume and electrolyte imbalance (hypokalemia, metabolic alkalosis) as a result of diarrhea. Associated endocrine abnormalities (MEN I syndrome) should be considered. A preoperative coagulation screen and liver

TABLE 14-4 ■ Causes of Increased Fasting Serum Gastrin

Hypochlorhydria and achlorhydria (± pernicious anemia)	*Helicobacter pylori* infection
G-cell hyperplasia	Retained gastric antrum
Renal insufficiency	Gastric outlet obstruction
Rheumatoid arthritis	Massive small bowel obstruction
Pheochromocytomas	Vitiligo
	Patients on antisecretory drugs
	Diabetes mellitus

function tests may be needed, as alterations in fat absorption could influence clotting factor formation. Intravenous administration of ranitidine is useful for preventing gastric acid hypersecretion during surgery.

IV. POSTGASTRECTOMY SYNDROMES

A. Dumping Symptoms. Nausea, epigastric discomfort, palpitations, reactive hypoglycemia, and, in extreme cases, dizziness or syncope occur immediately after a meal (early) or after 1 to 3 hours (late). Octreotide may be effective treatment.

B. Alkaline Reflux Gastritis. The clinical triad of postprandial epigastric pain, evidence of reflux of bile into the stomach, and associated histologic evidence of gastritis is called *alkaline reflux gastritis.* The only proven treatment is operative diversion of intestinal contents from contact with the gastric mucosa (Roux-en-Y gastrojejunostomy).

V. IRRITABLE BOWEL SYNDROME

Patients with irritable bowel syndrome complain of generalized bowel discomfort, usually confined to the left lower quadrant. Commonly the frequency of stools is increased and the stool is covered with mucus. Many patients have associated symptoms of vasomotor instability, including tachycardia, hyperventilation, fatigue, diaphoresis, and headaches. There is no known specific causative agent or structural or biochemical defect.

VI. INFLAMMATORY BOWEL DISEASE

Inflammatory bowel diseases are the most common chronic inflammatory disorders after rheumatoid arthritis.

A. Classification of Inflammatory Bowel Disease

1. **Ulcerative Colitis.** Ulcerative colitis is a mucosal disease involving the rectum and all or part of the colon. Major symptoms are diarrhea, rectal bleeding, tenesmus, passage of mucus, and crampy abdominal pain. Other signs and symptoms in moderate to severe disease include anorexia, nausea, vomiting, fever, and weight loss.
   a. ***Complications.*** Catastrophic illness, hemorrhage, toxic megacolon, perforation, peritonitis, and colonic obstruction may occur.
2. **Crohn's Disease (CD).** CD usually manifests as acute or chronic bowel inflammation. CD usually follows one of two patterns of disease: a penetrating-fistulous pattern or an obstructing pattern, each with different treatments and prognoses. Presentation is usually right lower quadrant pain with diarrhea but can mimic appendicitis. Obstruction, strictures, and fistulas all occur. Jejunal involvement can lead to malabsorption, steatorrhea, and nutritional deficiencies. Colitis and toxic megacolon can occur. Associated gastritis can

TABLE 14-5 ■ Extraintestinal Manifestations of Inflammatory Bowel Disease

Dermatologic	Erythema nodosum in 10%-15% of IBD; pyoderma gangrenosum in 1%-12%
Rheumatologic	Peripheral arthritis develops in 15%-20% of IBD patients
Ocular	1%-10% of IBD; conjunctivitis, anterior uveitis or iritis, and episcleritis
Hepatobiliary	Approximately 50% of IBD; hepatomegaly; fatty liver from chronic debilitating illness, malnutrition, and glucocorticoid therapy; cholelithiasis caused by malabsorption of bile acids; primary sclerosing cholangitis leading to biliary cirrhosis and hepatic failure
Urologic	Calculi in 10%-20%; ureteral obstruction
Others	Thromboembolic disease (pulmonary embolism, cerebrovascular accidents, and arterial emboli) caused by thrombocytosis; increased levels of fibrinopeptide A, factor V, factor VIII, and fibrinogen; accelerated thromboplastin generation; antithrombin III deficiency caused by increased gut losses or increased catabolism; free protein S deficiency, Endocarditis, myocarditis, pleuropericarditis Interstitial lung disease Secondary or reactive amyloidosis

IBD, Inflammatory bowel disease.

TABLE 14-6 ■ Surgical Indications: Inflammatory Bowel Disease

ULCERATIVE COLITIS
Massive hemorrhage, perforation, toxic megacolon, obstruction, intractable and fulminant disease, cancer
CROHN'S DISEASE
Stricture, obstruction, hemorrhage, abscess, fistulas, intractable and fulminant disease, cancer, and unresponsive perianal disease

result in nausea, vomiting, and epigastric pain. Patients with perianal CD are at higher risk of developing extraintestinal manifestations (Table 14-5).

B. Treatment of Inflammatory Bowel Disease

1. **Surgical Treatment** (Table 14-6)
2. **Medical Treatment** (Table 14-7)

VII. PSEUDOMEMBRANOUS ENTEROCOLITIS

Pseudomembranous enterocolitis is often associated with antibiotic therapy (especially clindamycin and lincomycin), bowel obstruction, uremia, congestive heart failure, and intestinal ischemia. Clinical manifestations include fever, watery diarrhea, dehydration, hypotension, cardiac dysrhythmias, skeletal muscle weakness, intestinal ileus, and metabolic acidosis.

VIII. CARCINOID TUMORS

A. Carcinoid Tumors. Carcinoid tumors can occur in almost any GI tissue, but most originate in a bronchus, the jejunoileum, or colon and rectum. Carcinoid tumors secrete a variety of amine and neuropeptide hormones (Table 14-8), which may be released in sufficient amounts to

TABLE 14-7 ■ Medical Treatment of Inflammatory Bowel Disease

Sulfasalazine	Antibacterial and antiinflammatory (5-acetylsalicylic acid). Effective at inducing remission in UC and CD, and maintains remission in UC. Newer agents include Asacol and Pentasa (mesalamine). About 30% of patients experience allergic reactions or side effects.
Sulfa-free aminosalicylate preparations	Mesalamine (Asacol, Pentasa); deliver drug to the site of bowel disease and have limited systemic toxicity.
Oral, topical, or parenteral glucocorticoids	Used in both UC and CD to induce remission. No role in maintenance therapy.
Antibiotics	Used to treat pouchitis in UC patients after colectomy (metronidazole or ciprofloxacin).
Immunomodulatory drugs	Azathioprine, 6-mercaptopurine (inhibit cell proliferation), methotrexate (inhibits dihydrofolate reductase, may decrease IL-1 production), cyclosporine (inhibits T-cell–mediated responses).

CD, Crohn's disease; *IL,* interleukin; *UC,* ulcerative colitis.

TABLE 14-8 ■ Substances Produced by Carcinoid Tumors at Various Locations

	FOREGUT	MIDGUT	HINDGUT
Serotonin (5HTP)	Low	High	Rarely
Other substances	ACTH, 5HTP, GRF	Tachykinins; rarely 5HTP, ACTH	Rarely 5HTP, ACTH; other numerous peptides
Carcinoid syndrome	Atypical	Typical	Rare

ACTH, Adrenocartico-tropic hormone; *GRF,* growth hormone releasing factor; *5HTP,* 5-hydroxyl-L-tryptophan.

TABLE 14-9 ■ Location and Presentation of Carcinoid Tumors

CARCINOID LOCATION	PRESENTATION
Small intestine	Abdominal pain (51%), intestinal obstruction (31%), tumor (17%), gastrointestinal bleed (11%)
Rectal	Bleeding (39%), constipation (17%), diarrhea (17%)
Bronchial	Asymptomatic (31%)
Thymic	Anterior mediastinal mass
Ovarian and testicular	Masses discovered on physical examination or ultrasonography
Metastatic	In the liver; often manifests as hepatomegaly

cause significant systemic symptoms (carcinoid syndrome). Most carcinoid tumors are found incidentally during surgery for suspected appendicitis (Table 14-9).

B. **Carcinoid Syndrome.** Carcinoid syndrome occurs in about 20% of patients. The two most common symptoms are flushing and diarrhea. Flushing may be associated with pruritus, lacrimation, diarrhea, or facial edema and may be precipitated by stress, alcohol, exercise, certain foods such as cheese, or agents such as catecholamines, pentagastrin, and serotonin reuptake inhibitors. Cardiac manifestations are caused by fibrosis involving the endocardium, primarily on the right side of the heart. The carcinoid triad is cardiac involvement with flushing and

TABLE 14-10 ■ Pharmacologic Agents Associated with Carcinoid Crisis

DRUGS THAT MAY PROVOKE MEDIATOR RELEASE
Succinylcholine, mivacurium, atracurium, and D-tubocurarine
Epinephrine, norepinephrine, dopamine, isoproterenol, and thiopental
DRUGS NOT KNOWN TO RELEASE MEDIATORS
Propofol, etomidate, vecuronium, cisatracurium, rocuronium, sufentanil, alfentanil, fentanyl, and remifentanil; all inhalation agents; desflurane may be the better choice in patients with liver metastasis because of its low rate of metabolism

diarrhea. Asthmalike wheezing can also occur. Carcinoid crisis, which can be fatal, is characterized by intense flushing, diarrhea, abdominal pain, and cardiovascular instability. Provocative events can include stress, biopsy, and certain drugs (Table 14-10).

1. **Diagnosis.** Diagnosis relies on measurement of urinary or plasma serotonin or seratonin metabolites in the urine.
2. **Management of Anesthesia.** Administration of octreotide, 150 to 250 mcg subcutaneously (SC) every 6 to 8 hours for 24 to 48 hours before anesthesia and throughout the procedure, will attenuate most adverse hemodynamic responses. Use of epidural analgesia in patients who have been adequately treated with octreotide is a safe technique, although the sympathetic blockade produced by epidural or spinal anesthesia may worsen hypotension. Awakening after general anesthesia may be delayed owing to high serotonin levels. Ondansetron, a serotonin antagonist, is a useful and logical antiemetic choice. Invasive arterial blood pressure monitoring may be necessary.
3. **Medical Treatment.** Medical treatment of carcinoid includes avoiding conditions that precipitate flushing, dietary supplementation with nicotinamide, treatment of heart failure and wheezing, and controlling the diarrhea (loperamide or diphenoxylate). 5-HT_3 receptor antagonists (ondansetron, tropisetron, alosetron) may control diarrhea and nausea. A combination of histamine H_1- and H_2-receptor antagonists (diphenhydramine and cimetidine or ranitidine) may control flushing in patients with foregut carcinoids. Somatostatin analogues octreotide and lanreotide control symptoms in most patients and are effective in treating carcinoid crises.
4. **Other Treatment.** Hepatic artery embolization alone or with chemotherapy (chemoembolization) has been used to control the symptoms of metastatic carcinoid tumors. Surgery is the only potentially curative therapy for nonmetastatic carcinoid tumors.

IX. ACUTE PANCREATITIS

Acute pancreatitis is characterized as an inflammatory disorder of the pancreas; pancreatic autodigestion is the most likely cause. Normal pancreatic function is restored after the acute event has resolved.

A. **Etiology.** Gallstones and alcohol abuse are causative factors in most patients with acute pancreatitis. Acute pancreatitis is common in patients with acquired immunodeficiency syndrome and those with hyperparathyroidism and associated hypercalcemia.

B. **Signs and Symptoms** (Table 14-11)

C. **Diagnosis.** The hallmark of acute pancreatitis is an increased serum amylase concentration. Contrast-enhanced computed tomography can document the morphologic changes associated with acute pancreatitis. The differential diagnosis includes a perforated duodenal ulcer, acute cholecystitis, mesenteric ischemia, and bowel obstruction.

D. **Prognosis.** Ranson's criteria can be used to estimate mortality (Table 14-12).

TABLE 14-11 ■ Signs and Symptoms of Acute Pancreatitis

Mid-epigastric abdominal pain radiating to the back, improved by leaning forward
Nausea and vomiting
Abdominal distention and ileus
Dyspnea caused by pleural effusions or ascites
Fever
Shock
Tetany (with development of hypocalcemia)
Obtundation and psychosis (if withdrawing from alcohol)

TABLE 14-12 ■ Ranson's Criteria for Acute Pancreatitis

CRITERIA
Age >55
White blood cell count >16,000/mm^3
Blood urea nitrogen >16 mmol/L
Aspartate transaminase >250 units/L
Arterial Po_2 (60 mm Hg)
Fluid deficit >6 L
Blood glucose >200 mg/dL, and no history of diabetes mellitus
Lactate dehydrogenase >350 International Units/L
Corrected calcium <8 mg/dL
Decrease in hematocrit of the more then 10
Metabolic acidosis with base deficit >4 mmol/L
(Note: Serum amylase is *not* a criterion.)
MORTALITY
0-2 criteria: >5%
3-4 criteria: 20%
5-6 criteria: 40%
7-8 criteria: 100%

E. Complications. Possible complications include shock, arterial hypoxemia, acute respiratory distress syndrome (20%), renal failure (25%), GI hemorrhage, coagulation defects from disseminated intravascular coagulation, and pancreatic infection (greater than 50% mortality).

F. Treatment. Treatment includes aggressive intravenous fluid administration (up to 10 L of crystalloid), resting the gut by stopping oral intake, opioids to manage the severe pain, prophylactic antibiotic therapy, endoscopic removal of obstructing gallstones within the first 24 to 72 hours of the onset of symptoms to decrease the risk of cholangitis, and parenteral nutrition if it is anticipated that the patient will experience a protracted course.

X. CHRONIC PANCREATITIS

Chronic pancreatitis is characterized by chronic inflammation that leads to irreversible damage to the pancreas.

A. Etiology. Chronic pancreatitis is most often caused by chronic alcohol abuse. Idiopathic chronic pancreatitis is the second most common form of this disease. Chronic pancreatitis occasionally occurs in association with cystic fibrosis or hyperparathyroidism (hypercalcemia) or as a hereditary disease transmitted by an autosomal dominant gene.

B. **Signs and Symptoms.** Chronic pancreatitis is often characterized by epigastric abdominal pain that radiates to the back and is often postprandial. Steatorrhea is present when at least 90% of the pancreas is lost. Diabetes mellitus eventually develops.

C. **Diagnosis.** Chronic pancreatitis is diagnosed based on the history of chronic alcohol abuse and presence of pancreatic calcifications. Serum amylase concentrations are usually normal. Ultrasonography may document the presence of an enlarged pancreas or identify a fluid-filled pseudocyst. Computed tomography demonstrates dilated pancreatic ducts and changes in the size of the pancreas. Endoscopic retrograde cholangiopancreatography is the most sensitive imaging test for detecting early changes in the pancreatic ducts caused by chronic pancreatitis.

D. **Treatment.** Treatment includes management of pain, malabsorption, and diabetes mellitus. Internal surgical drainage (pancreaticojejunostomy) or endoscopic placement of stents may be helpful in patients who are resistant to medical management of pain. Enzyme supplementation (lipase) allows fat digestion.

XI. MALABSORPTION AND MALDIGESTION

Malabsorption of nutrients is reflected by impaired absorption of fat (steatorrhea), though other substances may also be poorly absorbed. Steatorrhea is usually a result of small bowel, liver, or biliary tract disease or pancreatic exocrine insufficiency. Hypoalbuminemia may develop in small bowel disease and deficiencies in fat soluble vitamins, hypocalcemia, and Hypomagnesemia may develop with liver or biliary tract disease.

A. **Gluten-Sensitive Enteropathy.** Previously termed *celiac disease* and *nontropical sprue*, gluten-sensitive enteropathy is a disease of the small intestine resulting in malabsorption (steatorrhea), weight loss, abdominal pain, and fatigue. Treatment is removal of gluten (wheat, rye, barley) from the diet.

B. **Small Bowel Resection.** If the small intestinal surface area that remains for absorption is decreased below critical levels, small bowel resection may result in malabsorption (*short bowle syndrome*). Diarrhea, steatorrhea, trace element deficiencies, and electrolyte imbalances (*hyponatremia, hypokalemias*) can result. Total parenteral nutrition is needed if multiple small feedings are not effective.

XII. GASTROINTESTINAL BLEEDING (Table 14-13)

A. **Upper Gastrointestinal Bleeding.** Patients with acute upper GI bleeding may experience hypotension and tachycardia if blood loss exceeds approximately 25% of the total blood volume (1500 mL in adults). Most patients with evidence of acute hemorrhage (orthostatic hypotension characterized by decreases in systolic blood pressure of 10 to 20 mm Hg and corresponding increases in heart rate) have hematocrits less than 30%. The hematocrit may be normal early in the course of acute hemorrhage because of the insufficient time for equilibration of the plasma volume.

1. **Melena.** Usually melena indicates that bleeding has occurred at a site above the cecum. The blood urea nitrogen concentration is usually higher than 40 mg/dL because of the absorbed nitrogen load in the small intestine.
2. **Treatment.** For patients with bleeding peptic ulcers, endoscopic coagulation (thermotherapy, or injection with epinephrine or a sclerosant) is indicated when active bleeding is visible. Surgical treatment of nonvariceal upper GI bleeding (oversewing an ulcer, gastrectomy for diffuse hemorrhagic gastritis) is used in patients who continue to bleed despite optimal supportive therapy and in whom endoscopic coagulation is unsuccessful.

B. **Lower Gastrointestinal Bleeding.** Typically, lower GI bleeding manifests as abrupt passage of bright red blood and clots. Etiology includes diverticulosis, tumors, ischemic colitis, and infectious colitis. Sigmoidoscopy to exclude anorectal lesions is indicated as soon as patients are hemodynamically stable. If bleeding is persistent and brisk, angiography and embolic therapy may be attempted. Control of lower GI bleeding may require surgical intervention.

TABLE 14-13 ■ **Causes of Upper and Lower Gastrointestinal Bleeding**

CAUSES	INCIDENCE (%)
UPPER GASTROINTESTINAL BLEEDING	
Peptic ulcer	
Duodenal ulcer	36
Gastric ulcer	24
Mucosal erosive disease	
Gastritis	6
Esophagitis	6
Esophageal varices	6
Mallory-Weiss tear	3
Malignancy	2
LOWER GASTROINTESTINAL BLEEDING	
Colonic diverticulosis	42
Colorectal malignancy	9
Ischemic colitis	9
Acute colitis of unknown causes	5
Hemorrhoids	5

Adapted from Young HS. Gastrointestinal bleeding. *Sci Am Med.* 1998;1-10.

C. Occult Gastrointestinal Bleeding. Unexplained iron deficiency anemia or intermittent positive results of tests for blood in the feces may indicate occult GI bleeding. PUD and colonic neoplasm are the most common causes of occult GI bleeding.

XIII. DIVERTICULOSIS AND DIVERTICULITIS

Colonic diverticula, herniations of the mucosa and submucosa through the muscularis propria, occur most often in individuals who consume low-fiber diets. Diverticulitis occurs with inflammation of one or more diverticula, usually in the sigmoid or descending colon.

A. Signs and Symptoms. Signs and symptoms include fever and lower abdominal pain and tenderness. Nausea, vomiting, constipation, diarrhea, dysuria, tachycardia, and an elevated white blood cell count with a left shift may be noted. Right-sided colonic diverticulitis is usually indistinguishable from appendicitis. Severe diverticulitis can manifest with purulent peritonitis. Abdominal computed tomography is the most useful study for early evaluation of suspected diverticulitis.

B. Treatment. Treatment includes 7 to 10 days of broad-spectrum antimicrobial therapy, which includes anaerobic coverage. Intravenous fluids, bowel rest, and analgesics may also be needed. Surgical treatment (resection of diseased colon) may be required if the patient's condition does not improve within 48 hours despite maximal medical therapy.

XIV. APPENDICITIS

Appendicitis is often associated with obstruction of the lumen of the appendix by a fecalith, followed by bacterial invasion of the appendiceal wall and arterial compromise to the appendix because of high intraluminal pressures. Peak incidence is in the second and third decades of life.

A. Clinical Manifestations. Symptoms include mild, poorly localized abdominal pain, often cramping in nature. As inflammation spreads, pain becomes steadier, more severe, and localized to the right lower quadrant. Anorexia is very common, and nausea and vomiting occur in

TABLE 14-14 ■ Differential Diagnosis: Appendicitis

Mesenteric lymphadenitis	Ureteral calculus	Pelvic inflammatory disease
Ruptured graafian follicle	Acute cholecystitis	Corpus luteum cyst
Acute pancreatitis	Acute gastroenteritis	Strangulating intestinal obstruction
Perforated ulcer	Acute diverticulitis	No organic disease

TABLE 14-15 ■ Causes of Peritonitis

BOWEL PERFORATION
Trauma, iatrogenic causes (endoscopic perforation, ischemia, anastomotic leak, catheter perforation), ingested foreign body, inflammatory bowel disease, vascular causes (embolus, ischemia) strangulated hernia, volvulus, intussusception
OTHER ORGAN LEAK
Pancreatitis, cholecystitis, salpingitis, bile leak after biopsy, urinary bladder rupture
PERITONEAL DISRUPTION
Peritoneal dialysis, intraperitoneal chemotherapy, retained postoperative foreign body, penetrating fistula, trauma

50% to 60% of cases. The temperature is usually normal or slightly elevated (high temperature suggests perforation). For the differential diagnosis, see Table 14-14.

B. Treatment. Treatment is early surgery and appendectomy.

XV. PERITONITIS

Peritonitis is an inflammation of the peritoneum caused by spontaneous bacterial hematogenous spread or secondary to an intraabdominal process (Table 14-15).

A. Clinical Features. Signs and symptoms include acute abdominal pain and tenderness, often with rebound pain or rigidity of the abdominal wall, fever, absence of bowel sounds, and often tachycardia, hypotension, and signs of dehydration. Leukocytosis and acidosis are common laboratory findings. Ascites may show high numbers of neutrophils and increased protein and lactate dehydrogenase levels.

B. Treatment. Treatment is rehydration, correction of electrolyte abnormalities, antibiotics, and surgical correction of the underlying defect.

XVI. ACUTE COLONIC PSEUDO-OBSTRUCTION

Acute colonic pseudo-obstruction is a clinical syndrome characterized by massive dilation of the colon in the absence of mechanical obstruction. It occurs most often in hospitalized patients with medical or surgical disease. A current hypothesis is that an imbalance in neural input to the colon distal to the splenic flexure, with an excess of sympathetic stimulation and a paucity of parasympathetic input, results in spastic contraction of the distal colon and *functional* obstruction. Patients who fail conservative therapy (hydration, mobilization, enemas, nasogastric suction) for more than 48 hours should be considered for an active intervention. An intravenous administration of the cholinesterase inhibitor neostigmine at a dose of 2.0 to 2.5 mg given over 3 to 5 minutes, results in immediate colonic decompression in 80% to 90% of patients. Decompressive colonoscopy or placement of a cecostomy are other options.

CHAPTER 15

Inborn Errors of Metabolism

The presence of nutritional disorders or inborn errors of metabolism will significantly influence the management of anesthesia.

I. INBORN ERRORS OF METABOLISM (TABLE 15-1)

A. **Porphyrias.** Porphyrias are a group of inborn errors of metabolism characterized by the overproduction of porphyrins (essential for many vital physiologic functions, including oxygen transport and storage) and their precursors. The synthetic pathway involved in the production of porphyrins is determined by a sequence of enzymes. A defect in any of these enzymes results in accumulation of the preceding intermediaries and produces a form of porphyria (Figure 15-1). Heme is the most important porphyrin (hemoglobin and cytochrome P-450), and its production is controlled by aminolevulinic acid (ALA) synthetase, an inducible enzyme.

1. **Classification** (Table 15-2). Porphyrias are classified as either hepatic or erythropoietic depending on the primary site of production or accumulation of the precursors or porphyrins. Only acute forms of porphyria are relevant to the management of anesthesia, as they are the only forms of porphyria that may result in life-threatening reactions in response to certain drugs.
2. **Acute Porphyrias.** Acute attacks are most commonly precipitated by events that decrease heme concentrations, thus increasing the activity of ALA synthetase and stimulating the production of porphyrinogens (see Figure 15-1). Enzyme-inducing drugs are the most important triggering factors for the development of acute porphyrias.
   a. ***Signs and Symptoms.*** Acute attacks are characterized by severe abdominal pain, autonomic nervous system instability (tachycardia, hypertension), electrolyte disturbances, dehydration, skeletal muscle weakness, seizures, and other neuropsychiatric manifestations ranging from mild disturbances to fulminating life-threatening events. Complete and prolonged remissions are likely between attacks. Many individuals with the genetic defect never develop symptoms. Patients may experience their first symptoms in response to inadvertent administration of triggering drugs during the perioperative period. ALA synthetase concentrations are increased during all acute attacks of porphyria.
   b. ***Triggering Drugs.*** *See Table 15-3.*
   c. ***Types of Porphyria***
      i. ***Acute Intermittent Porphyria.*** This type of porphyria produces the most serious symptoms (systemic hypertension, renal dysfunction) and is the one most likely to be life-threatening.
      ii. ***Variegate Porphyria.*** Variegate porphyria is characterized by neurotoxicity and cutaneous photosensitivity in which bullous skin eruptions occur on exposure to sunlight as a result of the conversion of porphyrinogens to porphyrins.
      iii. ***Hereditary Coproporphyria.*** Acute attacks of hereditary coproporphyria are less common than acute intermittent porphyria or variegate porphyria. Neurotoxicity and cutaneous hypersensitivity are characteristic but less severe.

TABLE 15-1 ■ Inborn Errors of Metabolism

Porphyria
Purine metabolism disorders
Hyperlipidemia
Carbohydrate metabolism disorders
Amino acid disorders
Mucopolysaccharidoses
Gangliosidoses

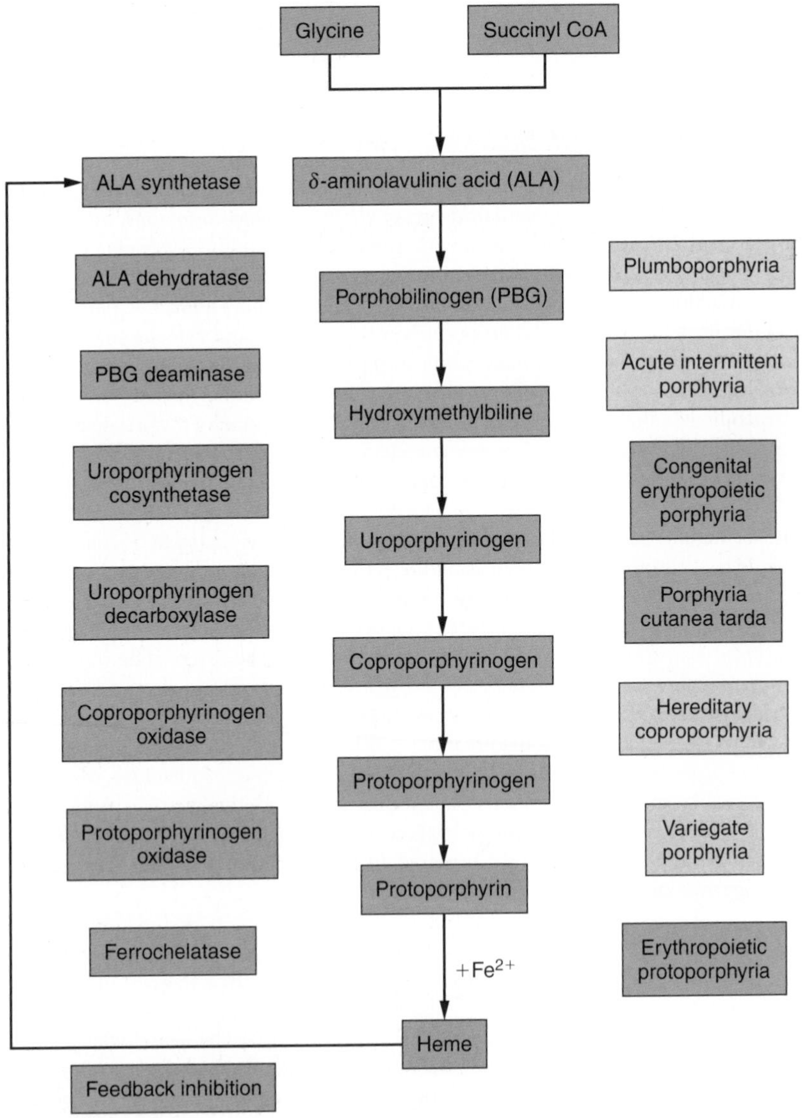

FIGURE 15-1 ■ Metabolic pathways for heme synthesis. Enzymes are noted on the feedback inhibition loop of the sequence, and the type of porphyria associated with the enzyme deficiency is designated on the right. Examples of acute porphyrias are indicated by the dark boxes. *CoA*, Coenzyme A. (Adapted from James MF, Hift RJ. Porphyrias. *Br J Anaesth*. 2000;85:143-153.)

TABLE 15-2 ■ **Classification of Porphyrias**

HEPATIC
Acute intermittent porphyria Variegate porphyria Hereditary coproporphyria Aminolevulinic acid dehydratase porphyria Porphyria cutanea tarda
ERYTHROPOIETIC
Congenital erythropoietic porphyrias Erythropoietic protoporphyria

TABLE 15-3 ■ **Recommendations Regarding the Use of Anesthetic Drugs in the Presence of Acute Porphyrias**

DRUG	RECOMMENDATION
INHALED ANESTHETICS	
Nitrous oxide	Safe
Isoflurane	Probably safe*
Sevoflurane	Probably safe*
Desflurane	Probably safe*
INTRAVENOUS ANESTHETICS	
Propofol	Safe
Ketamine	Probably safe*
Thiopental	Avoid
Thiamylal	Avoid
Methohexital	Avoid
Etomidate	Avoid
ANALGESICS	
Acetaminophen	Safe
Aspirin	Safe
Codeine	Safe
Morphine	Safe
Fentanyl	Safe
Sufentanil	Safe
Ketorolac	Probably avoid†
Phenacetin	Probably avoid†
Pentazocine	Avoid
NEUROMUSCULAR BLOCKING DRUGS	
Succinylcholine	Safe
Pancuronium	Safe

Continued

TABLE 15-3 ■ Recommendations Regarding the Use of Anesthetic Drugs in the Presence of Acute Porphyrias—cont'd

DRUG	RECOMMENDATION
Atracurium	Probably safe*
Cisatracurium	Probably safe*
Vecuronium	Probably safe*
Rocuronium	Probably safe*
Mivacurium	Probably safe*
OPIOID ANTAGONIST	
Naloxone	Safe
ANTICHOLINERGICS	
Atropine	Safe
Glycopyrrolate	Safe
ANTICHOLINESTERASE	
Neostigmine	Safe
LOCAL ANESTHETICS	
Lidocaine	Safe
Tetracaine	Safe
Bupivacaine	Safe
Mepivacaine	Safe
Ropivacaine	No data
SEDATIVES AND ANTIEMETICS	
Droperidol	Safe
Midazolam	Probably safe*
Lorazepam	Probably safe*
Cimetidine	Probably safe*
Ranitidine	Probably safe*
Metoclopramide	Probably safe*
Ondansetron	Probably safe*
CARDIOVASCULAR DRUGS	
Epinephrine	Safe
α-Agonists	Safe
β-Agonists	Safe
β-Antagonists	Safe
Diltiazem	Probably safe*
Nitroprusside	Probably safe*
Nifedipine	Probably avoid†

Adapted from James MFM, Hift RJ. Porphyrias. *Br J Anaesth.* 2000;85:143-153.

*Although safety is not conclusively established, the drug is unlikely to provoke acute porphyria.

†Use only if expected benefits outweigh the risks.

iv. ***Porphyria Cutanea Tarda.*** ALA synthetase activity is not important in this form of porphyria, and drugs capable of precipitating attacks of other forms of porphyria do *not* provoke an attack of porphyria cutanea tarda. Signs and symptoms most often appear as photosensitivity in men older than 35 years of age. Anesthesia is not a hazard, although the choice of drugs should take into consideration the likely presence of co-existing liver disease.

v. ***Erythropoietic Uroporphyria.*** In contrast to porphyrin synthesis in the liver, porphyrin synthesis in the erythropoietic system is responsive to changes in hematocrit and tissue oxygenation. Hemolytic anemia, bone marrow hyperplasia, and splenomegaly are often present. Repeated infections are common, and photosensitivity is severe. The urine of affected patients turns red when exposed to light. Neurotoxicity and abdominal pain do not occur.

vi. ***Erythropoietic Protoporphyria.*** A less debilitating form of erythropoietic porphyria, erythropoietic protoporphyria is characterized by photosensitivity, urticaria, and edema. Administration of barbiturates does not affect the course of the disease. Survival to adulthood is common.

d. ***Management of Anesthesia.*** Most patients with porphyria can be safely anesthetized, assuming that appropriate precautions are taken (short-acting drugs to limit exposure and reduce enzyme induction, avoidance of repeated or prolonged use). Exposure to multiple potential enzyme-inducing drugs may be more dangerous than exposure to any one drug. The American Porphyria Foundation maintains a drug database at www.drugs-porphyria.com.

i. ***Preoperative Evaluation.*** The evaluation includes a careful family history, examination for skin lesions, and notation of the presence of peripheral and/or autonomic neuropathy. If an acute attack is suspected, evaluation and treatment of fluid and electrolyte disorders should be undertaken. If prolonged fasting is anticipated, administration of a glucose-containing infusion should be considered (caloric restriction has been linked to the precipitation of acute porphyria attacks). If an acute attack is suspected in the perioperative period, important aspects of evaluation include muscle strength and cranial nerve function, because abnormalities may predict impending respiratory failure and pulmonary aspiration.

(a) ***Preoperative Medication.*** Benzodiazepines are often used. Aspiration prophylaxis with antacids and H_2-receptor antagonists is reasonable.

(b) ***Prophylactic Therapy.*** None has proven to be beneficial. Oral carbohydrate supplements or infusion of 10% glucose may be helpful.

ii. ***Regional Anesthesia.*** There is no absolute contraindication to the use of regional anesthesia, but it is essential to perform a neurologic examination before the block to minimize the likelihood that worsening of any preexisting neuropathy would be erroneously attributed to the regional anesthetic. Autonomic nervous system blockade induced by the regional anesthetic could unmask cardiovascular instability (autonomic neuropathy, hypovolemia, or both). There is no evidence that any local anesthetic has ever induced an acute attack of porphyria or caused neurologic damage in individuals with porphyria.

iii. ***General Anesthesia.*** The total dose of drugs administered and the length of exposure may influence the risk of triggering a porphyric crisis in vulnerable patients (see Table 15-3).

(a) ***Induction.*** Propofol has been used safely, although prolonged infusion is of unproven safety. Ketamine has been used safely. The use of etomidate is controversial. All barbiturates should be considered unsafe.

(b) ***Maintenance.*** Nitrous oxide is safe, as is isoflurane. Experience with sevoflurane and desflurane is limited. Opioids and neuromuscular blocking agents appear safe.

iv. ***Cardiopulmonary Bypass.*** Clinical experience does not support an increased incidence of porphyric crises in these patients when undergoing cardiopulmonary bypass.

v. ***Treatment of a Porphyric Crisis.*** Treatment includes removal of any known triggering factors; adequate hydration and carbohydrates; correction of electrolyte disturbances; sedation; treatment of pain, nausea, and vomiting; β-adrenergic blockers to control tachycardia and hypertension; and anticonvulsants to control seizures. Heme, as hematin, heme albumin, or heme arginine (3 to 4 mg/kg intravenously [IV] over 20 minutes) is the only specific form of therapy for an acute porphyric crisis. Somatostatin decreases the rate of formation of ALA synthetase and combined with plasmapheresis may effectively decrease pain and induce remission.

B. **Gout.** Gout is a disorder of purine metabolism characterized by hyperuricemia with recurrent episodes of acute arthritis caused by deposition of urate crystals in joints. The incidence of systemic hypertension, ischemic heart disease, and diabetes mellitus is increased in patients with gout.

1. **Treatment.** Treatment consists of decreasing serum concentrations of uric acid (probenecid, allopurinol) and colchicine to relieve joint pain, presumably by modifying leukocyte migration and phagocytosis.
2. **Management of Anesthesia.** Management of anesthesia focuses on prehydration to facilitate continued renal elimination of uric acid. Sodium bicarbonate alkalinizes the urine and facilitates excretion of uric acid. The increased incidence of systemic hypertension, ischemic heart disease, and diabetes mellitus in patients with gout is considered. Renal dysfunction is associated with increased clinical manifestations of gout. Probenecid and colchicine administration may be associated with decreased renal and hepatic function. Temporomandibular joint gout can be associated with difficult laryngoscopy.

C. **Lesch-Nyhan Syndrome.** Lesch-Nyhan syndrome is a genetically determined disorder of purine metabolism that occurs exclusively in males and is characterized by mental retardation, spasticity, and self-mutilation patterns that usually involve trauma to perioral tissues. Subsequent scarification may present difficulties with direct laryngoscopy for tracheal intubation. Anesthesia management may be affected by impaired drug metabolism and co-existing renal dysfunction. Sympathetic nervous system response to stress is enhanced.

D. **Disorders of Carbohydrate Metabolism.** Usually disorders of carbohydrate metabolism reflect genetically determined enzyme defects.

1. **Glycogen Storage Disease Type 1a (von Gierke's Disease).** This type of glycogen storage disease is caused by the deficiency or lack of the enzyme glucose-6-phosphatase. As a result, glycogen cannot be hydrolyzed so it accumulates intracellularly. Characteristics are severe hypoglycemia, metabolic acidosis, osteoporosis, mental retardation, growth retardation, seizures, hepatomegaly, and platelet dysfunction. Death usually occurs by age 2. Management of anesthesia includes provision of exogenous glucose, avoidance of lactate-containing solutions, and monitoring of arterial pH.
2. **Glycogen Storage Disease Type 1b.** Glycogen storage disease type 1b is deficiency of glucose-6-phosphate (a product of glycogen metabolism) transport that results in glycogen accumulation in the liver, kidneys, and intestinal mucosa. Hypoglycemia and lactic acidosis ensue. Clinical signs and symptoms resemble those described for glycogen storage disease type 1a. Preoperative fasting should be minimized, and perioperative glucose-containing infusions should be administered. Mechanical hyperventilation may stimulate release of lactate from skeletal muscle and worsen metabolic acidosis.

E. **Disorders of Amino Acid Metabolism.** There are more than 70 known disorders of amino acid metabolism, but most are extremely rare. Classic manifestations include mental retardation, seizures, and aminoaciduria (Table 15-4). Metabolic acidosis, hyperammonemia, hepatic failure, and thromboembolism can also occur. Management of anesthesia is directed toward maintenance of intravascular volume and acid-base homeostasis.

1. **Phenylketonuria.** The prototype of disorders caused by abnormal amino acid metabolism is phenylketonuria. Clinical features include mental retardation and seizures. Patients are more liable to develop vitamin B_{12} deficiency. They may also be more sensitive to narcotics.

TABLE 15-4 ■ **Disorders of Amino Acid Metabolism**

DISORDER	MENTAL RETARDATION	SEIZURES	METABOLIC ACIDOSIS	HYPERAMMONEMIA	HEPATIC FAILURE	THROMBOEMBOLISM	OTHER
Phenylketonuria	Yes	Yes	No	No	No	No	Friable skin
Homocystinuria	Yes/no	Yes	No	No	No	Yes	
Hypervalinemia	Yes	Yes	Yes	No	No	No	Hypoglycemia
Citrullinemia	Yes	Yes	No	Yes	Yes	No	
Branched-chain aciduria (maple syrup urine disease)	Yes	Yes	Yes	No		Yes	Hypoglycemia Neurologic deterioration during perioperative period
Methylmalonyl-coenzyme A mutase deficiency			Yes	Yes			Acidosis intraoperatively Avoid nitrous oxide?
Isoleucinemia	Yes	Yes	Yes	Yes	Yes	No	Hypovolemia
Methioninemia	Yes	No	No	No	No	No	Thermal instability
Histidinuria	Yes	Yes/no	No	No	No	No	Erythrocyte fragility
Neutral aminoaciduria (Hartnup's disease)	Yes/no		Yes	No	No	No	Dermatitis
Argininemia	Yes		No	Yes	Yes	No	

2. **Homocystinuria.** Manifestations include dislocation of the lens, osteoporosis, kyphoscoliosis, brittle light-colored hair, malar flush, and often mental retardation. Thromboembolism (caused by activation of the Hageman factor by homocysteine and increased platelet adhesiveness) can be life-threatening. Efforts to reduce the risk of thromboembolism during the perioperative period should include administration of pyridoxine or betaine (decreases platelet adhesiveness), hydration, infusion of dextran, and early ambulation.
3. **Maple Syrup Urine Disease.** A disorder in which a metabolic defect causes the urine to smell like maple syrup, maple syrup urine disease is associated with growth retardation and delayed psychomotor development. Infection or fasting often results in acute metabolic decompensation. Glucose-containing intravenous solutions should be administered intraoperatively. Measurement of arterial pH is helpful for detecting metabolic acidosis, which may necessitate treatment with intravenous sodium bicarbonate.
4. **Methylmalonyl-Coenzyme A Mutase Deficiency.** Methylmalonyl-coenzyme A mutase deficiency is caused by an inborn error of metabolism resulting in the formation of methylmalonic acidemia. Events during the perioperative period that increase protein catabolism (fasting, bleeding into the gastrointestinal tract, stress response, tissue destruction) predispose to acidosis. Clear fluid ingestion should be allowed up to 2 hours before scheduled induction of anesthesia. Anesthesia management involves minimizing hypovolemia and protein catabolism.

CHAPTER 16

Nutritional Diseases—Obesity and Malnutrition

Nutritional diseases are caused by underconsumption of essential nutrients or overconsumption of poor nutrients.

I. OBESITY

Obesity (body weight of 20% or more above ideal weight) is associated with increased morbidity and mortality and a wide spectrum of medical and surgical diseases (Tables 16-1 and 16-2). Risk of premature death is doubled in the obese population and risk of death resulting from cardiovascular disease is increased fivefold in the obese compared with the nonobese.

A. Pathophysiology. Obesity is a complex, multifactorial disease (mechanisms of fat storage, genetic, psychologic). Most simply, it occurs when net energy intake exceeds net energy expenditure over a prolonged period of time.

1. **Fat Storage.** Surplus calories are converted to triglycerides and stored in adipocytes, a process regulated by lipoprotein lipase. Central or *android* distribution of fat (more common in men) manifests as abdominal obesity. Abdominal fat deposits are metabolically more active than peripheral or *gynecoid* fat distribution (hips, buttocks, thighs) and are associated with a higher incidence of metabolic complications (dyslipidemias, glucose intolerance and diabetes mellitus, ischemic heart disease, congestive heart failure, stroke).
2. **Cellular Disturbances.** Fatty infiltration of the pancreas leads to decreased insulin secretion, and engorgement of adipocytes leads to insulin resistance. Engorged adipocytes secrete cytokines and tumor necrosis factor α, which worsen insulin resistance through secretion of adiponectin. Leptin, also secreted by adipose tissue, modulates hypothalamic secretion of neuropeptides regulating energy expenditure, food intake and decreases appetite. Leptin accelerates inflammatory changes. Ghrelin, a hormone opposing leptin, increases appetite via modulation of gastric vagal afferents. All of these substances stimulate the liver to produce very low-density lipoproteins and apolipoprotein B, stimulating the pancreas to produce more insulin and more pancreatic polypeptides, resulting in diffuse intracellular inflammatory changes.
3. **Genetic Factors.** Statistics suggest that more than half of the variations in BMI are genetically influenced.
4. **Environmental Factors.** Technologic advances have contributed to a decline in physical activity over the last 50 years. Consumption of high-calorie foods and aging contribute to obesity.
5. **Psychologic and Socioeconomic Factors.** Eating disorders associated with depression and obesity include binge-eating and night-eating syndromes (Table 16-3).

B. Diseases Associated with Obesity (see Table 16-1)

1. **Endocrine Disorders**

TABLE 16-1 ■ **Medical and Surgical Conditions Associated with Obesity**

ORGAN SYSTEM	SIDE EFFECTS
Respiratory system	Obstructive sleep apnea Obesity hypoventilation syndrome Restrictive lung disease
Cardiovascular system	Systemic hypertension Cardiomegaly Congestive heart failure Ischemic heart disease Cerebrovascular disease Peripheral vascular disease Pulmonary hypertension Deep vein thrombosis Pulmonary embolism Hypercholesterolemia Hypertriglyceridemia Sudden death
Endocrine system	Diabetes mellitus Cushing syndrome Hypothyroidism
Gastrointestinal system	Hiatal hernia Inguinal hernia Gallstones Fatty liver infiltration
Musculoskeletal system	Osteoarthritis of weight-bearing joints Back pain
Malignancy	Breast Prostate Cervical Uterine Colorectal

Adapted from Adams JP, Murphy PG. Obesity in anaesthesia and intensive care. *Br J Anaesth.* 2000;85:91-108.

a. ***Metabolic Syndrome (or Syndrome X).*** Metabolic syndrome is defined as the presence of at least three of the following: large waist circumference, high triglyceride levels, low levels of high-density lipoprotein cholesterol, glucose intolerance, and hypertension.
b. ***Diabetes Mellitus.*** Glucose tolerance curves are often abnormal, and the incidence of diabetes mellitus is increased severalfold in obese patients, as a result of the resistance of peripheral tissues to the effects of insulin in the presence of increased adipose tissue.
c. ***Endocrinopathies That Cause Obesity.*** Hypothyroidism and Cushing's disease may be underlying causes of obesity.

2. **Cardiovascular Disorders**

a. ***Systemic Hypertension.*** Obesity-induced hypertension is related to the effects of hyperinsulinemia on the sympathetic nervous system and extracellular fluid volume. Insulin also activates adipose tissue to release angiotensinogen. Increased circulatory cytokines cause vascular damage and fibrosis, increasing arterial stiffness. Left ventricular (LV) hypertrophy can develop. Pulmonary hypertension is common and most likely reflects the impact of chronic arterial hypoxemia or increased pulmonary blood volume (or both). Weight loss significantly improves, or even resolves, hypertension.

TABLE 16-2 ■ **Body Mass Index (BMI) Weight Categories**

CATEGORY	BMI RANGE (kg/m^2)
ADULTS	
Underweight	<18.5
Normal	18.5-24.9
Overweight	25-29.9
Obese class I	30-34.9
Obese class II	35-39.9
Obese class III (severe, morbid)	≥40
CHILDREN (2-18 yr)	
Overweight	85th-94th percentile
Obese	95th percentile or BMI ≥30
Severely obese	99th percentile

TABLE 16-3 ■ **Criteria for Common Eating Disorders**

BINGE-EATING DISORDER
Consumption of large meals rapidly and without control
Three or more of the following: rapid eating, solitary or secretive eating, eating despite fullness, eating without hunger, self-disgust, guilt, depression
Striking distress while eating
No compensatory features—that is, no excess exercise, purging, or fasting
Persistence for more than 2 days/wk for 6 mo
If vomiting is part of the disorder, it is classified as bulimia
NIGHT-EATING SYNDROME
Evening hyperphagia (>50% of daily intake occurs after the evening meal)
Guilt, tension, and anxiety while eating
Frequent waking with more eating
Morning anorexia
Consumption of sugars and other carbohydrates at inappropriate times
Persistence for >2 mo

Adapted from Stunkard AJ. Binge-eating disorder and the night-eating syndrome. In: Wadden TA, Stunkard AJ, eds. *Handbook of Obesity Treatment.* New York, NY: Guilford Press; 2002:107-121.

b. ***Coronary Artery Disease.*** Obesity seems to be an independent risk factor for the development of ischemic heart disease and is more common in individuals with central/android fat distribution.

c. ***Congestive Heart Failure*** *(Figure 16-1).* Systemic hypertension causes concentric LV hypertrophy and a progressively noncompliant left ventricle, which, when combined with hypervolemia, increases the risk of congestive heart failure. Obesity-induced cardiomyopathy is associated with hypervolemia and increased cardiac output. Insulin resistance also appears to play a role via cardiac steatosis, lipoapoptosis, and activation of cardiac genes that promote LV remodeling. Some of these structural and functional changes may reverse with significant weight loss.

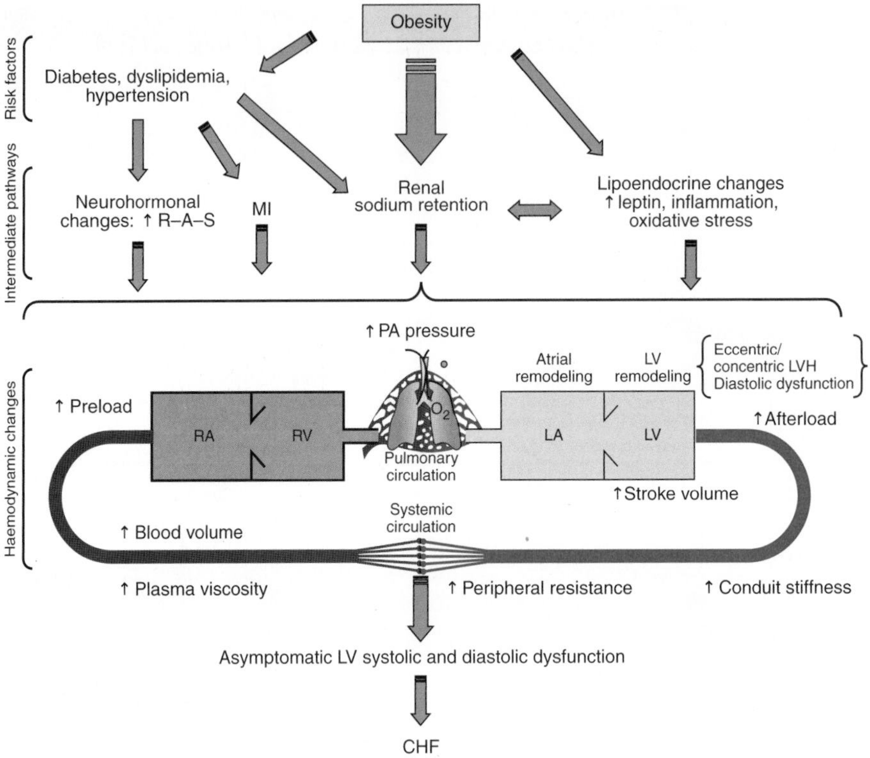

FIGURE 16-1 ■ Cardiac changes in obesity leading to heart failure. *LA*, left atrium; *LV*, left ventricle; *LVH*, left ventricular hypertrophy; *MI*, myocardial infarction; *PA*, pulmonary artery; *RA*, right atrium; *R-A-S*, renin-angiotensin-aldosterone; *RV*, right ventricle.

3. Respiratory Disorders

a. ***Lung Volumes.*** Obesity imposes a restrictive ventilatory defect because the weight of the thoracic cage and abdomen impedes the motion of the diaphragm and decreases functional residual capacity (FRC), especially in the supine position. These changes are accentuated by general anesthesia and impair the ability of obese patients to tolerate apnea (i.e., during direct laryngoscopy), resulting in rapid arterial oxygen desaturation after induction of anesthesia, often despite preoxygenation.

b. ***Gas Exchange and Work of Breathing.*** $PaCO_2$ and ventilatory response to carbon dioxide remain within a normal range in obese patients. Normocapnia is maintained by increased minute ventilation, resulting in increased work of breathing.

c. ***Lung Compliance and Resistance.*** Obesity is associated with a decrease in lung compliance and an increase in airway resistance that result in rapid, shallow breathing patterns and increased work of breathing that is most marked in the supine position.

d. ***Obstructive Sleep Apnea (OSA).*** OSA is cessation of breathing for more than 10 seconds during sleep, and hypopnea is a reduction in the size and number of breaths compared with normal breathing. OSA is present in about 5% of middle-aged adults and in about 40% of severely obese patients (Table 16-4).

i. ***Pathogenesis.*** Apnea occurs when the pharyngeal airways collapse. Increased inspiratory effort and response to arterial hypoxemia and hypercarbia cause arousal, which in turn restores upper airway tone. Repeated cycles occur during sleep.

ii. ***Risk Factors.*** Male gender, middle age, BMI over 30 kg/m^2, evening alcohol consumption, and use of pharmacologic sleep aids are risk factors.

TABLE 16-4 ■ Obstructive Sleep Apnea

Manifestations	Frequent episodes of (≥10 seconds, occurring ≥5 times/hr during sleep) or hypopnea (decrease in size and number of breaths) Snoring Daytime somnolence (concentration and memory problems, motor vehicle accidents) Physiologic changes; arterial hypoxemia, polycythemia, arterial hypercarbia, systemic hypertension, pulmonary hypertension, right ventricular failure
Risk factors	Male gender Middle age Obesity (BMI >30) Alcohol (evening ingestion) Drug-induced sleep

BMI, Body mass index.

iii. ***Treatment.*** Weight loss can result in significant improvement or resolution. Positive airway pressure, delivered through a nasal mask, is the initial treatment of choice for clinically significant OSA. Patients with mild sleep apnea who do not tolerate positive airway pressure may benefit from nighttime application of oral appliances designed to enlarge the airway by keeping the tongue in an anterior position or by displacing the mandible forward. Drug therapy (protriptyline, fluoxetine) has not been demonstrated to be effective. Nocturnal oxygen therapy is a consideration for individuals who experience severe arterial oxygen desaturation. Surgical treatment of OSA includes tracheostomy (in patients with severe apnea who do not tolerate positive airway pressure), palatal surgery (laser-assisted uvulopalatopharyngoplasty), and maxillofacial surgical procedures to enhance upper airway patency during sleep (genioglossal advancement).

iv. ***Obesity Hypoventilation Syndrome*** Apnea without respiratory efforts (obesity hypoventilation syndrome), is the long-term consequence of OSA. At its extreme, obesity hypoventilation syndrome culminates in the *pickwickian syndrome* (obesity, daytime hypersomnolence, arterial hypoxemia, polycythemia, hypercarbia, respiratory acidosis, pulmonary hypertension, right ventricular failure).

4. **Hepatobiliary Disease.** Abnormal liver function test results and fatty liver infiltration are common findings in obese patients. The risk of developing gallbladder and biliary tract disease is increased threefold.

   a. ***Nonalcoholic Fatty Liver Disease/Nonalcoholic Steatohepatitis (NAFLD/NASH).*** Accumulation of excess intrahepatic triglycerides, impaired insulin activity, and release of inflammatory cytokines leads to destruction of hepatocytes. NAFLD/NASH has become one of the most common causes of end-stage liver disease. In the United States, 85% of severely obese adults have NAFLD. NAFLD can progress to cirrhosis, portal hypertension, and/or hepatocellular carcinoma. Weight loss significantly improves and sometimes cures this form of hepatic inflammation.

   b. ***Gallbladder Disease.*** Supersaturation of bile with cholesterol predisposes to cholelithiasis. Women with BMI greater than 32 kg/m^2 have a threefold higher risk of gallstones, and those with a BMI greater than 45 kg/m^2 have a sevenfold higher risk, than the general population. Rapid weight loss *increases* the risk of gallstones.

   c. ***Gastric Emptying and Gastroesophageal Reflux Disease (GERD).*** Obesity is associated with *increased* gastric emptying, although obese patients have increased gastric volume.

5. **Inflammatory Syndrome of Obesity.** Obese patients have a higher rate of perioperative infections, which may be caused by impaired neutrophil function secondary to secretion of proinflammatory cytokines by adipocytes.
6. **Cancer.** Obesity appears to be associated with about 24% to 33% of breast, colon, endometrial, renal, and esophageal cancers. Peripheral conversion of sex hormones by aromatase in adipose tissue maybe partly responsible.
7. **Thromboembolic Disorders.** The risk of deep vein thrombosis in obese patients undergoing surgery is approximately double that of nonobese individuals due to polycythemia, increased intraabdominal pressure, and immobilization. Risk of stroke is also increased. For every 1 unit increase in BMI above normal, there is a 4% increase in risk of ischemic stroke and 6% increase in risk of hemorrhagic stroke.
8. **Musculoskeletal Disorders.** Degenerative arthritis (degenerative joint disease [DJD]) is increased in obese patients.
9. **Nervous System.** Autonomic nervous system dysfunction and peripheral neuropathy are increased in obese patients.

C. **Treatment.** A weight loss of only 5 to 20 kg has been associated with a decrease in systemic blood pressure and plasma lipid concentrations and enhanced control of diabetes mellitus.
1. **Lifestyle Changes.** Exercise and decreased calorie intake are beneficial.
2. **Medications.** Currently, pharmacologic therapy in addition to weight management programs is recommended in patients with BMI greater than 27 and persistent comorbid conditions such as diabetes or hypertension, and in patients with BMI greater than 30 without comorbidities. Currently, only phentermine (related to amphetamine) has been approved by the U.S. Food and Drug Administration (FDA). Addition of medications that bind gastric and pancreatic lipases in the gut (orlistat) can promote weight loss. Drugs that increase energy expenditure (ephedrine) are not FDA approved.
3. **Surgical Treatment.** Adult bariatric surgery is most effective in patients with BMI over 40 (or BMI over 35 with comorbidities) and results in significant, sustained weight loss and reduction of obesity-related comorbidities (hypertension, diabetes).
   a. ***Types of Surgery***
      i. ***Restrictive Bariatric Procedures.*** Laparoscopic adjustable gastric banding, sleeve gastrectomy, and vertical banded gastroplasty are procedures in which a small gastric pouch is created. The normal absorptive physiology of the entire small intestine is intact, so specific nutrient deficiencies are rare after surgery.
      ii. ***Malabsorptive Bariatric Procedures.*** These procedures include distal gastric or jejunoileal bypass, biliopancreatic diversion (BPD), and duodenal switch. Typically, gastric reduction is combined with bypass of various lengths of small intestine. The procedures are associated with a high incidence of anemia, deficiency of fat-soluble vitamins, and protein-calorie malnutrition in the first year after this surgery.
      iii. ***Combined Bariatric Procedures.*** Roux-en-Y gastric bypass (RYGB) includes both gastric restriction and some degree of malabsorption. RYGB results in the greatest weight loss and improvement in obesity-related health issues.
   b. ***Surgical Complications.*** Higher complication rates are associated with abdominal obesity, male gender, BMI of 50 or more, diabetes, OSA, older age, and lower-volume surgical centers. Thirty-day mortality is 0.1% to 2%, with gastric banding having the lowest complication rate. Mortality of RYGB is 0.5% to 1.5%. Complications include anastomotic leaks, stricture formation, pulmonary embolism, sepsis, gastric prolapse, and bleeding. Less common complications include wound dehiscence, hernia or seroma formation, lymphocele, lymphorrhea, and suture extrusion. Nutritional complications include deficiencies of iron, vitamin B_{12}, vitamin K (with coagulopathy), and folate. Subclinical microdeficiency is possible. Additional complications include dumping syndrome; major malnutrition, such as protein-calorie malnutrition; Wernicke's encephalopathy; and peripheral neuropathy. Fat malabsorption can lead to fat-soluble vitamin imbalances.

Metabolic bone disease is a potential long-term complication. Despite the risk of complications, there is a significant survival benefit in patients who undergo bariatric surgery.

c. ***Pediatric and Adolescent Patients.*** Bariatric surgery in adolescents appears safe and effective. Current guidelines for bariatric surgery include adolescent patients with BMI of 30 to 34.9 with comorbidities.

D. Management of Anesthesia

1. **Preoperative Evaluation.** The focus is on cardiovascular and respiratory systems and airway evaluation.

a. ***History.*** The history should focus on symptoms such as chest pain, syncope, exertional dyspnea, and symptoms suggestive of OSA. Other concerns include the presence of GERD, control of systemic hypertension, and the presence of diabetes (diagnosed or previously undiagnosed).

b. ***Physical Examination.*** Any signs of respiratory or cardiac compromise should be identified, and a detailed assessment of the airway performed. Intravenous access should be assessed.

c. ***Preoperative Diagnostic Testing.*** Tests may include electrocardiography (looking for signs of right heart strain or right or left ventricular hypertrophy), chest x-ray examination if congestive heart failure is suspected, transthoracic echocardiography to evaluate left and right ventricular function and pulmonary hypertension, and arterial blood gases if severe OSA is suspected.

d. ***Home Medications.*** Most medications should be continued perioperatively, with the exception of oral hypoglycemics, angiotensin-converting enzyme inhibitors, angiotensin receptor blockers, anticoagulants, and nonsteroidal antiinflammatory drugs. Proton pump inhibitors should be taken the morning of surgery, and deep venous thromboembolism prophylaxis should be considered (low-molecular-weight heparin or unfractionated heparin).

e. ***Continuous Positive Airway Pressure (CPAP) or Bi-Level Positive Airway Pressure (BiPAP).*** If such treatment is used at home, the patient should bring the mask so that this therapy can be continued in the perioperative period.

2. **Intraoperative Management**

a. ***Positioning.*** Specially designed operating room tables may be needed, and special transfer devices (such as air transfer mattresses) can minimize the risk of injury to patient or staff. "Ramping" the patient may allow better ventilator mechanics. Pressure points require special attention. Neutral arm position is preferred when possible.

b. ***Laparoscopic Surgery.*** Pneumoperitoneum during laparoscopy causes physiologic changes that may be accentuated in obesity (increased venous return if abdominal pressure is 10 mm Hg or less, and decreased venous return with abdominal pressure 20 mm Hg or more with decreased cardiac output; hypercarbia, acidosis, and increased pulmonary vascular resistance; higher myocardial oxygen demand). Trendelenburg positioning may further compromise ventilation.

c. ***Choice of Anesthesia.*** Local or regional anesthesia is preferable to general anesthesia if feasible.

i. ***Regional Anesthesia.*** In obese patients regional anesthesia may be technically difficult, as bony landmarks are obscured. Local anesthetic requirements for spinal and epidural anesthesia in obese patients may be as much as 20% lower than in nonobese patients.

ii. ***General Anesthesia***

(a) ***Premedication.*** Use of benzodiazepines is controversial owing to risk of upper airway obstruction.

(b) ***Airway Management.*** Difficulties with mask ventilation and tracheal intubation may occur (because of fat face and cheeks, short neck, large tongue, excessive palatal and pharyngeal soft tissue, restricted mouth opening, limited cervical and

TABLE 16-5 ■ **Recommended Weight Basis for Anesthetic Medication Dosing in Obesity**

DOSAGE BASED ON TOTAL BODY WEIGHT	DOSAGE BASED ON LEAN BODY WEIGHT
Propofol loading dose	Propofol maintenance dose
Midazolam	Thiopental
Succinyl choline	Vecuronium
Cisatracurium and atracurium loading doses	Cisatracurium and atracurium maintenance doses
Pancuronium*	Rocuronium
	Remifentanil
	Fentanyl
	Sufentanil

*Pancuronium requires higher doses to maintain 90% depression of twitch height in obese patients, but it will also have a longer duration of action at higher doses.

mandibular mobility, or large breasts). Emergency airway equipment should be readily available. Rapid decreases in arterial oxygenation may be seen with direct laryngoscopy and tracheal intubation, and adequate preoxygenation is critical. Awake intubation may be a consideration in some patients. Obese patients are traditionally presumed to be at increased risk of pulmonary aspiration during the induction of anesthesia, but the risk of pulmonary aspiration is related to difficult tracheal intubation rather than to BMI. Use of a laryngeal mask airway (LMA) is successful in aiding intubation in 96% of obese patients and is successful in establishing ventilation in less than 1 minute in almost 100% of obese patients.

(c) ***Management of Ventilation.*** Controlled ventilation using large tidal volumes is often applied in an attempt to offset the decreased FRC. Positive end-expiratory pressure may improve ventilation/perfusion matching and arterial oxygenation in obese patients, but adverse effects on cardiac output and oxygen delivery may offset these benefits. Patients should be maintained in a semi-upright position during spontaneous ventilation during emergence.

(d) ***Pharmacokinetics*** *(Table 16-5).* The dosage of injectable drugs is hard to predict. Total blood volume may be increased, but fat has relatively low blood flow, and doses based on total weight may be relatively excessive. In general, loading doses should be based on *lean body weight.* Lean body weight is total body weight minus fat weight. In clinically severe obesity, lean body weight accounts for 20% to 40% of excess body weight. *Cardiac output is increased, which can affect* drug distribution after intravenous injection. Repeat injections should be based on pharmacologic response but can result in cumulative drug effects owing to storage of drug in fat. Liver dysfunction may decrease drug clearance from the circulation. Awakening of obese patients is more prompt after exposure to desflurane or sevoflurane than after administration of either isoflurane or propofol. Ketamine and dexmedetomidine may be useful anesthetic adjuncts for patients who are susceptible to narcotic-induced respiratory depression.

(e) ***Monitoring.*** The technical difficulty of placing intravenous catheters and invasive monitors may be increased by the presence of obesity. Invasive arterial monitoring should be used for the morbidly obese with severe cardiopulmonary disease and for those patients in whom a poor fit of the noninvasive blood pressure cuff is likely because of the severe conical shape of the upper arms or unavailability of appropriately sized cuffs. Transesophageal echocardiography and/or pulmonary artery catheterization may be needed in patients with CHF or pulmonary hypertension. For surgeries performed with the patient under local or regional anesthesia, capnography is recommended to decrease the risk of undetected airway obstruction.

(f) ***Fluid Management.*** Fluid management should be based on lean body weight. Urinary output during laparoscopic surgery does not necessarily reflect volume status.

3. **Postoperative Management**
   a. ***Extubation.*** When obese patients are fully recovered from the depressant effects of anesthetics, extubation is considered. Ideally, obese patients should recover in a head-up to sitting position. A history of OSA or obesity hypoventilation syndrome mandates intense postoperative monitoring to ensure maintenance of a patent upper airway and acceptable oxygenation and ventilation.
   b. ***Transport.*** Transport should occur with the patient awake, in a semi-upright position, and receiving supplemental oxygen.
   c. ***Postoperative Analgesia.*** Opioid depression of ventilation in obese patients is a concern, and the intramuscular route of administration may be unreliable owing to the unpredictable absorption of drugs. Patient-controlled analgesia or neuraxial opioids are commonly used. Nonsteroidal antiinflammatory agents may reduce narcotic requirements. Intravenous acetaminophen has been recently approved by the FDA. Ketamine and dexmedetomidine may be useful. Patients with OSA are at risk for development of postoperative hypoxemia. Adequacy of ventilation should be assessed for 24 to 48 hours postoperatively.
   d. ***Respiratory Monitoring and Management.*** Adequacy of ventilation should be assessed for 24 to 48 hours postoperatively. CPAP or BIPAP, if used at home, should be resumed.
   e. ***Discharge to an Unmonitored Setting.*** When pain is controlled and patient is no longer at significant risk of postoperative respiratory depression, he or she may be discharged to an unmonitored setting.
   f. ***Postoperative Complications.*** Wound infection is twice as common in obese as in nonobese patients. Mechanical ventilation may be required in patients who have a history of CO_2 retention. Risks associated with OSA may extend for several days into the postoperative period. Likelihood of deep vein thrombosis and pulmonary embolism is increased.

II. MALNUTRITION AND VITAMIN DEFICIENCIES

A. **Malnutrition.** Malnutrition is a medically distinct syndrome that is responsive to caloric support provided by enteral or total parenteral nutrition (TPN) (hyperalimentation). Malnourished patients are identified by the presence of serum albumin concentrations below 3 g/dL, transferrin levels below 200 mg/dL, and prealbumin level of less than 15 mg/dL. Critically ill patients often experience negative caloric intake complicated by hypermetabolic states caused by increased caloric needs produced by trauma, fever, sepsis, and wound healing.

1. **Treatment.** It is often recommended that patients who have lost more than 20% of their body weight be treated nutritionally before undergoing elective surgery.
   a. ***Enteral Nutrition.*** When the gastrointestinal tract is functioning, enteral nutrition can be provided by means of nasogastric or gastrostomy tube feedings. Complications of enteral feedings are infrequent but may include hyperglycemia leading to osmotic diuresis and hypovolemia. Exogenous insulin administration is a consideration in such patients. Nasogastric and orogastric feedings should be discontinued 8 hours before surgery, and the stomach should be suctioned before the patient is taken to the operating room.
   b. ***Total Parenteral Nutrition.*** TPN is indicated when the gastrointestinal tract is not functioning. When daily caloric requirements exceed 2000 calories or prolonged nutritional support is required, a catheter is placed in the subclavian vein to permit infusion of hypertonic parenteral solutions (approximately 1900 mOsm/L) in a daily volume of approximately 40 mL/kg. Potential complications of TPN are numerous (Table 16-6).

B. **Vitamin Deficiencies** (Table 16-7)

TABLE 16-6 ■ Other Complications of Total Parenteral Nutrition and Peripheral Parenteral Nutrition

Hypokalemia Hypophosphatemia Bacterial translocation from the gastrointestinal tract Renal dysfunction Nonketotic hyperosmolar hyperglycemic coma	Hypomagnesemia Venous thrombosis Osteopenia Hyperchloremic metabolic acidosis	Hypocalcemia Infection or sepsis Elevated liver enzymes Fluid overload Refeeding syndrome*

*Hemolytic anemia, respiratory distress, tetany, paresthesias, and cardiac arrhythmias. More common in patients with anorexia or alcoholism and in rapid refeeding.

TABLE 16-7 ■ Vitamin Deficiencies

VITAMIN	CAUSES OF DEFICIENCY	SIGNS OF DEFICIENCY
Thiamine (B_1) (beriberi)	Chronic alcoholism causing decreased intake of thiamine	Low SVR; high CO; polyneuropathy (demyelination, sensory deficit, paresthesia); exaggerated blood pressure response to hemorrhage, change in body position, positive pressure ventilation
Riboflavin (B_2)	Almost always caused by dietary deficiency, photodegradation of milk, other dairy products	Magenta tongue, angular stomatitis, seborrhea, cheilosis
Niacin (B_3) (pellagra)	Nicotinic acid is synthesized from tryptophan; carcinoid tumor uses tryptophan to form serotonin instead of nicotinic acid, making these patients more susceptible	Mental confusion, irritability, peripheral neuropathy, achlorhydria, diarrhea, vesicular dermatitis, stomatitis, glossitis, urethritis, and excessive salivation
Pyridoxine (B_6)	Alcoholism; isoniazid therapy	Seborrhea, glossitis, convulsions, neuropathy, depression, confusion, microcytic anemia
Folate (B_9)	Alcoholism; sulfasalazine, pyrimethamine, triamterene therapy	Megaloblastic anemia, atrophic glossitis, depression, ↑ homocysteine
Cyanocobalamin (B_{12})	Gastric atrophy (pernicious anemia), terminal ileal disease, strict vegetarianism	Megaloblastic anemia, loss of vibratory and position sense, abnormal gait, dementia, impotence, loss of bladder and bowel control, ↑ homocysteine and methylmalonic acid levels
Biotin	Ingestion of *raw* egg whites; contain the protein avidin, which strongly binds the vitamin and reduces its bioavailability	Mental changes (depression, hallucinations), paresthesia; scaling rash around the eyes, nose, and mouth; alopecia

TABLE 16-7 ■ Vitamin Deficiencies—cont'd

VITAMIN	CAUSES OF DEFICIENCY	SIGNS OF DEFICIENCY
Ascorbic acid (C) (scurvy)	Smoking, alcoholism	Capillary fragility, petechial hemorrhage, joint and skeletal muscle hemorrhage, poor wound healing, catabolic state, loosened teeth and gangrenous alveolar margins, low potassium, iron
A	Dietary lack of leafy vegetables and animal liver, malabsorption	Loss of night vision, conjunctival drying, corneal destruction, anemia
D (rickets)	Limited sun exposure, inflammatory bowel disease and other fat malabsorption syndromes	Thoracic kyphosis could lead to hypoventilation; less calcium absorption; ↑ parathormone activity, which leads to increased osteoclastic activity and bone resorption
E	Occurs only with fat malabsorption or genetic abnormalities of vitamin E metabolism or transport	Peripheral neuropathy, spinocerebellar ataxia, skeletal muscle atrophy, retinopathy
K	Prolonged antibiotic therapy can eliminate the intestinal bacteria that synthesize this vitamin; fat malabsorption	Bleeding

CO, Cardiac output; *SVR,* systemic vascular resistance; ↑ increased.

CHAPTER 17

Renal Disease

The kidneys are responsible for, or contribute to, a number of essential functions, including water conservation, electrolyte homeostasis, acid-base balance, and several neurohumoral or hormonal functions. The kidneys receive 20% to 25% of the cardiac output. They contain approximately 1 million nephrons, each consisting of a glomerulus comprising Bowman's capsule, proximal tubule, distal tubule, and collecting duct. Plasma is filtered at a rate of 180 L/day.

I. CLINICAL ASSESSMENT OF RENAL FUNCTION

Renal function can be evaluated with laboratory tests that reflect glomerular filtration rate (GFR) and renal tubular function (Table 17-1).

A. Glomerular Filtration Rate. Alterations in the GFR are associated with predictable changes in erythropoietic activity. Clinical manifestations of uremia generally appear when the GFR is less than 15 mL/min/1.73 m^2 (normal value is at least 90 mL/min/1.73 m^2).

B. Creatinine Clearance. The creatinine clearance correlates with the GFR and is the most reliable measure of GFR. Creatinine clearance does not depend on corrections for age or the presence of a steady state. Preoperatively, patients with creatinine clearances of 10 to 25 mL/min must be considered at risk of developing prolonged or adverse responses to drugs that depend on renal excretion for their clearance from the plasma.

C. Serum Creatinine. Levels of serum creatinine can be used to estimate the GFR. Normal serum creatinine concentrations range from 0.6 to 1.0 mg/dL in women and 0.8 to 1.3 mg/dL in men. Serum creatinine values are slow to reflect acute changes in renal function.

D. Blood Urea Nitrogen. Blood urea nitrogen (BUN) concentrations vary with the GFR, dietary protein intake, co-existing disease, intravascular fluid, and increased protein catabolism (e.g., fever). BUN concentrations greater than 50 mg/dL usually reflect a decreased GFR.

E. Renal Tubular Function and Integrity

1. **Urine Concentrating Ability.** Renal tubular dysfunction is present if the kidneys do not produce appropriately concentrated urine in the presence of a physiologic stimulus for the release of antidiuretic hormone (ADH). In the absence of diuretic therapy or glycosuria, urine specific gravity greater than 1.018 suggests that the ability of renal tubules to concentrate urine is adequate.
2. **Proteinuria.** Transient proteinuria may be associated with fever, congestive heart failure, seizure activity, pancreatitis, and exercise, and resolves with the resolution of the underlying stimulus or illness. Orthostatic proteinuria is benign, occurring in up to 5% of adolescents while in the upright position and not in the recumbent position. In general, persistent proteinuria connotes significant renal disease.
3. **Fractional Urinary Sodium Excretion (Fe_{Na}).** Fe_{Na} is calculated as follows:

$$Fe_{Na}(\%) = [P_{Cr} \times U_{Na})/(P_{Na} \times U_{Cr})] \times 100$$

where urine and plasma creatinine are measured in mg/dL; P_{Cr} = plasma creatinine concentration; P_{Na} = plasma sodium concentration; U_{Cr} = urine creatinine concentration; and U_{Na} = urine sodium concentration.

TABLE 17-1 ■ Tests Used to Evaluate Renal Function

TEST	NORMAL VALUE
GLOMERULAR FILTRATION RATE	
Blood urea nitrogen	10-20 mg/dL
Serum creatinine	0.7-1.5 mg/dL
Creatinine clearance	110-150 mL/min
Proteinuria (albumin)	<150 mg/day
RENAL TUBULAR FUNCTION AND/OR INTEGRITY	
Urine specific gravity	1.003-1.030
Urine osmolality	38-1400 mOsm/L
Urine sodium excretion	<40 mEq/L
Glucosuria Enzymuria *N*-Acetyl-β-glucosaminidase α-Glutathione *S*-transferase	
FACTORS THAT INFLUENCE INTERPRETATION	
Dehydration Variable protein intake Gastrointestinal bleeding Catabolism Advanced age Skeletal muscle mass Accurate timed urine volume measurement	

An Fe_{Na} that is greater than 2% or a urinary sodium concentration that is greater than 40 mEq/L reflects decreased ability of the renal tubules to conserve sodium or drug-induced diuresis. Urine osmolarity is likely to be less than 350 mOsm/L. Drug-induced diuresis is associated with increased urinary excretion of sodium.

4. **Urinalysis.** Urinalysis can detect the presence of protein, glucose, acetoacetate, blood, and leukocytes. The urine pH and solute concentrations (specific gravity) are determined, and sediment microscopy is used to determine the presence of cells, casts, microorganisms, and crystals.
5. **Novel Biomarkers of Renal Function.** Cystatin C is produced by all nucleated cells and is freely filtered and not reabsorbed by the kidneys. Serum concentration is independent of gender, age, and muscle mass, and thus it may be a better marker of GFR than serum creatinine concentration. Neutrophil gelatinase-associated lipocalin is produced by renal tubular cells and may be an early marker of acute kidney injury (AKI).

II. ACUTE KIDNEY INJURY

AKI is characterized by deterioration of renal function over a period of hours to days, resulting in failure of the kidneys to excrete nitrogenous waste products and to maintain fluid and electrolyte homeostasis. AKI may be oliguric (urinary output below 400 mL/day) or nonoliguric (urinary output greater than 400 mL/day). The mortality rate of severe AKI requiring dialysis remains high. AKI is associated with a number of other systemic diseases, acute clinical conditions, drug treatments, and interventional therapies (Table 17-2).

TABLE 17-2 ■ Etiology of Acute Renal Failure

PRERENAL AZOTEMIA (DECREASED RENAL BLOOD FLOW)
Acute hemorrhage
Gastrointestinal fluid loss
Trauma
Surgery
Burns
Cardiogenic shock
Renal artery stenosis or renal artery or aortic clamping
Sepsis
Hepatic failure
Thromboembolism
RENAL AZOTEMIA (INTRINSIC)
Acute glomerulonephritis (5% of cases)
Vasculitis
Interstitial nephritis (drugs, infiltrative disease) (10% of cases)
Acute tubular necrosis (85% of cases)
• Ischemia (50% of cases)
• Nephrotoxic drugs (aminoglycosides, nonsteroidal antiinflammatory drugs)
• Solvents (carbon tetrachloride, ethylene glycol)
• Heavy metals (mercury, cisplatin)
• Radiographic contrast dye
• Myoglobinuria
• Intratubular crystals (uric acid, oxalate)
POSTRENAL AZOTEMIA (OBSTRUCTIVE)
Upper urinary tract obstruction (ureteral)
• Nephrolithiasis
Lower urinary tract obstruction (bladder outlet)
• Benign prostatic hypertrophy
• Clot retention
• Bladder carcinoma

Adapted from Klahr S, Miller SB. Acute oliguria. *N Engl J Med.* 1998;338:671-675; and Thadhani R, Pascual M, Bonventre JV. Acute renal failure. *N Engl J Med.* 1996;334:1148-1169.

A. Etiology

1. **Prerenal Azotemia.** Nearly half of hospital-acquired AKI cases consist of prerenal azotemia, which predisposes patients to ischemia-induced acute tubular necrosis (ATN). Prerenal azotemia is rapidly reversible if the underlying cause (hypovolemia, congestive heart failure) is corrected. Elderly patients are susceptible to prerenal azotemia because of their predisposition to hypovolemia (poor fluid intake) and high incidence of renovascular disease. Urinary indices may help distinguish prerenal from intrinsic AKI (Table 17-3).
2. **Renal Azotemia.** Intrinsic renal diseases that result in AKI are categorized according to the site of injury (renal tubules, interstitium, glomerulus, renal vasculature). Injury to the renal tubules is most often ischemic or nephrotoxic (aminoglycoside antibiotics, radiographic contrast agents). Ischemia and toxins often combine to cause AKI in severely ill patients with conditions such as sepsis or acquired immunodeficiency syndrome (AIDS). AKI resulting from acute interstitial nephritis is usually caused by allergic reactions to drugs.
3. **Postrenal Azotemia.** AKI occurs when urinary outflow tracts are obstructed (prostatic hypertrophy, cancer of the prostate or cervix). The potential for recovery is inversely related to the duration of the obstruction. Renal ultrasonography is the best diagnostic test.

TABLE 17-3 ■ **Characteristic Urinary Indices in Patients with Acute Oliguria Resulting from Prerenal or Renal Causes**

INDEX	PRERENAL CAUSES	RENAL CAUSES
Urinary sodium concentration (mEq/L)	<20	>40
Fractional excretion of sodium (%)	<1	>1
Urine osmolarity (mOsm/L)	>500	<400
Urine creatinine/plasma creatinine ratio	>40	<20
Urine/plasma osmolarity ratio	>1.5	<1.1
Sediment	Normal, occasional hyaline casts	Renal tubular epithelial cells, granular casts

Adapted from Klahr S, Miller SB. Acute oliguria. *N Engl J Med.* 1998;338:671-675; and Schrieir RW, Wang W, Poole B, et al. Acute renal failure: definition, diagnosis, pathogenesis, and therapy. *J Clin Invest.* 2004;114:5-14.

B. Risk Factors. Co-existing renal disease, advanced age, congestive heart failure, symptomatic cardiovascular disease, and major operative procedures (cardiopulmonary bypass, abdominal aneurysm resection) are risk factors for development of AKI. Sepsis and multiple organ system dysfunction caused by trauma introduce the risk of AKI. Iatrogenic causes include inadequate fluid replacement, delayed treatment of sepsis, and administration of nephrotoxic drugs or dyes.

C. Diagnosis. AKI is usually diagnosed based on an acute rise in serum creatinine; signs and symptoms are often absent early and are nonspecific (malaise, dyspnea, edema, hypertension). Urinalysis may be helpful in diagnosing whether AKI is likely to be prerenal, intrarenal, or postrenal. The sensitivity and specificity of urinary sodium below 20 mEq/L in differentiating prerenal azotemia from ATN are 90% and 82%, respectively (see Table 17-3).

D. Complications Associated with Acute Kidney Injury (Table 17-4)

E. Treatment. Treatment of AKI is aimed at limiting further renal injury and correcting the water, electrolyte, and acid-base derangements. Underlying causes should be sought and terminated or reversed, if possible.

1. **Fluids.** Prompt and adequate correction of hypovolemia and hypotension is much more important than the type of fluid used. Hetastarch may exacerbate injury, and normal saline may exacerbate hyperchloremic metabolic acidosis. Lactated Ringers or other bicarbonate-containing balanced salt solution may be the best choice.
2. **Vasopressors.** These agents may increase renal vasoconstriction and exacerbate AKI and should be used with caution. The use of dopamine to treat or prevent AKI is not supported by the literature. Vasopressin may be effective.
3. **Diuretics.** The practice of trying to convert oliguric to nonoliguric AKI with diuretics is not advised. Mannitol yields better outcomes in posttransplantation ATN and in combination with forced alkaline diuresis to prevent AKI in severe crush injuries.
4. ***N*-Acetylcysteine.** This agent may reduce AKI in high-risk patients exposed to radiocontrast dye.
5. **Activated Protein C and Steroid Replacement.** Steroids and activated protein C reduce mortality in patients with severe sepsis.
6. **Dialysis.** Dialysis (or hemofiltration) is still the mainstay of severe AKI.

F. Prognosis. For patients with hospital-acquired AKI the prognosis is poor, with current mortality rates of more than 20%, and 50% or more once dialysis is required. Only 15% of patients who develop AKI will fully recover their renal function.

G. Drug Dosage in Patients with Renal Impairment. The rate of elimination of drugs excreted by the kidneys is proportional to the GFR. If the patient is oliguric, use 5 mL/min for creatinine clearance.

TABLE 17-4 ■ **Complications of Acute Renal Failure**

Neurologic	Confusion Asterixis Somnolence Seizure
Cardiovascular	Hypertension Congestive heart failure Pulmonary edema Dysrhythmias Pericarditis Anemia
Hematologic	Anemia (hematocrit [Hct] 20%-30%) Platelet dysfunction (may be improved by administration of desmopressin perioperatively)
Metabolic	Hyperkalemia Metabolic acidosis Sodium and water retention
Gastrointestinal (GI)	Anorexia Nausea and vomiting Ileus GI bleeding
Infection	Respiratory tract Urinary tract

1. **Loading Dose Guidelines.** If extracellular fluid volume looks normal, use a normal loading dose. If extracellular fluid is contracted, reduce the loading dose; if extracellular fluid is expanded, use a higher loading dose.
2. **Repeat Dosing.** A combination of increasing the dosage interval and decreasing the dose is often used (e.g., analgesics; Table 17-5).
3. **Drugs Removed by Hemodialysis.** These agents are usually given at the end of the dialysis schedule to avoid the necessity of readministering them.

H. **Anesthetic Management.** Because of high morbidity and mortality, only life-saving surgery should be undertaken in patients with acute AKI. Principles are maintenance of an adequate mean systemic blood pressure and cardiac output and the avoidance of further renal insults including hypotension, hypovolemia, hypoxia, and nephrotoxic exposure. Invasive hemodynamic monitoring may be critical, as are frequent blood gas analysis and electrolyte determination. For patients undergoing renal replacement therapy, institute postoperative dialysis or hemodialysis as soon as the patient's condition is stable.

III. CHRONIC KIDNEY DISEASE

Chronic kidney disease (CKD) is progressive, irreversible deterioration of renal function that results from a wide variety of diseases (Table 17-6). Diabetes mellitus is the leading cause of end-stage renal disease (ESRD), followed by hypertension.

A. **Diagnosis.** Signs are often undetectable, and symptoms are nonspecific (fatigue, malaise, anorexia). In most patients the diagnosis is established through routine testing, such as serum creatinine level and urinary sediment analysis.

TABLE 17-5 ■ **Analgesic Dosage Adjustments in Patients with Renal Insufficiency**

DRUG	ADJUSTMENT METHOD	GFR >50 mL/min	GFR 10-50 mL/min	GFR <10 mL/min
Acetaminophen	↑ Interval	q4h	q6h	q8h
Acetylsalicylic acid	↑ Interval	q4h	q6-8h	Avoid
Alfentanil, remifentanil, sufentanil	↔ Dose	100%	100%	100%
Codeine	↓ Dose	100%	75%	50%
Fentanyl	↓ Dose	100%	75%	50%
Ketorolac*	↓ Dose	100%	50%	50%
Meperidine	↓ Dose	100%	75%	50%
Methadone	↓ Dose	100%	100%	50%-75%
Morphine	↓ Dose	100%	75%	50%

Adapted from Schrier RW: *Manual of Nephrology.* 6th ed. Philadelphia, PA: Lippincott Williams & Wilkins; 2005:268.
*Usually avoided because this class of drug may be associated with worsening of renal function.
↓, Decreases; ↑, increases; ↔, no change; GFR, glomerular filtration rate.

TABLE 17-6 ■ **Causes of Chronic Renal Failure**

Glomerulopathies
- Primary glomerular disease
- Focal glomerulosclerosis
- Membranoproliferative glomerulonephritis
- Membranous nephropathy
- Immunoglobulin A nephropathy
- Diabetes mellitus
- Amyloidosis
- Postinfective glomerulonephritis
- Systemic lupus erythematosus
- Wegener's granulomatosis

Tubulointerstitial disease
- Analgesic nephropathy
- Reflux nephropathy with pyelonephritis
- Myeloma kidney
- Sarcoidosis

Heredity disease
- Polycystic kidney disease
- Alport's syndrome
- Medullary cystic disease

Systemic hypertension
Renal vascular disease
Obstructive uropathy
Human immunodeficiency virus

Adapted from Tolkoff-Rubin NE, Pascual M. Chronic renal failure. *Sci Am Med.* 1998;1-12.

TABLE 17-7 ■ **Stages of Chronic Renal Failure**

STAGE OF FAILURE	FUNCTIONING NEPHRONS (% OF TOTAL)	GLOMERULAR FILTRATION RATE (mL/min)	SIGNS	LABORATORY ABNORMALITIES
Normal	100	125	None	None
Decreased renal reserve	40	50-80	None	None
Renal insufficiency	10-40	12-50	Nocturia	Increased blood urea nitrogen Increased serum creatinine
Renal failure	10	<12	Uremia	Increased blood urea nitrogen Increased serum creatinine Anemia Hyperkalemia Increased bleeding time

B. Progression. Stages of CKD are summarized in Table 17-7. Intrarenal hemodynamic changes (glomerular hypertension, glomerular hyperfiltration and permeability changes, glomerulosclerosis) are likely responsible for progression of renal disease.

1. **Systemic Hypertension.** A major risk factor is systemic hypertension. Administration of angiotensin-converting enzyme inhibitors (ACEIs) and/or angiotensin receptor blockers (ARBs) appears to be renoprotective (decreased proteinuria and slowed progression of glomerular sclerosis) compared with other antihypertensive regimens.
2. **Dietary Factors.** New guidelines call for moderate protein restriction in all patients with renal insufficiency.
3. **Strict Control of Blood Glucose Concentrations.** Strict control can delay the onset of proteinuria and slow the progression of nephropathy, neuropathy, and retinopathy.

C. Signs and Symptoms. Symptoms of CKD include general malaise and anorexia. Volume overload (peripheral edema, dyspnea, congestive heart failure) and electrolyte or acid-base disturbances are late signs of CKD. Other symptoms include cognitive impairment, peripheral neuropathy, infertility, and increased susceptibility to infection (Table 17-8).

D. Complications

1. **Uremic Syndrome.** Uremic syndrome is a constellation of signs and symptoms (anorexia, nausea, vomiting, pruritus, anemia, fatigue, coagulopathy) that reflect the kidney's progressive inability to perform its excretory, secretory, and regulatory functions. BUN concentration is a useful clinical indicator of the severity of the uremic syndrome and the patient's response to therapy (dietary protein restriction). Serum creatinine concentration correlates poorly with uremic symptoms.
2. **Renal Osteodystrophy.** A complication of CKD is renal osteodystrophy. As the GFR decreases, phosphate concentrations increase and serum calcium concentrations decrease, stimulating parathyroid hormone (PTH) secretion and causing bone resorption and calcium release. Treatment of renal osteodystrophy is restriction of dietary phosphate, administration of oral calcium supplements, and vitamin D therapy.
3. **Anemia.** Because of decreased erythropoietin production by the kidneys, anemia occurs. Treatment is recombinant human erythropoietin (epoetin), eliminating the need for blood transfusions and avoiding the symptoms of anemia in most patients. Blood transfusions are avoided if possible, as the resultant sensitization to human leukocyte antigens (HLAs) makes kidney transplantation less successful.

TABLE 17-8 ■ Manifestations of Chronic Renal Failure

Electrolyte imbalance
- Hyperkalemia
- Hypermagnesemia
- Hypocalcemia

Metabolic acidosis
Unpredictable intravascular fluid volume status
Anemia
- Increased cardiac output
- Oxyhemoglobin dissociation curve shifted to the right

Uremic coagulopathies
- Platelet dysfunction
- Increased bleeding time

Neurologic changes
- Autonomic dysfunction
- Encephalopathy
- Peripheral neuropathy

Cardiovascular changes
- Congestive heart failure
- Dyslipidemia
- Systemic hypertension
- Uremic pericarditis

Renal osteodystrophy
Pruritus

TABLE 17-9 ■ Treatment of Uremic Bleeding

DRUG	DOSE	ONSET OF EFFECT	PEAK EFFECT	DURATION OF EFFECT
Cryoprecipitate	10 units IV over 30 min	<1 hr	4-12 hr	12-18 hr
DDAVP (desmopressin)	0.3 mcg/kg IV or SC	<1 hr	2-4 hr	6-8 hr
Conjugated estrogen	0.6 mg/kg/day IV for 5 days	6 hr	5-7 days	14 days

Adapted from Tolkoff-Rubin NE, Pascual M. Chronic renal failure. *Sci Am Med.* 1998;1-12.
IV, Intravenously; SC, subcutaneously.

4. **Uremic Bleeding.** Patients with chronic renal failure have an increased tendency to bleed despite normal findings of laboratory coagulation studies (platelet count, prothrombin time, plasma thromboplastin time). Treatment of uremic bleeding may include the administration of cryoprecipitate to provide factor VIII–von Willebrand factor (vWF) complex (risk of transmission of viral diseases) or administration of 1-desamino-8-D-arginine vasopressin (DDAVP, desmopressin) (Table 17-9).

E. **Treatment.** Treatment of CKD includes aggressive treatment of the underlying cause (diabetes or hypertension if present), pharmacologic therapy to delay the progress, and renal replacement therapy as ESRD ensues.

1. **Hypertension.** ACEIs or ARBs are used to treat hypertension. For most patients the first drug of choice is an ACEI, which is then titrated upward into the moderate to high dose

TABLE 17-10 ■ Findings Suggestive of Inadequate Hemodialysis

CLINICAL
Anorexia, nausea, vomiting
Peripheral neuropathy
Poor nutritional status
Depressed sensorium
Pericarditis
Ascites
Minimal weight gain or weight loss between treatments
Fluid retention and systemic hypertension
CHEMICAL
Decrease in blood urea nitrogen concentration during hemodialysis of <65%
Albumin concentration <4 g/dL
Predialysis blood urea concentration <50 mg/dL (a sign of malnutrition)
Predialysis serum creatinine concentration <5 mg/dL (a sign of malnutrition)
Persistent anemia (hematocrit <30%) despite erythropoietin therapy

Adapted from Ifudu O. Care of patients undergoing hemodialysis. *N Engl J Med.* 1998;339:1054-1062.

range as tolerated. ARBs are the preferred choice in those with type 2 diabetes with CKD and proteinuria. β-Blockers and calcium channel blockers may also be useful.

2. **Diabetes.** The goal of treatment is to achieve less than 7% glycosylated hemoglobin (Hb). Euglycemia is associated with reversal of the typical lesions seen in diabetic nephropathy and a reduction in albuminuria. Dietary protein intake of 0.6 g/kg/day reduces the rate of progression of renal disease in patients with diabetes but should not be undertaken at the expense of nutrition in anorexic patients. Dietary phosphorus should be restricted to 800 to 1000 mg/day when serum phosphorus or PTH levels are elevated. Vitamin D supplementation may be helpful. Sodium intake should be restricted to less than 2.4 g/day.
3. **Anemia.** Anemia responds to treatment with erythropoietin in all stages of CKD. Hb, rather than hematocrit, is the preferred method for assessing anemia. Anemia is defined for males as an Hb level less than 13.0 g/dL, and for females as an Hb level less than 12.0 g/dL regardless of age.
4. **Renal Replacement Therapy.** When GFR approaches 30 mL/min/1.73 m^2, renal replacement therapy is considered.
   a. ***Hemodialysis.*** is usually instituted by the time GFR is 15 mL/min/1.73 m2. Objectives include adequate dialysis, adequate nutrition, maintenance of vascular access, correction of hormonal deficiencies, minimization of hospitalizations, and prolongation of life while enhancing its quality (Table 17-10). Vascular access for hemodialysis is established surgically (native atrioventricular fistula, grafts, or temporary hemodialysis intravenous catheters).
      i. ***Complications Associated with Hemodialysis***
         (a) ***Hypotension.*** During dialysis, hypotension and hypersensitivity reactions to polyacrylonitrile in dialysis membranes (most common in patients taking ACEIs) may occur.
         (b) ***Hypersensitivity Reactions.*** Reactions may occur to the ethylene oxide used to sterilize dialysis equipment or to polyacrylonitrile in dialysis membranes (reactions to the latter are most commonly seen in patients taking ACEIs).
         (c) ***Dialysis Disequilibrium Syndrome.*** This syndrome consists of nausea, headaches, and fatigue but can progress to seizures and coma. It is thought to result from

rapid changes in pH and solute concentrations in the central nervous system. Treatment includes reducing the rate of dialysis and blood flow.

(d) ***Muscle Cramps.*** Muscle cramps are likely caused by changes in potassium concentration.

(e) ***Fluid, Vitamin, and Electrolyte Balance.*** Patients on hemodialysis have decreased total body potassium and tolerance of hyperkalemia. Water-soluble vitamins are removed by hemodialysis and should be replaced. Between treatments, a weight gain of 3% to 4% of body mass in 2 days is appropriate. Insulin requirements may decrease owing to decreased catabolism of insulin.

(f) ***Cardiovascular Disease.*** Cardiovascular disease caused by accelerated atherosclerosis and impaired oxygen delivery during uremia accounts for nearly 50% of all deaths in patients on hemodialysis, Fluid retention is the most likely cause of systemic hypertension in most patients who require hemodialysis. Essential hypertension may require treatment with antihypertensive drugs in addition to hemodialysis. Pericarditis may result from inadequate hemodialysis.

(g) ***Bleeding.*** Bleeding caused by altered platelet function is partially correctable by hemodialysis.

(h) ***Infection.*** There is increased susceptibility to infection caused by impaired phagocytosis and chemotaxis. All patients on hemodialysis are vaccinated against pneumococcus and, if appropriate, hepatitis B. Tuberculosis (TB) is usually extrapulmonary; symptoms may be atypical, with anergy on skin testing. Unexplained weight loss with or without fever should prompt further testing to rule out TB. Actual hepatitis B and C infections may be asymptomatic. Many hemodialysis patients have antibodies to hepatitis C. Dose adjustments of drugs used to treat AIDS are not required for hemodialysis, and isolation of patients with AIDS or use of a dedicated hemodialysis machine is not necessary.

(i) ***Peritoneal Dialysis.*** This form of dialysis is simple to perform and may be useful in patients with severe vascular disease or congestive heart failure (more gradual fluid shifts, no need for vascular access). Peritonitis is the most common serious complication.

(j) ***Drug Clearance in Patients Undergoing Dialysis.*** Drug clearance may dictate adjustment of dosage intervals and supplemental administration if drugs are cleared by dialysis (e.g., low-molecular-weight compounds, water-soluble agents, non–protein-bound drugs).

(k) ***Perioperative Hemodialysis.*** Patients should undergo adequate hemodialysis before elective surgery to minimize the likelihood of uremic bleeding, pulmonary edema, and impaired arterial oxygenation.

F. Anesthetic Management of Patients with Chronic Kidney Disease (Table 17-11)

1. **Preoperative Evaluation.** Fluid status, electrolyte balance (particularly potassium), glucose management, and degree of anemia are evaluated preoperatively. Digoxin toxicity should be a concern in patients being treated with digoxin. Antihypertensive drug therapy is continued (except ACE inhibitors and ARBs, which may be withheld to reduce risk of intraoperative hypotension). Patients on hemodialysis should undergo dialysis during the 24 hours preceding elective surgery. Preoperative DDAVP may be considered. Perioperative H_2-receptor blockers should be dose-adjusted for renal failure.

2. **Intraoperative Considerations**

   a. ***Induction.*** Hypotension on induction is common, particularly in patients taking ACEIs. Decreased protein binding of drugs may result in the availability of more unbound drugs at receptor sites (see Table 17-11). Potassium release after administration of succinylcholine is not exaggerated in patients with CKD, but caution is indicated if preoperative serum potassium concentration is in the high-normal range.

TABLE 17-11 ■ **Drugs Used in Anesthesia Practice that Significantly Depend on Renal Elimination**

CLASS OF DRUG	ACTION TERMINATED BY RENAL EXCRETION	ACTION PARTIALLY TERMINATED BY RENAL EXCRETION
Induction agents	—	Barbiturates
Muscle relaxants	Gallamine, metocurine	Pancuronium, vecuronium
Cholinesterase inhibitors	—	Neostigmine, edrophonium
Cardiovascular drugs	Digoxin, inotropes	Atropine, glycopyrrolate, milrinone, hydralazine
Antimicrobials	Aminoglycosides, vancomycin, cephalosporin, penicillin	Sulfonamides

Adapted from Malhotra V, Sudheendra V, Diwan S. Anesthesia and the renal and genitourinary systems. In Miller RD, Fleischer LA, Johns RA, et al, eds. *Miller's Anesthesia.* 7th ed. Philadelphia, PA: Elsevier Churchill Livingstone, 2009.

b. ***Maintenance of Anesthesia.*** There is no evidence that patients with co-existing renal disease are at increased risk of renal dysfunction with sevoflurane. Selection of nondepolarizing muscle relaxants should consider the clearance mechanisms of these drugs. Clearance of vecuronium and rocuronium is slowed, whereas clearance of mivacurium, atracurium, and cisatracurium from plasma is independent of renal function. Lactated Ringer's solution (potassium 4 mEq/L) or other potassium-containing fluids should not be administered to anuric patients. In anuric (dialysis) patients, noninvasive operations require replacement of only insensible water losses with 5% glucose in water (5 to 10 mL/kg intravenously). Measuring the central venous pressure may be useful for guiding fluid replacement. Arterial cannulation should be avoided if possible, to avoid injury to vessels that may be required for future dialysis access. Patient positioning should include attention to protecting vascular access fistulas. Regional anesthesia is useful for placing the vascular shunts necessary for chronic hemodialysis.

c. ***Opioids.*** The use of opioids may minimize the need for volatile anesthetic agents. Morphine and meperidine undergo metabolism to potentially neurotoxic compounds that rely on renal clearance. Morphine metabolite morphine-6-glucuronide can accumulate in patients with CKD, resulting in respiratory depression. Hydromorphone may accumulate in CKD but is safely used with dose adjustment. Alfentanil, fentanyl, remifentanil, and sufentanil lack active metabolites, but fentanyl elimination may be delayed in CKD.

3. **Postoperative Management.** Attention must be given to inadequate reversal of muscle relaxant in anephric patients who show signs of skeletal muscle weakness during the postoperative period. Other considerations are sensitivity to opioids, arrhythmias related to hyperkalemia, and oxygen supplementation in anemic patients. Meperidine is avoided for postoperative analgesia because its metabolites may accumulate in patients with renal failure, causing seizures.

IV. RENAL TRANSPLANTATION

A. Management of Anesthesia

1. **General Anesthesia.** Renal function after kidney transplantation is not influenced by the volatile anesthetic administered. Goals are maintenance of cardiac output and tissue oxygen

delivery to promote renal perfusion. A high-normal systemic blood pressure is desirable to maintain adequate urine flow. Atracurium, cisatracurium, and mivacurium are reasonable muscle relaxants because of lack of dependence on renal clearance, although the transplanted kidney will clear muscle relaxants similarly to a normal kidney. Central venous pressure monitoring is useful to guide fluid infusions. Diuretics facilitate urine formation by the newly transplanted kidney. With release of the vascular clamps, potassium from the preservative solution and acid metabolites has been reported to lead to cardiac arrest. Hypotension results from the additional 300-mL capacity of the new kidney vascular bed. Treatment is fluid administration.

2. **Regional Anesthesia.** Blockade of the peripheral sympathetic nervous system can complicate control of systemic blood pressure.
3. **Postoperative Complications**
   a. ***Acute Rejection Affecting the Kidney Vasculature.*** Rejection can be so rapid that inadequate circulation is evident almost immediately after the blood supply to the kidney is established. The only treatment is removal of the transplanted kidney; disseminated intravascular coagulation occurs. Postoperative graft hematomas can cause vascular or ureteral obstruction.
   b. ***Delayed Graft Rejection.*** Signs include fever, local tenderness, and deterioration of urine output. Treatment is with high doses of corticosteroids and antilymphocyte globulin.
   c. ***Acute Tubular Necrosis.*** In the transplanted kidney, acute tubular necrosis secondary to prolonged ischemia usually responds to hemodialysis.
   d. ***Cyclosporine Toxicity.*** Cyclosporine toxicity may also cause AKI. Ultrasonography and needle biopsy are performed to differentiate between the possible causes of kidney malfunction.
   e. ***Opportunistic Infections.*** Infections caused by long-term immunosuppression are common after renal transplantation.
   f. ***Cancer.*** Large cell lymphoma is a well-recognized complication of renal transplantation and occurs almost exclusively in patients with evidence of Epstein-Barr virus (EBV) infection.

B. **Anesthetic Considerations for Renal Transplant Recipients.** Renal transplant recipients are often elderly and have co-existing cardiovascular disease and diabetes mellitus. The side effects of immunosuppressant drugs (systemic hypertension, lowered seizure thresholds, anemia, thrombocytopenia) must be considered. GFR and renal blood flow are likely to be lower than in healthy individuals, and the activity of drugs excreted by the kidneys may be prolonged. Drugs that are potentially nephrotoxic or dependent on renal clearance are avoided. Diuretics are administered only with careful evaluation of the patient's intravascular fluid volume status.

V. PRIMARY DISEASES OF THE KIDNEYS

A. **Glomerulonephritis.** Acute glomerulonephritis is usually caused by deposition of antigen-antibody complexes in the glomeruli. The source of antigens may be exogenous (poststreptococcal infection) or endogenous (collagen diseases). Clinical manifestations of glomerular diseases include hematuria, proteinuria, hypertension, edema, and increased plasma creatinine concentrations and the presence of red blood cell casts in the urine.

B. **Nephrotic Syndrome.** Nephrotic syndrome is defined by daily urinary protein excretion exceeding 3.5 g associated with sodium retention, hyperlipoproteinemia, and thromboembolic and infectious complications. Diabetic nephropathy is the most common cause of nephrotic proteinuria.

1. **Signs and Symptoms** (Table 17-12)
2. **Complications of Nephrotic Syndrome** (Table 17-13)

C. **Goodpasture's Syndrome.** A combination of pulmonary hemorrhage and glomerulonephritis, Goodpasture's syndrome occurs most often in young males. Prognosis is poor, with no

TABLE 17-12 ■ Features of Nephrotic Syndrome

Hypertension
Proteinuria, hematuria
Sodium retention
Edema
Hypovolemia
Thromboembolism
Hyperlipidemia
Infectious complications

TABLE 17-13 ■ Complications of Nephrotic Syndrome

Thromboembolic	Renal vein thrombosis Pulmonary embolism Deep vein thrombosis
Infectious	Pneumococcal peritonitis
Decreased plasma protein binding	Decreased levels of vitamins and hormones
Edema	Generalized; should be treated slowly with loop diuretics and thiazides

known effective therapy to prevent progression to renal failure, usually within 1 year of the diagnosis.

D. **Interstitial Nephritis.** Allergic reaction to drugs, including sulfonamides, allopurinol, phenytoin, and diuretics, can cause interstitial nephritis. Other, less common causes include autoimmune diseases (lupus erythematosus) and infiltrative diseases (sarcoidosis). Patients exhibit decreased urine-concentrating ability, proteinuria, and systemic hypertension.

E. **Hereditary Nephritis (Alport's Syndrome).** Hereditary nephritis is often accompanied by hearing loss and ocular abnormalities. Drug therapy has not proven successful, although ACEIs may slow progression of renal disease.

F. **Polycystic Renal Disease.** An autosomal dominant disease, polycystic renal disease typically progresses slowly until renal failure occurs during middle age. Mild systemic hypertension and proteinuria are common. Hemodialysis or renal transplantation is eventually necessary in most patients.

G. **Fanconi's Syndrome.** Fanconi's syndrome results from inherited or acquired disturbances of proximal renal tubular function, causing hyperaminoaciduria, glycosuria, and hyperphosphaturia. Symptoms include polyuria, polydipsia, metabolic acidosis caused by loss of bicarbonate ions, and skeletal muscle weakness related to hypokalemia. Dwarfism and osteomalacia, reflecting loss of phosphate, are prominent in these patients.

H. **Bartter's and Gitelman's Syndromes.** These are inherited renal salt-wasting disorders caused by defects in sodium, chloride, and potassium channels in the ascending limb of the distal convoluted tubule. Juxtaglomerular hyperplasia, hyperaldosteronism, and hypokalemic acidosis are pathognomonic. Treatment is with ACEIs, spironolactone, and sodium and potassium supplementation.

I. **Renal Tubular Acidosis (RTA).** RTA causes metabolic acidosis resulting from inappropriate acidification of the urine. Type 1 RTA is caused by impaired bicarbonate reabsorption in the

TABLE 17-14 ■ **Composition and Characteristics of Renal Stones**

TYPE OF STONE	INCIDENCE (%)	RADIOGRAPHIC APPEARANCE	ETIOLOGY
Calcium oxalate	65	Opaque	Primary hyperparathyroidism, idiopathic hypercalciuria, hyperoxaluria, hyperuricosuria
Magnesium ammonium phosphate (struvite)	20	Opaque	Alkaline urine (usually caused by chronic bacterial infection)
Calcium phosphate	7.5	Opaque	Renal tubular acidosis
Uric acid	5	Lucent	Acid urine, gout, hyperuricosuria
Cystine	1.5	Opaque	Cystinuria

proximal renal tubule. Type 2 RTA is caused by impaired secretion of hydrogen ion in the distal tubule. Both are characterized by hypokalemic, hyperchloremic metabolic acidosis and inappropriately basic urine. The conditions can be hereditary or acquired. Type 4 RTA is associated with hyperkalemia rather than hypokalemia and is often seen in patients with CKD.

J. Nephrolithiasis (Table 17-14). Renal stones passing down the ureter can produce intense flank pain, often radiating to the groin, associated with nausea and vomiting and mimicking an acute abdominal surgical emergency. Hematuria is common, and ureteral obstruction may cause signs and symptoms of renal failure.

1. Types of Stones

a. ***Calcium Oxalate Stones.*** Causes of hypercalcemia (hyperparathyroidism, sarcoidosis, cancer) must be considered in these patients.

b. ***Magnesium Ammonium Phosphate Stones.*** These stones may result from urinary tract infection with urea-splitting organisms that produce ammonia.

c. ***Uric Acid Stones.*** These stones occur in persons with persistently acidic urine (pH greater than 6.0), which decreases the solubility of uric acid. Approximately 50% of patients with uric acid stones have gout.

2. Treatment. Treatment depends on identifying the composition of the stone and correcting the predisposing factors, such as hyperparathyroidism, urinary tract infection, or gout. Extracorporeal shock wave lithotripsy is a noninvasive treatment.

K. Renal Hypertension. Renal disease is the most common cause of secondary systemic hypertension. The sudden onset of a marked increase in systemic blood pressure or the presence of hypertension before the age of 30 years should arouse suspicion of renovascular disease. A bruit may be audible on auscultation of the abdomen over the kidneys. Systemic hypertension caused by renovascular disease does not respond well to treatment with antihypertensive drugs. Treatment of renovascular hypertension is with renal artery endarterectomy or nephrectomy.

L. Uric Acid Nephropathy. This occurs when uric acid crystals are precipitated in the renal collecting tubules or ureters, producing acute oliguric renal failure. The condition is particularly likely to occur in patients with myeloproliferative disorders being treated with chemotherapeutic drugs.

M. Hepatorenal Syndrome. Hepatorenal syndrome is acute oliguria manifesting in patients with decompensated cirrhosis of the liver. Associated signs include deep jaundice, ascites, hypoalbuminemia, and hypoprothrombinemia. Treatment is directed at intravascular fluid volume replacement. In some patients a circulating toxin may be responsible for extreme renal vasoconstriction and AKI. Nevertheless, hemodialysis has not been reliable for eliminating suspected hepatic toxins.

TABLE 17-15 ■ **Signs and Symptoms of Transurethral Resection of the Prostate Syndrome**

SYSTEM	SIGNS AND SYMPTOMS	CAUSE
Cardiovascular	Hypertension, reflex bradycardia, pulmonary edema, cardiovascular collapse, hypotension, ECG changes (wide QRS, elevated ST segments, ventricular arrhythmias)	Rapid fluid absorption (reflex bradycardia may be secondary to hypertension or increased ICP); third spacing secondary to hyponatremia and hypo-osmolality; cardiovascular collapse, hyponatremia
Respiratory	Tachypnea, oxygen desaturation, Cheyne-Stokes breathing	Pulmonary edema
Neurologic	Nausea, restlessness, visual disturbances, confusion, somnolence, seizures, coma, death	Hyponatremia and hypo-osmolality causing cerebral edema and increased ICP, hyperglycinemia (inhibitory neurotransmitter, potentiates NMDA receptor activity), hyperammonemia
Hematologic	Disseminated intravascular hemolysis	Hyponatremia and hypo-osmolality
Renal	Renal failure	Hypotension, hyperoxaluria (metabolite of glycine)
Metabolic	Acidosis	Deamination of glycine to glyoxylic acid and ammonia

ECG, Electrocardiogram; *ICP,* intracranial pressure; *NMDA, N*-methyl-D-aminotransferase.

N. Benign Prostatic Hyperplasia. Benign Prostatic Hyperplasia (BPH) is a nonmalignant enlargement of the prostate. Transurethral resection of the prostate (TURP) and open prostatectomy have been the traditional treatments for men with symptomatic BPH. Laser ablation therapy is a recent technique allowing for brief operating times. Medical therapy consists of finasteride (inhibits 5α-reductase) to reduce prostate size and α-adrenergic antagonists (terazosin, doxazosin, tamsulosin) to decrease prostatic smooth muscle tone, improving urinary flow.

1. **TURP Syndrome** (Table 17-15) is characterized by intravascular fluid volume shifts and plasma solute effects caused by absorption of irrigation solution. Hypo-osmolality is the principal factor contributing to the neurologic and hypovolemic changes associated with TURP syndrome.
   a. ***Intravascular Fluid Volume Expansion.*** Rapid intravascular fluid volume expansion caused by systemic absorption of irrigating fluids (absorption rates may reach 200 mL/min) can cause systemic hypertension and reflex bradycardia. Patients with poor left ventricular function may develop pulmonary edema. The most widely used indicator of intravascular fluid volume gain is hyponatremia.
   b. ***Intravascular Fluid Volume Loss.*** Hyponatremia in association with systemic hypertension may result in water flux along osmotic and hydrostatic pressure gradients out of the intravascular space and into the lungs, with resultant pulmonary edema and hypovolemic shock.
   c. ***Hyponatremia.*** Hyponatremia caused by intravascular absorption of sodium-free irrigating fluids may cause confusion, agitation, visual disturbances, pulmonary edema, cardiovascular collapse, and seizures.
   d. ***Hypo-osmolality.*** The crucial physiologic derangement leading to central nervous system dysfunction during TURP is hypo-osmolality. Cerebral edema caused by acute

hypo-osmolality can result in increased intracranial pressure with resultant bradycardia and hypertension. Diuretics may accentuate hyponatremia and hypo-osmolality. No intervention is needed if the serum osmolality is near normal. When treatment is undertaken, serum osmolality should be monitored and corrected aggressively with hypertonic saline only until symptoms resolve substantially; then correction should be continued slowly (serum sodium concentrations increase 1.5 mEq/L/hr).

e. ***Hyperammonemia.*** Hyperammonemia is the result of systemic absorption of glycine and its oxidative deamination to glyoxylic acid and ammonia.

f. ***Hyperglycinemia.*** Glycine is the most likely cause of visual disturbances, including transient blindness, during TURP syndrome, reflecting the role of glycine as an inhibitory neurotransmitter in the retina. Vision returns to normal within 24 hours as serum glycine concentrations approach normal. Reassurance is the best treatment. Glycine may also exert toxic effects on the kidneys.

CHAPTER 18

Fluid, Electrolyte, and Acid-Base Disorders

Alterations in water and electrolyte content and distribution and acid-base disturbances can produce multiple organ system dysfunctions during the perioperative period. Impairment of central nervous system, cardiac, and neuromuscular function is especially likely in the presence of water, electrolyte (sodium, potassium, calcium, magnesium), and acid-base disturbances. In addition, numerous perioperative events can initiate or aggravate fluid, electrolyte, and acid-base disturbances (Table 18-1).

I. ABNORMALITIES OF WATER AND ELECTROLYTE HOMEOSTASIS

A. Water and Osmolal Homeostasis

1. **Total Body Water (TBW).** Water makes up 60% of body weight. TBW content is categorized as intracellular fluid (ICF) and extracellular fluid (ECF), according to the location of the water relative to cell membranes (Figure 18-1). ECF is primarily interstitial fluid (75% of ECF) and intravascular plasma (25% of ECF). Water shifts between compartments according to hydrostatic and oncotic pressure across membranes. The distribution and concentration of electrolytes differ greatly among fluid compartments. The electrophysiology of excitable cells is dependent on the intracellular and extracellular concentrations of sodium, potassium, and calcium. Unequal distribution of ions (more potassium inside and more sodium outside) produces electrochemical differences across the cell membrane. The normal kidney excretes urine with an osmolality that varies depending on serum osmolality. Regulators of water balance are osmolality sensors in the anterior hypothalamus that stimulate thirst and vasopressin (antidiuretic hormone). Vasopressin is released in response to an increase in serum osmolality and acts on the collecting ducts of the kidney, causing water retention. Many factors and drugs affect vasopressin secretion (Table 18-2).
2. **Osmolality**
   a. ***Normal Serum Osmolality.*** Normal osmolality is 280 to 290 mOsm/kg. A shorthand, indirect calculation of serum osmolality can be performed as follows:

   $$2[\text{Na}] + \text{glucose} / 18 + \text{BUN} / 2.8$$

   where BUN is blood urea nitrogen.

   b. ***"Osmolal Gap."*** The osmolal gap is the difference between the indirect calculation and measured serum osmolality. A significant difference may indicate the presence of unmeasured, osmotically active particles.

   c. ***Increased Osmolality.*** An increase can be caused by water depletion, ingestion of solutes such as ethanol or other toxins, hyperglycemia, or iatrogenic administration of osmolal loads such as mannitol or glycine. Administration of osmolal loads should take into

TABLE 18-1 ■ Etiology of Water, Electrolyte, and Acid-Base Disturbances During the Perioperative Period

DISEASE STATES
Endocrinopathies
Nephropathies
Gastroenteropathies
DRUG THERAPY
Diuretics
Corticosteroids
Nasogastric suction
SURGERY
Transurethral resection of the prostate
Translocation of body water as a result of tissue trauma
Resection of portions of the gastrointestinal tract
MANAGEMENT OF ANESTHESIA
Intravenous fluid administration
Alveolar ventilation
Hypothermia

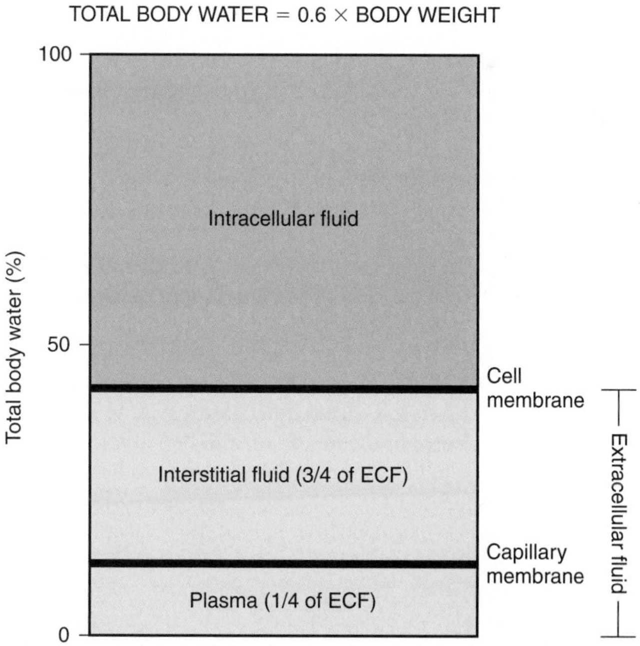

FIGURE 18-1 ■ Total body water (approximately 60% of total body weight) is designated as intracellular fluid (ICF) or extracellular fluid (ECF) depending on the location of the water relative to cell membranes. ECF is further divided into interstitial and plasma compartments depending on its location relative to vascular walls. Of total body water, two thirds is ICF. Of ECF, 75% is interstitial and 25% is intravascular

TABLE 18-2 ■ Factors and Drugs Affecting Vasopressin Secretion

STIMULATION OF VASOPRESSIN RELEASE	INHIBITION OF VASOPRESSIN RELEASE	DRUGS THAT STIMULATE VASOPRESSIN RELEASE AND/OR POTENTIATE THE RENAL ACTION OF VASOPRESSIN
Contracted ECF volume	Expanded ECF volume	Amitriptyline
Hypernatremia	Hyponatremia	Barbiturates
Hypotension	Hypertension	Carbamazepine
Nausea and vomiting		Chlorpropamide
Congestive heart failure		Clofibrate
Cirrhosis		Morphine
Hypothyroidism		Nicotine
Angiotensin II		Phenothiazines
Catecholamines		SSRIs
Histamine		
Bradykinin		

ECF, Extracellular fluid; *SSRIs*, selective serotonin reuptake inhibitors.

consideration preexisting osmolality to avoid extreme increases in serum osmolality (>320 mOsm/kg).

3. **Isotonic Changes in TBW.** Isotonic changes in TBW (e.g., changes in effective circulating volume) are detected by the kidney juxtaglomerular apparatus with resulting changes in kidney renin excretion. Renin converts angiotensinogen into angiotensin I, which is converted to angiotensin II in the lungs. Angiotensin II causes adrenal release of aldosterone. Aldosterone promotes sodium reabsorption and potassium loss in the distal renal tubule, as well as water resorption. Increases in circulating volume cause release of natriuretic peptide, promoting a return to water homeostasis.

B. Disorders of Sodium

1. **Hyponatremia.** When water retention or water intake exceeds the ability of the kidneys to excrete dilute urine, and serum sodium declines to less than 136 mEq/L, hyponatremia is present. (Normal serum sodium is 136 to 145 mEq/L.)
   a. ***Signs and Symptoms of Hyponatremia.*** Symptoms depend on the rate at which hyponatremia develops. Symptoms are rare with serum sodium concentration higher than 125 mEq/L (Table 18-3).
   b. ***Diagnosis*** (Figure 18-2). Hyponatremia usually co-exists with hypo-osmolality except in two circumstances. Glucose, mannitol, and glycine cause water to move from the intracellular space into the ECF with a resultant decrease in the serum sodium concentration without a change in total body sodium or TBW. In cases of severe hyperlipidemia or a paraproteinemic disorder, the measured sodium concentration will be falsely low (pseudohyponatremia). Once these two situations have been excluded, the approach to the diagnosis of hyponatremia is to first evaluate ECF volume from the clinical presentation.
      i. ***Hypervolemic Hyponatremia.*** This suggests renal failure, congestive heart failure, or a hypoalbuminemic state such as cirrhosis or nephrotic syndrome.
      ii. ***Normovolemic Hyponatremia.*** Normovolemic hyponatremia may be seen with syndrome of inappropriate antidiuretic hormone (SIADH) or habitual ingestion of hypotonic substances (e.g., psychogenic polydipsia).
      iii. ***Hypovolemic Hyponatremia.*** This suggests free water loss.
         (a) ***Renal losses.*** Diuretics, mineralocorticoid deficiency, and salt-wasting nephropathy cause renal losses.

TABLE 18-3 ■ **Symptoms and Signs of Hyponatremia**

SYMPTOMS	SIGNS
Anorexia	Abnormal sensorium
Nausea	Disorientation, agitation
Lethargy	Cheyne-Stokes breathing
Apathy	Hypothermia
Muscle cramps	Pathologic reflexes
	Pseudobulbar palsy
	Seizures
	Coma
	Death

(b) ***Extrarenal losses.*** Gastrointestinal (GI) losses and third spacing constitute extrarenal losses.

c. ***Treatment of Hyponatremia.*** Treatment depends on the volume status of the patient (Table 18-4) and whether the condition is acute or chronic.

i. ***Acute Symptomatic Hyponatremia.*** Treat promptly. Withhold solute-free solutions; administer hypertonic saline (3% NaCl) and furosemide, with frequent monitoring of serum electrolytes until symptoms disappear.

ii. ***Chronic Symptomatic Hyponatremia.*** Correct slowly to avoid the risk of osmotic demyelination. Guidelines for correction of chronic symptomatic hyponatremia call for an initial correction in the serum sodium of approximately 10 mEq/L; thereafter, correct 1 to 1.5 mEq/L/hr (daily maximum increase of 12 mEq/L).

iii. ***Chronic Asymptomatic Hyponatremia.*** Treatment includes appropriate sodium intake and volume restriction along with treatment of underlying cause.

d. ***Management of Anesthesia.*** Hyponatremia should be corrected before surgery whenever possible. If the surgery is urgent, then appropriate corrective treatment should continue throughout the surgery and into the postoperative period.

i. ***Vasopressors and/or Inotropes.*** These agents may be required to treat the hypotension and should be made available before the start of induction. Hypervolemic hyponatremic patients, particularly those with heart failure, may benefit from invasive hemodynamic monitoring.

ii. ***TURP Syndrome.*** Irrigating fluid used during transurethral resection of the prostate (TURP) (glycine, sorbitol, or mannitol) may be rapidly absorbed, with resulting volume overload, hyponatremia, and hypo-osmolality. This is more likely in prolonged surgery (>1 hour), if the fluid is suspended more than 40 cm above the operative field, or if the pressure in the bladder is more than 15 cm H_2O. TURP syndrome manifests with cardiovascular and neurologic signs and symptoms. Treatment consists of terminating the surgical procedure, diuretics for relief of cardiovascular symptoms, and hypertonic saline administration if severe neurologic symptoms are present or the serum sodium concentration is less than 120 mEq/L.

2. **Hypernatremia.** Defined as serum sodium greater than 145 mEq/L, hypernatremia is invariably accompanied by hyperosmolality and always causes cellular dehydration and shrinkage.

a. ***Signs and Symptoms of Hypernatremia*** *(Table 18-5)*

b. ***Diagnosis*** *(Figure 18-3)*

c. ***Treatment.*** The patient with euvolemic hypernatremia requires water replacement either orally or with 5% dextrose intravenously. Acute hypernatremia should be corrected over several hours. However, to avoid cerebral edema, chronic hypernatremia should be

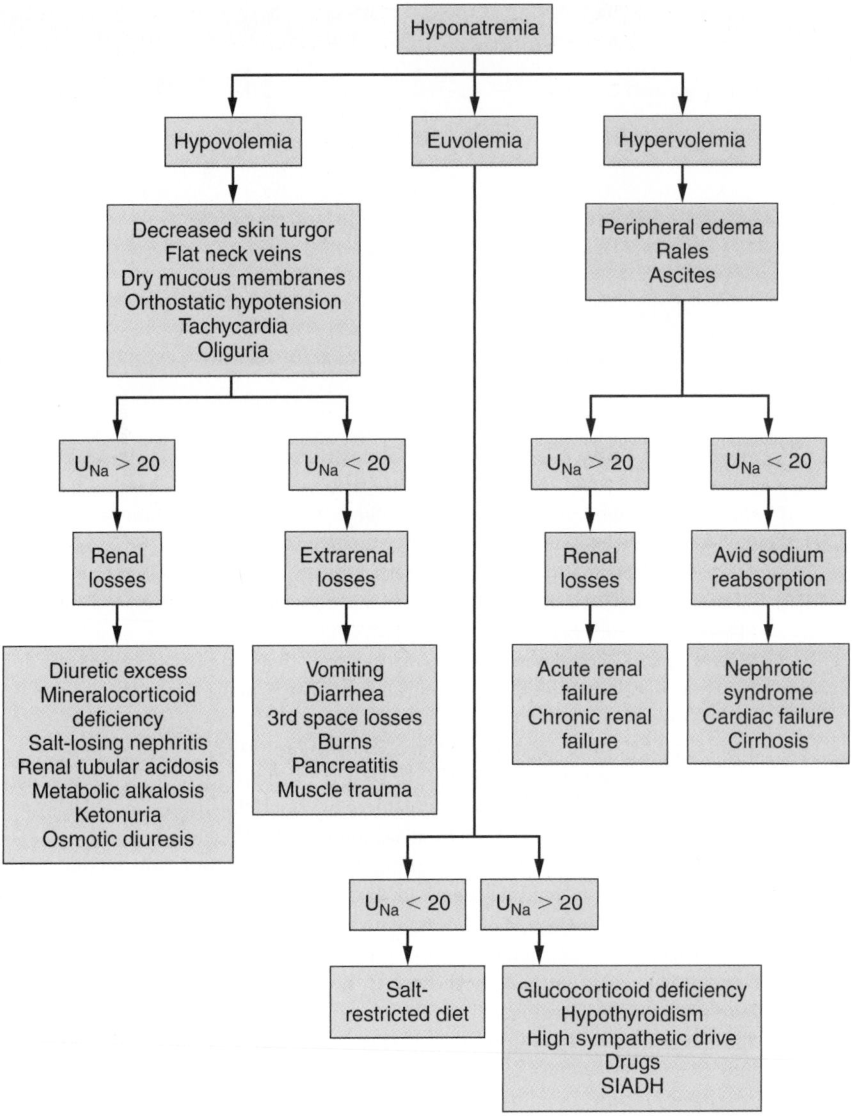

FIGURE 18-2 ■ Diagnostic algorithm for hyponatremia. Urinary sodium concentration *(U_{Na})* (mEq/L) in a spot urine sample. *SIADH,* Syndrome of inappropriate secretion of antidiuretic hormone. *(Adapted from Schrier RW:* Manual of Nephrology. *6th ed. Philadelphia, PA: Lippincott Williams & Wilkins, 2006.)*

TABLE 18-4 ■ **Treatment of Hyponatremia**

Hypovolemic hyponatremia	Volume resuscitation, usually with normal saline. Treatment of mineralocorticoid deficiency or adrenal insufficiency if present.
Euvolemic or hypervolemic hyponatremia	Withhold free water. Encourage free water excretion with loop diuretic. Saline administration seldom needed unless symptoms are present.

TABLE 18-5 ■ **Symptoms and Signs of Hypernatremia**

SYMPTOMS	SIGNS
Polyuria	Muscle twitching
Polydipsia	Hyperreflexia
Orthostasis	Tremor
Restlessness	Ataxia
Irritability	Muscle spasticity
Lethargy	Focal and generalized seizures
	Death

corrected more slowly, over 2 to 3 days. In patients with hypervolemic hypernatremia, treatment is diuresis.

d. ***Management of Anesthesia.*** Surgery should be delayed whenever possible until the hypernatremia has been corrected. Hypovolemia will be exacerbated by induction and maintenance of anesthesia, and prompt correction of hypotension with fluids, vasopressors, and/or inotropes may be required.

C. Disorders of Potassium

1. **Hypokalemia.** Hypokalemia is defined as a serum potassium concentration of less than 3.5 mEq/L (Table 18-6).

a. ***Signs and Symptoms.*** Signs of hypokalemia are generally restricted to the cardiac and neuromuscular systems and include dysrhythmias, muscle weakness, cramps, paralysis, and ileus.

b. ***Diagnosis.*** Diagnosis is made by testing the serum potassium concentration. A spot urinary potassium will guide the diagnosis toward either renal causes (urinary potassium >20 mEq/L) or extrarenal causes (urinary potassium <20 mEq/L).

c. ***Treatment.*** Treatment depends on the degree of potassium depletion and the underlying cause. If hypokalemia is profound or associated with life-threatening signs, potassium must be administered intravenously, and the amount depends on whether there are associated decreases in total body potassium. Typically, 20 mEq of potassium can be administered over 30 to 45 minutes, with administration repeated as needed. Such rapid repletion requires electrocardiographic monitoring.

d. ***Management of Anesthesia.*** The decision to treat hypokalemia before surgery depends on the chronicity and severity of the defect. The risk of perioperative dysrhythmias in these patients remains unclear. It may be prudent to correct significant hypokalemia in patients with other risk factors for dysrhythmias such as those with congestive heart failure or on digoxin therapy. It is also important to avoid further decreases in serum potassium concentration (e.g., as a result of administration of insulin, glucose, β-adrenergic agonists, bicarbonate, and diuretics; hyperventilation; and respiratory alkalosis).

2. **Hyperkalemia.** Hyperkalemia is defined as a serum potassium concentration greater than 5.5 mEq/L (Table 18-7).

a. ***Signs and Symptoms.*** Signs of hyperkalemia are dependent on the acuity of the increase. Chronic hyperkalemia is often asymptomatic, and dialysis-dependent patients can withstand considerable variations in serum potassium concentration. Acute or significant increases in potassium manifest as cardiac and neuromuscular changes and include weakness, paralysis, nausea, vomiting, and bradycardia or asystole.

b. ***Diagnosis.*** The first step is to rule out a spuriously high potassium level secondary to hemolysis of the specimen, thrombocytosis, or leukocytosis. If hyperkalemia is associated with increased total body potassium stores, then decreased renal excretion or increased extrarenal production of potassium is likely. The urinary potassium excretion rate can aid in the differential diagnosis.

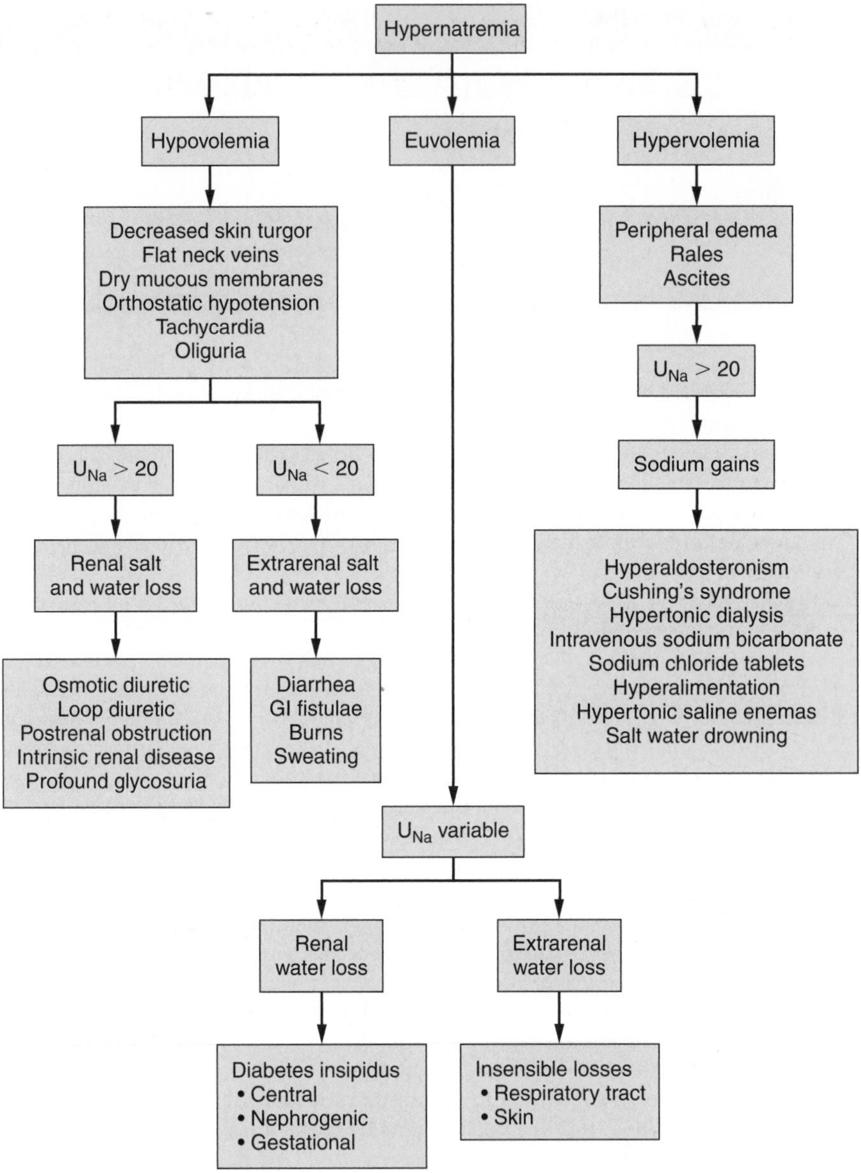

FIGURE 18-3 ■ Diagnostic algorithm for hypernatremia. *GI*, Gastrointestinal; U_{Na}, urinary sodium concentration (mEq/L) in a spot urine sample. *(Adapted from Schrier RW:* Manual of Nephrology. *6th ed. Philadelphia, PA: Lippincott Williams & Wilkins, 2006.)*

c. ***Treatment.*** Immediate treatment of hyperkalemia is required if life-threatening dysrhythmias or electrocardiographic changes are present. This treatment consists of intravenous calcium chloride or calcium gluconate to stabilize cellular membranes, insulin with or without glucose to help redistribute potassium into cells, and sodium bicarbonate and hyperventilation to promote alkalosis and movement of potassium intracellularly. Loop diuretics and sodium polystyrene sulfonate (Kayexalate) given either orally or by enema can promote potassium elimination from the body. Dialysis may be required to remove potassium in patients with poor renal function.

TABLE 18-6 ■ **Causes of Hypokalemia**

HYPOKALEMIA CAUSED BY INCREASED RENAL POTASSIUM LOSS
Thiazide diuretics
Loop diuretics
Mineralocorticoids
High-dose glucocorticoids
High-dose antibiotics (penicillin, nafcillin, ampicillin)
Drugs associated with magnesium depletion (aminoglycosides)
Surgical trauma
Hyperglycemia
Hyperaldosteronism
HYPOKALEMIA CAUSED BY EXCESSIVE GASTROINTESTINAL LOSS OF POTASSIUM
Vomiting and diarrhea
Zollinger-Ellison syndrome
Jejunoileal bypass
Malabsorption
Chemotherapy
Nasogastric suction
HYPOKALEMIA CAUSED BY TRANSCELLULAR POTASSIUM SHIFT
β-Adrenergic agonists
Tocolytic drugs (ritodrine)
Insulin
Respiratory or metabolic alkalosis
Familial periodic paralysis
Hypercalcemia
Hypomagnesemia

Adapted from Gennari JF. Hypokalemia. *N Engl J Med*. 1998;339:451-458.

TABLE 18-7 ■ **Causes of Hyperkalemia**

INCREASED TOTAL BODY POTASSIUM CONTENT
Acute oliguric renal failure
Chronic renal disease
Hypoaldosteronism
Drugs that impair potassium excretion
Triamterene
Spironolactone
Nonsteroidal antiinflammatory drugs
Drugs that inhibit the renin-angiotensin-aldosterone system
ALTERED TRANSCELLULAR POTASSIUM SHIFT
Succinylcholine
Respiratory or metabolic acidosis
Lysis of cells because of chemotherapy
Iatrogenic bolus
PSEUDOHYPERKALEMIA
Hemolysis of blood specimen
Thrombocytosis, leukocytosis

d. ***Management of Anesthesia.*** Serum potassium concentration should be below 5.5 mEq/L for elective surgery. Because succinylcholine increases serum potassium by approximately 0.5 mEq/L, it is best avoided. Respiratory and metabolic acidosis must be avoided because either will exacerbate the hyperkalemia and its effects. Intravenous fluids should be potassium free (avoid Ringer's lactate solution and Normosol).

D. Disorders of Calcium

1. **Hypocalcemia.** Hypocalcemia is defined as a reduction in serum ionized calcium concentration. Binding of calcium to albumin is pH dependent, and acid-base disturbances can change the fraction and therefore the concentration of ionized calcium without changing total body calcium. Alkalosis reduces the ionized calcium concentration, so ionized calcium may be significantly reduced after bicarbonate administration or with hyperventilation. Hypoalbuminemia results in decreases in bound calcium, which will reduce the serum calcium level. A corrected calcium level can be calculated as follows:

$$\text{Measured Ca (mg/dL)} + 0.8\,[4 - \text{albumin (mg/dL)}]$$

a. ***Signs and Symptoms.*** Symptoms depend on the rapidity and the degree of reduction in ionized calcium. They include paresthesias, irritability, seizures, hypotension, and myocardial depression. Laryngospasm can be life-threatening.

b. ***Diagnosis.*** The most common causes of hypocalcemia include a decrease in parathyroid hormone secretion, end-organ resistance to parathyroid hormone, or disorders of vitamin D metabolism. These are usually seen as complications of thyroid or parathyroid surgery, magnesium deficiency, and renal failure.

c. ***Treatment.*** Acute treatment is intravenous calcium and correction of metabolic or respiratory alkalosis. Treatment of hypocalcemia in the presence of hypomagnesemia is ineffective unless magnesium is also replenished. Less acute and asymptomatic hypocalcemia may be treated with oral calcium supplementation and vitamin D.

d. ***Management of Anesthesia.*** Symptomatic hypocalcemia must be treated before surgery. Alkalosis caused by hyperventilation or administration of bicarbonate should be avoided. Ionized calcium levels may decrease with massive transfusion of blood containing citrate or when citrate metabolism is impaired by hypothermia, liver disease, or renal failure. Sudden decreases in ionized calcium levels may occur postoperatively after thyroidectomy or parathyroidectomy and may cause laryngospasm.

2. **Hypercalcemia.** Hypercalcemia results from increased calcium absorption from the GI tract (milk alkali syndrome, vitamin D intoxication, granulomatous diseases such as sarcoidosis), decreased renal calcium excretion in renal insufficiency, and increased bone resorption of calcium (primary or secondary hyperparathyroidism, malignancy, hyperthyroidism, and immobilization).

a. ***Signs and Symptoms.*** Signs include confusion, hypotonia, depressed deep tendon reflexes, lethargy, abdominal pain, and nausea and vomiting, especially if the increase in serum calcium is relatively acute. Chronic hypercalcemia is often associated with polyuria, hypercalciuria, and nephrolithiasis.

b. ***Diagnosis.*** A workup for hyperparathyroidism or cancer is performed.

c. ***Treatment.*** Fluid deficits are corrected, and loop diuretics are given to enhance urinary excretion of sodium and calcium. Calcitonin, bisphosphonates, or mithramycin may be required in disorders associated with osteoclastic bone resorption. Dialysis may be required for life-threatening hypercalcemia. Surgical removal of the parathyroid glands may be necessary to treat primary or secondary hyperparathyroidism.

d. ***Management of Anesthesia.*** Hydration is performed before induction, and loop diuretics are given to increase urinary calcium excretion. (Avoid thiazide diuretics, which increase tubular reabsorption of calcium.)

E. Disorders of Magnesium

1. **Hypomagnesemia.** Hypomagnesemia occurs in up to 10% of hospitalized patients, particularly intensive care patients receiving parenteral nutrition or dialysis.
   a. ***Signs and Symptoms.*** Similar to those of hypocalcemia, signs and symptoms include dysrhythmias, weakness, muscle twitching, tetany, apathy, and seizures.
   b. ***Diagnosis.*** Hypomagnesemia caused by reduced GI uptake or renal wasting of magnesium can be differentiated by measuring the urinary magnesium excretion rate.
   c. ***Treatment.*** If cardiac dysrhythmias or seizures are present, magnesium is administered intravenously as a bolus (2 g of magnesium sulfate equals 8 mEq of magnesium), and the dose is repeated until symptoms abate.
   d. ***Management of Anesthesia.*** Ventricular dysrhythmias should be anticipated and treated as necessary. Muscle relaxation should be guided by the use of a peripheral nerve stimulator because hypomagnesemia can be associated with both muscle weakness and muscle excitation.
2. **Hypermagnesemia.** Defined as serum magnesium concentration over 2.5 mEq/L, hypermagnesemia is much less common than hypomagnesemia and is usually iatrogenic—that is, it occurs as a complication of magnesium sulfate therapy for preeclampsia or eclampsia.
   a. ***Signs and Symptoms.*** Signs of hypermagnesemia begin to occur at serum levels of 4 to 5 mEq/L and include lethargy, nausea and vomiting, and facial flushing. At levels above 6 mEq/L, a loss of deep tendon reflexes and hypotension are seen. Paralysis, apnea, and/or cardiac arrest are likely if the magnesium level exceeds 10 mEq/L.
   b. ***Diagnosis of Hypermagnesemia.*** Diagnosis involves determining renal function (creatinine clearance) and detecting any source of excess magnesium intake. Less common causes of hypermagnesemia include hypothyroidism, hyperparathyroidism, Addison's disease, and lithium therapy.
   c. ***Treatment.*** For acute clinical signs, treatment is intravenous calcium administration. Dialysis may be required.
   d. ***Management of Anesthesia.*** Management includes avoidance of acidosis and dehydration, maintenance of urine output, and recognition that response to muscle relaxants may be prolonged.

F. Acid-Base Disorders.

Acid-base balance is normally regulated within the range of 7.35 to 7.45 to ensure an optimal pH for cellular enzyme function. Values of arterial blood pH less than 7.35 are termed *acidosis* or *acidemia,* and values greater than 7.45 are termed *alkalosis* or *alkalemia.* The major buffer system participating in regulation of body pH is the bicarbonate–carbon dioxide system. Although the respiratory system (via CO_2 regulation) can provide some defense against acid-base disorders, the kidneys have a greater ability (via bicarbonate regulation) to normalize pH.

1. **The Henderson-Hasselbach Equation.** This equation describes the relationship between the pulmonary and renal regulation of pH by the following buffer system:

$$pH = 6.1 + \log(\text{serum bicarbonate concentration} / 0.03 \times Pa_{CO_2})$$

   Maintenance of a normal bicarbonate concentration relative to carbon dioxide tension results in an optimal ratio of approximately 20:1.
2. **Identification of an Acid-Base Disturbance.** Identification follows a series of steps (Figures 18-4, 18-5, and 18-6):
   a. Identify whether the pH is increased or decreased. An increase identifies an alkalosis, and a decrease identifies an acidosis.
   b. Identify the change in Pa_{CO_2} and bicarbonate from their normal levels of 40 mm Hg and 24 mEq/L, respectively.

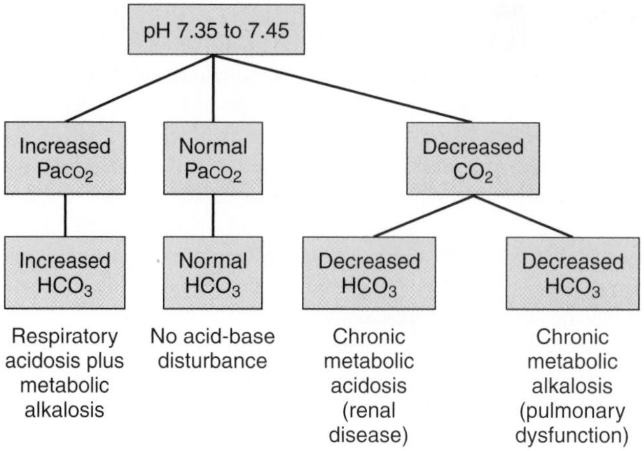

FIGURE 18-4 ■ Diagnostic approach to the interpretation of normal arterial pH based on $Paco_2$ and bicarbonate concentration.

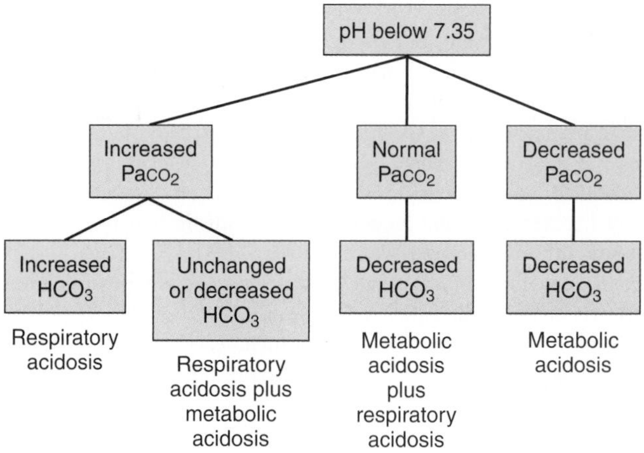

FIGURE 18-5 ■ Diagnostic approach to interpretation of an arterial pH less than 7.35 based on $Paco_2$ and bicarbonate concentration.

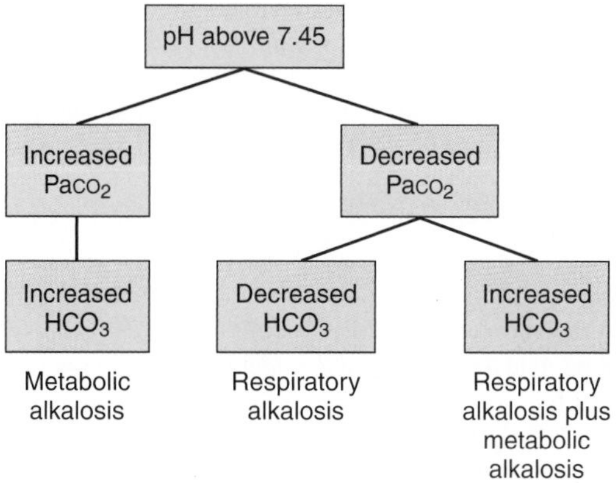

FIGURE 18-6 ■ Diagnostic approach to interpretation of an arterial pH greater than 7.45 based on $Paco_2$ and bicarbonate concentration.

TABLE 18-8 ■ Adverse Consequences of Severe Acidosis

NERVOUS SYSTEM
Obtundation Coma
CARDIOVASCULAR SYSTEM
Impaired myocardial contractility Decreased cardiac output Decreased arterial blood pressure Sensitization to cardiac dysrhythmias Decreased threshold for ventricular fibrillation Decreased responsiveness to catecholamines
VENTILATION
Hyperventilation Dyspnea Fatigue of respiratory muscles
METABOLISM
Hyperkalemia Insulin resistance Inhibition of anaerobic glycolysis

Adapted from Adrogué HJ, Madias NE. Management of life-threatening acid-base disorders. *N Engl J Med.* 1998;338:26-34.

c. If both $Paco_2$ and bicarbonate change in the same direction (i.e., both are increased or both are decreased), then there is a primary acid-base disorder with a compensatory secondary disorder that brings the ratio of bicarbonate/carbon dioxide tension back to 20:1.

d. If bicarbonate and $Paco_2$ change in opposite directions, there is a mixed acid-base disorder.

e. Determine the primary acid-base disorder by comparing the fractional change of the measured bicarbonate or carbon dioxide tension with the normal value.

f. There are equations and nomograms that calculate the expected change in one of the three parameters involved in acid-base determination (pH, bicarbonate, or carbon dioxide tension) for a given change in one of the other two parameters. If the actual change is markedly different from the expected change, then there is a mixed acid-base disorder.

g. Finally, calculate the anion gap to determine whether there is a hidden metabolic acidosis. Elevation in the anion gap requires subsequent identification of the unmeasured anion.

3. **Signs and Symptoms.** Major adverse consequences of severe systemic acidosis (pH <7.2) can occur independently of whether the acidosis is of respiratory, metabolic, or mixed origin (Table 18-8). Major adverse consequences of severe systemic alkalosis (pH >7.60) reflect impairment of cerebral and coronary blood flow because of arteriolar vasoconstriction (Table 18-9).

   a. ***Respiratory Acidosis.*** Respiratory acidosis is present when a decrease in alveolar ventilation results in an increase in the $Paco_2$ sufficient to decrease arterial pH to less than 7.35 (Table 18-10).

      i. ***Treatment.*** The disorder responsible for hypoventilation is corrected. Mechanical ventilation may be needed.

TABLE 18-9 ■ Adverse Consequences of Alkalosis

NERVOUS SYSTEM
Decreased cerebral blood flow
Seizures
Lethargy
Delirium
Tetany
CARDIOVASCULAR SYSTEM
Arteriolar vasoconstriction
Decreased coronary blood flow
Decreased threshold for angina pectoris
Predisposition to refractory dysrhythmias
VENTILATION
Hypoventilation
Hypercarbia
Arterial hypoxemia
METABOLISM
Hypokalemia
Hypocalcemia
Hypomagnesemia
Hypophosphatemia
Stimulation of anaerobic glycolysis

Adapted from Adrogué JH, Madias NE. Management of life-threatening acid-base disorders. *N Engl J Med.* 1998;338:107-111.

TABLE 18-10 ■ Causes of Respiratory Acidosis

Drug-induced ventilatory depression
Permissive hypercapnia
Upper airway obstruction
Status asthmaticus
Restriction of ventilation (rib fractures, flail chest)
Disorders of neuromuscular function
Malignant hyperthermia
Hyperalimentation solutions

ii. ***Hypokalemia and Hypochloremia.*** Both conditions are associated with metabolic alkalosis that may accompany respiratory acidosis and may require treatment.

b. ***Respiratory Alkalosis.*** Respiratory alkalosis is present when an increase in alveolar ventilation results in a decrease in $Paco_2$ sufficient to increase the pH to greater than 7.45 (Table 18-11).

i. ***Treatment.*** For respiratory alkalosis, treatment is directed at correcting the underlying disorder responsible for alveolar hyperventilation.

ii. ***Hypokalemia and Hypochloremia.*** Both conditions may co-exist with respiratory alkalosis and may also require treatment.

c. ***Metabolic Acidosis.*** Metabolic acidosis lowers blood pH, stimulating the respiratory center to lower carbon dioxide tension. Respiratory compensation does not in general fully

TABLE 18-11 ■ Causes of Respiratory Alkalosis

Iatrogenic (mechanical hyperventilation)
Decreased barometric pressure
Arterial hypoxemia
Central nervous system injury
Hepatic disease
Pregnancy
Salicylate overdose

TABLE 18-12 ■ Causes of Metabolic Acidosis

Lactic acidosis
Diabetic ketoacidosis
Renal failure
Hepatic failure
Methanol and ethylene glycol intoxication
Aspirin intoxication
Increased skeletal muscle activity
Cyanide poisoning
Carbon monoxide poisoning

compensate for increased acid production. "Normal anion gap" acidosis is the result of a net increase in chloride concentration, or *hyperchloremic metabolic acidosis.* A "high anion gap" occurs when a fixed acid is added to the extracellular space. Lactic acidosis, ketoacidosis, renal failure, and the acidosis associated with many poisonings are examples of forms of acidosis with a high anion gap.

i. ***Signs and Symptoms.*** Signs depend on the underlying disorder and the rate of development of the acidosis.

ii. ***Diagnosis.*** Analysis of arterial blood for pH, carbon dioxide tension, bicarbonate concentration, and anion gap is performed. Common causes of metabolic acidosis are listed in Table 18-12.

   (a) ***Metabolic Acidosis of Renal Origin.*** Metabolic acidosis occurs if the kidneys are unable to replace the bicarbonate that is lost by buffering normal endogenous acid production (distal renal tubular acidosis) or because an abnormally high fraction of bicarbonate is lost in the urine (proximal renal tubular acidosis or acetazolamide use).

   (b) ***Metabolic Acidosis of Extrarenal Origin.*** GI bicarbonate losses, ketoacidosis, and lactic acidosis can result in metabolic acidosis.

iii. ***Treatment.*** Treatment of metabolic acidosis includes treatment of the cause, and in some cases administration of sodium bicarbonate for acute treatment (e.g., if the pH is less than 7.1 or the bicarbonate concentration is less than 10 mEq/L). *Acute* changes in pH toward normal (or alkalosis) may result in increased hemoglobin affinity for oxygen and reduce oxygen tissue oxygen delivery. The 2005 American Heart Association Guidelines for Cardiopulmonary Resuscitation and Emergency Cardiovascular Care do not recommend administering sodium bicarbonate routinely during cardiac arrest and cardiopulmonary resuscitation unless life-threatening hyperkalemia or cardiac arrest associated with a preexisting metabolic acidosis has occurred.

TABLE 18-13 ■ Causes of Metabolic Alkalosis
Hypovolemia
Vomiting
Nasogastric suction
Diuretic therapy
Bicarbonate administration
Hyperaldosteronism
Chloride-wasting diarrhea

iv. ***Management of Anesthesia.*** Elective surgery should be postponed until acidosis has been treated. Invasive hemodynamic monitoring should be considered. Frequent laboratory measurement of acid-base parameters should be made throughout the perioperative period.

d. ***Metabolic Alkalosis.*** Metabolic alkalosis is an increase in pH, an increase in plasma bicarbonate concentration, and a compensatory increase in carbon dioxide tension. Common causes of metabolic alkalosis are noted in Table 18-13.

i. ***Treatment.*** Rarely is administration of an acid required; usually volume replacement is all that is needed.

ii. ***Management of Anesthesia.*** Management is directed at judicious volume replacement and adequate supplementation with chloride, potassium, and magnesium as needed.

CHAPTER 19

Endocrine Disease

I. DIABETES MELLITUS

Diabetes mellitus results from inadequate supply of insulin and/or inadequate tissue response to insulin with increased circulating glucose levels and eventual microvascular and macrovascular complications. Type 1a diabetes is caused by autoimmune destruction of pancreatic islet beta cells and complete absence or negligible circulating insulin levels. Type 1b diabetes is a rare nonautoimmune disease with absolute insulin deficiency. Type 2 diabetes is not immune mediated; it is caused by a relative deficiency of insulin coupled with an insulin receptor defect or defect(s) in its postreceptor intracellular signaling pathways.

A. Signs and Symptoms

1. **Type 1 Diabetes.** This type of diabetes (5% to 10% of all diabetes mellitus) manifests before age 40. It is caused by T cell–mediated autoimmune destruction of pancreatic beta cells. Viruses (e.g., enteroviruses), dietary proteins, and drugs or chemicals may initiate the autoimmune process in genetically susceptible hosts. After a long preclinical period (9 to 13 years), the onset of clinical disease (hyperglycemia, fatigue, weight loss, polyuria, polydipsia, blurring of vision, and volume depletion) is often sudden and severe. Diagnosis is based on a random blood glucose test result of more than 200 mg/dL and a hemoglobin A_{1c} (Hb A_{1c}) level greater than 7%. The presence of ketoacidosis indicates severe insulin deficiency and unrestrained lipolysis.
2. **Type 2 Diabetes.** Type 2 diabetes (90% of all diabetes mellitus) occurs typically in middle to older patients (more recently in younger patients and children as a result of obesity) and is caused by relative beta-cell insufficiency and insulin resistance. Three important defects in type 2 diabetes are (1) increased rate of hepatic glucose release, (2) impaired basal and stimulated insulin secretion, and (3) inefficient use of glucose by peripheral tissues (insulin resistance). Insulin resistance appears to be inherited. Acquired characteristics (obesity, sedentary lifestyle) are contributing factors.
3. **Metabolic Syndrome.** Insulin-resistance syndrome or metabolic syndrome (Table 19-1) is a combination of insulin resistance with other clinical characteristics (hypertension, dyslipidemia, a procoagulant state, obesity, premature atherosclerosis, and cardiovascular disease).

B. Diagnosis (Table 19-2).
The upper limit of normal for fasting plasma glucose is 100 mg/dL. Hyperglycemia that does not meet the criteria for diabetes is classified as either impaired fasting glucose or impaired glucose tolerance. Hb A_{1c} represents the percentage of hemoglobin molecules that has been glycosylated and reflects the average plasma glucose concentration during the previous 60 to 90 days. Normal range for Hb A_{1c} is 4% to 6%. Increased risk of microvascular and macrovascular disease begins at an Hb A_{1c} of 6.5%.

C. Treatment

1. **Considerations in Type 2 Diabetes**
   a. ***Diet.*** Reduction of body weight through diet and exercise is the first therapeutic measure in type 2 diabetes.

TABLE 19-1 ■ Metabolic Syndrome

At least three of the following must be present:
- Fasting plasma glucose ≥110 mg/dL
- Abdominal obesity (waist girth >40 inches [men], >35 inches [women])
- Serum triglycerides ≥150 mg/dL
- Serum high-density lipoprotein cholesterol <40 mg/dL (men), <50 mg/dL (women)
- Blood pressure ≥130/85 mm Hg

Adapted from Expert Panel on Detection, Evaluation, and Treatment of High Blood Cholesterol in Adults. Executive Summary of The Third Report of The National Cholesterol Education Program (NCEP) Expert Panel on Detection, Evaluation, and Treatment of High Blood Cholesterol in Adults (Adult Treatment Panel III). *JAMA*. 2001;285:2486-2497.

TABLE 19-2 ■ Diagnostic Criteria for Diabetes Mellitus

Symptoms of diabetes (polyuria, polydipsia, unexplained weight loss) plus a random plasma glucose concentration ≥200 mg/dL

or

Fasting (no caloric intake for ≥8 hr) plasma glucose ≥126 mg/dL

or

Two-hour plasma glucose >200 mg/dL during an oral glucose tolerance test

TABLE 19-3 ■ Second-Generation Sulfonylureas

DRUG	INITIAL DOSE (mg/day)	DAILY DOSE RANGE (mg/day)	DURATION (hr)	DOSES/DAY
Glyburide	1.25-2.5	1.25-20	18-24	1-2
Glipizide	2.5-5.0	2.5-40	12-18	1-2
Glimepiride	1-2	4-8	24	1

b. ***Oral Antidiabetic Agents.*** The four types of oral antidiabetic agents are used alone or in combination to maintain glucose control (fasting glucose, 90 to 130 mg/dL; peak postprandial glucose, <180 mg/dL; Hb A_{1c} <7%) in the initial stages of the disease.
   i. ***Secretagogues.*** Sulfonylureas and meglitinides increase insulin secretion from pancreatic beta cells and enhance tissue usage of glucose (Table 19-3). Hypoglycemia is the most common side effect.
   ii. ***Biguanides.*** Metformin suppresses excessive hepatic glucose release. Metformin is often combined with a sulfonylurea.
   iii. ***Thiazolidinediones.*** Thiazolidinediones, or glitazones (rosiglitazone, pioglitazone), improve insulin sensitivity.
   iv. ***α-Glucosidase Inhibitors.*** Acarbose and miglitol delay gastrointestinal glucose absorption.

c. ***Insulin Therapy in Type 2 Diabetes.*** An algorithm for treatment of type 2 diabetes, including oral agents, is summarized in Figure 19-1. Monotherapy with oral agents eventually usually fails, and combination therapy becomes necessary. If combination therapy is ineffective, a bedtime dose of intermediate-acting insulin is added. If oral agents plus single-dose insulin therapy is ineffective, patients with type 2 diabetes are switched to insulin exclusively. A combination of intermediate and regular insulin twice daily is commonly used

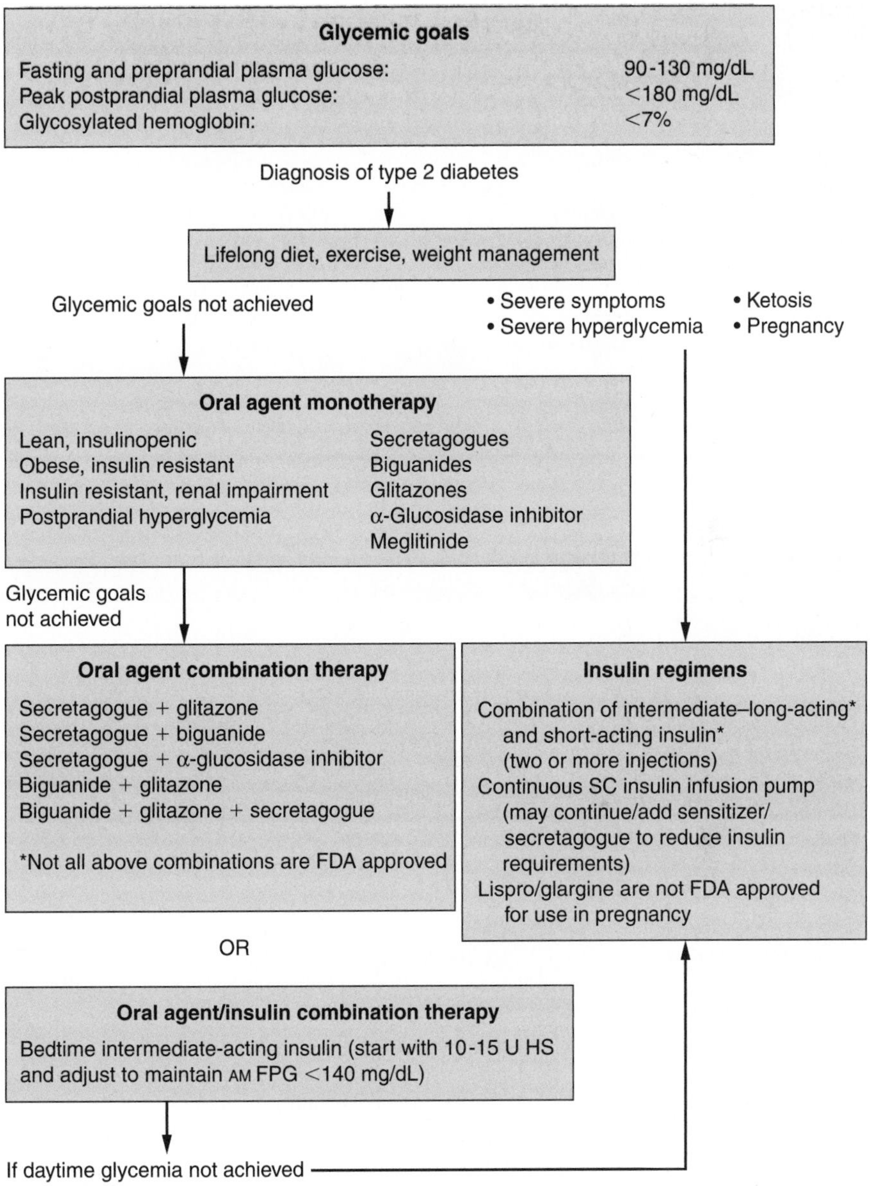

FIGURE 19-1 ■ Algorithm for treatment of type 2 diabetes. *FPG,* Fasting plasma glucose level; *HS,* at bedtime; *SC,* subcutaneous. *(Adapted from Inzucchi S [ed].* The Diabetes Mellitus Manual: A Primary Companion to Ellenberg and Rifkin's Sixth Edition. *New York, NY: McGraw-Hill; 2005: 193.)*

for optimal control. Goals of therapy include Hb A_{1c} less than 7%, low-density lipoprotein less than 100 mg/dL, high-density lipoprotein more than 40 mg/dL in men and more than 50 mg/dL in women, triglycerides less than 200 mg/dL, and blood pressure less than 130/80.

2. **Types of Insulin** (Table 19-4). Insulin is always necessary to manage type 1 diabetes (and is necessary for about 30% of patients with type 2 diabetes). Conventional insulin therapy involves twice-daily injections of combinations of intermediate-acting and short- or rapid-acting insulins.

TABLE 19-4 ■ **Insulin**

INSULINS	ONSET	PEAK	DURATION
SHORT-ACTING INSULINS			
Human regular	30 min	2-4 hr	5-8 hr
Lispro (Humalog)	10-15 min	1-2 hr	3-6 hr
Aspart (NovoLog)	10-15 min	1-2 hr	3-6 hr
INTERMEDIATE-ACTING INSULINS			
Human NPH	1-2 hr	6-10 hr	10-20 hr
Lente	1-2 hr	6-10 hr	10-20 hr
LONG-ACTING INSULINS			
Ultralente	4-6 hr	8-20 hr	24-48 hr
Glargine (Lantus)	1-2 hr	Peakless	24 hr

TABLE 19-5 ■ **Diagnostic Features of Diabetic Ketoacidosis**

Glucose (mg/dL)	≥300
pH	≤7.3
HCO_3^- (mEq/L)	≤18
SOsm (mOsm/L)	<320
Ketones	++-+++

SOsm, Serum osmolarity.

a. ***Basal Insulins.*** Basal insulins are intermediate-acting (NPH, lente, lispro protamine, aspart protamine) and given twice daily. A typical total daily basal dose of insulin equals weight (in kilograms) × 0.3.

b. ***Long-Acting Insulins (Ultralente and Glargine).*** These are given once daily.

c. ***Short-Acting Insulins.*** Short- (regular insulin) or rapid-acting insulins (lispro, aspart) provide glycemic control at mealtimes (prandial insulin).

3. **Hypoglycemia.** The most common and dangerous complication of insulin therapy, hypoglycemia can be exacerbated by simultaneous administration of alcohol, sulfonylureas, biguanides, thiazolidinediones, angiotensin-converting enzyme inhibitors (ACEIs), monoamine oxidase inhibitors, and nonselective β-blockers. β-Blockers may exacerbate hypoglycemia by inhibiting adipose tissue lipolysis, which provides alternate fuel during hypoglycemia. The diagnosis in adults requires a plasma glucose level less than 50 mg/dL. Symptoms are adrenergic (sweating, tachycardia, palpitations, restlessness, pallor) and neuroglycopenic (fatigue, confusion, headache, somnolence, convulsions, coma). Treatment is oral sugar in the form of sugar cubes, glucose tablets, or soft drinks (in unconscious patients, glucose 0.5 g/kg intravenously [IV] or glucagon 0.5 to 1.0 mg IV, intramuscularly [IM], or subcutaneously [SC]).

4. **Diabetic Ketoacidosis (DKA).** DKA occurs more commonly in type 1 diabetics and may be precipitated by infection or acute illness, insulin omission, and the new onset of diabetes mellitus (Table 19-5). Mortality is 5% to 10% overall.

TABLE 19-6 ■ Diagnostic Features of Hyperglycemic Hyperosmolar Syndrome	
Glucose (mg/dL)	≥600
pH	≥7.3
HCO_3^- (mEq/L)	≥15
SOsm (mOsm/L)	≥350

SOsm, Serum osmolarity.

a. *Characteristics*

i. ***Increased Ketoacid Production.*** Increased ketoacid production and metabolic acidosis are hallmarks of DKA. Acidosis is associated with an increased anion gap ($Na^+ - [Cl^- + HCO_3^-]$; normal, 8 to 14 mEq/L).

ii. ***Hyperglycemia***

iii. ***Osmotic Diuresis and Hypovolemia***

iv. ***Total Body Deficits in Water, Potassium, and Phosphorus.*** Deficits are present even if laboratory values are normal.

v. ***Hyponatremia***

vi. ***Hypokalemia.*** This is usually substantial: 3 to 5 mEq/kg.

b. *Treatment.*

i. ***Normal Saline.*** Large volumes of normal saline may be needed. Rehydration will lower plasma glucose by 30% to 50%.

ii. ***Insulin.*** Intravenous loading dose of 0.1 units of regular insulin per kilogram and an insulin infusion of 0.1 units/kg/hr should be given until normal acid-base status has been achieved. This may paradoxically require administration of glucose if hyperglycemia is corrected before acid-base status is normal.

iii. ***Electrolyte Supplementation.*** Potassium, phosphate, and magnesium supplementation is performed.

iv. ***Sodium Bicarbonate.*** For a pH of less than 7.1, sodium bicarbonate should be given.

4. Hyperglycemic Hyperosmolar Syndrome (Table 19-6). This syndrome consists of severe hyperglycemia, hyperosmolarity, and dehydration, usually in type 2 diabetics older than 60 years with an acute illness (infection, myocardial infarction, cerebrovascular accident, pancreatitis, intestinal obstruction, endocrinopathy, renal failure, burns). Mortality is 10% to 15%.

a. *Signs and Symptoms.* Signs include polyuria, polydipsia, hypovolemia, hypotension, tachycardia, organ hypoperfusion, obtundation (caused by hyperosmolarity >240 mOsm/L), and aketotic metabolic acidosis.

b. *Treatment*

i. ***Saline.*** If the plasma osmolarity is higher than 320 mOsm/L, large volumes (1000 to 1500 mL/hr) of 0.45% normal saline should be administered until the osmolarity is lower than 320 mOsm/L, at which time large volumes (1000 to 1500 mL/hr) of 0.9% normal saline are administered.

ii. ***Insulin.*** An intravenous bolus of 15 units of regular insulin is administered, followed by a 0.1-unit/kg/hr infusion. The infusion is decreased to 2 to 3 units/hr when the glucose decreases to 250 to 300 mg/dL.

iii. ***Electrolyte Supplementation***

5. Microvascular Complications

a. *Diabetic Nephropathy.* End-stage renal disease develops in 30% to 40% of type 1 diabetics and 5% to 10% of type 2 diabetics.

i. ***Clinical Progression.*** Progression is characterized by hypertension, albuminuria, peripheral edema, and progressive decrease in glomerular filtration rate (GFR). When

GFR is less than 15 to 20 mL/min, the ability of the kidneys to excrete potassium and acids is impaired.

ii. ***Treatment.*** Antihypertensive treatment (low-sodium diet, low-dose diuretics, and one of several antihypertensive agents, including a β_1-antagonist, ACEI, angiotensin II receptor blocker, calcium channel blocker, and/or an α_1-blocker) can slow progression. If end-stage renal disease develops, four treatment options are available: hemodialysis, peritoneal dialysis, continuous ambulatory peritoneal dialysis, and kidney or combined kidney-pancreas transplantation.

b. ***Peripheral Neuropathy.*** This condition develops in more than 50% of patients who have had diabetes for over 25 years. Distal symmetric diffuse sensorimotor polyneuropathy is most common, appearing in the toes or feet and progressing proximally in a "stocking-glove" distribution. Significant morbidity results from foot ulcers, recurrent infections, foot fractures (Charcot's joint), and subsequent amputations. Treatment of peripheral neuropathy includes optimal glucose control, nonsteroidal antiinflammatory agents, antidepressants, and anticonvulsants for pain control.

c. ***Retinopathy.*** Retinopathy results from hemorrhages, exudates, and growth of abnormal vessels and fibrous tissue. Visual impairment ranges from minor changes in color vision to total blindness. Strict glycemic control and blood pressure control can reduce the risk of development and progression of retinopathy.

d. ***Diabetic Autonomic Neuropathy (DAN).*** DAN can affect any part of the autonomic nervous system and depends on the duration of diabetes and the degree of metabolic control. Cardiovascular autonomic neuropathy is characterized by abnormalities in heart rate (resting tachycardia and loss of heart rate variability during sleep are early signs), systolic and diastolic dysfunction with reduced ejection fraction, and central and peripheral vascular dynamics (e.g., severe orthostatic hypotension). DAN may impair gastric motility, causing gastroparesis diabeticorum in up to 25% of patients.

6. Macrovascular Complications

a. ***Cardiovascular Disease.*** This is a major cause of morbidity and the leading cause of mortality in diabetics. Dyslipidemia is the major contributor to the initiation and development of atherosclerotic lesions. Statin therapy (3-hydroxy-3-methylglutaryl coenzyme A reductase inhibitors) should be considered for all diabetics. Prevention of coronary artery disease in diabetics includes aggressive management of elevated lipids, elevated glucose, and hypertension, as well as aspirin for thrombolysis.

D. Management of Anesthesia. Hyperglycemia appears to increase the risk of ischemic myocardial injury by decreasing coronary collateral blood flow and coronary vasodilator reserve, impairing coronary microcirculation, and causing endothelial dysfunction. Acute hyperglycemia causes dehydration, impaired wound healing, an increased rate of infection, worsening central nervous system and spinal cord injury with ischemia, and hyperviscosity with thrombogenesis. Tight control of serum glucose in the perioperative period is a primary goal.

1. Preoperative Evaluation. Evaluation includes assessment for possible cardiac and renal disease, control of hypertension, management of insulin and glucose control, and examination for limited joint mobility (especially neck) that may affect endotracheal intubation.

a. ***Management of Insulin in the Preoperative Period***

i. Two thirds of the usual bedtime dose of insulin (NPH and regular) should be given the night before surgery and half the usual NPH dose on the day of surgery. Regular insulin should be withheld the morning of surgery.

ii. A 5% dextrose with 0.45% normal saline ($D_5\frac{1}{2}$ NS) intravenous infusion at 100 mL/hr should be initiated preoperatively.

iii. With regard to the insulin pump, the overnight rate should be decreased by 30%. On the morning of surgery, the pump can be kept at the basal rate or replaced with an intravenous insulin infusion at the same rate, or the patient can be given subcutaneous glargine and the pump discontinued in 60 to 90 minutes.

iv. If the patient uses glargine and lispro or aspart for daily glycemic control, the patient should take two thirds of the glargine dose plus the entire lispro or aspart dose the night before surgery, and all morning insulin should be withheld.

v. Oral hypoglycemics should be discontinued 24 to 48 hours preoperatively.

2. **Intraoperative Management.** Goals are to minimize hyperglycemia (serum glucose 120 to 180 mg/dL) and avoid hypoglycemia. Management should be with continuous intravenous infusion of insulin. An initial hourly rate can estimated by dividing the patient's total daily insulin dose by 24. A typical rate is 0.02 units/kg/hr, or about 1.4 units/hr in a 70-kg patient. Subcutaneous insulin should not be used. Intraoperative serum glucose levels should be monitored at least hourly. $D_5\frac{1}{2}$ NS should also be infused to provide carbohydrate and inhibit hepatic glucose production and protein catabolism. Treatment of hypoglycemia consists of administration of 50 mL of 50% dextrose in water, which typically increases the serum glucose level by 100 mg/dL.

3. **Postoperative Care.** Postoperative care includes aggressive insulin therapy. Tight glucose control (80 to 110 mg/dL) is associated with better outcomes, possibly because of better neutrophil and macrophage function, beneficial changes to mucosal and skin barriers, enhanced erythropoiesis, reduced cholestasis, improved respiratory muscle function, and decreased axonal degeneration.

II. INSULINOMA

Insulinomas are rare, benign insulin-secreting tumors of pancreatic beta cells that may manifest in isolation or as part of multiple endocrine neoplasia (MEN) syndrome type I. The diagnosis is suggested by demonstrating Whipple's triad: (1) symptoms of hypoglycemia with fasting, (2) glucose level below 50 mg/dL with symptoms, and (3) relief of symptoms with administration of glucose. The diagnosis is confirmed by demonstrating an inappropriately high insulin level (>5 mU/mL) during a 48- to 72-hour fast. The principal anesthetic challenge during excision of an insulinoma is maintenance of a normal blood glucose concentration. Profound hypoglycemia can occur, particularly during manipulation of the tumor, and marked hyperglycemia can follow successful surgical removal of the tumor. Frequent (every 15 minutes) monitoring of glucose is mandatory.

III. THYROID DISEASE

A. **Physiology.** Thyroid hormones T_4 (thyroxine) and T_3 (triiodothyronine) stimulate virtually all metabolic processes, synthetic and catabolic. They influence growth and maturation of tissues, enhance tissue function, and stimulate protein synthesis and carbohydrate and lipid metabolism. Thyroid hormone increases myocardial contractility, decreases systemic vascular resistance, and increases intravascular volume. Production of normal quantities of thyroid hormones depends on the availability of exogenous iodine, the primary source of which is diet. Active thyroid hormones are T_3 (triiodothyronine) and T_4 (thyroxine). The normal ratio of T_4/T_3 in the blood is 10:1. The majority of hormone is bound to proteins in the blood (thyroid-binding globulin [TBG], prealbumin, and albumin). Only the free hormone is biologically active. T_3 is three to four times more active per weight than T_4. Regulation of thyroid function is via the hypothalamus, via thyrotropin-releasing hormone (TRH), and the pituitary via thyrotropin-stimulating hormone.

B. **Diagnosis**

1. **Hyperthyroidism and Hypothyroidism.** Free T_4 (FT_4) is elevated in 90% of patients with hyperthyroidism and is low in 85% of patients with hypothyroidism. The thyroid-stimulating hormone (TSH) level is now the single best test of thyroid hormone action at the cellular level. A low TSH level with normal levels of FT_3 and FT_4 is diagnostic of subclinical hyperthyroidism. An elevated TSH level with normal levels of FT_3 and FT_4 is diagnostic of subclinical hypothyroidism. Radioactive iodine uptake is sometimes used to

TABLE 19-7 ■ Signs and Symptoms of Hyperthyroidism and Hypothyroidism

HYPERTHYROIDISM	HYPOTHYROIDISM
Hypermetabolism	Hypometabolism
Anxiety, restlessness, hyperkinesis	Fatigue, lethargy, listlessness, apathy
Warm, moist skin	Dry, thickened, pale, cool skin
Increased sweating	Decreased sweating
Flushed face	Large tongue, hoarse voice
Fine hair, fragile nails	Dry hair
Upper-eyelid retraction	Periorbital edema
Heat intolerance	Cold intolerance
Proximal muscle weakness	Prolonged deep tendon reflexes
Sleep disturbance	Menorrhagia
Tremor	Hypercholesterolemia, hypertriglyceridemia
Weight loss, diarrhea	Weight gain, constipation
Tachycardia, arrhythmias, palpitations	Ventricular arrhythmias
Increased cardiac output, cardiomegaly	Pericardial effusion
Normal or high T_3 and T_4, reduced TSH	Reduced myocardial contractility
	Decreased T_3 and T_4, increased TSH

TSH, Thyroid-stimulating hormone.

confirm hyperthyroidism. Other tests include detection of antibodies directed toward thyroid antigens.

2. **Thyroid Nodules.** Thyroid scans using iodine-123 or technetium-99m evaluate nodules as "warm" or normal, "hot" or hyperfunctioning, or "cold" or hypofunctioning. Ultrasonography is 90% to 95% accurate for determining whether a lesion is cystic, solid, or mixed.

C. **Hyperthyroidism**

1. **Signs and Symptoms of Hyperthyroidism** (Table 19-7)
2. **Graves's Disease.** Graves's disease is characterized by a classic triad of hyperthyroidism, exophthalmos, and dermopathy. It appears to be a systemic autoimmune disease with thyroid-stimulating antibodies (long-acting thyroid stimulator [LATS]) binding to TSH receptors in the thyroid. Graves's ophthalmopathy includes upper-lid retraction, a wide-eyed stare, muscle weakness, proptosis, and an increase in intraocular pressure. Steroids, bilateral tarsorrhaphies, external radiation, or surgical decompression may be necessary in these cases.
   a. ***Diagnosis.*** Diagnosis of Graves's disease is confirmed by elevated thyroid hormone levels and radioactive iodine uptake. The TSH level is often low, and thyroid-stimulating antibodies are increased.
3. ***Toxic Multinodular Goiters.*** These usually arise from longstanding simple goiters and can produce extreme thyroid enlargements with signs and symptoms of airway obstruction. Hypermetabolism is usually less severe than with Graves's disease, and there is no associated ophthalmopathy or dermopathy. The diagnosis is confirmed by a thyroid scan and, occasionally, thyroid biopsy.
4. **A Solitary Toxic Nodule.** A solitary toxic nodule (toxic adenoma) is diagnosed with the same tests used for multinodular goiters.
5. **Treatment.** For hyperthyroidism, treatment is with an antithyroid drug—propylthiouracil (PTU) or methimazole (Tapazole), which interfere with thyroid hormone synthesis and peripheral conversion of T_4 to T_3. Iodide in high concentration inhibits release of hormones from the thyroid gland, and it is usually reserved for preparing hyperthyroid patients for surgery, managing patients with actual or impending thyroid storm, or treating patients with severe thyrocardiac disease. β-Adrenergic antagonists may relieve signs and symptoms (anxiety, sweating, heat intolerance, tremors, tachycardia). Ablative therapy with radioactive

iodine-131 (^{131}I) or surgery is recommended for patients with refractory Graves's disease and in patients with toxic multinodular goiter or a toxic adenoma. Surgery (subtotal thyroidectomy, total thyroidectomy) results in prompt control of disease and a lower incidence of hypothyroidism than radioactive iodine.

6. **Management of Anesthesia.** Euthyroidism should be established preoperatively (may require 6 to 8 weeks of therapy). In emergency cases, the use of an intravenous β-blocker, ipodate, cortisol, or dexamethasone and PTU is usually necessary. The anesthesiologist should be prepared to manage thyroid storm. Controlled studies demonstrate no clinically significant increase in anesthetic requirements.
   a. ***Thyroid Storm.*** Thyroid storm and malignant hyperthermia can manifest with similar signs and symptoms (hyperpyrexia, tachycardia, hypermetabolism). Treatment includes rapid alleviation of thyrotoxicosis, fluid resuscitation, cooling measures to counter fever, medications to control heart rate, and glucocorticoids. Antithyroid drugs (PTU 200 to 400 mg every 8 hours) may be given through a nasogastric tube, orally, or rectally. If circulatory shock is present, an intravenous direct vasopressor (phenylephrine) is indicated.

D. Hypothyroidism

1. **Signs and Symptoms** (see Table 19-7)
2. **Diagnosis**
   a. ***Primary Hypothyroidism.*** Primary hypothyroidism (decreased production of thyroid hormones despite increased levels of TSH) is confirmed by reduced thyroid hormone levels and elevated TSH level.
   b. ***Secondary Hypothyroidism.*** Secondary hypothyroidism (reduced levels of thyroid hormone levels caused by pituitary abnormality) is diagnosed by abnormal levels of free T_4, T_4 and T_3, with low TSH levels. Absent response to a TRH stimulation test can confirm a pituitary cause.
   c. ***Euthyroid Sick Syndrome.*** Euthyroid sick syndrome (abnormal thyroid function test results in critically ill patients with significant nonthyroid illness) is characterized by low T_3 and T_4 with a normal TSH (<5.0 mU/L). No treatment is necessary.
3. **Treatment.** Usually treatment is L-thyroxine (levothyroxine sodium). Alternative hormone preparations include thyroid extract USP, L-triiodothyronine (liothyronine sodium), and liotrix, a combination of T_4 and T_3 in a 4:1 ratio.
4. **Management of Anesthesia.** Patients with subclinical hypothyroidism usually present no anesthetic problems. Patients with mild to moderate disease should probably receive daily L-thyroxine (100 to 200 mcg/day) in the preoperative period. In an overtly hypothyroid patient, the potential for severe cardiovascular instability intraoperatively and myxedema coma in the postoperative period is high. If emergency surgery can be delayed for 24 to 48 hours, intravenous thyroid replacement therapy (L-thyroxine 300-500 mcg or L-triiodothyronine 25-50 mcg IV) is indicated. Other anesthetic considerations are summarized in Table 19-8.

E. Myxedema Coma.

This is a rare severe form of hypothyroidism characterized by delirium or unconsciousness, hypoventilation, hypothermia (80% of patients), bradycardia, hypotension, and a severe dilutional hyponatremia. Treatment is with L-thyroxine or L-triidothyronine, intravenous hydration with glucose-containing saline solutions, temperature regulation, ventilatory support, and hydrocortisone for possible adrenal insufficiency (AI).

F. Goiter and Thyroid Tumors

1. **Goiter.** Goiter results from compensatory hypertrophy and hyperplasia of follicular epithelium secondary to a reduction in thyroid hormone output. The cause may be a deficient intake of iodine, a dietary (i.e., cassava) or pharmacologic (i.e., phenylbutazone, lithium) goitrogen, or a defect in the hormonal biosynthetic pathway.
2. **Thyroid Tumors.** Surgical resection of benign nodules or carcinomas rarely creates problems for the anesthesiologist. However, the anesthetic management of a patient undergoing surgical removal of a large thyroid mass that compromises the airway presents a major

TABLE 19-8 ■ Anesthetic Considerations in Patients with Hypothyroidism

Airway compromise can occur because of edema—hold or reduce preoperative sedation.
Decreased gastric emptying.
Decreased cardiac output, SV, HR, baroreceptor reflexes, intravascular volume. Invasive monitors may be indicated—phosphodiesterase inhibitors (milrinone) may be the most effective inotrope because they do not depend on β receptors, which may be reduced in number and sensitivity.
Decreased ventilator responsiveness to hypoxia and hypercarbia.
Hypothermia occurs quickly.
Hematologic abnormalities include anemia, platelet dysfunction, coagulation factor abnormalities (especially factor VIII).
Electrolyte imbalance (hyponatremia).
Hypoglycemia—administer dextrose-containing fluids.
Depressed adrenal function—consider dexamethasone or cortisol.

HR, Heart rate; *SV,* stroke volume.

TABLE 19-9 ■ Multiple Endocrine Neoplasia (MEN)

SYNDROME	MANIFESTATIONS
MEN type IIA (Sipple syndrome)	Medullary thyroid cancer Parathyroid adenoma Pheochromocytoma
MEN type IIB	Medullary thyroid cancer Mucosal adenomas Marfan appearance Pheochromocytoma
von Hippel–Lindau syndrome	Hemangioblastoma of the central nervous system Pheochromocytoma

challenge. Awake intubation may be needed. Airway obstruction caused by extrinsic compression may occur with cessation of spontaneous respiration. Computed tomography (CT) scan and/or echocardiography may further delineate the thyroid mass.

G. Complications of Thyroid Surgery. Complications include recurrent laryngeal nerve injury and hypoparathyroidism caused by damage to the blood supply of the parathyroid glands (anxiety, circumoral numbness, tingling fingertips, muscle cramps, positive Chvostek's sign, and Trousseau's sign may point to hypocalcemia). Treatment is intravenous calcium gluconate or calcium chloride (1 g). A continued intravenous infusion of calcium is often necessary. Long-term therapy is with oral calcium and vitamin D_3, or autotransplantation of parathyroid tissue. Respiratory compromise as a result of tracheal compression caused by hematoma formation can also occur.

IV. PHEOCHROMOCYTOMA

Pheochromocytomas are catecholamine-secreting tumors that arise independently or as part of the MEN syndromes (Table 19-9). Patients with von Recklinghausen's disease, tuberous sclerosis, and Sturge-Weber syndrome have increased risk of pheochromocytoma.

A. Signs and Symptoms. Hypertension, headache, sweating, pallor, and palpitations are classic signs and symptoms. Hypertensive crises mimic the hemodynamic responses of acute catecholamine administration. Cardiomyopathy, cardiac hypertrophy, and electrocardiogram

TABLE 19-10 ■ Pattern of Catecholamine Production and Tumor Site

	ADRENAL	EXTRAADRENAL	ADRENAL + EXTRAADRENAL
Norepinephrine	61%	31%	8%
Epinephrine	100%	—	—
Norepinephrine + epinephrine	95%	—	5%

Adapted from Kaser H. Clinical and diagnostic findings in patients with chromaffin tumors: pheochromocytomas, pheochromoblastomas. *Recent Results Cancer Res*. 1990;118:97-105.

(ECG) abnormalities and arrhythmias can occur. The presentation of a pheochromocytoma may mimic thyrotoxicosis, malignant hypertension, diabetes mellitus, malignant carcinoid syndrome, or gram-negative septicemia. Hyperglycemia, but rarely frank diabetes, occurs in most patients owing to catecholamine stimulation of glycogenolysis and inhibition of insulin release.

B. Diagnosis. Diagnosis relies on demonstration of excess catecholamine secretion. The most sensitive test for high-risk patients (familial pheochromocytoma or classic symptoms) is a finding of plasma-free normetanephrine greater than 400 pg/mL and/or metanephrine greater than 220 pg/mL. A pheochromocytoma is excluded if normetanephrine is less than 112 pg/mL and metanephrine is less than 61 pg/mL. Determination of elevated urinary free catecholamine levels and their metabolites (i.e., metanephrine, normetanephrine, vanillylmandelic acid) is easy to perform and readily available and is sufficient for patients with a low probability of having a pheochromocytoma. Results of these tests are equivocal in 5% to 10% of patients, in which case a clonidine suppression test may be used (lowers plasma catecholamines in patients without pheochromocytoma but not in patients with pheochromocytoma). A positive glucagon stimulation test result is the safest and most specific provocative testing method (causes tumor release of catecholamines of at least three times baseline or >2000 pg/mL within 1 to 3 minutes), but the test should be limited to patients with diastolic blood pressure of less than 100 mm Hg. Tumor location can be predicted by the pattern of catecholamine production (Table 19-10). CT and magnetic resonance imaging (MRI) are the optimal noninvasive anatomic adrenal imaging studies. ^{131}I-MIBG (metaiodobenzylguanidine) scintigraphy localizes tumors via ^{131}I-MIBG uptake in catecholamine-secreting tumors.

C. Treatment. Treatment is surgical excision whenever possible. α-Methylparatyrosine (inhibits the rate-limiting step of the catecholamine synthetic pathway) may decrease catecholamine production by 50% to 80%. Usual doses range from 250 mg twice daily to 3 to 4 g/day. It is especially useful for malignant and inoperable tumors. Side effects include extrapyramidal reactions and crystalluria.

D. Management of Anesthesia (Table 19-11)

1. Preoperative Management. Most pheochromocytomas secrete predominantly norepinephrine. The therapeutic goal is normotension, resolution of symptoms, elimination of ST-T changes on the ECG, and elimination of arrhythmias.

a. α-Blockade. α-Blockade (with phenoxybenzamine, a noncompetitive α_1-antagonist, or alternatively prazosin, an α_1-competitive blocker) is used to lower blood pressure, increase intravascular volume, prevent paroxysmal hypertensive episodes, allow resensitization of adrenergic receptors, and decrease myocardial dysfunction. Because of the prolonged effect of phenoxybenzamine on α-receptors, it has been recommended that it be discontinued 24 to 48 hours before surgery or alternatively that only one half to two thirds of the morning dose be administered before surgery to avoid vascular unresponsiveness immediately after removal of the tumor. Hypertension usually occurs with manipulation of the tumor.

b. β-Adrenergic Blockade (Propranolol, Atenolol, Metoprolol). β-Adrenergic blockade is prescribed if tachycardia (i.e., heart rate >120 beats/min) or other arrhythmias result after

TABLE 19-11 ■ Anesthetic Considerations in Pheochromocytoma

Preoperative	α-Blockade; phenoxybenzamine, prazosin α-methylparatyrosine β-Blockade for tachycardia (propranolol, metoprolol, atenolol) Calcium channel blockers, ACEIs
Intraoperative	Avoid fear, stress, pain, shivering, hypoxia, hypercarbia (stimulate catecholamine release) Catecholamine release during induction, intubation, surgical incision, abdominal exploration, and tumor manipulation Monitoring: arterial catheter, CVP or PA catheter, Foley catheter Significant fluid administration possible to prevent hypotension after tumor removal All anesthetics are used Drugs to avoid: morphine and atracurium (histamine release can provoke catecholamine release), atropine, pancuronium, and succinylcholine (may stimulate the sympathetic nervous system), halothane (sensitizes the myocardium to catecholamine-induced arrhythmias), droperidol, chlorpromazine, metoclopramide, and ephedrine (hypertensive responses) Intraoperative hypertension: treat with sodium nitroprusside or phentolamine Antiarrhythmics to have available: lidocaine, esmolol, amiodarone Intraoperative blood salvage
After tumor removal	Hypotension caused by catecholamine decrease: give fluids, decrease anesthetic depth; administer vasopressors if these measures fail Hypoglycemia caused by increased insulin levels: monitor glucose, use dextrose-containing intravenous fluids Glucocorticoid therapy if bilateral adrenalectomy
Postoperative	Hypertension may persist for several days; consider persistent hypertension or residual tumor Hypotension is most common cause of death Hypoglycemia may persist ICU monitoring for at least 24 hours

ACEI, Angiotensin-converting enzyme inhibitor; *CVP,* central venous pressure; *ICU,* intensive care unit; *PA,* pulmonary arterial.

α_2-blockade with phenoxybenzamine. Esmolol has a fast onset and short elimination half-life and can be administered IV in the immediate preoperative period. A nonselective β-blocker should never be administered before α-blockade because blockade of vasodilatory β_2-receptors results in unopposed α-agonism, resulting in vasoconstriction and hypertensive crises.

c. ***α-Methylparatyrosine.*** In combination with phenoxybenzamine during the preoperative period, α-methylparatyrosine may facilitate intraoperative hemodynamic management.

d. ***Calcium Channel Blockers (Nifedipine, Diltiazem, Verapamil) and ACEIs (Captopril).*** These agents have all been used to control preoperative hypertension. An α_1-blocker plus a calcium channel blocker is an effective combination for resistant cases.

2. **Intraoperative Management.** Goals are avoidance of drugs or maneuvers that provoke catecholamine release or potentiate catecholamine action, and maintenance of cardiovascular stability. Hypertension can occur during pneumoperitoneum or tumor manipulation. Hypotension may follow ligature of the tumor's venous drainage. Hypoglycemia after tumor vein ligation can occur owing to increased insulin levels (see Table 19-11).

3. **Postoperative Management.** Plasma catecholamine levels do not return to normal for 7 to 10 days, and 50% of patients are hypertensive for several days after surgery. Hypotension is the most frequent cause of death in the immediate postoperative period.

V. ADRENAL GLAND DYSFUNCTION

The adrenal cortex is responsible for the synthesis of three groups of hormones: glucocorticoids (cortisol essential for life), mineralocorticoids (aldosterone), and androgens. These hormones are involved in blood pressure regulation, gluconeogenesis, sodium and potassium regulation, inhibition of inflammation, and fluid balance. The adrenal medulla synthesizes norepinephrine and epinephrine. Adrenal medulla insufficiency is not known to occur.

A. Hypercortisolism (Cushing's Syndrome). Cushing's syndrome is categorized as adrenocorticotropic hormone (ACTH)–dependent Cushing's syndrome (high ACTH concentrations stimulate the adrenal cortex to produce excess cortisol) and ACTH-independent Cushing's syndrome (excess production of cortisol by abnormal adrenocortical tissues causes the syndrome and suppresses secretion of corticotropic-releasing hormone [CRH] and ACTH). Cushing's disease is defined as Cushing's syndrome caused by high secretion of ACTH by pituitary adenomas.

1. **Diagnosis.** Symptoms and signs include weight gain, moon facies, facial telangiectasias, hypertension, glucose intolerance, oligomenorrhea or amenorrhea in premenopausal women, decreased libido in men, spontaneous ecchymoses, and skeletal muscle wasting and weakness. Diagnosis is confirmed by demonstrating cortisol hypersecretion based on 24-hour urinary secretion of cortisol. Determining whether a patient's hypercortisolism is ACTH dependent or ACTH independent requires reliable measurements of plasma ACTH using immunoradiometric assays. A high-dose dexamethasone suppression test distinguishes Cushing's disease from ectopic ACTH syndrome (complete resistance present).
2. **Treatment.** For patients with Cushing's disease, treatment is transsphenoidal microadenomectomy of the pituitary adenoma. Pituitary radiation and bilateral total adrenalectomy are necessary in some patients. Surgical removal of the adrenal gland is the treatment for adrenal adenoma or carcinoma.
3. **Management of Anesthesia**
   a. ***Preoperative Evaluation.*** Evaluation of systemic blood pressure, electrolyte balance, and the blood glucose concentration is especially important. Osteoporosis is a consideration when positioning patients for the operative procedure.
   b. ***Intraoperative.*** Etomidate may transiently decrease the synthesis and release of cortisol by the adrenal cortex. Mechanical ventilation is recommended to manage associated skeletal muscle weakness. A continuous infusion of cortisol (100 mg/day IV) may be initiated intraoperatively to prevent acute AI after tumor removal. Transient diabetes insipidus and meningitis may occur after microadenomectomy.

B. Primary Hyperaldosteronism (Conn's Syndrome). This syndrome involves excess secretion of aldosterone from a functional tumor (aldosteronoma) independent of a physiologic stimulus.

1. **Signs and Symptoms.** Signs include systemic hypertension (headache, sodium retention, increased extracellular fluid volume) or hypokalemia (polyuria, nocturia, skeletal muscle cramps, skeletal muscle weakness, metabolic alkalosis). Hypomagnesemia and abnormal glucose tolerance may be present.
2. **Diagnosis.** Spontaneous hypokalemia in patients with systemic hypertension is highly suggestive of aldosteronism. A plasma aldosterone concentration less than 9.5 ng/dL at the end of a saline infusion rules out primary aldosteronism.
3. **Treatment.** Treatment is supplemental potassium and administration of a competitive aldosterone antagonist, such as spironolactone. Definitive treatment for an aldosterone-secreting tumor is surgical excision. Bilateral adrenalectomy may be necessary if multiple aldosterone-secreting tumors are found.
4. **Management of Anesthesia**
   a. ***Preoperative.*** Goals are correction of hypokalemia and treatment of hypertension.
   b. ***Intraoperative.*** Hypokalemia may modify responses to nondepolarizing muscle relaxants. Bilateral mobilization of the adrenal glands to excise multiple functional tumors, however, may introduce the need for exogenous administration of cortisol. A continuous

TABLE 19-12 ■ **Steroid (Hydrocortisone) Supplementation**

Superficial surgery Dental procedures, biopsies	None
Minor surgery Inguinal hernia, colonoscopy	25 mg IV
Moderate surgery Cholecystectomy, colon surgery	50-75 mg IV, taper 1-2 days
Severe surgery Cardiovascular surgery, liver surgery, Whipple procedure	100-150 mg IV, taper 1-2 days
Intensive care unit Sepsis, shock	50-100 mg q6-8h for 2 days to 1 wk, taper

IV, Intravenously.

intravenous infusion of cortisol, 100 mg every 24 hours, may be initiated on an empirical basis if transient hypocortisolism caused by surgical manipulation is a consideration.

C. Hypoaldosteronism. Hyperkalemia in the absence of renal insufficiency suggests the presence of hypoaldosteronism. Hyporeninemic hypoaldosteronism typically occurs in patients older than 45 years with chronic renal disease and/or diabetes mellitus. Indomethacin-induced prostaglandin deficiency is a reversible cause of this syndrome. Treatment of hypoaldosteronism includes liberal sodium intake and daily administration of fludrocortisone.

D. Adrenal Insufficiency (AI)

1. **Signs and Symptoms.** In primary disease (Addison's disease), the adrenal glands are unable to elaborate sufficient quantities of glucocorticoid, mineralocorticoid, and androgen hormones. The most common cause is autoimmune disease. Addison's disease is characterized by fatigue, weakness, anorexia, nausea and vomiting, cutaneous and mucosal hyperpigmentation, cardiopenia secondary to chronic hypotension, hypovolemia, hyponatremia, and hyperkalemia. Secondary AI is caused by inadequate pituitary CRH or ACTH production. Unlike in Addison's disease, there is a glucocorticoid deficiency only with secondary disease. The most common cause is iatrogenic (pituitary surgery, pituitary irradiation, use of synthetic glucocorticoids).
2. **Diagnosis.** Critically ill patients with cortisol levels less than 20 mcg/dL have AI. The classic definition of AI includes a baseline plasma cortisol level below 20 mcg/dL and a cortisol level below 20 mcg/dL after an ACTH stimulation test. Absolute AI is characterized by a low baseline cortisol level and a positive ACTH stimulation test result. Relative AI has a higher baseline cortisol level but a positive ACTH stimulation test result.
3. **Treatment.** The most common cause of AI is exogenous steroids. For patients with a history of long-term steroid use, it may take 6 to 12 months after discontinuation of steroids for the adrenal glands to recover. Preoperative glucocorticoid coverage should be provided for patients who have a positive ACTH stimulation test result, who have Cushing's syndrome and AI, or who are at risk for AI because of prior glucocorticoid therapy. Patients with known or suspected adrenal suppression or AI should receive their baseline therapy plus supplementation in the perioperative period. Supplementation is individualized based on the surgery (Table 19-12).
4. **Management of Anesthesia.** Therapy includes glucocorticoid replacement and correction of water and sodium deficits. Glucocorticoid replacement may include intravenous hydrocortisone, methylprednisolone, or dexamethasone. Volume deficits may be substantial (2 to 3 L), and 5% glucose in normal saline is the fluid of choice. Hemodynamic support with vasopressors such as dopamine may be necessary. Metabolic acidosis and hyperkalemia usually resolve with fluids and steroids. Acute AI should be considered in the differential diagnosis of hemodynamic instability only after more common causes have been

TABLE 19-13 ■ **Signs and Symptoms of Hypercalcemia Caused by Hyperparathyroidism**

ORGAN SYSTEM	SIGNS AND SYMPTOMS
Neuromuscular	Skeletal muscle weakness
Renal	Polyuria and polydipsia Decreased glomerular filtration rate Kidney stones
Hematopoietic	Anemia
Cardiac	Prolonged PR interval Short QT interval Systemic hypertension
Gastrointestinal	Vomiting Abdominal pain Peptic ulcer Pancreatitis
Skeletal	Skeletal demineralization Collapse of vertebral bodies Pathologic fractures
Nervous	Somnolence Decreased pain sensation Psychosis
Ocular	Calcifications (band keratopathy) Conjunctivitis

treated or ruled out (hypovolemia, anesthetic overdose, cardiopulmonary disorders, surgical mechanical problems). Etomidate inhibits the synthesis of cortisol transiently in normal patients and should be avoided. Patients with untreated AI undergoing emergency surgery may require invasive monitoring.

5. **Intensive Care Unit Management.** The incidence of AI in high-risk, critically ill patients with hypotension, shock, and sepsis is approximately 30% to 40%. All patients suspected of having AI should be tested for serum cortisol and undergo an ACTH stimulation test, especially if the stress level is uncertain.

VI. PARATHYROID GLAND DYSFUNCTION

A. **Hyperparathyroidism.** When the secretion of parathormone is increased, hyperparathyroidism is present. Serum calcium concentrations may be increased, decreased, or unchanged. Hyperparathyroidism is classified as primary, secondary, or ectopic.

1. **Primary Hyperparathyroidism.** This results from excessive secretion of parathormone because of a benign parathyroid adenoma, carcinoma of a parathyroid gland, or hyperplasia of the parathyroid glands. Hyperparathyroidism caused by an adenoma or hyperplasia is the most common presenting symptom of MEN I syndrome.

   a. ***Diagnosis.*** Hypercalcemia (serum calcium concentration >5.5 mEq/L and ionized calcium concentration >2.5 mEq/L) is the hallmark of primary hyperparathyroidism. Measurement of serum parathormone concentrations is not always sufficiently reliable to confirm the diagnosis of primary hyperparathyroidism.

   b. ***Signs and Symptoms*** *(Table 19-13)*

   c. ***Treatment***

TABLE 19-14 ■ Etiology of Hypoparathyroidism

DECREASED OR ABSENT PARATHORMONE
Accidental removal of parathyroid glands during thyroidectomy
Parathyroidectomy to treat hyperplasia
Idiopathic (DiGeorge's syndrome)
RESISTANCE OF PERIPHERAL TISSUES TO EFFECTS OF PARATHORMONE
Congenital
Pseudohypoparathyroidism
Acquired
Hypomagnesemia
Chronic renal failure
Malabsorption
Anticonvulsive therapy (phenytoin)
Unknown
Osteoblastic metastases
Acute pancreatitis

i. ***Medical Management.*** Saline infusion (150 mL/hr) and loop diuretics (furosemide 40 to 80 mg IV every 2 to 4 hours) are administered. Bisphosphonates such as disodium etidronate are administered IV for life-threatening hypercalcemia. Hemodialysis can lower serum calcium concentrations, as can calcitonin, but the effects of this hormone are transient. Mithramycin inhibits the osteoclastic activity of parathormone, producing prompt lowering of serum calcium concentrations. The toxic effects (thrombocytopenia, hepatotoxicity, nephrotoxicity) limit its use.

ii. ***Surgical Management.*** Surgery is the definitive treatment, resulting in normalization of serum calcium concentration within 3 to 4 days. Postoperative complications include hypocalcemic tetany, hypomagnesemia, and acute arthritis.

iii. ***Management of Anesthesia.*** There is no evidence that any specific anesthetic drugs or techniques are necessary in patients with primary hyperparathyroidism undergoing elective surgical treatment for the disease.

2. **Secondary Hyperparathyroidism.** Secondary hyperparathyroidism reflects an appropriate compensatory response of the parathyroid glands to secrete more parathormone to counteract a disease process that produces hypocalcemia (e.g., chronic renal disease). Secondary hyperparathyroidism seldom produces hypercalcemia, and treatment is directed at controlling the underlying disease.

3. **Ectopic Hyperparathyroidism.** This is caused by secretion of parathormone (or a substance with similar endocrine effects) by tissues other than the parathyroid glands. Carcinoma of the lung, breast, pancreas, or kidney and lymphoproliferative disease are the most likely ectopic sites for parathormone secretion.

B. **Hypoparathyroidism.** When secretion of parathormone is absent or deficient or peripheral tissues are resistant to the effects of the hormone, hypoparathyroidism is present (Table 19-14). Pseudohypoparathyroidism is a congenital disorder in which the release of parathormone is intact but the kidneys are unable to respond to the hormone. Affected patients manifest mental retardation, calcification of the basal ganglia, obesity, short stature, and short metacarpals and metatarsals.

1. **Diagnosis.** A serum calcium concentration less than 4.5 mEq/L and an ionized calcium concentration less than 2.0 mEq/L indicate hypoparathyroidism.

2. **Signs and Symptoms.** Signs and symptoms of hypoparathyroidism depend on the rapidity of the onset of hypocalcemia.

a. ***Acute Hypocalcemia.*** This may manifest as perioral paresthesias, restlessness, and neuromuscular irritability, as evidenced by a positive Chvostek's sign or Trousseau's sign. A positive Chvostek's sign consists of facial muscle twitching produced by manual tapping over the area of the facial nerve at the angle of the mandible. A positive Trousseau's sign is carpopedal spasm caused by 3 minutes of limb ischemia produced by a tourniquet. Inspiratory stridor reflects neuromuscular irritability of the intrinsic laryngeal musculature.

b. ***Chronic Hypocalcemia.*** Chronic hypocalcemia is associated with fatigue and skeletal muscle cramps and possibly prolonged QT interval on the ECG. Neurologic changes include lethargy, cerebration deficits, and personality changes. Chronic hypocalcemia is associated with formation of cataracts, calcification involving the subcutaneous tissues and basal ganglia, and thickening of the skull. Chronic renal failure is the most common cause of chronic hypocalcemia.

3. **Treatment.** Infusion of calcium (10 mL of 10% calcium gluconate IV) is performed until signs of neuromuscular irritability disappear. For treatment of asymptomatic hypoparathyroidism, treatment is oral calcium and vitamin D.
4. **Management of Anesthesia.** Goals are to prevent further decreases in the serum calcium concentrations (avoid hyperventilation, rapid infusion of blood) and to treat the adverse effects of hypocalcemia.

VII. PITUITARY GLAND DYSFUNCTION

The pituitary gland, located in the sella turcica at the base of the brain, consists of the anterior pituitary and posterior pituitary. The anterior pituitary secretes six hormones under control of the hypothalamus (Table 19-15).

A. Acromegaly. Acromegaly is caused by excessive secretion of growth hormone in adults, most often by an adenoma in the anterior pituitary gland. Failure of plasma growth hormone concentrations to decrease 1 to 2 hours after ingestion of 75 to 100 g of glucose or growth hormone concentration greater than 3 ng/mL is presumptive evidence of acromegaly. Radiographic or CT evidence of enlargement of the sella turcica is characteristic of anterior pituitary adenomas.

1. **Signs and Symptoms** (Table 19-16)
2. **Treatment.** Transsphenoidal surgical excision of pituitary adenomas is the preferred initial therapy. When adenomas have extended beyond the sella turcica, surgery or radiation is no longer feasible; medical treatment with suppressant drugs (bromocriptine) may be an option.
3. **Management of Anesthesia.** For patients with acromegaly, considerations for anesthesia include potential changes in the upper airway (distorted facial anatomy, enlargement of the tongue and epiglottis, narrowed glottic opening, nasal turbinate enlargement) that can predispose to difficult intubation; the possible need to insert a smaller-diameter tracheal tube should be anticipated. When placing a catheter in the radial artery, it is important to consider the possibility of inadequate collateral circulation at the wrist. Monitoring blood glucose concentrations is useful if diabetes mellitus or glucose intolerance accompanies acromegaly.

B. Diabetes Insipidus. Diabetes insipidus reflects the absence of vasopressin (antidiuretic hormone [ADH]) caused by destruction of the posterior pituitary (neurogenic diabetes insipidus) or failure of renal tubules to respond to ADH (nephrogenic diabetes insipidus). Neurogenic and nephrogenic diabetes insipidus are differentiated based on the response to desmopressin, which concentrates urine in the presence of neurogenic, but not nephrogenic, diabetes insipidus.

1. **Treatment.** Intravenous infusion of electrolyte solutions is performed if oral intake cannot offset polyuria. Chlorpropamide potentiates the effects of ADH on renal tubules and may be useful for treating nephrogenic diabetes insipidus. Treatment of neurogenic diabetes

TABLE 19-15 ■ **Hypothalamic and Related Pituitary Hormones**

HYPOTHALAMIC HORMONE	ACTION	PITUITARY HORMONE OR ORGAN AFFECTED	ACTION
Corticotropin-releasing hormone	Stimulatory	Corticotropin	Stimulates secretion of cortisol and androgens
Thyrotropin-releasing hormone	Stimulatory	Thyrotropin	Stimulates secretion of thyroxine and triiodothyronine
Gonadotropin-releasing hormone	Stimulatory	Follicle-stimulating hormone	Stimulates secretion of estradiol*
		Luteinizing hormone	Stimulates secretion of progesterone,* stimulates ovulation,* stimulates secretion of testosterone,† stimulates spermatogenesis†
Growth hormone–releasing hormone	Stimulatory	Growth hormone	Stimulates production of insulin-like growth factor
Dopamine	Inhibitory	Prolactin	Stimulates lactation*
Somatostatin	Inhibitory	Growth hormone	
Vasopressin (antidiuretic hormone)	Stimulatory	Kidneys	Stimulates free-water reabsorption
Oxytocin	Stimulatory	Uterus	Stimulates uterine contractions*
		Breasts	Stimulates milk ejection*

Adapted from Vance ML. Hypopituitarism. *N Engl J Med*. 1994;330:1651-1662.
*Actions in females.
†Actions in males.

TABLE 19-16 ■ **Manifestations of Acromegaly**

Parasellar mass
Enlarged sella turcica
Headache
Visual field defects
Rhinorrhea
Excess growth hormone
Skeletal overgrowth (prognathism)
Soft tissue overgrowth (lips, tongue, epiglottis, vocal cords)
Connective tissue overgrowth (recurrent laryngeal nerve paralysis)
Peripheral neuropathy (carpal tunnel syndrome)
Visceromegaly
Glucose tolerance
Osteoarthritis
Osteoporosis
Hyperhidrosis
Skeletal muscle weakness

insipidus is with ADH administered intramuscularly every 2 to 4 days or by intranasal administration of DDAVP.

2. **Management of Anesthesia.** For patients with diabetes insipidus, management of anesthesia includes monitoring the urine output and serum electrolyte concentrations during the perioperative period.

C. **Syndrome of Inappropriate Secretion of Antidiuretic Hormone (SIADH).** SIADH can occur in many pathologic processes (intracranial tumors, hypothyroidism, porphyria, carcinoma of the lung).

1. **Diagnosis.** Inappropriately increased urinary sodium concentrations and osmolarity in the presence of hyponatremia and decreased serum osmolarity are highly suggestive of inappropriate ADH secretion. Abrupt decreases in serum sodium concentrations, especially less than 110 mEq/L, can result in cerebral edema and seizures.

2. **Treatment.** Treatment is restricted oral fluid intake (approximately 500 mL/day), antagonism of the effects of ADH on the renal tubules by administration of demeclocycline, and intravenous infusions of sodium chloride. In patients manifesting acute neurologic symptoms caused by hyponatremia, intravenous infusions of hypertonic saline sufficient to increase serum sodium concentrations 0.5 mEq/L/hr are recommended. Overly rapid correction of chronic hyponatremia has been associated with central pontine myelinolysis.

CHAPTER 20

Hematologic Disorders

ERYTHROCYTE DISORDERS

Disease states may be related to abnormal concentrations (anemia, polycythemia) or structures of hemoglobin (Hgb). Oxygen-carrying capacity and adequacy of tissue oxygen delivery are often the most important clinical manifestations of these derangements.

I. ANEMIA

A. **Physiology.** In adults, anemia is usually defined as Hgb concentrations below 11.5 g/dL (hematocrit [Hct] <36%) for women and below 12.5 g/dL (hematocrit <40%) for men. Adverse effects of anemia are decreased tissue oxygen delivery caused by decreases in arterial content of oxygen (Cao_2). Compensatory mechanisms for anemia are (1) rightward shift of the oxyhemoglobin dissociation curve, which facilitates release of oxygen from Hgb to tissues (see Figure 20-1), (2) increased cardiac output, and (3) increased release of erythropoietin to stimulate red blood cell (RBC) production.

B. **Symptoms.** Fatigue and decreased exercise tolerance are symptoms.

C. **The Transfusion Trigger.** During surgery, blood loss of 15% of total blood volume generally does not require replacement, and losses up to 30% can be replaced with crystalloid.

1. **Target Hct.** The traditional "10/30" rule (transfuse for Hgb <10 g/dL or Hct <30%) has little evidence to support it. The Transfusion Requirements in Critical Care trial found no difference in 30-day mortality, cardiac morbidity, or hospital length of stay between a group receiving a "restrictive" transfusion strategy (to keep Hgb at 7 to 8 mg/dL) and those receiving a "liberal" strategy (to keep Hgb at 10 to 12 g/dL).
2. **Complications.** Transmission of hepatitis B and C and human immunodeficiency virus (HIV) may occur. In intensive care unit (ICU) patients, transfusion is associated with longer ICU and hospital length of stay, higher mortality, and increased rates of ventilator-associated pneumonia. Cancer recurrence, postoperative bacterial infection, transfusion-related lung injury (TRALI), and hemolytic reactions have all been associated with RBC transfusion.
3. **Transfusion and Coronary Artery Disease.** Studies show myocardial ischemia can occur at Hgb levels of 7 g/dL. A transfusion trigger of Hct 28% to 30% should be used in patients with significant caronary artery disease, especially those with unstable caronary syndromes.

D. **Anesthetic Considerations.** In patients undergoing anesthesia who have chronic anemia, conditions that interfere with tissue oxygen delivery (decreased cardiac output, respiratory alkalosis, hypothermia) should be avoided. Normovolemic hemodilution and intraoperative blood salvage should be considered.

E. **Hemolytic Anemia.** Hemolytic anemia is accelerated destruction of RBCs, often caused by abnormalities of Hgb structure and immune disorders. Hemolytic anemia is characterized by reticulocytosis (>100,000 cells/mm^3), increased mean corpuscular volume (MCV), unconjugated hyperbilirubinemia, increased lactate dehydrogenase (LDH) levels, and decreased serum

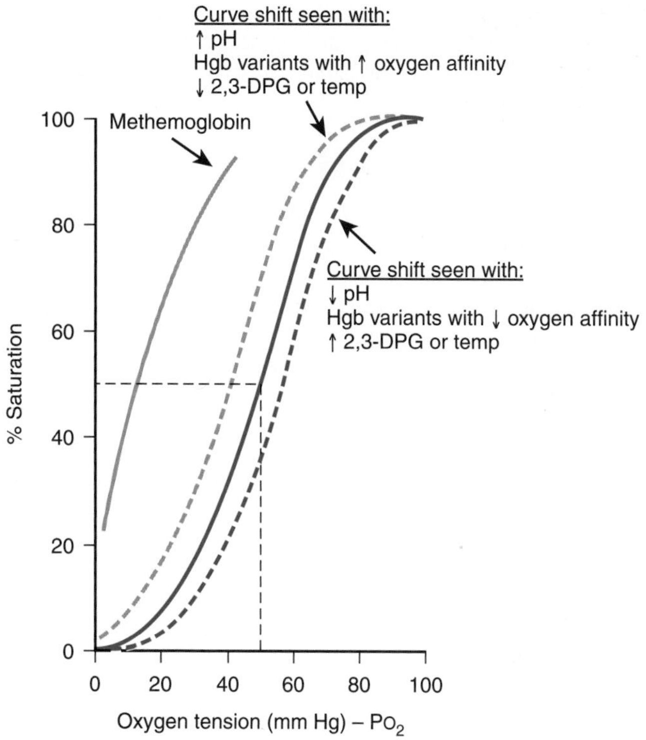

FIGURE 20-1 ■ Normal oxyhemoglobin dissociation curve and factors that result in alterations in O_2 dissociation. *2,3-DPG,* 2,3-Diphosphoglycerate; *Hgb,* hemoglobin.

haptoglobin. Diagnosis is via Coombs's test, examination of a peripheral blood smear, and Hgb electrophoresis.

II. DISORDERS OF RED CELL STRUCTURE

The mature RBC at rest takes the shape of a flexible biconcave disk. It lacks a nucleus or mitochondria, and intracellular energy requirements are supplied by glucose metabolism. Without a nucleus or protein metabolic pathway, the cell has a limited life span of 100 to 120 days.

A. Hereditary Spherocytosis (HS). HS is usually an autosomal dominant abnormality in membrane proteins spectrin and ankyrin. These cells show abnormal osmotic fragility and shortened circulation half-life. Hemolytic anemia can range from mild to severe. Hemolytic crises (hemolysis, jaundice, rare aplastic crisis) sometimes occur. Patients often have splenomegaly. The primary anesthetic consideration is the occurrence of episodic anemia.

B. Hereditary Elliptocytosis. An autosomal dominant abnormality in one of the membrane proteins, spectrin or glycophorin, makes the erythrocyte less pliable. Heterozygous patients rarely experience hemolysis, but homozygous or compound heterozygous patients may have significant hemolysis and anemia.

C. Acanthocytosis. This is a defect in membrane structure in patients with a congenital lack of β-lipoprotein (abetalipoproteinemia) and infrequently in patients with severe cirrhosis or pancreatitis. The membrane has a spiculated appearance. Hemolysis and anemia are the primary issues.

D. Paroxysmal Nocturnal Hemoglobinuria. This is a clonal disorder of hematopoietic cells involving abnormalities in or reductions of a membrane protein (glycosylphosphatidyl glycan).

Patients often have hemolytic anemia and are at increased risk of venous thrombosis due to initiation of coagulation by abnormal activation of the complement pathway. During anesthesia, factors that predispose to nocturnal hemolysis, such as hypoxemia, hypoperfusion, and hypercarbia, should be avoided.

III. DISORDERS OF RED CELL METABOLISM

The stability of the RBC membrane and the solubility of intracellular Hgb depend on four glucose-supported metabolic pathways. Anesthetic concerns involve avoiding triggering events for hemolysis and management of chronic anemia.

A. **The Embden-Meyerhof Pathway (Nonoxidative or Anaerobic Pathway).** This pathway generates adenosine triphosphate necessary for membrane function and maintenance of cell shape and pliability. Defects in anaerobic glycolysis are associated with increased cell rigidity and decreased survival, as well as hemolytic anemia. There are no characteristic morphologic changes. The severity of hemolysis is highly variable.

B. **The Phosphogluconate Pathway.** This pathway counteracts environmental oxidants and prevents globin denaturation. Lack of either of the two key enzymes, glucose-6-phosphate dehydrogenase (G6PD) or glutathione reductase, results in membrane damage and hemolysis.
   1. **G6PD Deficiency.** G6PD deficiency is one of the most prevalent disease-causing mutations and is encoded on the X chromosome. Manifestations are (1) chronic hemolytic anemia, (2) acute episodic hemolytic anemia, (3) hemolysis only with stressors, or (4) no apparent hemolysis. Events exacerbating anemia include infections, drugs (methylene blue), and fava bean ingestion. Anesthesia management is geared toward avoidance of oxidative drugs and management of anemia. Isoflurane, sevoflurane, and diazepam depress G6PD activity in vitro and should probably be avoided. Methylene blue is contraindicated and may be life-threatening. Drugs that can produce methemoglobinemia, such as lidocaine, prilocaine, and silver nitrate, should be avoided. Hypothermia, acidosis, hyperglycemia, and infection can precipitate hemolysis.
   2. **Pyruvate Kinase Deficiency.** The most common erythrocyte enzyme defect causing hemolytic anemia, pyruvate kinase deficiency is more likely than G6PD deficiency to cause chronic hemolytic anemia. Splenectomy decreases the rate of RBC destruction. Severity ranges from mild hemolysis without anemia to life-threatening hemolytic anemia that necessitates transfusion and is present at birth. Other clinical signs are chronic jaundice, pigmented gallstones, and splenomegaly.

C. **The Methemoglobin (MHb) Reductase Pathway.** This pathway maintains heme iron in its ferrous state. Mutation of the MHb reductase enzyme results in an inability to counteract oxidation of Hgb to MHb (which will not transport oxygen). Patients with type I enzyme deficiency accumulate small amounts of MHb in circulating red cells, whereas type II patients have severe cyanosis and mental retardation.

D. **The Luebering-Rapoport Pathway.** This pathway produces 2,3-DPG (also known as 2,3-disphosphoglycerate). A single enzyme, disphospheroglyceromutase, mediates both the synthase activity, resulting in 2,3-DPG formation, and the phosphatase activity that converts 2,3-DPG to 3-phosphoglycerate, returning it to the glycolytic pathway. Severe phosphate depletion results in a reduced 2,3-DPG production response.

IV. THE HEMOGLOBIN MOLECULE

Each heme group can bind an oxygen molecule. The respiratory motion (i.e., uptake and release of oxygen) involves a specific change in the molecular structure of Hgb. Oxygen binding by one of the heme groups increases the affinity of the other groups for oxygen. Inherited defects in Hgb structure can interfere with this respiratory motion. Some defects restrict the molecule to either a low- or high-affinity state, and others either change heme iron from ferrous to ferric or reduce the solubility of the Hgb molecule. Hgb S (sickle cell disease) results in reduced solubility and precipitation of the abnormal Hgb.

A. Disorders of Hemoglobin

1. **Sickle S Hemoglobin.** In the deoxygenated state, Hgb S undergoes conformational changes exposing a hydrophobic region of the molecule. These regions aggregate, distorting and damaging the erythrocyte membrane, causing deformation and a shortened life span. Sickle cell anemia (homozygous Hgb S disease) manifests early in life as severe hemolytic anemia and vasoocclusive disease involving the marrow, spleen, kidney, and central nervous system. Other clinical manifestations are painful crises (bone and joint pain, recurrent splenic infarction [functional asplenia], renal medullary infarcts [chronic renal failure], and acute chest syndrome [new pulmonary infiltrate and at least one of the following: chest pain, fever higher than 38.5° C, tachypnea, wheezing, or cough]) and neurologic complications (stroke).
   a. ***Anesthetic Considerations.*** Risk factors for perioperative complications include older age, frequent hospitalizations and/or transfusions for episodes of crisis, and evidence of organ damage. There is no benefit in aggressive preoperative transfusion to decrease the *ratio* of Hgb S to normal Hgb, Rather, the goal is to achieve a preoperative Hct of 30% for moderate or high-risk surgery. Anesthetic technique does not affect the risk. Avoiding dehydration, acidosis, and hypothermia during anesthesia should reduce perioperative sickling. Acute chest syndrome may develop, typically 2 to 3 days into the postoperative period.
2. **Sickle C Hemoglobin.** Much less prevalent than Hgb S, sickle C Hgb causes the erythrocyte to lose water via enhanced activity of the potassium-chloride co-transport system and is associated with a mild-to-moderate hemolytic anemia. The presence of both Hgb S and Hgb C (Hgb SC) produces a tendency toward sickling and its associated complications approaching that of Hgb SS disease. Transfusions may reduce the incidence of sickle complications in this subset.
3. **Hemoglobin Sickle–β-Thalassemia.** Clinical presentation is largely determined by whether it is associated with reduced amounts of Hgb A (sickle cell–β-thalassemia) or complete absence of Hgb A (sickle cell–β^0-thalassemia). In the latter, patients experience acute vasoocclusive crises, acute chest syndrome, and other sickling complications at rates approaching those of Hgb SS. Anesthetic considerations are the same as those for homozygous sickle S Hgb.

B. Unstable Hemoglobins. Structural changes can destabilize Hgb molecules and reduce their solubility or make them more susceptible to oxidation. Destabilizing mutations typically impair globin folding or heme-globin binding that holds the heme moiety within the globin pocket. Once freed from the pocket, heme binds nonspecifically to other regions of the globin chains, causing them to form a precipitate containing globin chains, chain fragments, and heme (Heinz body). Heinz bodies reduce red cell deformability and favor their removal by splenic macrophages. Anesthetic management involves transfusion for severe hemolysis and avoidance of oxidizing agents.

C. Thalassemias. In adults, 96% to 97% of Hgb consists of two α-globin and two β-globin chains (Hgb A) with minor components of Hgb F and A_2. An inherited defect in globin chain synthesis, thalassemia, is one of the leading causes of microcytic anemia.

1. **Thalassemia Minor.** This occurs in individuals who are heterozygotes for an α-globin (α-thalassemia trait) or β-globin (β-thalassemia trait) gene mutation. The anemia is usually modest (Hgb 10 to 14 g/dL), and morbidity is rare.
2. **Thalassemia Intermedia.** Patients with thalassemia intermedia have more severe anemia and prominent microcytosis and hypochromia. They may have hepatosplenomegaly, cardiomegaly, and skeletal changes secondary to marrow expansion. These patients have either a milder form of homozygous β-thalassemia, a combined α- and β-thalassemia defect, or β-thalassemia with high levels of Hgb F.
3. **Thalassemia Major.** Patients with thalassemia major develop severe, life-threatening anemia during childhood and require long-term transfusion therapy. Complications of iron

overload (cirrhosis, right-sided heart failure, and endocrinopathy) often require chelation therapy. In the most severe forms of thalassemia major, patients exhibit three defects that markedly depress their oxygen-carrying capacity: (1) ineffective erythropoiesis, (2) hemolytic anemia, and (3) hypochromia with microcytosis. Other features of severe thalassemia include those attributable to severe bone marrow hyperplasia (frontal bossing, maxillary overgrowth, stunted growth, osteoporosis) and extramedullary hematopoiesis (hepatomegaly). Bone marrow transplantation is a therapeutic option.

V. DISORDERS OF HEMOGLOBIN RESULTING IN REDUCED OR INEFFECTIVE ERYTHROPOIESIS: MACROCYTIC OR MEGALOBLASTIC ANEMIA

Disruption of the red cell maturation sequence by vitamin deficiencies, chemotherapy, or preleukemic states results in macrocytic anemia and megaloblastic bone marrow morphology.

A. **Folic Acid and Vitamin B_{12} Deficiencies.** These deficiencies are primary causes of macrocytic anemia in adults. Marrow precursors appear much larger than normal and are unable to complete cell division. The marrow becomes megaloblastic, and macrocytic red cells are released into the circulation.

B. **Other Causes.** Alcoholism, tropical and nontropical sprue (malabsorption), and chronic nitrous oxide exposure are other causes.

C. **Macrocytic Anemia.** Macrocytic anemia caused by folate or vitamin B_{12} deficiency may result in Hgb levels less than 8 to 10 g/dL, a mean red cell volume of 110 to 140 fL (normal = 90 fL), a normal reticulocyte count, and increased levels of lactate dehydrogenase and bilirubin. Vitamin B_{12} deficiency is associated with bilateral peripheral neuropathy (degeneration of the lateral and posterior spinal cord columns), memory impairment, and depression.

D. **Anesthetic Management.** Anesthetic management is aimed at maintaining oxygen delivery to tissues. Regional techniques might be avoided because of the presence of neuropathy. Even relatively short exposures to nitrous oxide may produce megaloblastic changes.

VI. DISORDERS OF HEMOGLOBIN RESULTING IN REDUCED OR INEFFECTIVE ERYTHROPOIESIS: MICROCYTIC ANEMIA

A. **Iron Deficiency Anemia.** This is caused by chronic blood loss in nonpregnant adults. Nutritional deficiency of iron causes anemia only in infants and small children. Parturients are susceptible to iron deficiency anemia caused by increased RBC mass and the needs of the fetus for iron.
   1. **Diagnosis.** Diagnosis is made by evidence of mild microcytic, hypochromic anemia (Hgb 9 to 12 g/dL) and decreased serum ferritin concentrations (<30 ng/mL).
   2. **Treatment.** Ferrous iron salts (oral ferrous sulfate) are administered. Appropriate response to iron therapy is an increase in Hgb concentration of 2 g/dL in 3 weeks or return of Hgb concentrations to normal in 6 weeks. Recombinant human erythropoietin may be used to treat drug-induced anemia or to improve Hgb concentrations before elective surgery.

VII. HEMOGLOBINS WITH INCREASED OXYGEN AFFINITY

These Hgbs bind oxygen more readily than normal and deliver less oxygen to tissues at normal capillary Po_2 levels. Blood returns to the lungs still saturated with oxygen. Mild tissue hypoxia results, with increased erythropoietin production and polycythemia. Patients with mild erythrocytosis do not need treatment. Patients with high Hct (>55% to 60%), whose blood viscosity may further compromise oxygen delivery, may require exchange transfusion and careful avoidance of hemoconcentration both preoperatively and intraoperatively. Hemodilution and blood loss, however, may cause critical decreases in the tissue oxygen delivery, even at Hcts tolerated by patients with normal Hgb levels.

VIII. METHEMOGLOBINEMIA

A. Formation of Methemoglobin. MHb is formed when iron in the Hgb is oxidized from the ferrous (Fe^{2+}) state to the ferric (Fe^{3+}) state. The normal erythrocyte maintains MHb levels of 1% or less. MHb has high oxygen affinity and delivers little oxygen to the tissues. When MHb is 30% to 50% of the total Hgb, symptoms of oxygen deprivation occur, and at more than 50%, coma and death can ensue. Methemoglobinemias result from (1) mutations that favor formation of MHb, (2) mutations impairing the MHb reductase system, and (3) toxic exposures that oxidize normal Hgb iron at a rate exceeding the capacity of normal reducing mechanisms. MHb has a brownish-blue color that does not change to red on exposure to oxygen, giving patients a cyanotic appearance independent of their $Pa{O_2}$.

1. Patients with methemoglobinemia may be asymptomatic, if their MHb levels do not exceed 30% of their total Hgb.
2. Mutations impairing the MHb reductase system rarely result in methemoglobinemia levels greater than 25%.
3. Exposure to chemical agents may produce an acquired methemoglobinemia in which life-threatening amounts of MHb accumulate.

B. Emergency Treatment. A total of 1 to 2 mg/kg of intravenous methylene blue is infused over 3 to 5 minutes. Methylene blue acts through the reduced nicotinamide adenine dinucleotide phosphate reductase system and accordingly requires the activity of G6PD. Patients who are G6PD deficient and patients severely affected by methemoglobinemia may require exchange transfusions.

C. Anesthetic Management. Oxidizing agents should be avoided, and blood pH and MHb levels such as local anesthetics, nitrates, and nitrous oxide are measured as needed.

IX. DISORDERS OF RED CELL PRODUCTION

A. Hypoproliferation

1. **Constitutional Aplastic Anemia (Fanconi Anemia).** This is an autosomal recessive disorder that causes severe pancytopenia usually in the first two decades of life and often progresses to acute leukemia.
2. **Drug-Associated and Radiation-Associated Marrow Damage Anemia.** This type of anemia is a predictable side effect of chemotherapy and radiation therapy. Recovery is usually full, provided there is a sufficient infection-free period. Long-term exposure to low levels of external radiation or ingested radioisotopes and certain drugs can cause aplastic anemia (Table 20-1).
3. **Infection-Associated Marrow Damage Anemia.** Marrow damage can result from direct invasion of the marrow itself by an infectious agent (miliary tuberculosis) or by immunosuppression of stem cell growth. Aplastic anemia is seen after viral illnesses (hepatitis, Epstein-Barr virus infection, HIV infection, rubella, parvovirus infection).
4. **Anemia Caused by Hematologic or Other Marrow-Involving Malignancy.** Anemia may be caused by any leukemia, by solid tumor metastases to the marrow (breast, lung, prostate), and by clonal expansion of other marrow constituents (myelodysplastic syndromes, myeloproliferative disorders). By contrast, clonal expansion of erythroid cells in the marrow (erythrocytosis), may produce polycythemia vera (PV), discussed in the next section.
5. **Anesthetic Management.** Patients undergoing surgery may have anemia and thrombocytopenia that necessitate transfusion. Immunocompromise may affect the need for and choice of antibiotic coverage.

B. Polycythemia. Sustained hypoxia causes a rise in the RBC mass and Hct. At Hct levels over 55%, blood viscosity can be increased to a point at which blood flow to key organs such as the brain can be significantly reduced.

TABLE 20-1 ■ Classes of Drugs Associated with Marrow Damage

Antibiotics (chloramphenicol, penicillin, cephalosporins, sulfonamides, amphotericin B, streptomycin, pyrimethamine)
Antidepressants (lithium, tricyclics)
Antiepileptics (phenytoin, carbamazepine, valproic acid, phenobarbital)
Antiinflammatory drugs (phenylbutazone, nonsteroidals, salicylates, gold salts)
Antiarrhythmics (lidocaine, quinidine, procainamide)
Antithyroid drugs (propylthiouracil)
Diuretics (thiazides, furosemide)
Antihypertensives (captopril)
Antiuricemics (allopurinol, colchicine)
Antimalarials (quinacrine, chloroquine)
Hypoglycemics (tolbutamide)
Platelet inhibitors (ticlopidine)
Tranquilizers (prochlorperazine, meprobamate)

1. **Physiology.** Polycythemia can be relative (reduction in plasma volume, no change in red cell mass) or absolute (increased red cell mass). Clinical signs and symptoms vary but Hct values of 55% to 60% or higher can cause headaches, easy fatigability, compromised organ perfusion, and venous and arterial thrombosis.
2. **Primary Polycythemia (Polycythemia Vera [PV]).** PV is a clonal stem cell disorder, which is nearly always caused by a mutation in the *JAK-2* gene. Platelets and leukocytes may also be increased. Diagnostic criteria for PV are an elevated Hgb (>18.5 g/dL in men and >16.5 g/dL in women) or elevated RBC mass, normal arterial oxygenation, and splenomegaly not attributable to another cause. Thrombosis (especially cerebral thrombosis) may be the presenting sign. Treatment is regular phlebotomy to an Hct of 45% for men and 38% to 40% for women. Alternative treatment is administration of hydroxyurea.
   a. ***Anesthesia Management.*** PV patients are at increased risk of perioperative thrombosis and, paradoxically, hemorrhage. Bleeding associated with PV is caused by acquired von Willebrand disease (vWD) resulting from hyperviscosity-related changes in von Willebrand factor (vWF). Phlebotomy and avoidance of extreme dehydration lower the risk of both thrombosis and hemorrhage in the PV patient in the perioperative period.
3. **Secondary Polycythemia Caused by Hypoxia.** Secondary polycythemia can occur in individuals who live at high altitude, those with chronic tissue hypoxia caused by significant cardiopulmonary disease (e.g., cyanotic congenital heart disease, low cardiac output states), and inherited defects in Hgb, such as high-affinity Hgb and defects in 2,3-DPG amount or function (impaired delivery of oxygen causing tissue hypoxia). Anesthetic considerations include oxygen therapy, preoperative phlebotomy when indicated, and appreciation of perioperative hypercoagulability and potential for bleeding diatheses.
4. **Secondary Polycythemia Caused by Increased Erythropoietin Production.** Renal disease (hydronephrosis, polycystic renal disease, benign and malignant renal tumors) and erythropoietin-secreting tumors have been associated with secondary polycythemia. Nonrenal tumors (uterine myomas, hepatomas, cerebellar hemangiomas) sometimes secrete erythropoietin. Treatment is management of the underlying disorder and phlebotomy when necessary.

DISORDERS OF HEMOSTASIS

Disorders of hemostasis can be acquired or hereditary (Table 20-2). Activation of coagulation can be divided into three phases.

TABLE 20-2 ■ **Categorization of Coagulation Disorders**

HEREDITARY
Hemophilia A
Hemophilia B
von Willebrand's disease
Afibrinogenemia
Factor V deficiency
Factor VIII deficiency
Hereditary hemorrhagic telangiectasia
Protein C deficiency
Antithrombin III deficiency
ACQUIRED
Disseminated intravascular coagulation
Perioperative anticoagulation
Intraoperative coagulopathies
Dilutional thrombocytopenia
Dilution of procoagulants
Massive blood transfusion
Type of surgery (cardiopulmonary bypass, brain trauma, orthopedic surgery, urologic surgery, obstetric delivery)
Drug-induced hemorrhage
Drug-induced platelet dysfunction
Idiopathic thrombocytopenic purpura
Thrombotic thrombocytopenic purpura
Catheter-induced thrombocytopenia
Vitamin K deficiency

1. *Initiation phase.* Blood is exposed to a source of tissue factor (TF), usually on subendothelial cells after damage to a blood vessel. TF binds factor VIIa in the circulating blood, catalyzing the conversion of factor X to Xa, which then generates thrombin.
2. *Amplification phase.* Platelets, factor V, and factor XI are activated by a small amount of thrombin.
3. *Propagation phase.* Thrombin activates platelets and factors V and VIII, with formation of factor VIIIa-IXa complex. This complex turns on a "switch" in coagulation, from the TF-VIIa catalyzed reaction to the Xase (intrinsic) pathway. This pathway is much more efficient in producing Xa, and explosive thrombin generation occurs.

Common laboratory tests of soluble coagulation factors (prothrombin time [PT] and activated partial thromboplastin time [PTT]) measure only the kinetics of the initiation phase. These tests are sensitive at detecting severe deficiencies in clotting factors—for example, hemophilia—and in guiding warfarin or heparin therapy; they do not necessarily predict the risk of intraoperative bleeding.

I. HEMOSTATIC DISORDERS AFFECTING COAGULATION FACTORS OF THE INITIATION PHASE

A. Factor VII Deficiency. Factor VII deficiency is a rare autosomal recessive disease with highly variable clinical severity. Only homozygous deficient patients have factor VII levels low enough (<15%) to have symptomatic bleeding. The unique laboratory pattern is a prolonged PT with a normal PTT.

1. Anesthetic Considerations. Treatment depends on the severity of the deficiency. Patients with mild to moderate deficiency can be treated with infusions of fresh frozen plasma (FFP). Patients with factor VII levels less than 1% require treatment with a concentrated source of factor VII, such as Proplex T (factor IX complex, with a high level of factor VII). In the case of active bleeding, activated recombinant factor VIIa should be used, beginning with a dose of 20 to 30 mcg/kg, with readministration directed by PT results.

B. Congenital Deficiencies in Factors X and V and Prothrombin (II). These deficiencies are autosomal recessive disorders. Severe deficiencies are rare. Patients with severe deficiencies of any of these factors demonstrate prolongations of both PT and PTT. Patients with congenital factor V deficiency may also have a prolonged bleeding time because of the relationship between factor V and platelet function in supporting clot formation.

1. **Anesthetic Considerations.** Deficiencies in factors X and V and prothrombin can be corrected with FFP, but large volumes are needed (4 to 6 units or 800 to 1200 mL to increase factor level 20% to 30%). Factor V is stored in platelet granules, and in a bleeding patient, platelet transfusion is an alternative way to replace factor V. For patients with severe deficiencies, several prothrombin complex concentrates (PCCs) are available; these lower the risk of volume overload but may be associated with thrombosis, thromboembolism, and disseminated intravascular coagulation (DIC).

II. HEMOSTATIC DISORDERS AFFECTING COAGULATION FACTORS OF THE PROPAGATION PHASE

Not all deficiencies causing prolongation of the PTT are associated with bleeding. Deficiencies of factor XII, high-molecular-weight kininogen, and prekallikrein, for example, do not increase the risk of bleeding. Patients with deficiencies of these particular factors require no special management except alteration of their coagulation testing to allow accurate measurement of physiologic factors critical to in vivo hemostasis.

A. Hemophilia A and Hemophilia B

1. **Congenital Factor VIII Deficiency: Hemophilia A.** This is an X-linked recessive genetic disorder. Clinical severity of hemophilia A is best correlated with the factor VIII activity level. Severe hemophiliacs have factor VIII activity levels less than 1% of normal and are usually diagnosed during childhood because of frequent, spontaneous hemorrhages into joints, muscles, and vital organs. Factor levels only 1% to 5% of normal reduce severity of the disease, but these patients are at increased risk of hemorrhage with surgery or trauma. Patients with factor levels of 6% to 30% are only mildly affected and may go undiagnosed into adult life. They are also at risk for excessive bleeding with a major surgical procedure. Female carriers of hemophilia A can also be at risk with surgery.
   a. ***Diagnosis.*** Patients with severe hemophilia A are male and have a significantly prolonged PTT (in milder disease, the PTT may be only a few seconds longer than normal). The PT is normal. Factor VIII levels are necessary to distinguish hemophilia A from hemophilia B.
   b. ***Anesthetic Considerations.*** The factor VIII level must be brought to near normal (100%) for major surgery in patients with severe hemophilia A. This requires an initial infusion of 50 to 60 units/kg (3500 to 4000 units in a 70-kg patient) of factor VIII concentrate. Repeat infusions of 25 to 30 units/kg every 8 to 12 hours are needed to keep the plasma factor VIII level greater than 50%. In children, the half-life of factor VIII may be shorter, necessitating more frequent infusions. Peak and trough factor VIII levels should be measured to confirm the appropriate dosage and administration interval. Therapy must be continued for up to 2 weeks to avoid postoperative bleeding that disrupts wound healing. Longer periods of therapy (4 to 6 weeks) may be required in patients who undergo bone or joint surgery. Up to 30% of severe hemophilia A patients exposed to factor VIII concentrate or recombinant product develop factor VIII inhibitors. FFP, desmopressin, and fibrinolytic inhibitors, such as ε-aminocaproic acid and tranexamic acid, may be useful adjunct therapy.
2. **Congenital Factor IX Deficiency: Hemophilia B.** This disease is clinically similar to hemophilia A. Factor IX levels of less than 1% are associated with severe bleeding. Moderate disease occurs in patients with levels of 1% to 5%. Patients with factor IX levels of 5% to 40% have

mild disease and this disease may not be detected until surgery is performed or the patient has a dental extraction. Hemophilia B patients also have a prolonged PTT and a normal PT.

a. ***Anesthetic Considerations.*** Recombinant or purified factor IX or factor IX PCC is used to treat mild bleeding episodes or as prophylaxis for minor procedures. However, these factor preparations are associated with increased risk of thromboembolic complications. Therefore higher doses should be used only in patients undergoing major orthopedic surgery and those with severe traumatic injuries or liver disease. Purified factor IX concentrates or recombinant IX is used over several days to treat bleeding in hemophilia B. A dose of 100 units/kg (7000 units in a 70-kg patient) is administered, followed by repeated infusions at 50% of the original dose every 12 to 24 hours to keep factor IX plasma levels above 50%. Doses of 30 to 50 units/kg will give mean factor IX levels of 20% to 40% (adequate to control less severe bleeding).

3. **Acquired Factor VIII or IX Inhibitors.** Approximately 30% to 40% of patients with severe deficiency of factor VIII develop circulating inhibitors to factor VIII. Hemophilia B patients are less likely to develop an inhibitor to factor IX (3% to 5% incidence). A severe hemophilia-like syndrome can occur in genetically normal individuals secondary to the appearance of an acquired autoantibody to either factor VIII or, factor IX. These patients are usually middle-aged or older with no personal or family history of abnormal bleeding; they develop sudden, severe, spontaneous hemorrhage.

a. ***Diagnosis.*** The presence of an inhibitor is diagnosed by a mixing study in which the patient's plasma and normal plasma are mixed in a 1:1 ratio to determine whether the prolonged PTT shortens. In classic hemophilia A with no circulating factor VIII inhibitor, PTT usually shortens to within 4 seconds of normal or less, whereas little or no correction will occur in the presence of an inhibitor. Inhibitors are measured in Bethesda units. Factor VIII inhibitor patients fall into one of two groups. High responders (>10 Bethesda units/mL) have a marked inhibitor response after any factor infusion and dramatic anamnestic responses to therapy. Their inhibitor levels cannot be neutralized by replacement therapy. Low responders (5 to 10 Bethesda units/mL) develop and maintain relatively low levels of inhibitor and do not show anamnestic responses to factor VIII concentrates.

b. ***Anesthetic Management.*** Management of hemophilia A patients with inhibitors depends on whether the patient is a high or low responder. Low responders can usually be managed with factor VIII concentrates. In high responders, treatment with factor VIII concentrates is not feasible. Major life-threatening bleeding can be treated with bypass products such as activated PCCs or recombinant factor VIIa. Because of increased risk of thrombosis with PCCs, recombinant factor VIIa is now the treatment of choice for acquired inhibitors. For active bleeding, a dose of 90 to 120 mcg/kg intravenously (IV) is recommended every 2 to 3 hours until hemostasis has been achieved. Usually, factor IX inhibitor patients can be managed acutely using recombinant VIIa or PCC products. Patients who develop autoantibody to factor VIII or IX with no history of hemophilia can have life-threatening hemorrhage and may exhibit very high inhibitor levels. Treatment with recombinant factor VIIa or an activated prothrombin concentrate is required; factor VIII or IX alone will not be effective.

B. **Factor XI Deficiency (Rosenthal's disease).** The only other defect causing an isolated prolongation of the PTT and a bleeding tendency is factor XI deficiency (Rosenthal's disease). The bleeding tendency is quite mild and may be apparent only after a surgical procedure. Hematomas and hemarthroses are very unusual.

1. **Anesthetic Considerations.** Treatment depends on the severity of the deficiency and bleeding history. Most patients' factor XI deficiency can be treated with infusions of FFP. Treatment of factor XI deficiency with active bleeding is either PCCs or recombinant factor VIIa (20 to 30 mcg/kg, with readministration according to PTT results). Management of factor XI inhibitors is comparable to that of hemophilia A and B inhibitors.

C. **Congenital Abnormalities in Fibrinogen Production.** Congenital abnormalities will obviously interfere with the final step in the generation of a fibrin clot.

1. **Decreased Levels of Fibrinogen (Hypofibrinogenemia, Afibrinogenemia).** Deficiencies of fibrinogen are rare. Patients with afibrinogenemia have a severe bleeding diathesis with both spontaneous and posttraumatic bleeding. Hypofibrinogenemic patients usually do not have spontaneous bleeding but may have difficulty with surgery. Severe bleeding can be anticipated in patients with plasma fibrinogen levels below 50 to 100 mg/dL.
2. **Dysfibrinogenemia (Production of Abnormal Fibrinogen).** This is a more common defect. Clinical presentation is highly variable. Patients who demonstrate both a reduced amount and a dysfunctional fibrinogen (hypodysfibrinogenemia) usually exhibit excessive bleeding. Most dysfibrinogenemic patients do not have a bleeding tendency despite abnormal coagulation test results. Some patients have a paradoxically increased risk of thrombosis.
   a. ***Diagnosis.*** Laboratory evaluation includes measurement of both fibrinogen concentration and function. Both thrombin time (TT) and clotting time are sensitive to fibrinogen dysfunction. Definitive diagnosis and subclassification of dysfibrinogenemia require fibrinopeptide chain analysis and amino acid sequencing.
3. **Anesthetic Considerations.** Most patients have no clinical disease and do not require therapy. For those who are symptomatic or are at risk of bleeding with surgery, cryoprecipitate therapy is warranted. To increase the fibrinogen level by at least 100 mg/dL in the average-size adult, 10 to 12 units of cryoprecipitate should be infused, followed by 2 to 3 units each day. Dysfibrinogenemia patients with a thrombotic tendency require long-term anticoagulation.

D. **Factor XIII Deficiency.** Factor XIII is involved in clot stability. Factor XIII deficiency manifests at birth (persistent umbilical or circumcision bleeding). Adults have a severe bleeding diathesis (recurrent soft tissue bleeding, poor wound healing, intracranial hemorrhage, spontaneous abortion). Typically, bleeding is delayed because clots form but are weak and unable to maintain hemostasis.

1. **Diagnosis.** Factor XIII deficiency should be suspected in a patient with a severe bleeding diathesis who has otherwise normal coagulation screening test results (PT, PTT, fibrinogen level, platelet count, bleeding time). Clot dissolution in 5M urea can be used as a screen, and definitive diagnosis is by enzyme-linked immunosorbent assay. Patients at risk of severe hemorrhage have factor XIII levels of 1% of normal.
2. **Anesthetic Considerations.** Factor XIII–deficient patients can be treated with FFP, cryoprecipitate, or a plasma-derived factor XIII concentrate (Fibrogammin P). Factor XIII has a long half-life (7-12 days) and adequate hemostasis if achieved with a plasma concentration of 1% to 3%.

ARTERIAL COAGULATION

I. DISORDERS AFFECTING PLATELET NUMBER

For relatively minor procedures (catheter insertions, biopsies, lumbar puncture) the platelet count should be more than 20,000 to 30,000/mcL. For major surgery the platelet count should, if possible, be 50,000 to 100,000/mcL. Each unit of apheresis platelets or 6 units of random donor platelets should increase the platelet count in a normal-sized adult by about 50,000/mcL. One unit of single-donor apheresis platelets is equivalent to a random donor pool of 4 to 8 units. Random and single-donor platelets do not need to be ABO compatible. However, Rh-negative women of childbearing age should receive platelets from Rh-negative donors or be treated with RhoGAM after transfusion of Rh-positive product. Patients with very low platelet counts (<15,000/mcL) may have significant bleeding from multiple sites, including the nose, mucous membranes, gastrointestinal tract, skin, and vessel puncture sites. One sign of thrombocytopenia is a petechial rash of the skin or mucous membranes.

A. Disorders Resulting in Platelet Production Defects

1. Congenital

a. ***Congenital Hypoplastic Thrombocytopenia with Absent Radii (TAR Syndrome).*** This is an autosomal recessive disorder with thrombocytopenia in the third trimester of fetal development or early after birth. Thrombocytopenia is often initially severe (<30,000/mcL) but slowly improves over time, nearing normal by age 2.

b. ***Fanconi Syndrome.*** Hematologic manifestations do not usually appear until about age 7. The bone marrow shows reduced cellularity and reduced numbers of megakaryocytes. Stem cell transplantation is curative in the majority of children.

c. ***May-Hegglin Anomaly.*** This anomaly is typically associated with giant platelets in the circulation and Döhle's bodies (basophilic inclusions) in white blood cells. One third of patients have significant thrombocytopenia and risk of bleeding.

d. ***Wiskott-Aldrich Syndrome.*** This is an X-linked disorder that manifests with eczema, immunodeficiency, and thrombocytopenia. Circulating platelets are smaller than normal, function poorly because of granule defects, and have a reduced survival.

e. ***Autosomal Dominant Thrombocytopenia.*** This disorder involves increased megakaryocyte mass, ineffective production, and in some cases the release of macrocytic platelets into the circulation. Many of these patients have nerve deafness and nephritis (Alport's syndrome).

2. Acquired. A failure in platelet production can result from marrow damage (radiation and/or chemotherapy; insecticide or benzene exposure; reactions to thiazides, alcohol, estrogens, and viral hepatitis), neoplastic marrow infiltration (multiple myeloma, acute leukemia, lymphoma), and myeloproliferative disorders. Ineffective thrombopoiesis is also seen in patients with vitamin B_{12} or folate deficiency, including patients with alcoholism and defective folate metabolism. This failure in platelet production is rapidly reversed by appropriate vitamin therapy.

a. ***Anesthetic Considerations.*** Platelet transfusions are the mainstay of therapy. Ineffective thrombopoiesis associated with either vitamin B_{12} or folate deficiency should be immediately treated with appropriate vitamin therapy. Recovery of the platelet count to normal occurs within a matter of days, making platelet transfusion unnecessary in all but the most acute situations.

B. Disorders Caused by Platelet Destruction

1. Nonimmune Destruction

a. ***Thrombotic Thrombocytopenic Purpura (TTP).*** Signs may include fever, thrombocytopenia with an otherwise negative DIC screen (normal PT, PTT, and fibrinogen levels), multiple small vessel occlusions in multiple sites (kidney, central nervous system, skin, distal extremities), and a microangiopathic hemolytic anemia with schistocytosis due to mechanical fragmentation of RBCs flowing past intraarteriolar platelet thrombi.

i. ***Diagnosis.*** The presence of thrombocytopenia and microangiopathic hemolytic anemia (anemia, schistocytosis, reticulocytosis, decreased haptoglobin level, increased LDH and negative Coombs's test result as evidence of hemolysis) is considered diagnostic. TTP can be familial, sporadic (idiopathic), a chronic relapsing condition, a complication of marrow transplantation or drug therapy (quinine, ticlopidine, mitomycin C, interferon-α, pentostatin, gemcitabine, tacrolimus, or cyclosporine), or a complication of preeclampsia. Plasma exchange may be effective treatment in some cases.

b. ***Hemolytic-Uremic Syndrome (HUS).*** HUS is most often seen in children with bloody diarrhea secondary to *Escherichia coli* or related bacteria and progresses to acute renal failure; thrombocytopenia and anemia are less pronounced than with TTP. Most young children spontaneously recover with hemodialysis support, but mortality in adults and older children is high, and they should be treated with both plasma exchange and hemodialysis, regardless of the pattern of illness.

c. ***HELLP Syndrome.*** Up to 50% of preeclamptic mothers will develop a DIC-like picture with severe thrombocytopenia (platelet counts of 20,000 to 40,000/mcL) at the time of delivery. This is referred to as *HELLP syndrome* when the combination of red cell hemolysis (H), elevated liver enzymes (EL), and low platelet count (LP) is present. Treatment is control of hypertension and delivery of the baby. A few patients will have full-blown TTP-HUS after delivery, which can be a life-threatening.

d. ***Anesthetic Considerations.*** In patients with nonimmune destruction, platelet and plasma transfusions are supportive. The only truly effective therapy is the treatment of the underlying cause. Surgery should be delayed whenever possible until the underlying disorder has been brought under control.

2. **Autoimmune Platelet Destruction.** Severity of the thrombocytopenia is highly variable. With some conditions, the platelet count falls to as low as 1000 to 2000/mcL. Diagnosis can usually be made from the clinical presentation, an increase in the reticulated (RNA-containing) platelets in blood, and demonstration of an increase in marrow megakaryocytes (high rate of platelet production is required because of shortened survival of platelets in the circulation).

   a. ***Thrombocytopenic Purpura in Adults.*** Adults can develop posttransfusion purpura after exposure to a blood product, most often RBCs or platelets. Usually a potent alloantibody with platelet antigen A1 specificity is readily detected in the patient's plasma.

   b. ***Drug-Induced Autoimmune Thrombocytopenic Purpura.*** This condition is best known following quinine, quinidine, and sedormid exposure. Thrombocytopenia can be severe (platelets <20,000/mcL).

   c. ***Heparin-Induced Thrombocytopenia (HIT)***

      i. ***HIT type I (Nonimmune).*** HIT type I is a modest decrease in the platelet count seen in a majority of patients within the first day of full-dose unfractionated heparin (UH) therapy. It is caused by passive heparin binding to platelets, with modest shortening of platelet life span. It is transient and clinically insignificant.

      ii. ***HIT type II (Immune).*** HIT type II can occur in patients receiving heparin for longer than 5 days. Antibodies to the heparin-platelet complex form and induce platelet activation and aggregation. In addition, heparin-platelet complex binding to endothelial cells stimulates thrombin production. The result is increased clearance of platelets (thrombocytopenia) and venous and/or arterial thrombus formation involving severe organ damage and thrombosis in unusual sites (adrenal gland, portal vein, skin). Incidence is higher with bovine heparin than with porcine heparin. Patients on full-dose UH for longer than 5 days or who have previously received heparin should be monitored with every-other-day platelet counts. A decrease of more than 50% in platelet count may signal the appearance of an HIT type II antibody and mandates stopping the heparin and substituting a direct thrombin inhibitor (lepirudin, argatroban). An acute form of HIT type II can occur in patients restarted on heparin within 20 days of a previous exposure. When an HIT antibody is already present, a patient restarted on heparin can exhibit an acute drug reaction (severe dyspnea, shaking chills, diaphoresis, hypertension, tachycardia). Such patients are at extreme risk of a fatal thromboembolism if heparin is continued. Diagnosis is based on a method called the "4Ts system," which is summarized in Table 20-3.

   d. ***Anesthetic Considerations for Drug-Induced Thrombocytopenia.*** Treatment is platelet transfusion if the patient is experiencing a life-threatening hemorrhage or is bleeding into a closed space as with an intracranial hemorrhage. If thrombocytopenia is related to a drug reaction, the most important step is to discontinue the drug. Corticosteroid therapy may speed recovery in patients with an idiopathic thrombocytopenic purpura (ITP). HIV-infected thrombocytopenic patients may benefit from treatment with zidovudine well before (1 to 2 months) surgery. Corticosteroids, intravenous immunoglobulin (Ig), and intravenous anti-D (WinRho) have also been used in patients with acquired immunodeficiency syndrome.

      i. In patients with HIT, all heparin forms must be stopped immediately. Substitution of low-molecular-weight heparin (LMWH) is *not* an option because there is significant antibody cross-reactivity. When continued anticoagulation is required, HIT patients should be started on a direct thrombin inhibitor (lepirudin, argatroban). Lepirudin

TABLE 20-3 ■ **The 4Ts Scoring System for Heparin-Induced Thrombocytopenia***

CATEGORY	2 POINTS	1 POINT	0 POINTS
Thrombocytopenia	Platelet count decreased >50% from baseline *and* platelet nadir ≥20,000/mm^3	Platelet count decreased 30%-50% from baseline *or* platelet nadir 10,000-19,000/mm^3	Platelet count decreased <30% from baseline *or* platelet nadir <10,000/mm^3
Timing of the platelet decrease	Clear onset between days 5 and 10 of heparin exposure, *or* platelet decrease in less than a day with heparin exposure within the prior 30 days	Decrease in platelet counts consistent with onset between days 5 and 10 of heparin exposure but timing is not clear because of missing platelet counts, *or* onset after day 10 of heparin exposure, *or* decrease in platelet counts in less than a day with prior heparin exposure between 30 and 100 days earlier	Platelet count decrease within 4 days of heparin exposure
Thrombosis or other sequelae	New thrombosis, skin necrosis, or acute systemic reaction after unfractionated heparin exposure	Progressive or recurrent thrombosis or unconfirmed but clinically suspected thrombosis	No thrombosis or previous heparin exposure
Other causes of Thrombocytopenia	None apparent	Possible other causes present	Probable other causes present

Data from Crowther MA, Cook DJ, Albert M, et al. The 4Ts scoring system for heparin-induced thrombocytopenia in medical-surgical intensive care unit patients. *J Crit Care*. 2010;25:287-293.
*The scores are divided into high (6 - 8 points), intermediate (4 - 5 points), and low (≤3 points) groups.

is given as an intravenous bolus of 0.4 mg/kg, followed by a continuous infusion at 0.15 mg/kg/hr, adjusted to keep the PTT between 1.5 and 2.5 times normal. Argatroban is given as an infusion of approximately 2.0 mcg/kg/min, titrated to keep the PTT between 1.5 and 3 times normal. Oral anticoagulants should never be started until there is continuous successful anticoagulation with a direct thrombin inhibitor. The immediate reduction in protein C (PC) levels with warfarin therapy can cause worsening thrombosis. If this occurs, warfarin should be discontinued and vitamin K given to reverse the effect.

3. **Idiopathic Thrombocytopenic Purpura.** ITP is thrombocytopenia unrelated to a drug, infection, or autoimmune disease. This diagnosis can be made only by excluding all other causes of nonimmune and immune destruction. Typically, thrombocytopenia must be severe before bleeding becomes a problem. ITP patients with platelet counts even as low as 2000/mcL are usually not at great risk of a major organ or intracerebral bleed. Patients with chronic ITP generally show less severe thrombocytopenia, with platelet counts of 20,000 to 100,000/mcL.
   a. ***Anesthetic Considerations.*** Severe ITP with bleeding manifestations in adults should be treated as a medical emergency with high-dose corticosteroids for the first 3 days. For emergency surgery or clinical evidence of intracranial hemorrhage, the patient should also be given intravenous Ig and platelet transfusions at least every 8 to 12 hours, regardless of the effect on the platelet count. Splenectomy should be considered for chronic ITP.

b. ***Chronic ITP in Pregnancy.*** This can often be managed without medication, small doses of prednisone, or intermittent use of intravenous immunoglobulin. When thrombocytopenia is severe, therapeutic options include higher-dose steroid therapy (0.5 to 1 mg of prednisone per kilogram per day) and intravenous Ig during the last 2 to 3 weeks of pregnancy. Infants born to mothers with ITP may experience thrombocytopenia and should be monitored. Prophylactic cesarean section is still recommended by some obstetricians to decrease the chance of intracranial hemorrhage in infants born to mothers with ITP.

C. Qualitative Platelet Disorders

1. Congenital Disorders of Platelet Function

a. ***von Willebrand's Disease (vWD).*** Symptomatic vWD's disease is typically manifested by epistaxis, menorrhagia, easy bruising, and gingival and gastrointestinal bleeding.

i. ***Diagnosis.*** Full evaluation of vWD patients requires measurement of factor VIII coagulant activity, vWF antigen, vWF activity, and vWF multimer distribution. These studies are of diagnostic importance in the classification of vWD, which in turn is important in planning clinical management.

ii. ***Type 1 Disease.*** Type 1 vWD results from a defect in vWF release, rather than reduced platelet or endothelial stores. Administration of DDAVP improves vWF release. Clinical severity of the disease is variable. In patients and families with repeated and severe bleeding episodes, vWF antigen and vWF activity are usually less than 15% to 25% of normal. These patients should be treated aggressively for bleeding and given prophylactic treatment for even minor surgical procedures. A moderately low vWF level (<50%) by itself does not make the diagnosis of vWD. The majority of such individuals will not have an increased bleeding tendency and should not be labeled as having vWD.

iii. ***Type 2 Disease.*** Type 2 vWD results from a qualitative defect in plasma vWF causing a disproportionate decrease in vWF activity (ristocetin cofactor activity) when compared with vWF antigen.

iv. ***Type 3 Disease.*** Tye 3 vWD is characterized by a virtual absence of circulating vWF antigen and very low levels of both vWF activity and factor VIII (3% to 10% of normal). These patients experience severe bleeding with mucosal hemorrhage, hemarthroses, and muscle hematomas reminiscent of hemophilia A or B. However, unlike in classic hemophilia, the bleeding time is very prolonged.

v. ***Anesthetic Considerations.*** Useful therapeutic agents are DDAVP (stimulates release of endogenous vWF) and blood products that contain vWF in high concentrations (cryoprecipitate). Patients with type 1 vWD are the best responders to DDAVP. DDAVP can be administered IV (0.3 mcg/kg). A concentrated nasal spray of DDAVP can be self-administered (300 mcg total dose) by patients with type 1 vWD for management of menorrhagia and for tooth extractions or minor surgery. Because of the short duration of action and tachyphylaxis to DDAVP, vWF replacement is a more reliable therapy for severe bleeding and surgical prophylaxis. This is accomplished by transfusion of cryoprecipitate or purified concentrates containing the vWF–factor VIII complex. The recommended doses (expressed in International Units [IU] of both vWF and factor VIII) for bleeding management and surgical prophylaxis are an initial loading dose of 40 to 75 IU/kg IV, followed by repeat doses of 40 to 60 IU/kg at 8- to 12-hour intervals. Once bleeding has been controlled, a single daily dose of concentrate is sufficient. Both vWF and factor VIII must be provided to reliably treat bleeding in type 3 vWD.

D. Acquired Abnormalities of Platelet Function

1. **Myeloproliferative Disease.** Myeloproliferative disease (i.e., polycythemia vera, myeloid metaplasia, idiopathic myelofibrosis, essential thrombocythemia, and chronic myelogenous leukemia) is commonly associated with abnormal platelet function. The bleeding time may be prolonged but is a poor predictor of abnormal bleeding. The most consistent laboratory abnormalities in bleeding patients are defects in epinephrine-induced aggregation and dense granule and α-granule function.

2. **Dysproteinemias.** Dysproteinemias can be associated with defects in platelet adhesion, aggregation, and procoagulant activity. Almost one third of patients with Waldenström macroglobulinemia or IgA myeloma will have a demonstrable defect; IgG multiple myeloma patients are less commonly affected. The concentration of the monoclonal protein spike appears to correlate with the abnormalities in platelet function.
3. **Uremia.** Platelet adhesion, activation, and aggregation are abnormal, and thromboxane A_2 generation is decreased. Bleeding time is prolonged but corrected by hemodialysis. For acute bleeding episodes, DDAVP therapy can improve platelet function transiently.
4. **Liver Disease.** Liver disease is associated with a multifaceted defect in coagulation. Thrombocytopenia related to hypersplenism and a diminished thrombopoietin response is common. Platelet dysfunction is secondary to high levels of circulating fibrin degradation products. Reduced production of factor VII and low-grade chronic DIC with increased fibrinolysis are additional factors.
5. **Inhibition by Drugs.** Many drugs can affect platelet function (Table 20-4).
6. **Anesthetic Considerations.** Because the platelets are dysfunctional, absolute platelet number does not predict bleeding risk. Treatment with DDAVP may "overcome" a mild to moderate platelet defect, or platelet transfusions may be required. The bleeding time results of platelet function analysis, or the thromboelastogram will not guarantee adequacy of platelet function for the challenge of surgery. Hypothermia and acidosis adversely affect the function of both native and transfused platelets.

II. HYPERCOAGULABLE DISORDERS

A. Heritable Causes of Hypercoagulability (Table 20-5)

1. **Thrombophilia Caused by Decreased Antithrombotic Proteins**
   a. ***Hereditary Antithrombin (AT) Deficiency.*** This is an autosomal dominant inherited trait. Homozygosity is a fatal fetal defect; heterozygotes have AT III levels between 40% to 70% of normal. Risk of venous thromboembolism is increased twentyfold in these patients.

TABLE 20-4 ■ Drugs that Inhibit Platelet Function

STRONG ASSOCIATION
Aspirin (and aspirin-containing medications)
Clopidogrel, ticlopidine
Abciximab (ReoPro)
Nonsteroidal antiinflammatory drugs: naproxen, ibuprofen, indomethacin, phenylbutazone, piroxicam, ketorolac
MILD TO MODERATE ASSOCIATION
Antibiotics, usually only in high doses
Penicillin, carbenicillin, penicillin G, ampicillin, ticarcillin, nafcillin, mezlocillin
Cephalosporins
Nitrofurantoin
Volume expanders: dextran, hydroxyethyl starch
Heparin
Fibrinolytic agents: ε-aminocaproic acid
WEAK ASSOCIATION
Oncologic drugs: daunorubicin, mithramycin
Cardiovascular drugs: β-blockers, calcium channel blockers, nitroglycerin, nitroprusside, quinidine
Alcohol

b. ***Hereditary Protein C (PC) and Protein S (PS) Deficiencies.*** These deficiencies interfere with mechanisms that limit rates of thrombin generation. This results in an overabundance of thrombin and clinically the same effect as AT deficiency. Synthesis of PC and PS is vitamin K dependent, and PC-deficient individuals are at particular risk of thrombosis if warfarin therapy is initiated without prior protective anticoagulation with heparin. In patients with PC deficiency, purified PC concentrate and activated protein C (APC) can be used.

2. **Thrombophilia Caused by Increased Prothrombotic Proteins**

a. ***Factor V_{Leiden}.*** This is an abnormal factor V that is resistant to the normal cleavage and inactivation by APC. Accordingly, factor V_{Leiden} has prolonged action, fostering increased thrombin generation. Heterozygotes for the gene for factor V_{Leiden} have a fivefold to sevenfold increased risk of deep venous thrombosis (DVT), whereas the risk in homozygous carriers is increased up to eightyfold. Up to 1 in 20 patients undergoing routine surgery may have increased risk of deep vein thrombosis attributable to this gene.

b. ***Prothrombin G20210A Gene Mutation.*** This gene leads to increased levels of prothrombin. Alone, it has only modest effects on DVT risk. The importance of this thrombophilia resides in the frequency of this gene, rather than its potency.

B. **Acquired Causes of Hypercoagulability**

1. **Myeloproliferative Disorders.** These disorders are associated with an increased incidence of thrombophlebitis, pulmonary embolism (PE), and arterial occlusions, although the pathogenesis of the thrombosis in these patients is not clear.

2. **Malignancies.** Patients with certain adenocarcinomas (pancreas, colon, stomach, ovaries) may first demonstrate a single or multiple episodes of DVT or migratory superficial thrombophlebitis. The pathogenesis appears to be a combination of release of procoagulant factor(s) by the tumor, endothelial damage by tumor invasion, and blood stasis.

3. **Pregnancy and Oral Contraceptive Use.** Pregnancy and oral contraceptives increase the risk of thrombosis fivefold to sixfold. The risk of PE is highest during the third trimester of pregnancy and in the immediate postpartum period. PE is a leading cause of maternal death. AT III–deficient women are at the greatest risk and should be anticoagulated throughout pregnancy. Factor V_{Leiden} and the prothrombin G20210A mutation are associated with much less risk, and these patients do not need to be anticoagulated unless they have a history of a PE or recurrent DVT. Women who take oral contraceptives and who also smoke, have a history of migraine headaches, or carry an inherited hypercoagulable defect are at increased risk (thirtyfold) of venous thrombosis, PE, and cerebrovascular thrombosis.

4. **Nephrotic Syndrome.** Patients with nephrotic syndrome are at risk of thromboembolic disease, including renal vein thrombosis. The reasons are unclear but may include

TABLE 20-5 ■ **Major Hereditary Conditions Linked to Hypercoagulability**

	PREVALENCE IN HEALTHY CONTROLS	PREVALENCE IN PATIENTS WITH FIRST DVT (%)	DVT LIKELIHOOD BY AGE 60 (%)
Antithrombin deficiency*	0.2	1.1	62
Protein C deficiency*	0.8	3	48
Protein S deficiency*	1.3	1.1	33
Factor V_{Leiden}*	3.5	20	6
Prothrombin G20210A*	2.3	18	<5

*All numbers pertain to heterozygous state.
DVT, Deep venous thrombosis.

lower-than-normal levels of antithrombin III or PC, factor XII deficiency, platelet hyperactivity, abnormal fibrinolytic activity, and higher-than-normal levels of other coagulation factors. Hyperlipidemia and hypoalbuminemia have also been proposed as possible causative factors.

5. **Antiphospholipid Antibodies.** Antiphospholipid antibodies (e.g., lupus anticoagulant) are associated with increased tendency for both venous and arterial thrombosis. The term *anticoagulant* is therefore a clinical misnomer. The mechanism of action is not known; the antibodies may activate endothelial cells to increase the expression of vascular adhesion molecule-1 and E-selectin, increasing binding of white blood cells and platelets to the endothelial surface, leading to thrombus formation.
6. **Anesthetic Considerations for Venous Hypercoagulability.** Current antithrombotic strategies range from simple management (early ambulation) to the combination of subcutaneous heparin with compression stockings followed by conversion to outpatient warfarin with laboratory monitoring.
   a. ***Drugs for DVT Prophylaxis.*** Drugs include heparin (unfractionated or LMWH), warfarin, direct thrombin inhibitors (hirudin), and factor Xa inhibitors (fondaparinux). Administration of heparin confers a 60% to 70% risk reduction. Graded compression elastic stockings have a 40% to 45% risk reduction, and intermittent pneumatic compression stockings show a risk reduction that approaches that of heparin when used as the only prophylactic method.
   b. ***Regional Anesthesia.*** Although studies have shown that regional anesthesia decreases DVT, risk remains unacceptably high even when regional anesthesia is combined with early ambulation and intraoperative antiembolism stockings. With routine antithrombotic prophylaxis, the advantages of regional over general anesthesia are unclear, raising the question whether, for patients receiving pharmacologic perioperative thromboprophylaxis, neuraxial anesthesia still reduces the risk of DVT. As a result, postoperative prophylactic anticoagulation with drugs such as warfarin and subcutaneous heparin is now the standard of care for high-risk operations, such as knee and hip surgery.
   c. ***Vena Caval Filters.*** These can be used to prevent recurrent pulmonary emboli in patients who have an absolute contraindication to anticoagulation or have a major bleeding complication.
7. **Anesthetic Considerations for Patients on Long-Term Anticoagulation.** Most anticoagulated patients are managed on warfarin. In high-risk patients, bridging therapy with UH or LMWH should be considered. Bridging therapy reduces the risk of venous thromboembolism by up to 80%. Warfarin should be stopped 5 days before surgery and heparin therapy started 36 hours after the last dose of warfarin. Patients given LMWH should receive the last dose no less than 18 hours preoperatively for a twice-daily regimen and 30 hours for a once-daily regimen. UH by continuous infusion should be discontinued 6 hours before surgery. The effects of warfarin are delayed, and therefore warfarin should be resumed as soon as possible after surgery except in patients at high bleeding risk; consideration can be given to bridging therapy until the INR becomes therapeutic. In patients receiving regional anesthesia, anticoagulants usually need to be discontinued for some period of time before nerve block or epidural placement (Table 20-6).

C. Acquired Hypercoagulability of the Arterial Vasculature

1. **Atrial Fibrillation (AF).** Patients with AF, particularly those with valvular disease, a dilated atrium, and evidence of heart failure or a previous embolus, require moderate-dose warfarin therapy indefinitely (Tables 20-7 and 20-8). Patients with acute anterior wall infarctions who, because of a wall motion abnormality, are likely to form a mural thrombus need to receive warfarin for 2 to 3 months, after which there is little risk of embolism.
2. **Antiphospholipid Antibodies.** See the discussion of acquired causes of hypercoagulability.

TABLE 20-6 ■ **Management of Neuraxial Anesthesia in Patients Receiving Thromboprophylaxis**

ANTICOAGULANT DRUG	RECOMMENDATION
Subcutaneous unfractionated heparin	No contraindication with twice-daily dosing and total daily dose ≤10,000 units. Consider delaying heparin dose until after block if technical difficulty is anticipated.
Intravenous unfractionated heparin to be given during surgery	Heparinize 1 hr after neuraxial block. Remove catheter 24 hr after last heparin dose. No mandatory surgical delay if block placement is traumatic.
LMWH	*Twice-daily dosing:* Delay neuraxial block for at least 24 hr after last preoperative dose of heparin. First postoperative dose of LMWH should not be given sooner than 24 hr after surgery, regardless of anesthetic technique. Remove neuraxial catheter 2 hr before first postoperative LMWH dose. *Once-daily dosing:* Delay neuraxial block for at least 12 hr after last preoperative heparin dose. First postoperative LMWH dose can be given 6-8 hr after surgery and next dose 24 hr later. Indwelling neuraxial catheters can be maintained. Remove neuraxial catheter 12 hr after last LMWH dose.
Warfarin	INR should be normal before neuraxial anesthesia is induced. Remove catheter when INR is <1.5 during re-initiation of warfarin therapy.
Fondaparinux	Use neuraxial blockade only if it can be accomplished with a single pass of an atraumatic needle and without an indwelling catheter.
Direct thrombin inhibitors	Avoid neuraxial techniques.

Adapted from Horlocker TT, Wedel DJ, Rowlingson JC, et al. Regional anesthesia in the patient receiving antithrombotic or thrombolytic therapy: American Society of Regional Anesthesia and Pain Medicine Evidence-Based Guidelines (third edition). *Reg Anesth Pain Med*. 2010;35:64-101.
INR, International normalized ratio; *LMWH,* low-molecular-weight heparin.

TABLE 20-7 ■ **$CHADS_2$ Scoring System to Estimate Stroke Risk in Nonrheumatic Atrial Fibrillation***

	CONDITION	POINTS
C	Congestive heart failure	1
H	Hypertension	1
A	Age ≥75 yr	1
D	Diabetes mellitus	1
S_2	Prior stroke or transient ischemic attack	2

*For risk stratification based on $CHADS_2$ score, see Table 20-8.

TABLE 20-8 ■ **Risk Stratification for Perioperative Thromboembolic Events**

RISK CATEGORY	MECHANICAL HEART VALVE	ATRIAL FIBRILLATION	VTE
High	Any mitral valve prosthesis Caged-ball or tilting-disk aortic valve prosthesis Recent (within 6 mo) stroke or TIA	$CHADS_2$ score of 5 or 6 Recent (within 3 mo) stroke or TIA Rheumatic heart disease	Recent (within 3 mo) VTE Severe thrombophilia (e.g., deficiency of protein C, protein S, or antithrombin III); presence of antiphospholipid antibodies; or multiple abnormalities
Moderate	Bileaflet aortic valve prosthesis and one of the following: atrial fibrillation, prior stroke or TIA, hypertension, diabetes, congestive heart failure, age >75 yr	$CHADS_2$ score of 3 or 4	VTE within the past 3 to 12 mo Mild to moderate thrombophilic condition Recurrent VTE Active cancer (treated within 6 mo or with palliative care)
Low	Bileaflet aortic valve prosthesis without atrial fibrillation and no other risk factors for stroke	$CHADS_2$ score of 0 to 2 No prior stroke or TIA	Single VTE occurring >12 mo earlier, no other risk factors

Data from Douketis JD, Berger PB, Dunn AS, et al. The perioperative management of antithrombotic therapy: American College of Chest Physicians Evidence-Based Clinical Practice Guidelines (8th edition). *Chest.* 2008;133(6 Suppl):299S-339S.

TIA, Transient ischemic attack; *VTE,* venous thromboembolism.

CHAPTER 21

Skin and Musculoskeletal Diseases

Diseases of the skin and musculoskeletal system manifest with obvious clinical signs, but less visible systemic effects of many of these disorders are also important.

SKIN AND CONNECTIVE TISSUE DISEASE

I. EPIDERMOLYSIS BULLOSA

Epidermolysis bullosa (EB) is a group of genetic diseases of mucous membranes and skin, particularly the oropharynx and esophagus.

A. **Signs and Symptoms.** EB is characterized by bulla formation (blistering) caused by separation within the epidermis followed by fluid accumulation. Bulla formation is typically initiated when lateral shearing forces are applied to the skin. Pressure applied perpendicular to the skin is not as great a hazard. EB is classified as simplex, junctional, or dystrophic.
   1. EB simplex has a benign course.
   2. Junctional EB is associated with high mortality in early childhood as a result of sepsis. Junctional EB is characterized by blistering beginning at birth, absence of scar formation, and generalized mucosal involvement.
   3. Dystrophic EB is also associated with high early childhood mortality. It is associated with severe scarring, fusion of the digits, microstomia, esophageal strictures, and dental dysplasia. Chronic infection is associated with malnutrition, anemia, electrolyte imbalance, and hypoalbuminemia.

B. **Treatment.** EB treatment is symptomatic and supportive, often including corticosteroids.

C. **Management of Anesthesia** (Table 21-1)

II. PEMPHIGUS

Pemphigus refers to a group of chronic autoimmune blistering (vesiculobullous) diseases that may involve extensive areas of the skin and mucous membranes. Cutaneous pemphigus closely resembles the oral manifestations of EB dystrophica (eating is painful; malnutrition may develop). Pemphigus may be associated with underlying malignancy, especially lymphoreticular cancer.

A. **Treatment.** Treatment of pemphigus is with corticosteroids. Mycophenolate mofetil, rituximab, azathioprine, methotrexate, and cyclophosphamide have also been used successfully for early treatment of pemphigus. Immune globulin has replaced high-dose corticosteroids as a rescue therapy.

B. **Management of Anesthesia.** Management is similar to that of patients with EB. Preoperative evaluation must include consideration of current drug therapy. Electrolyte derangements and dehydration may be present because of chronic fluid losses through bullous skin lesions. Airway management may be difficult because of bullae in the oropharynx. Airway manipulation, including direct laryngoscopy and endotracheal intubation, can result in acute bulla formation, upper airway obstruction, and bleeding.

TABLE 21-1 ■ **Anesthesia Considerations in Epidermolysis Bullosa**
Consider preoperative treatment with corticosteroids
Avoid trauma to skin and mucous membranes (e.g., hold IV equipment in place with gauze wrap or suture; pad blood pressure cuffs; gel pad should be placed under patient; use nonadhesive pulse oximeter; remove adhesive from ECG pads—petroleum jelly gauze can help hold them in place).
Minimize upper airway instrumentation, avoid esophageal stethoscopes, lubricate the laryngoscope blade.
Endotracheal intubation appears safe (laryngeal involvement is rare).
Succinylcholine appears safe.
Avoid oropharyngeal suctioning.
Regional anesthesia techniques may be useful.

Adapted from Greaves MW. Chronic urticaria. *N Engl J Med.* 1995;332:1767-1772.
ECG, Electrocardiogram; *IV,* intravenous.

III. PSORIASIS

Psoriasis is a common chronic dermatologic disorder affecting 1% to 3% of the world's population and is characterized by accelerated epidermal growth resulting in inflammatory erythematous papules covered with loosely adherent scales *(chronic plaque psoriasis)*. An asymmetric arthropathy occurs in approximately 5% to 8% of patients.

A. Treatment. Psoriasis treatment is directed at slowing the rapid proliferation of epidermal cells Topical treatments include coal tar, salicylic acid, topical corticosteroids, calcipotriene ointment, and tazarotene. Systemic therapy with methotrexate or cyclosporine and biologic therapy with etanercept (a tumor necrosis factor inhibitor), infliximab (a monoclonal antibody to tumor necrosis factor), alefacept (an immunomodulatory fusion protein), or efalizumab (a monoclonal antibody to CD11a) may be required for severe cases. Toxic effects of these drugs include cirrhosis, renal failure, hypertension, and pneumonitis.

B. Management of Anesthesia. Management includes evaluation of the drugs being used for the treatment of psoriasis, including topical corticosteroids and chemotherapeutic drugs. Patients with psoriasis often have a marked increase in skin blood flow that can contribute to altered thermoregulation.

IV. MASTOCYTOSIS

Mastocytosis is a rare disorder of mast cell proliferation that can occur in a cutaneous form (urticaria pigmentosa) or in a systemic form.

A. Signs and Symptoms. Signs reflect degranulation of mast cells with anaphylactoid responses characterized by pruritus, urticaria, and flushing. These changes may be accompanied by hypotension (sometimes life-threatening) and tachycardia. H_1-receptor and H_2-receptor antagonists are not always protective, and the incidence of bronchospasm is low. Bleeding is unusual in these patients even though mast cells contain heparin.

B. Management of Anesthesia. Although anesthesia is usually uneventful, there are reports of life-threatening anaphylactoid reactions with even minor surgical procedures (epinephrine should be immediately available). Preoperative administration of H_1- and H_2-receptor antagonists may be considered. Monitoring serum tryptase concentration during the perioperative period may be useful for detecting the occurrence of mast cell degranulation.

V. ATOPIC DERMATITIS

Atopic dermatitis is the cutaneous manifestation of the atopic state (dry, scaly, eczematous, pruritic patches on the face, neck, and flexor surfaces of the arms and legs). Pruritus is the

TABLE 21-2 ■ **Features of Common Types of Chronic Urticaria**

TYPE OF URTICARIA	AGE RANGE (yr)	CLINICAL FEATURES	ANGIOEDEMA	DIAGNOSTIC TEST
Chronic idiopathic	20-50	Pink or pale edematous papules or wheals; wheals often annular; pruritus	Yes	
Symptomatic dermatographism	20-50	Linear wheals with a surrounding bright-red flare at sites of stimulation; pruritus	No	Light stroking of skin causes wheal.
Physical urticarias				
Cold	10-40	Pale or red swelling at sites of contact with cold surfaces or fluids; pruritus	Yes	Application of ice pack causes a wheal within 5 min of removing the ice (cold stimulation test).
Pressure	20-50	Swelling at sites of pressure (soles, palms, waist) lasting ≥2-24 hr; painful; pruritus	No	Application of pressure perpendicular to skin produces persistent red swelling after a latent period of 1-4 hr.
Solar	20-50	Pale or red swelling at site of exposure to ultraviolet or visible light; pruritus	Yes	Radiation by a solar simulator for 30-120 sec causes wheals in 30 min.
Cholinergic	10-50	Monomorphic pale or pink wheals on trunk, neck, and limbs; pruritus	Yes	Exercise or hot shower elicits wheals.

primary symptom. Systemic antihistamines and corticosteroids are effective. Pulmonary manifestations of the atopic state (asthma, hay fever, otitis media, sinusitis) affect anesthetic management.

VI. URTICARIA

Urticaria may be characterized as acute urticaria, chronic urticaria, or physical urticaria (Table 21-2). Anesthesia management is avoidance of triggering drugs and events, H_1- and H_2-receptor antagonists and corticosteroids when appropriate, and, in the case of cold urticaria, warming intravenous (IV) fluids and IV injectable agents and increasing the ambient temperature in the operating room.

TABLE 21-3 ■ **Signs and Symptoms of Scleroderma**

Skin and musculoskeletal	Contractures (fingers, mouth) Proximal muscular weakness
Nervous system	Nerve compression by thickened connective tissue Trigeminal neuralgia Keratoconjunctivitis sicca
Cardiovascular system	Dysrhythmias Conduction abnormalities Congestive heart failure Peripheral vasospasm (Raynaud's phenomenon)
Lungs	Pulmonary fibrosis Pulmonary hypertension Cor pulmonale Arterial hypoxemia
Kidneys	Renal artery stenosis Accelerated systemic hypertension
Gastrointestinal	Dysphagia Xerostomia Hypomotility Reflux

VII. ERYTHEMA MULTIFORME

Erythema multiforme is a recurrent disease of the skin and mucous membranes characterized by lesions ranging from edematous macules and papules to vesicular or bullous lesions that may ulcerate.

A. Stevens-Johnson Syndrome. Erythema multiforme major (Stevens-Johnson syndrome) is a severe manifestation associated with multisystem dysfunction (fever, tachycardia, tachypnea). Drugs associated with the onset of this syndrome include antibiotics, analgesics, and certain over-the-counter medications. Corticosteroids are used in the management of severe cases. Anesthetic considerations are similar to those encountered in anesthetizing patients with EB.

VIII. SCLERODERMA

Scleroderma (systemic sclerosis) is characterized by inflammation, vascular sclerosis, and fibrosis of the skin and viscera. In some patients, the disease evolves into the CREST syndrome (*c*alcinosis, *R*aynaud's phenomenon, *e*sophageal hypomotility, *s*clerodactyly, *t*elangiectasia). Prognosis is poor and related to the extent of visceral involvement. No drugs or treatments have proved safe and effective in changing the course of the disease.

A. Signs and Symptoms (Table 21-3)

B. Anesthesia Considerations. Difficult intubation, difficult IV access, intravascular volume depletion due to chronic hypertension, and regurgitation and pulmonary aspiration are possible. Patients are sensitive to the respiratory depressant effects of opioids, and postoperative ventilatory support may be required in patients with severe pulmonary disease. Renal dysfunction affects the selection of anesthetic drugs. Measures to minimize peripheral vasoconstriction include maintenance of the operating room temperature at more than 21° C and administration of warmed IV fluids. The eyes should be protected to prevent corneal abrasions.

TABLE 21-4 ■ Anesthesia Considerations in Ehlers-Danlos Syndrome

- Avoid intramuscular injections or instrumentation of the nose or esophagus (bleeding propensity).
- Hematoma formation may be excessive at instrumentations sites.
- Extravasation of intravenous fluids may go undetected because of skin laxity.
- Maintain low airway pressures during positive pressure ventilation to avoid pneumothorax.
- Regional anesthesia should be avoided.
- Surgical complications are bleeding and wound dehiscence.

IX. PSEUDOXANTHOMA ELASTICUM

Pseudoxanthoma elasticum is a rare hereditary disorder of elastic tissue (degeneration and calcification) leading to loss of visual acuity, gastrointestinal hemorrhage, systemic hypertension, and ischemic heart disease.

A. Management of Anesthesia. Management is based on an appreciation of the abnormalities associated with this disease. Cardiovascular derangements are probably the most important considerations. There are no specific recommendations regarding the choice of anesthetic drugs or techniques.

X. EHLERS-DANLOS SYNDROME

Ehlers-Danlos syndrome consists of a group of inherited connective tissue disorders caused by abnormal production of procollagen and collagen. The only form of this syndrome associated with an increased risk of death is type IV (vascular). This form may be complicated by rupture of large blood vessels or disruption of the bowel.

A. Signs and Symptoms. Joint hypermobility, skin fragility or hyperelasticity, bruising and scarring, musculoskeletal discomfort, and susceptibility to osteoarthritis are signs. The gastrointestinal tract, uterus, and vasculature have a lot of type III collagen, accounting for such complications as spontaneous rupture of the bowel, uterus, or major arteries. Dilation of the trachea is often present, and the risk of pneumothorax is increased. Patients may exhibit extensive ecchymoses with minimal trauma, although a specific coagulation defect has not been identified.

B. Management of Anesthesia (Table 21-4)

XI. MARFAN'S SYNDROME

Marfan's syndrome, an autosomal dominant connective tissue disorder, is associated with skeletal abnormalities (high-arched palate, pectus excavatum, kyphoscoliosis, hyperextensibility of the joints), ocular changes (lens dislocation, myopia, retinal detachment), and cardiovascular abnormalities (aortic dilation, dissection, or rupture; mitral valve prolapse; heightened risk of endocarditis; cardiac conduction abnormalities).

A. Management of Anesthesia. Preoperative evaluation concentrates on cardiopulmonary abnormalities. It is prudent to avoid any sustained increase in systemic blood pressure to help avoid the risk of aortic dissection.

XII. MUSCULAR AND SKELETAL DISEASES

A. Polymyositis and Dermatomyositis Polymyositis and dermatomyositis are multisystem diseases of unknown cause that manifest as inflammatory myopathies. Dermatomyositis causes characteristic skin changes (upper lid discoloration, periorbital edema, malar rash, atrophic changes over extensor surfaces of joints) in addition to muscle weakness.

TABLE 21-5 ■ Signs and Symptoms of Polymyositis

- Proximal skeletal muscle weakness (neck, shoulders, hips); difficulty climbing stairs
- Dysphagia and aspiration (paresis of pharyngeal muscles)
- Ventilatory insufficiency (paresis of respiratory muscles)
- Increased serum creatine kinase
- Heart block
- Left ventricular dysfunction
- Myocarditis
- Associated with systemic lupus erythematosus, scleroderma, rheumatoid arthritis

TABLE 21-6 ■ Anesthetic Considerations in Pseudohypertrophic Muscular Dystrophy

Patient is at increased risk of aspiration (weak laryngeal reflexes, gastrointestinal hypomotility).
Succinylcholine is contraindicated (rhabdomyolysis, hyperkalemia, cardiac arrest).
Response to nondepolarizing muscles relaxants is prolonged.
Volatile agents may be associated with rhabdomyolysis.
Increased incidence of malignant hyperthermia is seen (dantrolene should be available).
Regional anesthesia is acceptable.
Monitors should be used to detect malignant hyperthermia and cardiac dysfunction.
Anticipate postoperative pulmonary dysfunction.

1. **Signs and Symptoms** (Table 21-5)
2. **Diagnosis.** When proximal skeletal muscle weakness, an increased serum creatine kinase concentration, and a characteristic skin rash are present, diagnosis is considered.
3. **Treatment.** Usually treatment is corticosteroids. Immunosuppressive therapy (methotrexate, azathioprine, cyclophosphamide, mycophenolate, cyclosporine) may be effective. IV immunoglobulin may be useful in refractory cases.
4. **Management of Anesthesia.** The vulnerability of patients with polymyositis to pulmonary aspiration must be considered. Responses to nondepolarizing muscle relaxants and succinylcholine are normal.

B. Muscular Dystrophy Muscular dystrophy is a group of hereditary diseases characterized by painless degeneration and atrophy of skeletal muscles.

1. **Pseudohypertrophic Muscular Dystrophy (Duchenne's Muscular Dystrophy).** This is the most common and severe form of childhood progressive muscular dystrophy. The disease is caused by an X-linked recessive gene and becomes apparent in 2- to 5-year-old boys (waddling gait, frequent falling, difficulty climbing stairs). Serum creatine kinase concentrations are 20 to 100 times normal.
   a. ***Cardiopulmonary Dysfunction.*** Degeneration of cardiac muscle invariably accompanies this muscular dystrophy. Characteristic electrocardiographic changes are tall R waves in V_1, deep Q waves in the limb leads, a short PR interval, and sinus tachycardia. Chronic weakness of the respiratory muscles and a decreased ability to cough result in loss of pulmonary reserve and accumulation of secretions.
   b. ***Management of Anesthesia*** *(Table 21-6)*
2. **Limb-Girdle Muscular Dystrophy.** This is a slowly progressive but relatively benign disease with only shoulder or hip muscles involved.
3. **Facioscapulohumeral Muscular Dystrophy.** This condition is characterized by a slowly progressive wasting of facial, pectoral, and shoulder girdle muscles that begins during

TABLE 21-7 ■ Signs and Symptoms of Myotonia Dystrophy

Facial muscle weakness (expressionless facies)
Ptosis
Dysarthria
Dysphagia, slowed gastric emptying, pulmonary aspiration
Inability to relax hand grip
Mental retardation
Endocrine dysfunction (gonadal atrophy, diabetes mellitus, hypothyroidism, adrenal insufficiency)
Central sleep apnea
Cardiomyopathy (dysrhythmias, cardiac conduction abnormalities)

adolescence. There is no involvement of cardiac muscle, and serum creatine kinase concentration is seldom increased.

4. **Nemaline Rod Muscular Dystrophy.** This is an autosomal dominant disease characterized by slowly progressive or nonprogressive symmetric dystrophy of skeletal and smooth muscle. Micrognathia and dental malocclusion are common. Restrictive lung disease may result from the myopathy and/or scoliosis. Cardiac failure resulting from dilated cardiomyopathy has been described.
   a. ***Anesthesia Considerations.*** Included are possible difficult intubation, exaggerated respiratory depression, regurgitation risk (bulbar palsy), unpredictable response to muscle relaxants (succinylcholine appears safe), and myocardial depression.
5. **Oculopharyngeal Dystrophy.** This is a rare variant of muscular dystrophy characterized by progressive dysphagia and ptosis. These patients may be at risk of aspiration during the perioperative period, and their sensitivity to muscle relaxants may be increased.
6. **Emery-Dreifuss Muscular Dystrophy.** An X-linked recessive disorder, this condition is characterized by development of skeletal muscle contractures that precede the onset of skeletal muscle weakness. Cardiac involvement may be life-threatening and may manifest as congestive heart failure, thromboembolism, or bradycardia. In contrast to the other muscular dystrophies, female carriers of this disorder may have cardiac impairment.

C. **Myotonic Dystrophy** Myotonic dystrophy comprises a group of hereditary degenerative diseases of skeletal muscle characterized by persistent contracture (myotonia) after voluntary contraction of a muscle or following electrical stimulation. Peripheral nerves and the neuromuscular junction are not affected.

1. **Myotonia Dystrophica.** This is the most common and most serious form of myotonic dystrophy affecting adults. Death from pneumonia or heart failure often occurs by the sixth decade of life. Treatment is symptomatic and may include use of phenytoin.
   a. ***Signs and Symptoms*** *(Table 21-7)*
   b. ***Management of Anesthesia*** *(Table 21-8)*
2. **Myotonia Congenita.** Myotonia congenita does not involve other organ systems, does not progress, and does not result in a decreased life expectancy. Patients respond to phenytoin, mexiletine, or quinine therapy. The response to succinylcholine administration is abnormal.
3. **Paramyotonia Congenita.** This condition is characterized by generalized myotonia that is exacerbated by exercise and cold. Treatment is similar to that of myotonia congenita.
4. **Schwartz-Jampel Syndrome.** A rare childhood disorder, Schwartz-Jampel syndrome is associated with progressive skeletal muscle stiffness; myotonia; and ocular, facial, and skeletal abnormalities, including micrognathia. Tracheal intubation is predictably difficult. These children may be susceptible to malignant hyperthermia.

TABLE 21-8 ■ Anesthesia Considerations in Patients with Myotonia Dystrophica

Exaggerated myocardial depression can be produced by volatile agents.
Succinylcholine produces prolonged muscle contraction.
Response to nondepolarizing muscle relaxants is normal.
Reversal of neuromuscular blockade does not usually cause muscle contraction.
Sensitive to respiratory-depressant drugs.
Postoperative shivering may induce myotonia.

TABLE 21-9 ■ Clinical Features of Familial Periodic Paralysis

TYPE	SERUM POTASSIUM CONCENTRATION DURING SYMPTOMS (mEq/L)	PRECIPITATING FACTORS	OTHER FEATURES
Hypokalemic	<3.0	Large carbohydrate meal, strenuous exercise, glucose infusion, stress, menstruation, pregnancy, anesthesia, hypothermia	Cardiac dysrhythmias Electrocardiographic signs of hypokalemia
Hyperkalemic	>5.5	Exercise, potassium infusion, metabolic acidosis, hypothermia	Skeletal muscle weakness may be localized to tongue and eyelids

D. **Periodic Paralysis** Periodic paralysis is a spectrum of diseases characterized by intermittent acute attacks of skeletal muscle weakness or paralysis associated with hypokalemia or hyperkalemia (Table 21-9). Muscle strength is normal between attacks.

1. **Management of Anesthesia.** A principal goal is avoidance of events that precipitate skeletal muscle weakness (hypothermia, electrolyte abnormalities, carbohydrate loading in hypokalemic paralysis patients). Shorter-acting neuromuscular blockers are preferable if skeletal muscle relaxation is required. Glucose-containing solutions should be avoided because of potassium shifts into cells. Succinylcholine is acceptable in patients with hypokalemic paralysis but should be avoided in patients with hyperkalemic paralysis. Perioperative potassium depletion with diuretics should be considered in patients with hyperkalemia periodic paralysis. Frequent monitoring of potassium is indicated.

E. **Myasthenia Gravis** Myasthenia gravis is a chronic autoimmune disorder caused by a decrease in functional acetylcholine receptors at the neuromuscular junction because of their destruction or inactivation by circulating antibodies. The hallmarks of the disease are weakness and rapid exhaustion of voluntary muscle strength with repetitive use followed by partial recovery with rest. Skeletal muscles innervated by cranial nerves (ocular, pharyngeal, and laryngeal muscles) are especially vulnerable, as reflected by the appearance of ptosis, diplopia, and dysphagia, often the initial symptoms of the disease. Other conditions that cause weakness of the cranial and somatic musculature must be considered in the differential diagnosis of myasthenia gravis (Table 21-10).

1. **Classification** (Table 21-11)
2. **Signs and Symptoms** (Table 21-12)
3. **Treatment** (Table 21-13)
4. **Management of Anesthesia** (Table 21-14)

TABLE 21-10 ■ Differential Diagnosis of Myasthenia Gravis

CONDITION	SYMPTOMS AND CHARACTERISTICS	COMMENTS
Congenital myasthenic syndromes	Rare, early onset, not autoimmune	Electrophysiologic and immunocytochemical tests required for diagnosis
Drug-induced myasthenia gravis		
Penicillamine	Triggers autoimmune myasthenia gravis	Recovery within weeks of discontinuing the drug
Nondepolarizing muscle relaxants	Increased sensitivity to their effects	Recovery after drug discontinuation
Aminoglycosides		
Procainamide		
Eaton-Lambert syndrome	Small cell lung cancer, fatigue	Incremental response on repetitive nerve stimulation, antibodies to calcium channels
Hyperthyroidism	Exacerbation of myasthenia gravis	Thyroid function abnormal
Graves's disease	Diplopia, exophthalmos	Thyroid-stimulating immunoglobulin present
Botulism	Generalized weakness, ophthalmoplegia	Incremental response on repetitive nerve stimulation, mydriasis
Progressive external ophthalmoplegia	Ptosis, diplopia, generalized weakness in some cases	Mitochondrial abnormalities
Intracranial mass compressing cranial nerves	Ophthalmoplegia, cranial nerve weakness	Abnormalities on computed tomography or magnetic resonance imaging

Adapted from Drachman DB. Myasthenia gravis. *N Engl J Med*. 1994;330:1797-1810.

TABLE 21-11 ■ Classification of Myasthenia Gravis

Type I	Limited to extraocular muscles
Type IIa	Slowly progressive, spares muscles of respiration; response to anticholinesterase therapy is good
Type IIb	Severe, rapidly progressive, may involve muscles of respiration, response to anticholinesterase therapy may not be good
Type III	Abrupt onset, rapid deterioration (within 6 months), high mortality rate
Type IV	Severe muscle weakness resulting from progression of type I or type II disease

TABLE 21-12 ■ Signs and Symptoms of Myasthenia Gravis

Ptosis and diplopia (most common initial complaints)
Dysphagia, dysarthria, drooling
Asymmetric skeletal muscle weakness with exercise
Lack of muscle atrophy
Myocarditis (cardiomyopathy, atrial fibrillation, heart block)
Hyperthyroidism (in 10% of patients)
Occasionally isolated respiratory failure
Associated rheumatologic disease (rheumatoid arthritis, systemic lupus erythematosus, pernicious anemia)
Muscle weakness may be aggravated by aminoglycoside antibiotics

TABLE 21-13 ■ Treatment of Myasthenia Gravis

Anticholinesterase drugs	Pyridostigmine 60 mg PO (onset of effect in 30 min; peak effect in 2 hr). Treatment effects may wane after weeks or months of therapy.
Thymectomy	Induces remission or decreases doses of immunosuppressive drugs required. If vital capacity <2 L, preoperative plasmapheresis may help improve likelihood of adequate spontaneous ventilation postoperatively. Full benefit of thymectomy make take months to occur.
Immunosuppressive therapy	Corticosteroids, azathioprine, cyclosporine, mycophenolate. Used when muscle weakness not adequately controlled by anticholinesterase drugs.
Short-term immunotherapy	Plasmapheresis (removes antibodies, benefit is transient). Immunoglobulin.

PO, Orally.

TABLE 21-14 ■ Anesthesia Management in Patients with Myasthenia Gravis

Preoperative	Avoid opioids.
Muscle relaxants	Increased sensitivity to nondepolarizing muscle relaxants. Initial dose should be titrated to response according to peripheral nerve stimulator. Patients may be resistant to succinylcholine.
Induction	Use short-acting intravenous drugs. Consider intubation without muscle relaxants.
Maintenance	Administer nitrous oxide plus volatile agents (decreases dose of muscle relaxants needed). Short- or intermediate-acting muscle relaxants are used; decrease initial dose by half to two thirds.
Postoperative	May require postoperative ventilation (higher risk with disease duration >6 years, presence of COPD, daily dose of pyridostigmine >750 mg, vital capacity <2.9 L).

COPD, Chronic obstructive pulmonary disease.

TABLE 21-15 ■ Comparison of Myasthenic Syndrome and Myasthenia Gravis

PARAMETER	MYASTHENIC SYNDROME	MYASTHENIA GRAVIS
Manifestations	Proximal limb weakness (legs more than arms), exercise improves strength, muscle pain common, reflexes absent or decreased	Extraocular, bulbar, and facial muscle weakness, fatigue with exercise; muscle pain uncommon; reflexes normal
Gender	Males more often than females	Females more often than males
Co-existing pathology	Small cell lung cancer	Thymoma
Response to muscle relaxants	Sensitive to succinylcholine and nondepolarizing muscle relaxants Poor response to anticholinesterases	Resistant to succinylcholine, sensitive to nondepolarizing muscle relaxants Good response to anticholinesterases

F. **Myasthenic Syndrome (Eaton-Lambert Syndrome)** Myasthenic syndrome is a disorder of neuromuscular transmission that resembles myasthenia gravis (Table 21-15). This syndrome has been described in patients with small cell carcinoma of the lung, as well as in patients without cancer. Myasthenic syndrome is an acquired autoimmune disease with IgG antibodies to voltage-sensitive calcium channels that cause a deficiency of these channels at the motor nerve terminal. Anticholinesterase drugs are not effective therapy in patients with myasthenic syndrome. Patients are sensitive to both depolarizing and nondepolarizing muscle relaxants.

G. **Osteoarthritis** Osteoarthritis is a degenerative process that affects articular cartilage and involves minimal inflammatory reaction in joints, especially the knees, hips, and spine. Degenerative changes are most significant in the mid to lower cervical spine and in the lower lumbar area.

1. **Treatment.** Physical therapy and exercise programs are used to maintain muscle function. Pain relief can also be achieved by application of heat, simple analgesics such as acetaminophen, and antiinflammatory drugs (NSAIDs). Systemic corticosteroids have *no* place in the treatment of osteoarthritis. Joint replacement surgery may be recommended when pain from osteoarthritis is persistent and disabling or significant limitation of joint function is present.

H. **Kyphoscoliosis** Kyphoscoliosis is a spinal deformity characterized by anterior flexion (kyphosis) and lateral curvature (scoliosis) of the vertebral column.

1. **Signs and Symptoms.** Restrictive lung disease and pulmonary hypertension progressing to cor pulmonale are associated with kyphoscoliosis with a spinal curvature greater than 40 degrees.
2. **Management of Anesthesia.** Pulmonary function tests reflect the magnitude of restrictive lung disease. Arterial blood gases are helpful for detecting unrecognized hypoxemia or acidosis that could cause pulmonary hypertension. No specific anesthetic drug or drug combination can be recommended as optimal for patients with kyphoscoliosis. Nitrous oxide may increase pulmonary vascular resistance. Controlled hypotension may be used to help minimize intraoperative blood loss during extensive spine surgery. A "wake-up test" or monitoring of somatosensory and/or motor evoked potentials is often employed to detect spinal cord compression or ischemia that can occur during spine straightening surgery, and these may influence the choice of anesthetic agents (total IV anesthesia is a common choice). Postoperative mechanical ventilation may be necessary in some patients with severe kyphoscoliosis.

I. **Back Pain** Low back pain is the most common musculoskeletal complaint requiring medical attention (Table 21-16).

TABLE 21-16 ■ Causes of Low Back Pain

MECHANICAL LOW BACK OR LEG PAIN (97%)
Idiopathic low back pain (lumbar sprain or strain) (70%)
Degenerative processes of discs and facets (age-related) (10%)
Herniated disc (4%)
Spinal stenosis (3%)
Osteoporotic compression fractures (4%)
Spondylolisthesis (2%)
Traumatic fracture (<1%)
Congenital disease (<1%)
Severe kyphosis
Severe scoliosis
Spondylolysis
NONMECHANICAL SPINAL CONDITIONS (1%)
Cancer (0.7%)
Multiple myeloma
Metastatic cancer
Lymphoma and leukemia
Spinal cord tumors
Retroperitoneal tumors
Primary vertebral tumors
Infection (0.01%)
Osteomyelitis
Paraspinal abscess
Epidural abscess
Inflammatory arthritis
Ankylosing spondylitis
Psoriatic spondylitis
Reiter's syndrome
Inflammatory bowel disease
VISCERAL DISEASE (2%)
Disease of pelvic organs
Prostatitis
Endometriosis
Pelvic inflammatory disease
Renal disease
Nephrolithiasis
Pyelonephritis
Perinephric abscess
Aortic aneurysm
Gastrointestinal disease
Pancreatitis
Cholecystitis
Penetrating ulcer

Percentages indicate the estimated incidence of these conditions in adult patients.
Adapted from Deyo RO, Weinstein JN. Low back pain. *N Engl J Med.* 2001;344:363-370.

TABLE 21-17 ■ **Comparison of Rheumatoid Arthritis and Ankylosing Spondylitis**

PARAMETER	RHEUMATOID ARTHRITIS	ANKYLOSING SPONDYLITIS
Family history	Rare	Common
Gender	Female (30-50 years old)	Male (20-30 years old)
Joint involvement	Symmetric polyarthropathy	Asymmetric oligoarthropathy
Sacroiliac involvement	No	Yes
Vertebral involvement	Cervical	Total (ascending)
Cardiac changes	Pericardial effusion, aortic regurgitation, cardiac conduction abnormalities, cardiac valve fibrosis, coronary artery arteritis	Cardiomegaly, aortic regurgitation, cardiac conduction abnormalities
Pulmonary changes	Pulmonary fibrosis, pleural effusion	Pulmonary fibrosis
Eyes	Keratoconjunctivitis sicca	Conjunctivitis, uveitis
Rheumatoid factor	Positive	Negative
HLA-B27	Negative	Positive

1. **Acute Low Back Pain.** Pain improves within 30 days in 90% of patients. NSAIDs are often effective for analgesia for acute back pain. Pain arising from inflammation initiated by mechanical or chemical insult to a nerve root may be responsive to epidural administration of corticosteroids. A herniated disc should be considered in patients with radiculopathy (L4-5, L5-S1) that is suggested by pain radiating down a leg or by symptoms reproduced by straight leg raising. Surgical intervention is indicated in patients with persistent radiculopathy or neurologic deficits.
2. **Lumbar Spinal Stenosis.** Lumbar spinal stenosis is narrowing of the spinal canal or its lateral recesses because of hypertrophic degenerative changes in spinal structures, most often in elderly patients with chronic back pain and sciatica. The diagnosis is confirmed by magnetic resonance imaging or myelography. Surgical decompression and fusion are needed for those with progressive functional deterioration.

J. **Rheumatoid Arthritis** Rheumatoid arthritis, the most common chronic inflammatory arthritis, affects approximately 1% of adults (women more often than men) and is characterized by morning stiffness, symmetric polyarthropathy, and significant systemic involvement (Table 21-17). Involvement of the proximal interphalangeal and metacarpophalangeal joints of the hands and feet distinguish rheumatoid arthritis from osteoarthritis (which typically affects weight-bearing joints and distal interphalangeal joints). The course of the disease is characterized by exacerbations and remissions.

1. **Signs and Symptoms**
   a. ***Joint Involvement.*** Joints of the hands, wrists, knees, and feet are symmetrically affected. Temporomandibular joint involvement can produce marked limitation of mandibular motion. Cervical spine involvement may include atlantoaxial subluxation and consequent separation of the atlanto-odontoid articulation. Cricoarytenoid arthritis with hoarseness is common.
   b. ***Systemic Involvement.*** In the cardiovascular system, rheumatoid arthritis may manifest as pericarditis, myocarditis, coronary artery arteritis, accelerated coronary atherosclerosis, cardiac valve fibrosis, and formation of rheumatoid nodules in the cardiac conduction

system. Patients may demonstrate a neuropathy (mononeuritis multiplex), skin ulcerations, and purpura. Pulmonary manifestations include pleural effusion, pulmonary nodules, and pulmonary fibrosis. Costochondral involvement may produce restrictive lung changes with decreased lung volumes and vital capacity. Anemia and dry eyes and dry mouth *(Sjögren's syndrome)* are also seen. Mild abnormalities of liver function can occur, and renal dysfunction may result from amyloidosis, vasculitis, or drug therapy.

c. ***Treatment.*** Goals are relief of pain, preservation of joint function and strength, prevention of deformities, and attenuation of systemic complications. Drug therapy is used to provide analgesia, control inflammation, and produce immunosuppression.

   i. ***Nonsteroidal Antiinflammatory Drugs.*** NSAIDs including aspirin are important for symptomatic relief of rheumatoid arthritis but have little role in changing the underlying disease process.

   ii. ***Corticosteroids.*** The use of corticosteroids decreases joint swelling, pain, and morning stiffness but is often associated with significant long-term side effects (osteoporosis, osteonecrosis, increased susceptibility to infection, myopathy, hyperglycemia, poor wound healing).

   iii. ***Disease-Modifying Antirheumatic Drugs (DMARDs).*** DMARDs include methotrexate, sulfasalazine, leflunomide, antimalarials, D-penicillamine, azathioprine, and minocycline. These drugs generally take 2 to 6 months to achieve their effects. Cytokines play a central role in the pathogenesis of rheumatoid arthritis. Drugs such as infliximab (Remicade) and etanercept (Enbrel), which are tumor necrosis factor inhibitors, are effective therapies, although long-term toxicities such as infection (tuberculosis) and demyelinating syndromes are a concern. Anakinra, an interleukin-1 receptor antagonist, is effective but has a slower onset of action. Gold is extremely effective therapy but is not commonly used because of its toxicities.

   iv. ***Surgery.*** Indications for surgery include intractable pain, impairment of joint function, or the need for joint stabilization.

d. ***Management of Anesthesia.*** Compromise of the airway may occur at the cervical spine, temporomandibular joints, and cricoarytenoid joints. Atlantoaxial subluxation (confirmed by radiographic examination) may predispose to cervical cord compression with neck motion. Awake, sedated endotracheal intubation by fiberoptic laryngoscopy may be indicated if preoperative evaluation suggests that direct visualization of the glottic opening will be difficult. Postoperative ventilatory support might be needed in patients with rheumatoid pulmonary involvement. The effect of aspirin or NSAIDs on platelet function must be considered. Corticosteroid supplementation may be indicated in patients undergoing long-term treatment with these drugs. Postextubation laryngeal obstruction may occur in patients with cricoarytenoid arthritis.

K. **Systemic Lupus Erythematosus** (Table 21-18) Systemic lupus erythematosus (SLE) is a multisystem chronic inflammatory disease, usually of young women, characterized by antinuclear antibody production (95% of SLE patients). SLE can be drug induced or naturally occurring. The natural history of SLE is highly variable, but the presence of nephritis and hypertension is associated with a worse prognosis. Pregnancy, especially in patients with nephritis and hypertension, is associated with a substantial risk of disease exacerbation and poor fetal outcome. Corticosteroids are the principal treatment for severe manifestations of lupus. Anesthesia management is dictated by the magnitude of organ dysfunction and drugs used in treatment.

L. **Spondyloarthropathies** Spondyloarthropathies are a group of nonrheumatic arthropathies that include ankylosing spondylitis, reactive arthritis (Reiter's syndrome), juvenile chronic polyarthropathy, psoriatic arthritis, and enteropathic arthritis. These diseases are characterized by involvement of the spine and absence of rheumatoid nodules or detectable circulating rheumatoid factor (see Table 21-17). There are predilections for new bone formation (joint ankylosis) and ocular inflammation.

TABLE 21-18 ■ Manifestations of Systemic Lupus Erythematosus

Dermatitis, malar rash
Symmetric arthritis
Pericarditis, myocarditis, heart failure
Pleuritis, restrictive lung disease
Nephritis, hypertension, hematuria
Abnormal liver function tests (30% of patients)
Cognitive dysfunction, psychologic changes, cerebritis
Antiphospholipid antibodies
Myopathy
Hematologic: anemia, hemolytic anemia, thrombocytopenia, leukopenia, functional asplenia, and thromboembolism, are all reported

1. **Ankylosing Spondylitis.** Ankylosing spondylitis is a chronic, usually progressive, inflammatory disease involving the articulations of the spine and adjacent soft tissues. Cardiomegaly, aortic regurgitation, cardiac conduction abnormalities, pulmonary fibrosis, and unilateral uveitis may be present.
   a. ***Treatment.*** Treatment consists of exercises designed to maintain joint mobility and posture plus antiinflammatory drugs (indomethacin, diclofenac). Topical corticosteroid eye drops are used to treat uveitis.
   b. ***Management of Anesthesia.*** Awake fiberoptic tracheal intubation may be needed because of cervical spine disease. Restrictive lung disease from costochondral rigidity and flexion deformity of the thoracic spine must be appreciated. Sudden or excessive increases in systemic vascular resistance are poorly tolerated if significant aortic regurgitation is present. Neurologic monitoring is a consideration for patients undergoing corrective spinal surgery. Regional anesthesia is acceptable but may be technically difficult because of limited joint mobility and closed interspinous spaces.
   c. ***Reactive Arthritis.*** This is an *aseptic* arthritis that occurs after an extraarticular infection, especially infection with *Chlamydia, Salmonella,* and *Shigella* species. Management consists of antibiotic treatment for the initial infection and NSAIDs or sulfasalazine for symptomatic relief of the arthritis.
   d. ***Juvenile Chronic Polyarthropathy.*** Juvenile chronic polyarthropathy is similar to adult rheumatoid arthritis. An acute form of polyarthritis (fever, rash, lymphadenopathy, splenomegaly in young children who are negative for rheumatoid factor and HLA-B27) is designated *Still's disease.*
   e. ***Enteropathic Arthritis.*** This is an inflammatory polyarthritis, most often involving the large joints of the lower extremities that may develop in patients with Crohn's disease or ulcerative colitis.

M. **Paget's Disease** Paget's disease of bone is characterized by excessive osteoblastic and osteoclastic activity, resulting in abnormally thick but weak bones. Bone pain is the most common symptom.
   1. **Complications.** Complications involve bones (fractures and neoplastic degeneration), joints (arthritis), and the nervous system (nerve compression, paraplegia). Hypercalcemia and renal calculi may also occur.
   2. **Treatment.** Paget's disease treatment is calcitonin and bisphosphonates.

N. **Dwarfism** Dwarfism can occur in two forms: *proportionate dwarfism,* in which the limbs, trunk, and head size are in the same relative proportions as a normal adult, and *disproportionate dwarfism,* in which the limbs, trunk, and head size are not in the usual proportions of a normal adult.

1. **Achondroplasia.** The most common cause of disproportionate dwarfism, achondroplasia occurs more often in females. The anticipated height of achondroplastic males is 132 cm (52 inches) and of females is 122 cm (48 inches). Premature fusion of the bones at the base of the skull may result in a stenotic foramen magnum. There may also be functional fusion of the atlantooccipital joint, atlantoaxial instability, and severe cervical kyphosis.
   a. ***Central Sleep Apnea.*** In achondroplastic dwarfs, central sleep apnea may be a result of brainstem compression caused by foramen magnum stenosis. Pulmonary hypertension leading to cor pulmonale is the most common cardiovascular disturbance that develops in dwarfs.
   b. ***Management of Anesthesia.*** Management is influenced by potential airway difficulties, cervical spine instability, the potential for spinal cord trauma with neck extension, and sleep apnea. Hyperextension of the neck during direct laryngoscopy should be avoided. Weight rather than age is the best guide for selecting the proper-size endotracheal tube. IV access may be technically difficult. Regional anesthesia might be considered for cesarean section but may be technically difficult because of kyphoscoliosis and a narrow epidural space and spinal canal.
2. **Russell-Silver Syndrome.** This is a form of dwarfism characterized by intrauterine growth retardation, dysmorphic facial features (including mandibular and facial hypoplasia), limb asymmetry, congenital heart defects, and a constellation of endocrine abnormalities, including hypoglycemia, adrenocortical insufficiency, and hypogonadism.
   a. ***Management of Anesthesia.*** Preoperative evaluation should consider the serum glucose concentration, especially in neonates at risk of hypoglycemia. IV infusions containing glucose may be indicated preoperatively. Intubation may be difficult, and an endotracheal tube smaller than the predicted size may be needed.

O. **Tumoral Calcinosis** Tumoral calcinosis is a rare genetic disorder that manifests as metastatic calcifications adjacent to large joints. The principal anesthetic consideration is that involvement of the hyoid bone, hypothyroid ligament, or cervical intervertebral joints may lead to difficult intubation.

XIII. OTHER MUSCULOSKELETAL SYNDROMES

A. **Rotator Cuff Tear.** This is the most common pathologic entity involving the shoulders. As many as half of individuals older than 55 years of age have arthrographically detectable rotator cuff tears.
   1. **Treatment.** Corticosteroid injection into the subacromial space may provide symptomatic relief. Arthroscopic release or manipulation under anesthesia may be used in an attempt to restore shoulder motion.
   2. **Anesthesia Management.** Brachial plexus anesthesia via the interscalene approach with continuous infusion of local anesthetic can provide anesthesia for shoulder surgery and postoperative analgesia.

B. **Floppy Infant Syndrome.** Infants who have weak, hypotonic skeletal muscles are said to have *floppy infant syndrome.* A diminished cough reflex and difficulty swallowing predispose to aspiration, and recurrent pneumonia is common.
   1. **Management of Anesthesia.** Anesthesia, such as for skeletal muscle biopsy to confirm the diagnosis, is influenced by increased sensitivity to nondepolarizing muscle relaxants, hyperkalemia and cardiac arrest after administration of succinylcholine, and susceptibility to malignant hyperthermia.

C. **Tracheomegaly.** Tracheomegaly is characterized by marked dilation of the trachea and bronchi because of a congenital defect in elastin and smooth muscle fibers in the tracheobronchial tree or their destruction after radiotherapy.

D. **Alcoholic Myopathy.** Acute and chronic forms of proximal skeletal muscle weakness commonly occur in alcoholic patients. Distinguishing alcoholic myopathy from alcoholic neuropathy is based on proximal, rather than distal, skeletal muscle involvement, an increased serum creatine kinase concentration, myoglobinuria in acute cases, and rapid recovery after cessation of alcohol consumption.

E. **Prader-Willi Syndrome.** Prader-Willi syndrome manifests at birth as hypotonia, which may be associated with a weak cough, swallowing difficulties, and upper airway obstruction.
   1. **Anesthesia Concerns.** Concerns center on hypotonia and altered metabolism of fat and carbohydrates (hypoglycemia). Weak skeletal musculature is associated with a poor cough and an increased incidence of aspiration pneumonia. Disturbances in thermoregulation, often characterized by intraoperative hyperthermia and metabolic acidosis, occur, but a relationship to malignant hyperthermia has not been established.

F. **Prune-Belly Syndrome.** This condition is characterized by congenital agenesis of the lower central abdominal musculature and the presence of urinary tract anomalies.

G. **Mitochondrial Myopathies.** A heterogeneous group of disorders of skeletal muscle energy metabolism, mitochondrial myopathies are characterized by abnormal fatigability with sustained exercise, skeletal muscle pain, and progressive weakness.
   1. **Kearns-Sayre Syndrome.** This is a rare mitochondrial myopathy accompanied by heart block. Dilated cardiomyopathy and congestive heart failure may be present.

H. **Multicore Myopathy.** Multicore myopathy is a heterogeneous group of diseases characterized by proximal skeletal muscle weakness and musculoskeletal abnormalities (scoliosis, high-arched palate). Cardiomyopathy may accompany this myopathy. It is important to recognize the potential relationship between multicore myopathy and malignant hyperthermia.

I. **Centronuclear Myopathy.** This type of myopathy is characterized by progressive muscle weakness of extraocular, facial, neck, and limb muscles. Development of scoliosis with restrictive lung disease is an important manifestation of disease severity. Management of anesthesia is influenced by the degree of skeletal muscle weakness, the presence of restrictive lung disease, and gastroesophageal reflux. Muscle relaxants are often avoided, and a nontriggering general anesthetic technique is used.

J. **Meige Syndrome.** Meige syndrome is an idiopathic dystonic disorder that manifests as blepharospasm and oromandibular dystonia affecting middle-aged to elderly women.

K. **Spasmodic Dysphonia.** A laryngeal disorder characterized by adductor or abductor dystonic spasms of the vocal cords, spasmodic dysphonia manifests as abnormal phonation but on rare occasions is associated with respiratory distress.
   1. **Anesthesia Concerns.** The presence of laryngeal stenosis may necessitate the use of smaller-than-usual tracheal tubes. The risk of pulmonary aspiration may be increased by vocal cord dysfunction caused by therapeutic interventions such as botulinum toxin injection or interruption of the recurrent laryngeal nerve.

L. **Juvenile Hyaline Fibromatosis.** This is a rare syndrome characterized by the presence of numerous dermal and subcutaneous nodules. Resistance to the effects of succinylcholine has been described in these patients.

M. **Chondrodysplasia Calcificans Punctata.** This disorder manifests as erratic cartilage calcification resulting in bone and skin lesions, cataracts, cardiac malformations, dwarfism, kyphoscoliosis, and subluxation of the hips. Tracheal stenosis can occur, which may complicate perioperative airway management.

N. **Erythromelalgia.** Erythromelalgia literally means red, painful extremities. Erythema, intense, burning pain, and increased temperature of the involved extremities are hallmarks of the disease. Neuraxial opioids and local anesthetics may provide some pain relief.

O. **Farber's Lipogranulomatosis.** Farber's lipogranulomatosis is associated with accumulation of ceramide in tissues (pleura, pericardium, synovial lining of joints, liver, spleen, lymph nodes). Progressive arthropathy, psychomotor retardation, and nutritional failure result. Difficult airway management is a common problem because of granuloma formation in the pharynx or larynx. Tracheal intubation is best avoided if possible because laryngeal edema or bleeding from the granulomas may occur.

P. **McCune-Albright Syndrome.** This syndrome consists of a triad of physical signs: osseous lesions (polyostotic fibrous dysplasia), melanotic cutaneous macules (café au lait spots), and sexual precocity (autonomous ovarian steroid secretion). Conductive and neural deafness occur along with endocrine dysfunction (hyperthyroidism, acromegaly, hypophosphatemia).

Q. **Klippel-Feil Syndrome.** Klippel-Feil syndrome is characterized by a short neck resulting from a reduced number of cervical vertebrae or fusion of several vertebrae. Movement of the neck is limited, and associated skeletal abnormalities include spinal stenosis and kyphoscoliosis.

R. **Osteogenesis Imperfecta.** An inherited disease of connective tissue, osteogenesis imperfecta affects bones, the sclera, and the inner ear. Bones are *extremely* brittle because of defective collagen production.

   1. **Anesthetic Implications** (see Table 21-19)

S. **Fibrodysplasia Ossificans.** This is a rare inherited autosomal dominant disease characterized by myositis and proliferation of connective tissue. Cervical spine involvement is common, and temporomandibular joint involvement may have implications for tracheal intubation.

T. **Deformities of the Sternum.** Pectus carinatum (outward protuberance of the sternum) and pectus excavatum (inward concavity of the sternum) produce cosmetic problems, but functional impairment is unusual. Obstructive sleep apnea is more common in young children with pectus excavatum.

U. **Macroglossia.** Macroglossia is an uncommon but potentially lethal postoperative complication that is most often associated with posterior fossa craniotomy performed in the sitting position. Possible causes are arterial compression, venous compression caused by excessive neck flexion or a head-down position, and mechanical compression of the tongue by the teeth, an oral airway, or an endotracheal tube. When the onset of macroglossia is immediate, it is easily recognized; airway obstruction does not occur because tracheal extubation is delayed. However, the development of macroglossia may be delayed for 30 minutes or longer, and there is then the risk of complete airway obstruction occurring at an unexpected time during the postoperative period.

TABLE 21-19 ■ **Anesthetic Considerations in Osteogenesis Imperfecta**
Brittle bones (cervical and mandibular fractures can occur with airway manipulation)
Defective dentition (prone to damage during tracheal intubation)
Predisposition to fractures (succinylcholine-induced fasciculations and blood pressure cuff inflations can cause fractures)
Kyphoscoliosis and pectus excavatum (decreased vital capacity, arterial hypoxemia)
Platelet dysfunction (desmopressin may be effective treatment)
Increased serum thyroxine concentration and oxygen consumption
Mild hyperthermia is not a forerunner to malignant hyperthermia

CHAPTER 22

Infectious Diseases

I. ANTIBIOTIC RESISTANCE

In recent decades infectious diseases that were presumably eradicated, such as tuberculosis, are having a resurgence, and some pathogens, such as multidrug-resistant (MDR) tuberculosis and extensively drug-resistant (XDR) tuberculosis, have resistance to previously successful antibiotic therapies. MDR organisms are responsible for an increasing number of hospital-acquired infections. Much attention is presently focused on gram-positive organisms, such as methicillin-resistant *Staphylococcus aureus* (MRSA), but there is little development of antibiotics active against resistant gram-negative bacteria.

II. SURGICAL SITE INFECTIONS

Surgical site infections (SSIs) occur at a rate of 2% to 5% for extraabdominal surgeries and up to 20% for intraabdominal surgeries. They account for 15% of all nosocomial infections.

A. **Types of Infection** (Table 22-1 and Figure 22-1)
B. **Who Is at Risk?** (Table 22-2)
C. **Signs and Symptoms.** SSIs usually manifest within 30 days of surgery with surgical site inflammation and poor healing. Fever and malaise may occur.
D. **Diagnosis** (Table 22-3)
E. **Management of Anesthesia**
   1. **Preoperative.** Elective surgery should be postponed until infection has resolved. Cessation of smoking for 4 to 8 weeks before orthopedic surgery decreases the incidence of wound-related complications. One month of preoperative abstinence from alcohol reduces postoperative morbidity in alcohol abusers. Optimization of diabetes may decrease perioperative infection. Appropriate diet and weight loss may be beneficial before major surgery. Topical mupirocin applied to the anterior nares has been successful in eliminating carriage of *S. aureus* and decreasing postoperative infections (may promote mupirocin resistance, however). Hair clipping should be used instead of shaving to remove hair from the surgical site. Preoperative skin cleaning with chlorhexidine may reduce the incidence of SSIs.
   2. **Intraoperative**
      a. ***Prophylactic Antibiotics.*** Postoperative wound infections may be prevented by prophylactic antibiotics when bacterial counts are high (e.g., in colonic or vaginal surgery) or when there is insertion of an artificial device such as a hip prosthesis or heart valve. Antibiotic prophylaxis should ideally be given within 60 minutes before incision. Prolonged surgery (longer than 4 hours) may necessitate a second dose. Prophylactic antibiotics should be discontinued within 24 hours of the procedure, except for cardiac surgery, for which they should be continued for 48 hours. A first-generation cephalosporin (cefazolin) is effective for many types of surgery. Vancomycin is indicated for MRSA. Coverage

TABLE 22-1 ■ Types of Surgical Site Infections

1. Superficial infections: skin and subcutaneous tissue
2. Deep infections: fascia and muscle organ or tissue space infection

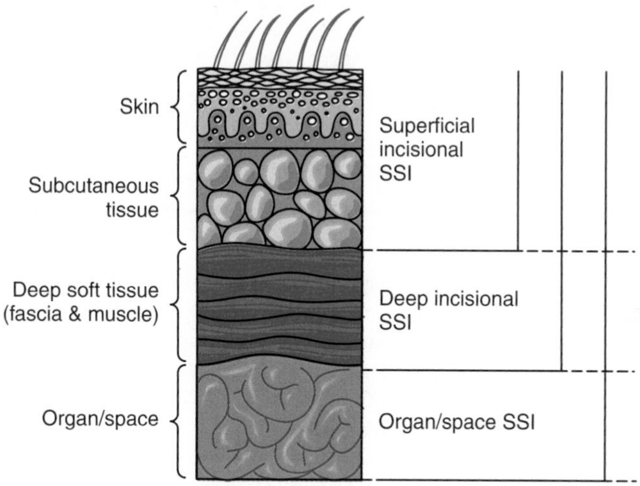

FIGURE 22-1 ■ Cross-section of abdominal wall showing the Centers for Disease Control and Prevention classification of surgical site infection (SSI). *(From Horan TC, Gaynes RP, Martone WJ, et al. CDC definitions of nosocomial surgical site infections, 1992: a modification of CDC definitions of surgical wound infections. Infect Control Hosp Epidemiol. 1992;13:606-608.)*

TABLE 22-2 ■ Risk Factors for Surgical Site Infection

PATIENT-RELATED FACTORS	MICROBIAL FACTORS	WOUND-RELATED FACTORS
Extremes of age	Enzyme production	Devitalized tissue
Poor nutritional status	Polysaccharide capsule	Dead space
American Society of Anesthesiologists (ASA) class 2 or higher	Bind to fibronectin	Hematoma
Diabetes mellitus	Biofilm and slime formation	Contamination
Smoking		Foreign material
Obesity		
Co-existing infections		
Colonization		
Immunocompromise		
Longer preoperative hospital stay		

TABLE 22-3 ■ **Diagnosis of Surgical Site Infections**

TYPE OF SSI	TIME COURSE	CRITERIA (AT LEAST ONE)
Superficial incisional SSI	Within 30 days of surgery	Superficial pus drainage Organisms from superficial tissue or fluid Signs and symptoms (pain, redness, swelling, heat)
Deep incisional SSI	Within 30 days of surgery or within 1 yr if prosthetic implant	Deep pus drainage Dehiscence or wound opened by surgeon (for fever >38° C, pain, tenderness) Abscess (e.g., radiographically diagnosed)
Organ or organ space SSI	Within 30 days of surgery or within 1 yr if prosthetic implant	Pus from a drain in the organ or organ space Organisms from aseptically obtained culture of fluid or tissue in the organ or organ space Abscess involving the organ or organ space

SSI, Surgical site infection.

for gram-negative organisms (ertapenem, cefotetan) is important during large bowel and gynecologic surgery, particularly in high-risk patients. Some patients may require specific prophylaxis to prevent subacute bacterial endocarditis, that is, those with prosthetic heart valves, congenital heart disease, previous episodes of infective endocarditis, or cardiac transplantation recipients with valvopathy.

b. *Physical and Physiologic Preventive Measures*

i. ***Oxygen.*** An inverse correlation has been demonstrated between subcutaneous tissue oxygen tension and the rate of wound infections. Tissue hypoxia increases vulnerability to infection.

ii. ***Normothermia.*** Hypothermia is associated with increased infection rates.

iii. ***Analgesia.*** Good postoperative analgesia is associated with increased oxygen tension at wound sites and decreased rates of infection.

iv. ***Carbon Dioxide.*** Mild intraoperative hypercapnia increases subcutaneous and colonic oxygen tension, which may be associated with a reduction in SSIs.

v. ***Supplemental Perioperative Fluid Administration.*** This increases tissue perfusion and tissue oxygen partial pressure, but excess fluids may be associated with increased morbidity, especially pulmonary complications.

vi. ***Glucose.*** The goal is to maintain glucose in the narrow physiologic range; increased blood sugar may inhibit leukocyte function and promotes bacterial growth. Administration of glucose, insulin, and potassium may restore immunocompetence in diabetic patients.

vii. ***Wound-Probing Protocols.*** It appears that infection of contaminated wounds can be decreased by following wound-probing protocols.

III. BLOODSTREAM INFECTION

Central venous catheters (CVCs) are the predominant cause of nosocomial bacteremia and fungemia. A mortality rate of 12% to 25% is attributable to such infections.

A. Signs and Symptoms. Signs are typically nonspecific (mental status change, hemodynamic instability, altered tolerance for nutrition, malaise), with no obvious candidate source other than an indwelling catheter. A sudden change in a patient's condition should alert the clinician to the possibility of a bloodstream infection (BSI).

B. Diagnosis. *Catheter-associated BSI* is defined as bacteremia or fungemia in a patient with an intravascular catheter and at least one positive blood culture obtained from a peripheral vein, clinical manifestations of infection, and no apparent source for the BSI except the

TABLE 22-4 ■ Most Common Pathogens Associated with Bloodstream Infections (1992-1999)

Coagulase-negative staphylococci (37%)
Staphylococcus aureus (13%)
Enterococcus (13%)
Gram-negative bacilli (14%)
· *Escherichia coli* (2%)
· *Enterobacter species* (5%)
· *Pseudomonas aeruginosa* (4%)
· *Klebsiella pneumoniae* (3%)
Candida species (8%)

From National Nosocomial Infections Surveillance (NNIS) system report, data from January 1990–May 1999, issued June 1999. *Am J Infect Control.* 1999;27(6):520-532.

catheter. The diagnosis is more compelling if, when a catheter is removed, the same organisms that grew from blood grow from the catheter tip. Table 22-4 lists some pathogens associated with BSI.

C. **Treatment.** The best treatment is prevention. The source of the infection, usually a CVC, should be removed and broad-spectrum empiric antimicrobial therapy should be initiated pending the results of cultures, at which point therapy should be appropriately targeted.

D. **Anesthesia Management**

1. **Preoperative Management.** Many CVCs are placed by anesthesiologists who are unaware of BSIs that occur days later. The subclavian and internal jugular routes carry less risk of infection than the femoral route. Hand washing, full-barrier precautions during CVC insertion, cleaning the skin with chlorhexidine, avoiding the femoral site if possible, and removing unnecessary catheters all are effective in reducing catheter-related BSIs. Sterility must be maintained when accessing catheter ports. CVCs that are coated or impregnated with antimicrobial or antiseptic agents have been associated with lower rates of BSIs.
2. **Intraoperative Management.** Blood transfusions are associated with immunosuppression and the potential for transmission of infectious agents (hepatitis virus, human immunodeficiency virus [HIV]).
   a. ***Immunosuppression.*** Immunosuppression from blood transfusion may be decreased by leukodepletion of blood products.
   b. ***Transmission of Infectious Agents.*** During early viral infection with HIV and hepatitis C virus, there is a "window period" during which circulating antibodies are not yet present but there is a significant viral count. Bacterial contamination of blood products is highest with platelet units (about 1 in 1000 to 3000 platelet units). Infectious organisms include coagulase-negative staphylococci, *S. aureus, Bacillus cereus, Serratia marcescens,* streptococci, and *Pseudomonas aeruginosa*. The prevalence of severe episodes of transfusion-associated bacterial sepsis is approximately 1 in 50,000 for units of packed platelet units and 1 in 500,000 for units of packed red blood cells. Only organisms that grow at cold temperatures, such as *Yersinia enterocolitica,* are able to grow in refrigerated blood. The best way to avoid the infectious complications of transfusion is to avoid transfusion.
3. **Postoperative Management.** Remove central lines and pulmonary artery catheters as soon as they are no longer needed. Avoid unnecessary parenteral nutrition and even dextrose-containing fluids because these may be associated with increased risk of BSI.

IV. SEPSIS

Sepsis is a spectrum of disorders, with localized inflammation at one end and a severe generalized inflammatory response with multiorgan failure at the other (Figure 22-2). Surgery and anesthesia

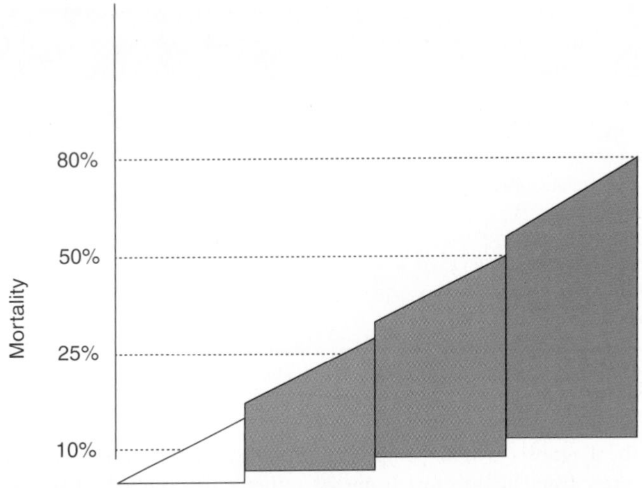

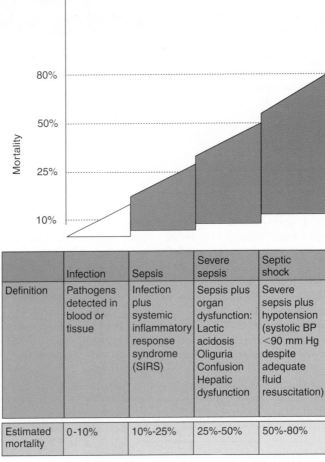

	Infection	Sepsis	Severe sepsis	Septic shock
Definition	Pathogens detected in blood or tissue	Infection plus systemic inflammatory response syndrome (SIRS)	Sepsis plus organ dysfunction: Lactic acidosis Oliguria Confusion Hepatic dysfunction	Severe sepsis plus hypotension (systolic BP <90 mm Hg despite adequate fluid resuscitation)
Estimated mortality	0-10%	10%-25%	25%-50%	50%-80%

FIGURE 22-2 ■ Continuum of sepsis with definitions and approximate mortality rates. *(Adapted from Bone RC. Toward an epidemiology and natural history of systemic inflammatory response syndrome.* JAMA. *1992;268:3452-3455.)*

TABLE 22-5 ■ Systemic Inflammatory Response Syndrome

Two or more of the following:
- White blood count >12,000/mm^3 or <4000/mm^3 or >10% immature forms
- Heart rate >90 beats/min
- Temperature >38° C or <36° C
- Respiratory rate >20 breaths/min or $Paco_2$ <32 mm Hg

should be postponed until sepsis is at least partially treated. However, sometimes the underlying cause of sepsis (abscess, endocarditis, bowel perforation, necrotizing fasciitis) requires urgent surgical intervention.

A. Signs and Symptoms. Signs of sepsis are often nonspecific. The systemic inflammatory response syndrome (Table 22-5) is an important component of sepsis. Sepsis may result in multiple organ system failure. Classically, hypotension, bounding pulses, and wide pulse pressure are present.

B. Diagnosis. Diagnosis is surmised from history, signs, and symptoms. Confirmation is based on the isolation of specific causative pathogens from blood, urine, sputum, cerebrospinal fluid (CSF), or tissue samples.

C. Treatment (Figure 22-3)

1. **Rapid Initiation of Broad Antimicrobial Coverage.** This is the initial treatment. Therapy should be tailored to the specific organism and its sensitivities. In addition to their antimicrobial spectrum, antibiotics should be chosen for their ability to penetrate various tissues, including bone, CSF, lung tissue, and abscess cavities.
2. **Supportive Treatment.** Supportive treatment relating to organ system dysfunction is essential. Support should be directed at optimizing oxygen delivery and cardiac output. Mixed venous or central venous saturation may be useful guides for therapeutic end points. Early fluid resuscitation is usually indicated. Appropriate use of inotropes and vasoconstrictors may be important (see Figure 22-3).

D. Prognosis. The prognosis depends on the virulence of the infecting pathogen(s), the stage at which appropriate treatment is initiated, the inflammatory response of the patient, the immune status of the patient, and the extent of organ system dysfunction.

E. Management of Anesthesia

1. **Preoperative.** The most important questions are whether the surgery may be postponed pending treatment of sepsis and whether, if surgery is urgent, the patient's condition may be improved before surgery. Preoperative resuscitation should aim to achieve mean arterial pressure greater than 65 mm Hg, central venous pressure of 8 to 12 mm Hg, adequate urine output, a normal pH without a metabolic (lactic) acidosis, and mixed venous or central venous saturation above 70%.
2. **Intraoperative.** Invasive monitoring (arterial blood pressure, central venous pressure, or pulmonary artery pressure) is usually indicated. Sufficient intravenous (IV) access is needed to allow volume resuscitation and transfusion of blood and blood components. Prophylactic antibiotics should be administered within 30 minutes before skin incision. Normothermia and normoglycemia are a priority. Inotropes (e.g., epinephrine) and vasoconstrictors (e.g., norepinephrine and vasopressin) should be available. IV steroids may be indicated for refractory shock.
3. **Postoperative.** Continued hemodynamic monitoring and support are provided as needed (see Figure 22-3).

V. *CLOSTRIDIUM DIFFICILE*

C. difficile is an anaerobic, gram-positive, spore-forming bacterium that is the major identifiable cause of antibiotic-associated diarrhea and pseudomembranous colitis. *C. difficile* produces two toxins (A and B) that cause diarrhea.

A. Risk Factors (Table 22-6)

B. Signs and Symptoms. Most commonly, signs and symptoms are diarrhea and abdominal pain. Patients may be febrile with abdominal tenderness and distention.

C. Diagnosis. The most common confirmatory study is an enzyme immunoassay for *C. difficile* toxins A and B in the stool.

D. Treatment. Treatment is fluid and electrolyte replacement, withdrawal of current antibiotic therapy if possible, and targeted antibiotic treatment to eradicate *C. difficile* (oral metronidazole 400 mg three times daily, or oral vancomycin 125 mg four times daily). Treatment is typically administered for at least 10 days but should be continued until symptoms and diarrhea resolve.

E. Management of Anesthesia

1. **Preoperative.** In general, the sickest patients with *C. difficile* colitis, including those who do not improve with conventional therapy, undergo surgery, such as subtotal colectomy and ileostomy. Surgery carries a high mortality.

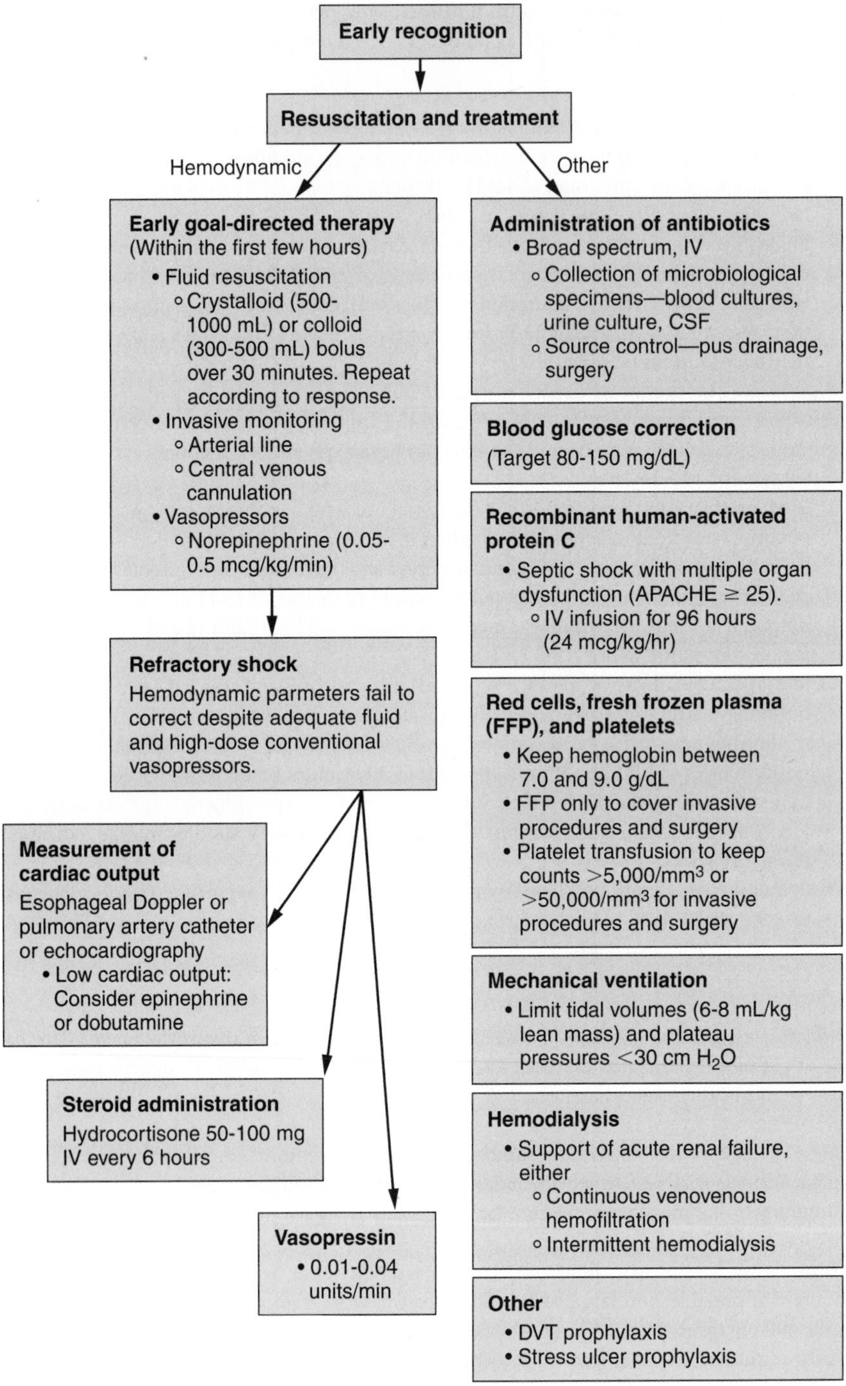

FIGURE 22-3 ■ Management of sepsis. *APACHE,* Acute Physiology and Chronic Health Evaluation II; *DVT,* deep vein thrombosis.

TABLE 22-6 ■ Risk Factors for Developing *Clostridium difficile*–Associated Diarrhea

Increasing age (except infants)
Severe underlying disease
Gastrointestinal surgery
Presence of a nasogastric tube
Use of antiulcer medication
Admission to an intensive care unit
Long duration of hospital stay
Long duration of antibiotic course (risk doubles after 3 days)
Multiple antibiotic therapy
General immunocompromise
Immunosuppressive therapy
Recent surgical procedure
Sharing hospital room with a *C. difficile*–infected patient

2. **Intraoperative.** Hemodynamic instability is likely, and invasive monitoring may guide fluid administration and the use of inotropes and vasopressors. Dehydration, acid-base, and electrolyte abnormalities may occur after episodes of diarrhea. Opiates decrease intestinal motility, which may exacerbate toxin-mediated disease.
3. **Postoperative.** One of the most important considerations is prevention of the spread of *C. difficile;* therefore contact and isolation precautions are essential, and routine use of disposable gloves and gowns is important. Vigorous hand washing with soap and water may remove spores.

VI. NECROTIZING SOFT TISSUE INFECTION

Necrotizing infection includes diagnoses such as gas gangrene, toxic shock syndrome, Fournier's gangrene, severe cellulitis, and flesh-eating infection. Severity may be underappreciated at the time of presentation. The organisms responsible are highly virulent, the clinical course is rampant, and mortality is high (up to 75%).

A. **Signs and Symptoms.** Signs include general features of infection, including malaise, fever, sweating, and altered mental status. Pain is always present and may be out of proportion to physical signs. Because the infection begins in deep tissue planes, cutaneous signs are often surprisingly mild and are not reflective of the extent of tissue necrosis or the severity of the disease. Hypotension is an ominous sign.

B. **Diagnosis.** Patients with a history of alcohol abuse, malnutrition, obesity, trauma, cancer, burns, older age, vascular disease, diabetes, and immunocompromise are more susceptible. There may be a high white blood cell count, thrombocytopenia, coagulopathy, electrolyte abnormalities, acidosis, hyperglycemia, elevated markers of inflammation such as C-reactive protein, and radiographic evidence of extensive necrotic inflammation with subcutaneous air. Computed tomography or magnetic resonance imaging may delineate the extent of necrotic tissue. Blood, urine, and tissue samples should be sent to the laboratory for culture.

C. **Treatment.** Extensive surgical débridement of necrotic tissue is coupled with appropriate antimicrobial therapy, which typically includes coverage of gram-positive, gram-negative, and anaerobic organisms.

D. **Prognosis.** The mortality rate is high, and if patients survive the initial insult, they may remain vulnerable to secondary infection.

E. **Management of Anesthesia**

1. **Preoperative.** The anesthesiologist should treat such patients as having severe sepsis and try to resuscitate preoperatively. However, surgical débridement should not be postponed because delay is associated with increased mortality.

2. **Intraoperative.** Concern has been raised about the use of etomidate when patients have septic shock because they may already have adrenal insufficiency, and this may theoretically be worsened by even a single dose of etomidate. Major fluid shifts, blood loss, and release of cytokines may occur intraoperatively. Good IV access is essential, and invasive arterial and central venous monitoring may be useful. Blood should be cross-matched and readily available. Patients are at risk of developing both hypovolemic and septic shock.
3. **Postoperative.** As with sepsis, patients are at risk of developing multiorgan failure. Postoperative admission to an intensive care unit (ICU) is advisable. Antibiotic therapy should be continued in the postoperative period and should be targeted to the organisms that grow from tissue specimens.

VII. TETANUS

The neurotoxin tetanospasmin, produced by vegetative forms of *Clostridium tetani* organisms, causes the clinical manifestations of tetanus. Tetanospasmin suppresses inhibitory internuncial neurons in the spinal cord, resulting in generalized skeletal muscle contractions (spasms). In the brain, the fourth ventricle is believed to have selective permeability for tetanospasmin, resulting in early manifestations of trismus and neck rigidity. Sympathetic nervous system hyperactivity may develop.

A. **Signs and Symptoms** (Table 22-7)

B. **Treatment**

1. **Control of Skeletal Muscle Spasms.** Control is achieved by use of diazepam, muscle relaxants, and mechanical ventilation.
2. **Prevention of Sympathetic Nervous System Hyperactivity.** Prevention is possible with use of β-blockers.
3. **Ventilatory Support.** Tracheal intubation is used to control secretions, and ventilatory support includes prevention of airway obstruction caused by laryngospasm.
4. **Neutralize Circulating Exotoxin.** This is accomplished with intramuscular administration of human antitetanus immunoglobulin.
5. **Surgical Débridement.** The source of the exotoxin can be eliminated via surgical débridement.
6. **Antibiotic Treatment.** Penicillin destroys the exotoxin-producing vegetative forms of *C. tetani.*

C. **Management of Anesthesia.** General anesthesia with volatile agents (to decrease sympathetic nervous system activity) and tracheal intubation (because of increased potential for

TABLE 22-7 ■ **Symptoms and Signs of Tetanus**
Trismus (75%)
Laryngospasm
Facial muscle rigidity ("risus sardonicus")
Dysphagia
Abdominal and lumbar muscle rigidity (opisthotonic posture)
Excruciating skeletal muscle spasms precipitated by external stimulation, such as sudden exposure to light, unexpected noise, or tracheal suction
Increased body temperature caused by increased skeletal muscle work
Hypotension (myocarditis) or transient hypertension
Tachydysrhythmias
Peripheral vasoconstriction
Diaphoresis
Inappropriate antidiuretic hormone secretion with hyponatremia and decreased plasma osmolality

laryngospasm) is the usual approach. Surgical débridement is delayed for several hours after the patient has received antitoxin because tetanospasmin will be mobilized into the systemic circulation during surgical resection. Invasive blood pressure and central venous pressure monitoring is often indicated. Drugs such as lidocaine, esmolol, metoprolol, magnesium, nicardipine, and nitroprusside should be readily available.

VIII. PNEUMONIA

A. Types of Pneumonia.

1. **Community-Acquired Pneumonia.** This is one of the 10 leading causes of death in the United States. *Streptococcus pneumoniae* is the most common cause of bacterial pneumonia in adults *(typical pneumonia).* Other common organisms include *Haemophilus influenzae, Mycoplasma pneumoniae, S. aureus, Legionella pneumophila, Klebsiella pneumoniae, Chlamydia pneumoniae,* and influenza virus *(atypical pneumonias).*
2. **Aspiration Pneumonia.** Risks include depressed consciousness (alcohol abuse, drug abuse, head trauma, seizures and other neurologic disorders, administration of sedatives), abnormalities of deglutition or esophageal motility resulting from placement of nasogastric tubes, esophageal cancer, bowel obstruction, repeated vomiting, poor oral hygiene and periodontal disease, and induction and recovery from anesthesia. Clinical manifestations depend on the nature and volume of aspirated material and can include fulminating arterial hypoxemia, airway obstruction, atelectasis, and pneumonia.
3. **Postoperative Pneumonia.** This occurs most often in patients undergoing major thoracic, esophageal, or upper abdominal surgery but is rare in other procedures in previously fit patients. Chronic lung disease increases the incidence of postoperative pneumonia three fold.
4. **Lung Abscess.** Lung abscesses may develop after bacterial pneumonia. The finding of an air-fluid level on the chest radiograph signifies rupture of the abscess into the bronchial tree, and foul-smelling sputum is characteristic. Surgery is indicated only when complications such as empyema occur.

B. Diagnosis. An initial chill, followed by abrupt onset of fever, chest pain, dyspnea, fatigue, rigors, cough, and copious sputum production characterizes bacterial pneumonia. Nonproductive cough is a feature of atypical pneumonias. Patient history may suggest possible causative organisms, such as exposure to hotels and whirlpools *(L. pneumophila),* cave exploration *(Histoplasma capsulatum),* diving *(Scedosporium apiospermum),* contact with birds *(Chlamydia psittaci),* contact with sheep *(Coxiella burnetii),* alcoholism *(K. pneumoniae),* and immunocompromise such as in acquired immunodeficiency syndrome (AIDS) (*Pneumocystis jiroveci* pneumonia [PCP]). Chest radiograph, microscopic examination of sputum and cultures, urine testing for the presence of *L. pneumophila* antigen, blood antibody titers for *M. pneumoniae,* sputum polymerase chain reaction for *Chlamydia,* and serum testing for HIV infection can be helpful.

C. Treatment. For severe pneumonia, treatment is empiric therapy (typically a combination such as a cephalosporin plus a macrolide antibiotic such as azithromycin or clarithromycin). Therapy should be narrowed and targeted when the pathogen has been identified.

D. Prognosis (Table 22-8)

E. Management of Anesthesia. Anesthesia and surgery should ideally be deferred with acute pneumonia. Fluid management is challenging; fluid overload may worsen hypoxia. During general anesthesia, ventilation should generally be with tidal volumes of 6 to 8 mL/kg ideal body mass and mean airway pressures less than 30 cm H_2O.

IX. VENTILATOR-ASSOCIATED PNEUMONIA

Ventilator-associated pneumonia (VAP) is the most common nosocomial infection in the ICU and makes up one third of all nosocomial infections. Mortality is 15% to 50%. Several simple

TABLE 22-8 ■ Elements of the Pneumonia Severity Index
Age in years
Gender
Nursing home resident
Neoplastic disease history
Liver disease
Congestive heart failure
Cerebrovascular disease
Renal disease
Altered mental status
Respiratory rate > 29 breaths/min
Systolic blood pressure < 90 mm Hg
Temperature < 35° C or > 39.9° C
Pulse > 124 beats/min
pH < 7.35
Blood urea nitrogen > 29 mg/dL
Sodium < 130 mmol/L
Glucose > 249 mg/dL
Hematocrit < 30%
Pao_2 < 60 mm Hg
Pleural effusion on radiograph

interventions may decrease the occurrence of VAP, including meticulous hand hygiene, oral care, limiting patient sedation, positioning patients semiupright, suctioning subglottic secretions, limiting intubation time, and considering the appropriateness of noninvasive ventilation support.

A. Diagnosis (Table 22-9). The National Nosocomial Infections Surveillance (NISS) System uses a standardized diagnostic algorithm for VAP and a clinical pulmonary infection score to promote diagnostic consistency among clinicians and investigators. A clinical pulmonary infection score greater than 6 is consistent with a diagnosis of VAP. Both the NNIS System and the clinical pulmonary infection score are relatively sensitive for VAP (>80%) but nonspecific.

B. Treatment (Figure 22-4)

C. Management of Anesthesia. Patients with VAP often require anesthesia for tracheostomy. Major surgery should be deferred until the pneumonia has resolved and respiratory function has improved. Patients with respiratory failure may be positive end-expiratory pressure (PEEP) dependent. Ideally, the same ventilator settings that were used in the ICU should be used in the operating room, including the same mode of ventilation and the same amount of PEEP. The lowest inspired oxygen necessary to achieve adequate oxygen saturation (Spo_2 >95%) should be administered.

X. SEVERE ACUTE RESPIRATORY SYNDROME AND INFLUENZA

Influenza A and severe acute respiratory syndrome (SARS)–associated viruses are examples of viruses that have rampant courses, high virulence, and high mortality.

A. Signs and Symptoms. Signs and symptoms include nonspecific complaints (cough, sore throat, headache, diarrhea, arthralgia, muscle pain). In more severe cases, patients may have respiratory distress, confusion (encephalitis), and hemoptysis. Other signs include fever, tachycardia, sweating, conjunctivitis, rash, tachypnea, use of accessory respiratory muscles, cyanosis, and pulmonary features of pneumonia, pleural effusion, or pneumothorax. A chest radiograph may be helpful.

B. Diagnosis. In the context of an outbreak, history, symptoms, and presentation are usually sufficient to suggest a diagnosis. The incubation period for SARS coronavirus (SARS-CoV) and

TABLE 22-9 ■ **Clinical Pulmonary Infection Score**

PARAMETER	OPTIONS	SCORE
Temperature (°C)	≥36.5 and ≤38.4	0
	≥38.5 and ≤38.9	1
	≥39 or ≤36	2
Blood leukocytes (mm^3)	≥4000 and ≤11,000	0
	<4000 or >11,000	1
	+ band forms ≥50%	Add 1
Tracheal secretions	Absence of tracheal secretions	0
	Presence of nonpurulent tracheal secretions	1
	Presence of purulent tracheal secretions	2
Oxygenation: PaO_2/FIO_2 (mm Hg)	>240 or ARDS	0
	≤240 and no ARDS	2
Pulmonary radiography	No infiltrate	0
	Diffuse (or patchy) infiltrate	1
	Localized infiltrate	2
Progression of pulmonary infiltrate	No radiographic progression	0
	Radiographic progression (after cardiac failure and ARDS excluded)	2
Culture of tracheal aspirate	Pathogenic bacteria cultured in rare or light quantity	0
	Pathogenic bacteria cultured in moderate or heavy quantity	1
	Same pathogenic bacteria seen on Gram stain	Add 1

Reproduced from Luyt CE, Chastre J, Fagon JY. Value of the clinical pulmonary infection score for the identification and management of ventilator-associated pneumonia. *Intensive Care Med.* 2004;30:844-852; with permission.
ARDS, Acute respiratory distress syndrome.

H5N1 influenza A, "bird flu," is about 1 week. For influenza the range is 2 to 17 days. Serologic testing is not usually helpful because it may take 2 to 3 weeks for seroconversion after infection. Polymerase chain reaction tests can be useful for diagnosing SARS-CoV infection and H5N1 influenza A infection.

C. Treatment. Vaccine development is key in prevention of widespread infection and reduction of morbidity and mortality. No vaccine currently exists for the SARS-CoV or for the H5N1 influenza A virus. In the case of influenza, neuraminidase inhibitors (zanamivir, oseltamivir) may decrease the severity of infection. Amantadine and rimantadine may also be used. These drugs are of only modest benefit and are helpful only if administered within the first 48 hours of symptoms. The mainstay of treatment for influenza and SARS is supportive care.

D. Prognosis. The prognosis depends on the pathogenicity of the infecting virus as well as the susceptibility of the infected person.

E. Management of Anesthesia

1. Preoperative. Ideally, infected patients should be cared for in rooms with negative pressure to decrease aerosolized spread and contagion. Barrier precautions should be used with patients infected with SARS-CoV and newly evolved virulent influenza strains, including full-body disposable oversuits, double gloves, goggles, and powered air-purifying respirators with high-efficiency particulate air (HEPA) filters. If these are not available, N95 masks (block 95% of particles) should be used rather than regular surgical masks. Filters should be placed in both limbs of breathing circuits to protect ventilators and anesthesia

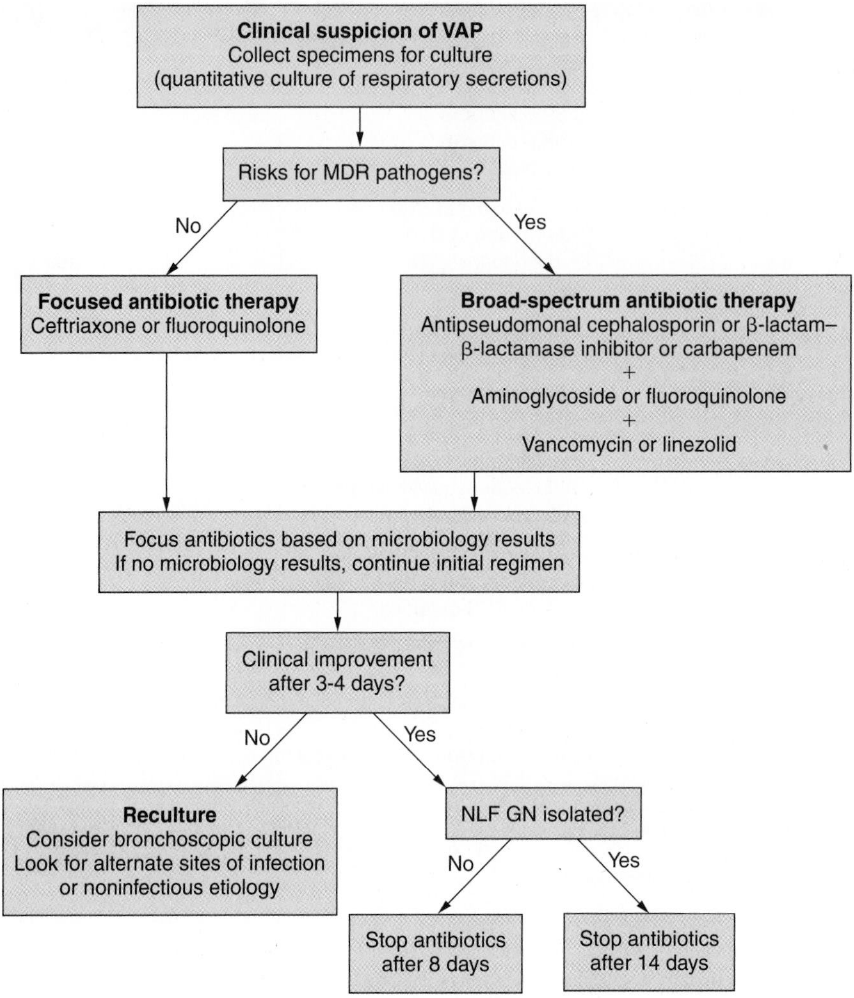

FIGURE 22-4 ■ Management of ventilator-associated pneumonia. *NLF GN*, Non lactose fermenting gram negative bacteria. *(Adapted from Porzecanski I, Bowton DL. Diagnosis and treatment of ventilator-associated pneumonia.* Chest. *2006;130:597-604.)*

machines from contamination. All surfaces should be sterilized with alcohol, and ideally rooms should not be used for other patients (if practical) for up to 48 hours after a person with SARS-CoV infection or H5N1 influenza A has been in the room.

2. **Intraoperative.** Fears about contagion should not blind anesthesiologists to the high level of care required for these vulnerable patients. When appropriate precautions are taken, spread of infection may be prevented. If mechanical ventilation is required, protective ventilation as for acute respiratory distress syndrome is indicated. Tidal volumes should be limited to 6 to 8 mL/kg lean body mass and mean airway pressure should be less than 30 cm H_2O.
3. **Postoperative.** Precautions to prevent spread of infection should be ongoing.

XI. TUBERCULOSIS

Mycobacterium tuberculosis is an obligate aerobe responsible for TB, which survives most successfully in tissues with high oxygen concentrations. At present, most cases of TB in the United States occur in racial and ethnic minorities, foreign-born individuals from areas where TB is endemic (Asia and Africa), IV drug abusers, and those with HIV infection or AIDS. Any patient with TB should be tested for HIV. The appearance of MDR strains of *M. tuberculosis* has contributed to the resurgence of TB worldwide. In addition, XDR TB is resistant to second-line therapeutic agents, including fluoroquinolones and at least one of three injectable second-line drugs used to treat TB (amikacin, kanamycin, or capreomycin).

A. **Diagnosis.** Diagnosis of TB is based on the presence of clinical signs and symptoms (persistent nonproductive cough, anorexia, weight loss, chest pain, hemoptysis, night sweats), the epidemiologic likelihood of infection, and results of diagnostic tests. The most common test for TB is the tuberculin skin (Mantoux's) test. The result of this test may be positive if people have received a bacille Calmette-Guérin (BCG) vaccine or if they have been exposed to TB, even if there are no viable mycobacteria present at the time of the skin test. Two interferon release assays (QuantiFERON-TB Gold In-Tube test and the T-SPOT.*TB* test) are considered equivalent to, and perhaps better than, the TB skin test in sensitivity and specificity. Both are blood tests, and neither is affected by prior BCG vaccination. Chest radiographs show apical or subapical infiltrates, or bilateral upper lobe infiltration with the presence of cavitation. Patients with AIDS may demonstrate a less classic picture on chest radiography. Tuberculous vertebral osteomyelitis (Pott's disease) is a common manifestation of extrapulmonary TB. Sputum smears may show acid-fast bacilli.

B. **Increased Risk of Anesthesiologists.** Anesthesiologists are at increased risk of nosocomial TB and should participate in annual tuberculin screening so that those who develop a positive skin test result may be offered chemotherapy.

C. **Treatment.** Chemotherapy with isoniazid is the treatment. Other drugs include pyrazinamide, rifampicin, and ethambutol. In order to be curative, treatment for pulmonary TB is recommended for 6 months. Extrapulmonary TB usually requires a longer course.

D. **Management of Anesthesia**

1. **Preoperative Assessment.** A detailed history is taken, including the presence of a persistent cough and the tuberculin status. Elective surgical procedures should be postponed until patients are no longer infectious (i.e., they have received antituberculous chemotherapy, are improving clinically, and have had three consecutive negative sputum smears). If surgery cannot be delayed, limit the number of involved personnel. High-risk procedures (bronchoscopy, tracheal intubation, tracheal suctioning) should be performed in a negative-pressure environment. Patients should be transported wearing a tight-fitting N95 face mask, and staff should also wear N95 masks.
2. **Intraoperative.** Special precautions should be taken not to injure the spine during airway manipulation in patients with TB of the spine. A HEPA filter should be placed between the Y connector and the mask, laryngeal mask airway, or tracheal tube. Bacterial filters should be placed on the exhalation limb of the anesthesia delivery circuit to decrease the discharge of tubercle bacilli into the ambient air. Use of a dedicated anesthesia machine and ventilator is recommended.
3. **Postoperative.** Care should take place in an isolation room, preferably with negative pressure.

XII. INFECTIOUS DISEASES IN SOLID ORGAN TRANSPLANT RECIPIENTS

Immunosuppression after solid organ transplantation is variable and depends on the immunosuppressant dosage and duration and the time since transplantation. Immunosuppression is most intense the first few months following transplantation, and becomes less intense as therapy is withdrawn over time. In addition to drug effects on the immune system, metabolic abnormalities, damage to mucocutaneous barriers, and the possible presence of immunomodulating viruses (cytomegalovirus [CMV], HIV) can affect immunosuppression. The time period during which infectious disease processes affect posttransplant patients can be divided into the first month after transplantion, months 2 to 6, and beyond month 6.

A. **Important Infection Periods and Factors**
   1. **First Month.** Active infections may be harbored in the allograft and are typically bacterial or fungal. The most common viral infection during the first month after transplant is reactivated herpes simplex virus.
   2. **Months 2 to 6.** Unusual infections occur, either community-acquired or opportunistic infections. Trimethoprim-sulfamethoxazole is often given for *Pneumocystis* pneumonia prophylaxis during the first 6 months after solid organ transplant, and for longer after heart and lung transplant. Reactivation of latent recipient infections can occur: TB is common and occurs in about 1% of transplant recipients.
   3. **Beyond Month 6.** Most infections parallel those seen in the community at large. However, some individuals have progressive infections with hepatitis B, hepatitis C, CMV, or Epstein-Barr virus (EBV). The most common viral infection is varicella-zoster, manifesting as herpes zoster.
   4. **Cases of Chronic Rejection.** Patients are predisposed to opportunistic infections because of higher doses of immunosuppressants. Posttransplant patients with HIV and/or AIDS need close following for evidence of infection, both common and opportunistic. HIV highly active retroviral therapeutic regimens must be maintained.

B. **Anesthesia Management**
   1. **Preoperative.** Assessment focuses on degree of immunosuppression and allograft function. Laboratory evaluation includes complete blood count (CBC) with differential, metabolic panel, liver function tests, viral panels as indicated, chest radiograph, and electrocardiogram (ECG). Blood levels of immunosuppressants may be appropriate. Evidence of active rejection is a contraindication to elective surgery. All antimicrobial agents and immunosuppressive drugs should be continued throughout the perioperative period.
   2. **Intraoperative.** Selection of anesthetic technique is based on the surgery, patient's comorbidities, presence of specific anesthetic contraindications, and potential for interaction between immunosuppressants and anesthetic drugs. Although concerns about possible infection due to regional anesthetic techniques have been raised, the evidence is scant. Nasal intubation is not preferred owing to the bacteremia that is associated with this procedure. Cyclosporine may delay metabolism of neuromuscular blocking agents, especially pancuronium and vecuronium. Strict use of aseptic technique for invasive line placement is critical.
   3. **Postoperative.** A major consideration is to monitor for deterioration in graft function or potential infection. All antibiotic regimens should be strictly followed. Be aware that signs and symptoms of infection may be blunted and hard to detect.

XIII. ACQUIRED IMMUNODEFICIENCY SYNDROME

It is estimated that more than 40 million people worldwide are infected with HIV, which is thought to have caused more than 25 million deaths to date. The predominant mode of HIV transmission is heterosexual sex. There is a variable period during which the patient remains healthy but is viremic.

A. **Pathogenesis.** Acute seroconversion illness occurs with a high viral load soon after infection. After several months, there is a decrease in the viremia as the patient's immune response is stimulated. Then gradual involution of lymph nodes occurs, with a concomitant decrease in T-helper lymphocytes (CD4 T cells) and an increase in viral load as the inexorable onset of AIDS occurs. *Pneumocystis* pneumonia does not usually occur until the CD4 count is less than 200 cells/mL.

B. **Signs and Symptoms** (Table 22-10)

C. **Diagnosis.** Diagnosis is via an enzyme-linked immunosorbent assay (ELISA); the result usually becomes positive when the antibodies to HIV increase 4 to 8 weeks after infection. During

TABLE 22-10 ■ **Signs and Symptoms of and Systemic Involvement in Acquired Immunodeficiency Syndrome (AIDS)**

Constitutional	Night sweats, weight loss
Respiratory	Breathlessness, abnormal chest radiograph Opportunistic pneumonia, pneumothorax Kaposi's sarcoma and lymphoma with hemoptysis HIV-induced pulmonary syndrome (similar to emphysema) Disseminated TB
Lymph nodes	Diffuse adenopathy
Neurologic	Dementia Cerebral toxoplasmosis CNS lymphoma Progressive multifocal leukoencephalopathy Meningitis (*Cryptococcus,* HIV, tuberculosis) Peripheral neuropathy
Cardiac	Often silent involvement Abnormal echocardiogram in up to 50% of patients Pericardial effusion in up to 25% of patients Cardiac disease (especially premature atherosclerosis) may be exacerbated by HAART Myocarditis; caused by toxoplasmosis, cryptococcosis, Coxsackie B virus, CMV, lymphoma, aspergillosis, and HIV
Generalized vascular disease	Abdominal aortic aneurysms and aortic dissection
Adrenal insufficiency	Hypotension
Kaposi's sarcoma	Skin and endobronchial involvement; may cause hemoptysis
Hematologic	Lymphocytosis ($CD8^+$ T lymphocytes) Bone marrow involvement with HIV or infection Leukopenia, lymphopenia, thrombocytopenia Bone marrow suppression caused by zidovudine therapy
Renal	Toxic acute tubular necrosis and nephrolithiasis caused by HAART Nephrotic syndrome Nephrolithiasis

CMV, Cytomegalovirus; *CNS,* central nervous system; *HAART,* highly active antiretroviral therapy; *HIV,* human immunodeficiency virus; *TB,* tuberculosis.

this period, patients are more infectious. Infection may be confirmed with a Western blot test or by measurement of HIV viral load in the blood. If a patient is tested very shortly after initial infection, the ELISA test result can be negative or inconclusive. Nucleic acid testing of HIV RNA is the most specific and sensitive test for HIV. $CD4^+$ cell levels are indicative of the degree of HIV progression, initially declining dramatically, then rising again, and over the course of 8 to 12 years undergoing slow decline. The diagnosis of AIDS in HIV-positive patients is established when *one* of the AIDS-defining diagnoses is present (Table 22-11).

D. Treatment. Six major classes of antiretroviral agents are currently in use (Table 22-12). A typical antiretroviral regimen consists of three agents: a protease inhibitor (PI) or nonnucleoside reverse transcriptase inhibitor (NNRTI) combined with two nucleoside reverse transcriptase inhibitors (NRTIs). Numerous side effects (hypersensitivity reactions, severe myopathy, respiratory muscle dysfunction) and drug interactions complicate treatment and decrease

TABLE 22-11 ■ AIDS-Defining Diagnoses in HIV-Seropositive Patients

Bacterial infection, multiple or recurrent
Burkitt's lymphoma
Candidiasis of the bronchi, trachea, lungs, or esophagus
$CD4^+$ T-lymphocyte cell count <200 cells/mm^3
Cervical cancer, invasive
Coccidiomycosis, disseminated or extrapulmonary
Cryptococcosis, extrapulmonary
Cryptosporidiosis, chronic intestinal (>1 mo)
Cytomegalovirus retinitis or cytomegalovirus infection (with loss of vision)
Herpes simplex with chronic ulcers (>1 mo), bronchitis, pneumonitis, or esophagitis
HIV-related encephalopathy
Histoplasmosis, disseminated or extrapulmonary
Isosporiasis, chronic (>1 mo)
Immunoblastic lymphoma
Kaposi's sarcoma
Lymphoma of the brain, primary
Mycobacterium avium-intracellulare complex or *Mycobacterium kansasii* infection, disseminated or extrapulmonary
Mycobacterium infection, any other species, pulmonary or extrapulmonary
Mycobacterium tuberculosis infection, any site
Pneumocystis jiroveci (Pneumocystis carinii) pneumonia (PCP)
Pneumonia, recurrent
Progressive multifocal leukoencephalopathy (PML)
Recurrent *Salmonella* septicemia
Toxoplasmosis of the brain
Wasting syndrome resulting from HIV

compliance. Of particular importance to anesthesiologists is the fact that patients are subject to long-term metabolic complications, including lipid abnormalities and glucose intolerance, which may result in the development of diabetes, coronary artery disease, and cerebrovascular disease. IRIS (immune reconstitution inflammatory syndrome) can develop as a reaction to highly active antiretroviral therapy (HAART) and leads to paradoxical deterioration of general clinical status in the context of improving $CD4^+$ counts and reduced viral load. IRIS is marked by the appearance and/or exacerbation of previously silent diseases such as hepatitis A, B, and C; PCP; TB; and other opportunistic infections.

E. **Prognosis.** The continued development of antiretroviral drugs has turned AIDS from a rapidly fatal disease to a chronic illness with many long-term survivors.

F. **Management of Anesthesia**

1. **Preoperative.** HAART can affect multiple organ systems: CBC, metabolic panel, renal function studies, liver function tests, and coagulation studies may be appropriate. Chest x-ray examination and ECG may be appropriate. The utility of $CD4^+$ cell count and viral load determinations is unproven.

2. **Intraoperative**

   a. ***Universal Precautions.*** Every patient must be regarded as potentially infected with a blood-borne virus. After an accident with a high-risk body fluid, such as a (hollow) needlestick injury, postexposure prophylaxis should begin as soon as possible after the injury, ideally within 1 to 2 hours, but can be considered up to 1 to 2 weeks after the injury. A recommended postexposure prophylaxis regimen for a duration of 4 weeks is zidovudine 250 mg every 12 hours, lamivudine 150 mg every 12 hours, and indinavir 800 mg every 8 hours.

TABLE 22-12 ■ **Highly active antiretroviral therapy (HAART) drug interactions**

CLASS	COMMON DRUG-HAART INTERACTIONS	ANESTHETIC-SPECIFIC DRUG-HAART INTERACTIONS
Nucleoside reverse transcriptase inhibitors (NRTIs)	Interactions with: *Anticonvulsant:* phenytoin *Antifungals:* ketoconazole, dapsone Alcohol *H_2 blocker:* cimetidine	HAART potentially changes drug clearance and effects of: *Opiate:* methadone
Nonnucleoside reverse transcriptase inhibitors (NNRTIs)	Interactions with: *Anticoagulant:* warfarin *Anticonvulsants:* carbamazepine, phenytoin, phenobarbital *Anti-TB drug:* rifampin, *Herbal:* St. John's wort	HAART prolongs half-life and/or effects of: *Sedatives:* diazepam, midazolam, triazolam *Opiates:* fentanyl, meperidine, methadone
Protease inhibitors (PIs)	Interactions with: *Anticoagulant:* warfarin *Anticonvulsants:* carbamazepine, phenytoin, phenobarbital *Antidepressant:* sertraline *Calcium channel blockers* *Anti-TB drug:* rifampin, *Herbal:* St. John's wort *Immunosuppressant:* cyclosporine	HAART prolongs half-life and/or effects of: *Antiarrhythmics:* amiodarone, digoxin, quinidine *Sedatives:* diazepam, midazolam, triazolam *Opiates:* fentanyl, meperidine, methadone *Local anesthetic:* lidocaine
Integrase strand transfer inhibitors (INSTIs)	Interactions with: *Proton pump inhibitor:* omeprazole *Anti-TB drug:* rifampin	None
Entry inhibitors	Interactions with: *Anticonvulsant:* carbamazepine *Anti-TB drug:* rifampin *Oral contraceptives* *Proton pump inhibitor:* omeprazole *Herbal:* St. John's wort	HAART potentially changes drug clearance and effects of: *Sedative:* midazolam

TB, Tuberculosis.

b. *Focal Neurologic Lesions.* These lesions may increase intracerebral pressure, precluding neuraxial anesthesia. Neurologic involvement may make the use of succinylcholine hazardous. Steroid supplementation should be considered for unexplained hypotension.

3. Postoperative. HIV infection does not increase the risk of postprocedural complications including death up to 30 days postoperatively. Little information exists concerning the overall risk of anesthesia and surgery in the HIV-seropositive patient. In studies of HIV-seropositive parturients who were given regional anesthesia, no neurologic or infectious complications occurred related to the anesthetic or obstetric course. In the immediate postpartum period, immune function measurements remained essentially unchanged, as did the severity of the disease. The safety of epidural blood patches for treatment of postdural puncture headache has been reported in HIV-seropositive patients, but, given the theoretic risk of introducing virus into the central nervous system, other treatment strategies should be tried first.

CHAPTER 23

Cancer

Cancer is the second most common cause of death in the United States, exceeded only by heart disease.

I. MECHANISM

Cancer results from an accumulation of mutations in genes that regulate cellular proliferation (oncogenes). An example of a critical gene is tumor suppressor *p53.* This gene is critical in monitoring damage to DNA and essential for cell viability. Inactivation of *p53* is an early step in the development of many types of cancer. Stimulation of oncogene formation by carcinogens (tobacco, alcohol, sunlight) is estimated to be responsible for 80% of cancers in the United States. Evidence of a protective role of the immune system in fighting cancer is the increased incidence of cancer in immunosuppressed patients, such as those with acquired immunodeficiency syndrome and those receiving organ transplants.

II. DIAGNOSIS

Cancer often becomes evident when tumor bulk compromises the function of vital organs. The initial diagnosis is often by aspiration cytology or biopsy (needle, incisional, excisional). Monoclonal antibodies against specific cancers (prostate, lung, breast, ovarian) may aid in the diagnosis. A commonly used staging system for solid tumors is the TNM system based on tumor size (T), lymph node involvement (N), and distant metastasis (M). This system further groups patients into stages I to IV. Stage I has the best prognosis and stage IV the worst. Imaging techniques, including computed tomography and magnetic resonance imaging, are used for further delineation of tumor presence and spread.

III. TREATMENT

Treatment of cancer includes chemotherapy, radiation, and surgery. Surgery is often necessary for the initial diagnosis of cancer (biopsy) and subsequent definitive treatment. Palliative and rehabilitative therapy may involve surgery. Adequate relief of acute and chronic pain associated with cancer is a mandatory part of treatment.

A. **Chemotherapy.** Cancer chemotherapy may produce significant side effects (Table 23-1) that may have important implications for anesthesia management.
   1. **Traditional chemotherapy** involves the use of cytotoxic drugs that target rapidly dividing cells and interfere with all replication
   2. **Targeted chemotherapy** utilizes a set of chemotherapeutic drugs directed against specific processes involved in tumor cell proliferation and migration. Such therapies include those that bind to estrogen receptors in breast cancer, those that inhibit endothelial or vascular endothelial growth factors, and those that angiogenesis in a tumor

B. **Surgery.** Often surgery is needed for the initial diagnosis of cancer (biopsy) as well as for definitive treatment and may be required for tumor palliation.

C. **Radiation Therapy.** Radiation works by causing damage to tumor cell DNA. Radiation can be delivered via external beam or via implantable pellets in the target organ.

TABLE 23-1 ■ Toxicities of Commonly Used Chemotherapeutic Agents

AGENT	ADVERSE EFFECTS
Doxorubicin	Cardiac toxicity, myelosuppression
Arsenic	Leukocytosis, pleural effusion, QT interval prolongation
Asparaginase	Coagulopathy, hemorrhagic pancreatitis, hepatic dysfunction, thromboembolism
Bevacizumab	Bleeding, congestive heart failure, gastrointestinal perforation, hypertension, impaired wound healing, pulmonary hemorrhage, thromboembolism
Bleomycin	Pulmonary hypertension, pulmonary toxicity
Busulfan	Cardiac toxicity, myelosuppression, pulmonary toxicity
Carmustine	Myelosuppression, pulmonary toxicity
Chlorambucil	Myelosuppression, pulmonary toxicity, SIADH
Cisplatin	Dysrhythmias, magnesium wasting, mucositis, ototoxicity, peripheral neuropathy, SIADH, renal tubular necrosis, thromboembolism
Cyclophosphamide	Encephalopathy/delirium, hemorrhagic cystitis, myelosuppression, pericarditis, pericardial effusion, SIADH, pulmonary fibrosis
Erlotinib	Deep vein thrombosis, pulmonary toxicity
Etoposide	Cardiac toxicity, myelosuppression, pulmonary toxicity
Fluorouracil	Acute cerebellar ataxia, cardiac toxicity, gastritis, myelosuppression
Ifosfamide	Cardiac toxicity, hemorrhagic cystitis, renal insufficiency, SIADH
Methotrexate	Encephalopathy, hepatic dysfunction, mucositis, platelet dysfunction, pulmonary toxicity, renal failure, myelosuppression
Mitomycin	Myelosuppression, pulmonary toxicity
Mitoxantrone	Cardiac toxicity, myelosuppression
Paclitaxel	Ataxia, autonomic dysfunction, myelosuppression, peripheral neuropathy, arthralgias, bradycardia
Sorafenib	Cardiac ischemia, hypertension, impaired wound healing, thromboembolism
Sunitinib	Adrenal insufficiency, cardiac ischemia, hypertension, thromboembolism
Tamoxifen	Thromboembolism
Thalidomide	Bradycardia, neurotoxicity, thromboembolism
Tretinoin	Myelosuppression, retinoic acid syndrome
Vinblastine	Cardiac toxicity, hypertension, myelosuppression, pulmonary toxicity, SIADH
Vincristine	Autonomic dysfunction, cardiac toxicity, peripheral neuropathy, SIADH, pulmonary toxicity

SIADH, Syndrome of inappropriate secretion of antidiuretic hormone.

IV. EFFECTS OF CANCER TREATMENT

A. Cardiovascular

1. **Cardiotoxicity.** Adriamycin (doxorubicin) and idarubicin are associated with cardiotoxicity and cardiomyopathy, particularly if total accumulative dose is high (i.e., >300 mg/m^2 for doxorubicin). Acute toxicity arises early in treatment (prolonged QT, dysrhythmias,

cardiomyopathy) and generally reverses with cessation of therapy. Chronic toxicity can occur as early onset (within 1 year of therapy) or late onset (years to decades after therapy). Risks are increased in patients who underwent concomitant radiation therapy or therapy with other cardiotoxic drugs. The use of free radical preparations (dexrazoxane) or liposomal preparations may decrease toxicity. Other drugs associated with cardiomyopathy include mitoxantrone, cyclophosphamide, clofarabine, and tyrosine kinase inhibitors.

2. **Myocardial Ischemia.** This effect is associated with fluorouracil and capecitabine.
3. **Miscellaneous Cardiac Effects of Chemotherapy.** Pericarditis, angina, coronary vasospasm, electrocardiogram (ECG) changes, and conduction defects can occur. Paclitaxel and thalidomide can cause severe bradycardia and require pacemaker implantation. Arsenic, lapatinib, and nilotinib can prolong QT.
4. **Hypertension.** This effect is associated with bevacizumab, trastuzumab, sorafenib, and sunitinib. It occurs in 35% to 45% of patients.
5. **Miscellaneous Cardiac Effects of Radiation Therapy.** Myocardial fibrosis, valvular fibrosis, pericarditis, conduction abnormalities, and accelerated coronary artery disease may occur.

B. Respiratory

1. **Chemotherapy.** Pulmonary toxicity of chemotherapy is well recognized with bleomycin therapy (3% to 20%). Pulmonary fibrosis can develop decades later. Exposure to high oxygen concentrations in the operating room predisposes to postoperative pulmonary failure; perioperative steroids may mitigate this effect. Pulmonary damage can occur with busulfan, cyclophosphamide, methotrexate, lomustine, carmustine, mitomycin, and vinca alkaloids. Epidermal growth factor (EGF) receptor blockade is believed to underlie alveolar damage from erlotinib and gefitinib. Type II pneumocytes possess EGF receptors that play a role in alveolar repair.
2. **Radiation Therapy.** Pulmonary effects of radiation therapy include interstitial pneumonitis and pulmonary fibrosis. Symptoms often occur within 2 to 3 months of therapy and often regress within 12 months of treatment completion. "Radiation recall" can occur in patients with prior radiation treatment who are later exposed to a second pulmonary toxin.

C. Renal

1. **Nephrotoxicity.** Cisplatin, high-dose methotrexate, and ifosfamide may cause nephrotoxicity. Hypomagnesemia is may be present. Leucovorin therapy may be helpful with methotrexate-related renal failure.
2. **Syndrome of Inappropriate Secretion of Antidiuretic Hormone (SIADH).** SIADH can occur after cyclophosphamide therapy.
3. **Hemorrhagic Cystitis.** This condition is associated with cyclophosphamide therapy.
4. **Hyperuricemia and Acute Renal Failure.** These effects can occur after induction chemotherapy or high-dose radiation owing to tumor lysis and release of large amounts of uric acid.
5. **Glomerulonephritis.** Glomerulonephritis can occur, after radiation exposure.

D. Hepatic

1. **Acute Liver Dysfunction.** Methotrexate, asparaginase, arabinoside, plicamycin, and streptozocin may cause acute liver dysfunction. Chronic liver disease is uncommon. Radiation-related dysfunction is typically dose dependent and reversible.
2. **Sinusoidal Obstruction Syndrome.** The most severe form of liver dysfunction, this syndrome usually follows total body irradiation but can be associated with busulfan, cyclophosphamide, vincristine, and dactinomycin. Mortality ranges from 20% to 50%.

E. Airway and Oral Cavity

1. **Mucositis.** Mucositis is relatively common after high-dose chemotherapy, particularly with anthracyclines, taxanes, platinum-based compounds, methotrexate, and fluorouracil. Onset is usually within a week of initiation of treatment, and resolution occurs after chemotheraphy has been terminated.
2. **Radiation-Related Tissue Fibrosis.** Tissue fibrosis can restrict the airway, mouth opening, and neck and tongue mobility.

F. **Gastrointestinal (GI).** Nausea, vomiting, diarrhea, and enteritis are common. Radiation may produce adhesions and stenotic lesions in the GI tract. Hemorrhagic pancreatitis is associated with asparaginase.

G. **Endocrine.** Hyperglycemia is related to glucocorticoid therapy. Adrenal suppression can occur. SIADH is seen with some agents, although symptomatic hyponatremia is uncommon. Total body irradiation and head and neck irradiation can cause panhypopituitarism and/or hypothyroidism and thyroid cancer.

H. **Hematologic.** Myelosuppression (anemia, leukopenia, thrombocytopenia, and platelet dysfunction with bleeding) may occur. Bevacizumab therapy should be withheld before surgery due to angiogenesis inhibitor–related bleeding. Hypercoagulability and a high risk of venous thromboembolism can result from release of tumor factors and use of the chemotherapeutic agents thalidomide, lenalidomide, cisplatin, and tamoxifen. Postradiation bleeding can occur due to necrosis of the vascular endothelium.

I. **Nervous System**

1. **Peripheral Neuropathy and Autonomic Neuropathy.** These effects are associated with vincristine. They are usually reversible.
2. **Large Fiber Neuropathy.** Cisplatin causes large fiber neuropathy. It can damage dorsal root ganglia and decrease proprioception; these effects take several months to resolve after treatment. Paclitaxel is associated with dose-dependent ataxia.
3. **Corticosteroids.** Corticosteroids are associated with neuromyopathy of proximal limb and neck muscles.
4. **Central Nervous System (CNS).** Encephalopathy, delirium, and cerebellar ataxia (high-dose cyclophosphamide and methotrexate) may occur. Methotrexate can cause permanent dementia after prolonged administration.

J. **Tumor Lysis Syndrome.** This syndrome is caused by release of large amounts of uric acid, potassium, and phosphate after chemotherapy and radiation, most often after treatment for hematologic neoplasms. Acute renal failure, hyperkalemia, cardiac dysrhythmias, hypocalcemia (secondary to hyperphosphatemia), muscle spasms, and tetany can occur.

V. IMMUNOLOGY OF CANCER CELLS

Tumor cells are antigenically different from normal cells and may therefore elicit immune reactions similar to those that cause rejection of allografts. Antigens present in cancer cells but not in normal cells are designated *tumor-specific antigens.* Tumor-associated antigens (α-fetoprotein, prostate-specific antigen [PSA], carcinoembryonic antigen [CEA]) are present in both cancer cells and normal cells, but concentrations are higher in tumor cells. Antibodies to tumor-associated antigens can be used for the immunodiagnosis of cancer. Most spontaneously occurring tumors appear to be weakly antigenic.

A. **Cancer Vaccines.** Two preventative vaccines are currently marketed—one against human papillomavirus (HPV) types 6, 11, 16, and 18, and the other against hepatitis B. HPV types 16 and 18 are responsible for about 70% of cervical cancers, as well as being involved in cancer of the vagina, vulva, anus, penis, and oropharynx. Chronic hepatitis B infection is a risk factor for hepatocellular cancer.

VI. PARANEOPLASTIC SYNDROMES (Table 23-2)

Paraneoplastic syndromes manifest as pathophysiologic disturbances that may accompany cancer.

A. **Fever and Cachexia.** Fever may reflect tumor necrosis, inflammation, the release of toxic products by cancer cells, or the production of endogenous pyrogens. Cachexia is related to psychologic effects of cancer, deprivation of nutrients in normal tissue by tumor cells, and GI effects of cancer and therapy.

TABLE 23-2 ■ Pathophysiologic Manifestations of Paraneoplastic Syndromes

Fever
Anorexia
Weight loss
Anemia
Thrombocytopenia
Coagulopathy
Neuromuscular abnormalities
Ectopic hormone production
Hypercalcemia
Hyperuricemia
Tumor lysis syndrome
Adrenal insufficiency
Nephrotic syndrome
Ureteral obstruction
Pulmonary hypertrophic osteoarthropathy (digital clubbing)
Pericardial effusion
Pericardial tamponade
Superior vena cava obstruction
Spinal cord compression

TABLE 23-3 ■ Ectopic Hormone Production

HORMONE	ASSOCIATED CANCER	MANIFESTATIONS
Corticotropin	Lung cancer (small cell), thyroid cancer (medullary), thymoma, carcinoid, islet cell tumor	Cushing's syndrome
Antidiuretic hormone	Lung cancer (small cell), pancreatic cancer, lymphoma	Water intoxication
Gonadotropin	Lung (large cell), ovarian, adrenal cancer	Gynecomastia, precocious puberty
Parathyroid hormone	Lung, kidney, pancreatic, ovarian cancer	Hyperpigmentation, hyperparathyroidism
Thyrotropin	Choriocarcinoma, testicular (embryonal) cancer	Hyperthyroidism
Thyrocalcitonin	Thyroid (medullary)	Hypocalcemia
Insulin	Retroperitoneal tumors	Hypoglycemia

B. **Neuromuscular Abnormalities.** These occur in 5% to 10% of patients. The most common is the skeletal muscle weakness (myasthenic syndrome) associated with lung cancer. About 80% of paraneoplastic neurologic syndromes manifest *before* the diagnosis of cancer. Eaton-Lambert syndrome and myasthenia gravis can occur in association with lung cancer and thymoma.

C. **Endocrine Abnormalities and Ectopic Hormone Production.** Active hormones are produced by a number of tumors, resulting in predictable physiologic effects (Table 23-3), including SIADH.

D. **Hypercalcemia.** In hospitalized patients, hypercalcemia is most often caused by cancer, reflecting local osteolytic activity from bone metastases (especially breast cancer) or the ectopic parathyroid hormonal activity associated with tumors of the kidneys, lungs, pancreas, or ovaries. Hypercalcemia occurring in patients with cancer may manifest as lethargy and coma, polyuria, and/or dehydration.

E. Cushing's Syndrome. Often associated with neuroendocrine tumors of the lung, Cushing's syndrome is caused by excess secretion of adrenocorticotropic hormone (ACTH) or corticotropin-releasing factor (CRF). Symptoms include hypertension, weight gain, central obesity, and edema. Diagnosis is via serum levels of ACTH or CRF and performance of a dexamethasone suppression test, in which dexamethasone administration fails to suppress cortisol production. Treatment is with agents that block steroid production (ketoconazole, mitotane).

F. Hypoglycemia. Hypoglycemia occurs with insulin-producing islet cell tumors of the pancreas or non–islet cell tumors of the pancreas that produce insulin-like growth factor 2 (IGF-2).

G. Renal Abnormalities. Membranous glomerulonephritis, nephrotic syndrome, and amyloidosis (most often associated with renal cell carcinoma) may occur.

H. Dermatologic and Rheumatologic Abnormalities

a. Acanthosis nigricans: thickening and hyperpigmentation of the skin. When found on the palms, it is always associated with cancer, usually adenocarcinoma.

b. Dermatomyositis: skin changes (including rash on the eyelids and hands) and proximal muscle weakness. It is most often associated with ovarian, breast, lung, prostate, and colorectal cancer.

c. Hypertrophic osteoarthropathy (clubbing): subperiosteal bone deposition. It is usually associated with intrathoracic tumors.

d. Hematologic abnormalities: eosinophilia is related to production of specific interleukins (ILs), most often seen in lymphoma and leukemia. Granulocytosis can occur with solid tumors, particularly large cell cancer. Pure red cell aplasia is associated with thymoma, and also leukemia and lymphoma. Thrombocytosis (platelet count >400,000/mm^3) is associated with underlying malignancy in one third of cases and is caused by tumor-released cytokines (IL-6).

VII. LOCAL TUMOR EFFECTS

A. Superior Vena Cava Obstruction. This complication is caused by spread of cancer into the mediastinum or directly into the caval wall, resulting in engorgement of veins above the level of the heart, edema of the arms and face, and sometimes dyspnea, hoarseness, and airway obstruction. Increased intracranial pressure (ICP)caused by increased cerebral venous pressure may cause nausea, seizures, and decreased levels of consciousness. Treatment is prompt radiation or chemotherapy to decrease the size of the tumor and relieve venous and airway obstruction. Bronchoscopy and/or mediastinoscopy to obtain a tissue diagnosis may be very hazardous in the presence of co-existing airway obstruction and increased pressure in the mediastinal veins.

B. Spinal Cord Compression. Tumor or metastases in the epidural space (breast, lung, prostate, lymphoma) may cause spinal cord compression. Radiation therapy is most useful when neurologic deficits are only partial or evolving. Corticosteroids can minimize inflammation and edema. After total paralysis is present, treatment results are poor.

C. Increased ICP. Increased ICP caused by metastatic tumors can manifest as mental deterioration, focal neurologic deficits, or seizures. Treatment includes corticosteroids, diuretics, mannitol, radiation therapy, and, in the case of single metastatic lesions, surgical resection. Intrathecal chemotherapy is needed if the tumor involves the meninges.

VIII. TREATMENT OF ACUTE AND CHRONIC PAIN

Pain can result from pathologic fractures, tumor invasion, surgery, radiation, and chemotherapy. Treatment of pain is an essential part of cancer management.

1. **Pathophysiology.** Cancer pain may be subdivided into nociceptive and neuropathic pain.

a. ***Nociceptive Pain.*** This category includes somatic and visceral pain and refers to pain caused by the stimulation of nociceptors in somatic (bones, muscle) or visceral structures. It typically responds to both nonopioids and opioids.
b. ***Neuropathic Pain.*** Neuropathic pain involves peripheral or central afferent neural pathways, is commonly described as burning or lancinating, and responds poorly to opioids.
c. ***Trauma Associated with Surgery.*** Surgery for removal of cancerous tissue may cause both acute and chronic pain. Multimodal analgesia with local anesthetics and gabapentin may be used for treatment. Gabapentin has been shown to reduce analgesic requirements for acute postoperative pain but does not significantly affect the development of chronic pain.

2. **Drug Therapy**
   a. ***Nonsteroidal Antiinflammatory Drugs (NSAIDs).*** NSAIDs and acetaminophen are often initial therapy. NSAIDs are especially effective for managing bone pain, the most common cause of cancer pain.
   b. ***Codeine.*** Codeine or one of its analogues is often the next step in management of moderate to severe pain.
   c. ***Opioids.*** Often-used opioids include morphine (routes of administration include oral, intravenous, subcutaneous, epidural, intrathecal, transmucosal, transdermal) and fentanyl (transdermal, transmucosal). There is no limit in dosing morphine and other μ-agonist opioids to treat cancer pain. Tolerance to these drugs occurs, but addiction is rare when these drugs are used correctly.
   d. ***Tricyclic Antidepressant Drugs (TCAs).*** TCAs are recommended for depression and appear to have direct analgesic effects that potentiate those of opioids.
   e. ***Anticonvulsants.*** Anticonvulsants are useful for management of chronic neuropathic pain.
   f. ***Corticosteroids.*** These agents can decrease pain perception, have a sparing effect on opioid requirements, improve mood, increase appetite, and lead to weight gain.
   g. ***Adjunct Agents.*** Ketamine and gabapentin are adjunct agents.
3. **Neuraxial Analgesia.** Neuraxial analgesia provides effective pain control after cancer surgery. Neuraxial analgesia with local anesthetics provides immediate pain relief in patients whose pain cannot be relieved with oral or intravenous analgesics. Morphine may be administered intrathecally or epidurally. Spinal opioids may be delivered for weeks to months via a long-term, subcutaneously tunneled, exteriorized catheter or an implanted intrathecal or epidural drug delivery system. Some patients require an additional low concentration of neuraxial local anesthetic to achieve adequate pain control.
4. **Neurolytic Procedures.** Neurolytic procedures intended to destroy sensory components of nerves may help control pain but also destroy motor and autonomic nervous system fibers. Constant pain is more amenable to destructive nerve blocks than is intermittent pain. Neurolytic celiac plexus block (alcohol, phenol) has been used to treat pain originating from abdominal viscera—for example, from pancreatic cancer—and may last as long as 6 months.
5. **Neurosurgical Procedures.** Neuroablative or neurostimulatory procedures are reserved for patients unresponsive to other, less invasive procedures. Cordotomy (interruption of the spinothalamic tract in the spinal cord) is considered for unilateral pain involving the lower extremity, thorax, or upper extremity. Dorsal rhizotomy (interruption of sensory nerve roots) is used when pain is localized to specific dermatomal levels. Dorsal column stimulators or deep brain stimulators may be used in selected patients.

IX. MANAGEMENT OF ANESTHESIA

Preoperative evaluation of patients with cancer includes consideration of the pathophysiologic effects of the disease (see Tables 23-2 and 23-3) and recognition of the potential adverse effects of cancer chemotherapeutic drugs (see Table 23-1). Preoperative tests to detect side effects of chemotherapy are listed in Table 23-4.

TABLE 23-4 ■ Preoperative Tests in Patients with Cancer

Hematocrit
Platelet count
White blood cell count
Prothrombin time
Electrolytes
Liver function tests
Renal function tests
Blood glucose concentrations
Arterial blood gases
Chest radiography
Electrocardiography

A. Side Effects of Chemotherapy

1. **Pulmonary and Cardiac Toxicity.** A history of drug-induced pulmonary fibrosis (dyspnea, nonproductive cough) or congestive heart failure will influence anesthesia management. Bleomycin-treated patients are vulnerable to the development of interstitial pulmonary edema because of impaired lymphatic drainage from the pulmonary fibrosis. Bleomycin therapy may increase the risk of oxygen toxicity in the presence of high inspired oxygen concentrations, and it is prudent to use the minimum oxygen concentration that provides the desired Spo_2. The myocardial depressant effects of anesthetic drugs may be enhanced in patients with drug-induced cardiac toxicity.

B. Preoperative Preparation. Correction of nutrient deficiencies, anemia, coagulopathy, and electrolyte abnormalities may be necessary. The presence of hepatic or renal dysfunction may influence the choice of anesthetic drugs and muscle relaxants.

C. Intraoperative Considerations. Attention to aseptic technique is critical because immunosuppression occurs with most chemotherapeutic agents. Cancer patients may have life-threatening airway difficulties and upper airway obstruction with head, neck, and chest tumors. Those who have been receiving corticosteroids for longer than 3 weeks are at risk of adrenal suppression. Steroid replacement (hydrocortisone 100 mg intravenously [IV] at induction and every 8 hours for 24 hours) should be considered. Anesthetics may have immunomodulatory properties (see Chapter 24), some of which may promote the proliferation of tumor cells. Baseline peripheral neuropathies should be documented, particularly if regional anesthetic techniques are used. Infectious and thromboembolic prophylaxis should be considered.

D. Postoperative Considerations. Postoperative mechanical ventilation may be required, particularly after invasive or prolonged operations and in patients with drug-induced pulmonary fibrosis. Patients with drug-induced cardiac toxicity are more likely to experience postoperative cardiac complications.

X. COMMON CANCERS ENCOUNTERED IN CLINICAL PRACTICE

A. Lung Cancer. Lung cancer is the leading cause of adult cancer deaths and accounts for nearly one third of all cancer deaths in the United States. It is largely a preventable disease, because more than 90% of lung cancer deaths are related to cigarette smoking.

1. **Etiology.** In addition to cigarette smoking, lung cancer is associated with marijuana smoking, ionizing radiation, asbestos exposure, and exposure to radon gas.
2. **Signs and Symptoms.** Symptoms usually reflect features related to the extent of the disease, including local and regional manifestations, signs and symptoms of metastatic disease, and various paraneoplastic syndromes related indirectly to the cancer (see Table 23-2).

3. **Histologic Subtypes.** Clinical manifestations of lung cancer vary with the histologic subtype. *Squamous cell cancer* arise in major bronchi or their primary divisions (central origin) and tend to grow slowly. *Adenocarcinomas* usually originate in the lunch periphery and have a tendency to invade the pleura. *Large cell carcinomas* are usually peripheral in origin and metastasize early, especially to the central nervous system. *Small cell carcinomas* are of bronchial origin, invade the lymphatic system early, and metastasize widely. They are often associated with paraneoplastic syndromes.
4. **Diagnosis.** Cytologic analysis of sputum is often sufficient for the diagnosis. Flexible fiberoptic bronchoscopy with biopsy, brushings, or washings may be used in initial evaluation. Peripheral lung lesions can be diagnosed by percutaneous fine-needle aspiration guided by fluoroscopy, ultrasonography, or computed tomography. Video-assisted thoracoscopic surgery is useful for diagnosing peripheral lung lesions and pleura-based tumors. Mediastinoscopy and video-assisted thoracoscopy are employed to perform biopsy of the lymph nodes and stage the tumor.
5. **Treatment.** Surgical resection (lobectomy, pneumonectomy) is the most effective treatment. Pulmonary function testing can help determine candidacy for surgery ($FEV_1 > 2$ L, and DLCO > 80% are favorable predictors; predicted postoperative $FEV_1 < 0.8$ L predicts poor outcome). Surgery has little effect on survival when the disease has spread to unilateral mediastinal lymph nodes. The 5-year survival is unaffected by radiation, chemotherapy, immunotherapy, and combinations of these treatments. Radiotherapy is effective in palliating symptoms from tumor invasion in most patients. Radiation therapy with adjunct chemotherapy is preferred for small cell carcinoma.
6. **Management of Anesthesia.** In patients with lung cancer, anesthesia management includes preoperative consideration of tumor-induced effects such as malnutrition, pneumonia, pain, and ectopic endocrine effects, including hyponatremia (see Table 23-3). When resection of lung tissue is planned, it is important to evaluate underlying pulmonary and cardiac function, especially for the presence of pulmonary hypertension.
   a. ***Mediastinoscopy.*** Hemorrhage and pneumothorax are the most commonly encountered complications of mediastinoscopy. The mediastinoscope can exert pressure on the right innominate artery, with loss of the distal pulse and an erroneous diagnosis of cardiac arrest. Compression of the right innominate artery, of which the right carotid artery is a branch, may manifest as a postoperative neurologic deficit. Bradycardia can occur because of stretching of the vagus nerve or tracheal compression by the mediastinoscope.

B. **Colorectal Cancer.** Colon cancer is second only to lung cancer as a cause of cancer death in the United States.
1. **Etiology.** Most colorectal cancers arise from premalignant adenomatous polyps. Colorectal cancer appears to be increased by high intake of animal fat. Familial history of colon cancer, history of inflammatory bowel disease, and cigarette smoking all increase the risk of colon cancer.
2. **Diagnosis.** Early detection and removal of localized superficial tumors and precancerous lesions in asymptomatic individuals increase the cure rate. Screening programs (digital rectal examination, examination of the stool for occult blood, colonoscopy) are particularly useful for persons with a family history of colon cancer.
3. **Signs and Symptoms.** Signs and symptoms of colorectal cancer reflect the anatomic location of the cancer, ranging from anemia and fatigue (ascending colon) to obstruction (descending colon). Colorectal cancers initially spread to regional lymph nodes and then through the portal venous circulation to the liver, which is the most common visceral site of metastases.
4. **Treatment.** Radical surgical resection, including the blood vessels and lymph nodes draining the involved bowel, offers the best potential for cure. Radiation therapy is a consideration in patients with rectal tumors because the risk of recurrence after surgery is significant.

5. **Management of Anesthesia.** For surgical resection of colorectal cancers, anesthesia may be influenced by anemia and the effects of metastatic lesions in liver, lung, bone, or brain. Blood transfusion during surgical resection of colorectal cancers appears to be associated with a *decrease* in the length of patient survival, possibly because of immunosuppression produced by transfused blood. For this reason, careful review of the risks and benefits of blood transfusion in these patients is prudent.

C. **Prostate Cancer.** Prostate cancer is the second leading cause of cancer death among men.

1. **Diagnosis.** Increased serum PSA concentration (particularly levels >10 ng/mL) may indicate the presence of prostate cancer in asymptomatic men and prompt a digital rectal examination. Rectal examination can evaluate only the posterior and lateral aspects of the prostate. If the rectal examination indicates the possible presence of cancer, transrectal ultrasonography and biopsy are needed regardless of the PSA concentration.
2. **Treatment.** Focal, well-differentiated prostate cancers are usually cured by transurethral resection. If lymph nodes are involved, radical prostatectomy or definitive radiation therapy may be recommended. Radiation therapy can be delivered either by an external beam or by implantation of radioactive seeds. Hormone therapy is indicated for management of metastatic prostate cancer because most of these tumors are under the trophic influence of androgens. When advanced prostate cancers become resistant to hormone therapy, incapacitating bone pain often develops. Systemic chemotherapy with mitoxantrone plus corticosteroids or estramustine plus a taxane may be effective in palliating pain. In the terminal phases of the disease, high doses of prednisone for short periods may produce subjective improvement.

D. **Breast Cancer.** Women in the United States have a 12% lifetime risk of developing breast cancer.

1. **Risk Factors.** The principal risk factors for development of breast cancer are increasing age and family history. Other risk factors are early menarche, late menopause, late first pregnancy, and nulliparity. Two breast cancer susceptibility genes *(BRCA1, BRCA2)* are mutations that are inherited as autosomal dominant traits.
2. **Screening Strategies.** For breast cancer, screening strategies include the triad of breast self-examination, clinical breast examination by a professional, and screening mammography.
3. **Prognosis.** Axillary lymph node invasion and tumor size are the two most important determinants of outcome in patients with early breast cancer. The absence of estrogen and progesterone receptor expression in the tumor is associated with a poorer prognosis.
4. **Treatment**
   a. ***Surgery.*** Breast conservation therapy (lumpectomy with radiation therapy), simple mastectomy, and modified radical mastectomy provide similar survival rates. Distant micrometastatic disease is correlated with the number of lymph nodes containing tumor invasion. Morbidity associated with breast cancer surgery is largely related to side effects of lymph node dissection (lymphedema, restricted arm motion).
   b. ***Radiation.*** This is an important component of breast conservation therapy because lumpectomy alone is associated with a high incidence of recurrence. High-dose radiation therapy may be associated with brachial plexopathy or nerve damage, pneumonitis, pulmonary fibrosis, and cardiac injury.
   c. ***Systemic Treatment.*** Many women with early-stage breast cancer already have distant micrometastases at the time of diagnosis. Tamoxifen therapy, chemotherapy, and ovarian ablation are intended to prevent or delay recurrence of the disease. The most serious late sequelae of chemotherapy are leukemia and doxorubicin-induced cardiac impairment.
   d. ***Supportive Treatment.*** In advanced breast cancer, supportive treatment includes administration of bisphosphonates (pamidronate, clodronate) in addition to hormone therapy or chemotherapy to decrease bone pain. Adequate pain control is usually achieved with sustained-release oral and/or transdermal opioid preparations.
5. **Management of Anesthesia.** Preoperative evaluation includes a review of potential side effects related to chemotherapy. Placement of intravenous catheters in the arm at risk of

lymphedema is avoided because of exacerbation of lymphedema and susceptibility to infection. The arm should also be protected from compression (as with a blood pressure cuff) and heat exposure. The presence of bone pain and pathologic fractures is noted when considering regional anesthesia and when positioning patients. If isosulfan blue dye is injected during the surgical procedure, pulse oximetry may demonstrate a transient spurious decrease in the measured Spo_2 value.

XI. LESS COMMON CANCERS ENCOUNTERED IN CLINICAL PRACTICE

A. **Cardiac Tumors.** These may be primary or secondary and benign or malignant. Metastatic cardiac involvement, usually from adjacent lung cancer, occurs 20 to 40 times more often than a primary malignant cardiac tumor.

1. **Cardiac Myxomas.** Most benign cardiac tumors that occur in adults are cardiac myxomas.
   a. ***Signs and Symptoms.*** Symptoms reflect interference with filling and emptying of the involved cardiac chamber (heart failure, syncope, dysrhythmias, pulmonary hypertension) and emboli composed of myxomatous material or thrombi that have formed on the tumor.
   b. ***Diagnosis.*** Echocardiography can determine the location, size, shape, attachment, and mobility of cardiac myxomas.
   c. ***Treatment.*** Surgical resection of cardiac myxomas is usually curative.
   d. ***Management of Anesthesia.*** The possibility of low cardiac output and arterial hypoxemia caused by obstruction at the mitral or tricuspid valve are considered. Symptoms of obstruction may be exacerbated by changes in body position. The presence of a right atrial myxoma prohibits placement of right atrial or pulmonary artery catheters.

B. **Head and Neck Cancers.** These cancers account for approximately 5% of all cancers in the United States, with a predominance in men older than 50 years of age. Most patients have a history of excessive alcohol use and cigarette smoking. The most common sites of metastases are lung, liver, and bone. Preoperative nutritional therapy may be indicated before surgical resection of the tumor.

C. **Thyroid Cancer.** Papillary and follicular thyroid cancers are among the most curable cancers. Medullary thyroid cancers may be associated with pheochromocytomas in an autosomal dominant disorder known as *multiple endocrine neoplasia type 2.* Subtotal or total thyroidectomy is the primary treatment, and external beam radiation can be used for palliative treatment of obstruction and bony metastases.

D. **Esophageal Cancer.** Excessive alcohol consumption and cigarette smoking are risk factors for development of *squamous cell carcinoma* of the esophagus. Barrett's esophagus, a complication of gastroesophageal reflux disease, is the primary risk factor for *adenocarcinoma.* The likelihood of underlying alcohol-induced liver disease, chronic obstructive pulmonary disease from cigarette smoking, and cross-tolerance with anesthetic drugs in alcohol abusers is a consideration during anesthetic management of patients with esophageal cancer.

E. **Gastric Cancer.** Achlorhydria (loss of gastric acidity), pernicious anemia, chronic gastritis, and *Helicobacter* infection contribute to the development of gastric cancer. Gastric cancer is usually far advanced when signs such as weight loss, palpable epigastric mass, jaundice, or ascites appear. Complete surgical resection is the only treatment that may be curative.

F. **Liver Cancer.** Liver cancer occurs most often in men with liver disease caused by hepatitis B or hepatitis C virus, alcohol consumption, or hemochromatosis. Radical surgical resection or liver transplantation offers the only hope for survival, but most patients with liver cancer are not surgical candidates because of extensive cirrhosis, impaired liver function, and the presence of extrahepatic disease.

G. **Pancreatic Cancer.** Abdominal pain, anorexia, and weight loss are the usual initial symptoms. Pain suggests retroperitoneal invasion, and jaundice reflects biliary obstruction in patients with tumor in the head of the pancreas. Complete surgical resection (total pancreatectomy and pancreaticoduodenectomy or Whipple's procedure) is the only effective treatment of ductal pancreatic cancer. The median survival for patients with unresectable tumors is 5 months. Celiac plexus block with alcohol or phenol is the most effective intervention for treating the pain associated with pancreatic cancer.

H. Renal Cell Cancer. This type of cancer most often manifests itself as hematuria, mild anemia, and flank pain. Risk factors include a family history of renal cancer and cigarette smoking. Paraneoplastic syndromes, especially hypercalcemia resulting from ectopic parathyroid hormone secretion and erythrocytosis caused by ectopic erythropoietin production, are common.

I. Bladder Cancer. Bladder cancer is associated with cigarette smoking and chronic exposure to chemicals used in the dye, leather, and rubber industries. The most common presenting feature is hematuria. Treatment of noninvasive bladder cancer includes endoscopic resection and intravesical chemotherapy.

J. Testicular Cancer. This is the most common cancer in young men and represents a tumor that can be cured even when distant metastases are present. Testicular cancer usually manifests as a painless testicular mass and is diagnosed at the time of orchiectomy.

K. Uterine Cervix Cancer. This is the most common gynecologic cancer in girls and women 15 to 34 years old. HPV infection of the uterine cervix is the principal cause. Carcinoma in situ as detected by a Papanicolaou smear is treated with a cone biopsy, whereas more extensive local disease or disease that has metastasized is treated with some combination of surgery, radiation therapy, and chemotherapy.

L. Uterine Cancer. Most often, uterine cancer manifests as postmenopausal or irregular bleeding. Initial evaluation is usually fractional dilation and curettage. In the absence of metastatic disease, a total abdominal hysterectomy and bilateral salpingo-oophorectomy with or without radiation is the treatment.

M. Ovarian Cancer. Advanced disease is usually present by the time the cancer is discovered. Aggressive surgical tumor debulking, even if all cancer cannot be removed, improves the length and quality of survival. Intraperitoneal chemotherapy is indicated postoperatively in most women and is usually well tolerated.

N. Cutaneous Melanoma. The initial treatment of a suspected lesion is wide and deep excisional biopsy, often with sentinel node mapping. Melanoma can metastasize to virtually any organ. Treatment of metastatic melanoma is directed at palliation and can include resection of a solitary metastasis, simple or combination chemotherapy, and immunotherapy.

O. Bone Cancer

1. **Multiple Myeloma.** Multiple myeloma (plasma cell myeloma, myelomatosis) is characterized by poorly controlled growth of a single clone of plasma cells that produce a monoclonal immunoglobulin.
   a. ***Signs and Symptoms.*** Signs and symptoms are bone pain (often from vertebral collapse), anemia, thrombocytopenia, neutropenia, hypercalcemia (from bone destruction), renal failure (from deposition of Bence Jones protein in renal tubules or renal amyloidosis), and recurrent bacterial infection (caused by bone marrow invasion by tumor cells and decreased cell-mediated immunity).
   b. ***Treatment.*** Autologous stem cell transplantation and chemotherapy are treatments. Palliative radiation is limited to patients who have disabling pain and a well-defined focal process that has not responded to chemotherapy. Hypercalcemia requires prompt treatment with intravenous saline infusion and administration of furosemide.
   c. ***Management of Anesthesia.*** The presence of compression fractures requires caution when positioning these patients. Pathologic fractures of the ribs may impair ventilation and predispose to development of pneumonia.
2. **Osteosarcoma.** This type of cancer occurs most often in adolescents and typically involves the distal femur and proximal tibia. Treatment consists of combination chemotherapy followed by surgical excision or amputation.

3. **Ewing's Tumor.** Ewing's tumor or sarcoma usually occurs in children and young adults and most often involves the pelvis, femur, and tibia. Ewing's sarcoma is highly malignant, and metastatic disease is often present at the time of diagnosis. Treatment consists of surgery, local radiation, and combination chemotherapy.
4. **Chondrosarcoma.** Chondrosarcoma usually involves the pelvis, ribs, or upper end of the femur or humerus in young or middle-aged adults. This tumor is treated by radical surgical excision of larger lesions and radiation of smaller lesions.

XII. LYMPHOMAS AND LEUKEMIAS

A. **Hodgkin's Disease.** Hodgkin's disease is a lymphoma that appears to have infective (Epstein-Barr virus), genetic, and environmental associations. Impaired immunity as seen in patients after organ transplantation or in patients who are human immunodeficiency virus (HIV) positive appears to predispose to lymphoma.
   1. **Signs and Symptoms.** These include lymphadenopathy, night sweats, and unexplained weight loss. Moderately severe anemia is often present. Peripheral neuropathy and spinal cord compression may occur as a direct result of tumor growth.
   2. **Treatment.** Radiation therapy is curative for localized early-stage Hodgkin's disease. Bulkier or more advanced Hodgkin's disease is treated by combination chemotherapy.

B. **Non-Hodgkin's Lymphoma.** Non-Hodgkin's lymphoma can be of B-cell, T-cell or natural killer cell origin. Chemotherapy is the first-line treatment. Stem cell transplantation may be considered in refractory cases.

C. **Leukemia.** The uncontrolled production of leukocytes due to cancerous mutation of lymphogenous cells or myelogenous cells is called *leukemia.* Lymphocytic leukemias begin in lymph nodes, whereas myeloid leukemia begins in the bone marrow with spread to extramedullary organs. Bone marrow failure is the cause of fatal infection or hemorrhage as a result of thrombocytopenia. Leukemia cells may also infiltrate the liver, spleen, lymph nodes, and meninges, producing organ dysfunction.
   1. **Acute Lymphoblastic Leukemia.** This form of leukemia accounts for approximately 15% of all leukemias in adults. CNS dysfunction is common. Up to 80% of children and 40% of adults can be cured by chemotherapy.
   2. **Chronic Lymphocytic Leukemia.** Chronic lymphocytic leukemia rarely occurs in children and accounts for approximately 25% of all leukemias. Signs and symptoms are highly variable, with the extent of bone marrow infiltration often determining the clinical course. Corticosteroid therapy, splenectomy, and single or combination chemotherapy are usual treatments. Radiation therapy is used to treat localized nodal masses or splenomegaly. The 5-year survival rate is 75%.

3. **Acute Myeloid Leukemia.** This type of leukemia is characterized by an increase in the number of myeloid cells in bone marrow and arrest of their maturation, resulting in hematopoietic insufficiency (granulocytopenia, thrombocytopenia, anemia). Many patients have life-threatening infections on presentation. Other presenting signs and symptoms include fatigue, bleeding gums or nosebleeds, pallor, and headache. Hyperleukocytosis (>100,000 cells/mm^3) can result in signs of leukostasis with ocular and cerebrovascular dysfunction or bleeding. Chemotherapy and bone marrow transplantation are usual treatments. Retinoic acid syndrome is a potentially lethal combination of induction therapy in patients with acute promyelocytic leukemia, who are treated with all-*trans* retinoic acid (tretinoin). Respiratory distress, pulmonary infiltrates, fever, and hypotension are common. High-dose corticosteroids are the most common treatment.
   4. **Chronic Myeloid Leukemia.** Chronic myeloid leukemia manifests as myeloid leukocytosis with splenomegaly. Cytoreduction therapy with hydroxyurea, chemotherapy, leukapheresis, and splenectomy may be necessary. Bone marrow transplantation may be considered.

TABLE 23-5 ■ Manifestations of Acute Graft-Versus-Host Disease

Desquamation, erythroderma, maculopapular rash
Interstitial pneumonitis
Gastritis, diarrhea, abdominal cramping
Mucosal ulceration and mucositis
Hepatitis with coagulopathy
Glomerulonephritis, nephrotic syndrome
Immunodeficiency and pancytopenia

D. Treatment of Leukemia

1. **Chemotherapy.** Chemotherapy is intended to decrease the number of tumor cells so organomegaly regresses and function of the bone marrow improves. Drugs used for chemotherapy are principally those that depress bone marrow activity. Therefore hemorrhage and infection will determine the maximum doses of the chemotherapeutic drugs. Destruction of tumor cells by chemotherapy produces a uric acid load that may result in urate nephropathy and/or gouty arthritis.
2. **Bone Marrow Transplantation.** Bone marrow transplantation offers a potential cure for several otherwise fatal diseases. Autologous bone marrow transplantation entails collection of the patient's own bone marrow for subsequent reinfusion, and allogeneic transplantation uses bone marrow or peripheral blood elements from an immunocompatible donor. Recipients undergo a combination of total body radiation and chemotherapy to achieve bone marrow ablation prior to infusion of the marrow elements.
   a. ***Anesthesia for Bone Marrow Transplantation.*** General or regional anesthesia is required during aspiration of bone marrow from the iliac crests. Nitrous oxide might be avoided in the donor because of potential bone marrow depression associated with this drug. However, there is no evidence that nitrous oxide administered during bone marrow harvesting adversely affects marrow engraftment and subsequent function. Blood replacement may be necessary, either with autologous blood transfusion or by reinfusion of separated erythrocytes obtained during the harvest.
   b. ***Complications of Bone Marrow Transplantation***
      i. ***Graft-versus-Host Disease*** *(GVHD; Table 23-5).* GVHD is a life-threatening complication of bone marrow transplantation in which the donor cells attack antigens on the recipient's cells. It manifests as organ system dysfunction, most often involving the skin (rash, desquamation), liver (jaundice), and GI tract (diarrhea). Acute GVHD occurs 30 to 60 days after transplant and is usually treated with high-dose corticosteroids. *Extracorporeal photopheresis* involves removing a patient's white blood cells, exposing them to ultraviolet light, and reinfusing them. This induces apoptosis and an acute inflammatory response that reduces risk of graft rejection. Chronic GVHD has autoimmune features such as dermal sclerosis, xerostomia, fasciitis, myositis, transaminitis, pericarditis, nephritis, and restrictive lung disease.
      ii. ***Graft Rejection.*** Rejection occurs when immunologically competent cells of host origin destroy the cells of donor origin.
      iii. ***Pulmonary Complications.*** Infection, adult respiratory distress syndrome, chemotherapy-induced lung damage, and interstitial pneumonia (often cytomegalovirus or fungal infection) may occur.
      iv. ***Venoocclusive Disease of the Liver.*** This may manifest as jaundice, tender hepatomegaly, ascites, and weight gain. Progressive hepatic failure and multiorgan failure can develop, and mortality is high.

CHAPTER 24

Diseases Related to Immune System Dysfunction

The effects of the immune system can be divided into *innate immunity* (rapid response consisting of neutrophils, macrophages, monocytes, killer cells, the complement system, acute-phase proteins, and contact activation pathways), which has no specific memory, and *adaptive or acquired immunity* (delayed response, mediated by B cells, antibodies, and cellular response via T cells), which has memory for previous exposures. Defects specific to each of these types of immunity generally predispose to infection with a characteristic subset of pathogenic organisms (Table 24-1). Both innate and acquired immunity exhibit defects that can be divided into three injury categories: those caused by (1) an inadequate immune response, (2) an excessive immune response, and (3) misdirection of the immune response.

I. INADEQUATE INNATE IMMUNITY

A. **Neutropenia.** An absolute granulocyte count below $1500/mm^3$ is neutropenia. Infectious risk increases when the granulocyte count is less than $500/mm^3$ and increases dramatically if the count decreases to less than $100/mm^3$ (Table 24-2).

B. **Abnormalities of Phagocytosis.** Abnormalities include chronic granulomatous disease (high rate of staphylococcal infection), neutrophil glucose 6-phosphate dehydrogenase (G6PD) deficiency (infections with catalase-positive bacteria), Chédiak-Higashi syndrome (partial albinism, frequent bacterial infections, mild bleeding disorder, neuropathy, cranial nerve defects), specific granule deficiency syndrome (impaired neutrophil chemotaxis and bactericidal activity—recurrent abscesses and fungal infections) and leukocyte adhesion deficiency.

C. **Management of Patients with Neutropenia or Abnormal Phagocytosis.** Recombinant granulocyte colony-stimulating factor (G-CSF) reduce the duration of neutropenia in patients undergoing chemotherapy and treatment of HIV infection. It also shortens the length of antibiotic therapy and reduces the risk of life-threatening bacteremia or fungemia in neutropenic patients.

D. **Deficiencies in Components of the Complement System** (Table 24-3)

E. **Hyposplenism.** Splenectomy is the most common cause of splenic dysfunction, but various clinical conditions (e.g., sickle cell anemia) may lead to impaired systemic function. Hyposplenism predisposes patients to infection with *Streptococcus pneumoniae, Neisseria meningitides, Escherichia coli,* and *Haemophilus influenzae,* and malaria. Treatment is prevention via immunization against *S. pneumoniae, H. influenzae* type b, and *N. meningitides.* Penicillin prophylaxis after splenectomy in children younger than age 5 is now being questioned due to emergence of antibiotic-resistant bacteria and the effectiveness of immunization in most patients.

II. EXCESSIVE INNATE IMMUNITY

A. **Neutrophilia.** An absolute granulocyte count higher than $7000\,mm^3$ defines neutrophilia. An increase in the granulocyte count does not produce signs or symptoms unless the count exceeds $100{,}000/mm^3$. Major causes of neutrophilia are listed in Table 24-4. Such marked

TABLE 24-1 ■ **Pathogens Associated with Specific Immune Defects**

ORGANISM	PHAGOCYTE DEFECT	COMPLEMENT DEFECT	B-CELL DEFECT AND ANTIBODY DEFICIENCY	T-CELL DEFECT OR DEFICIENCY	COMBINED B- AND T-CELL DEFICIENCY
Bacteria	Staphylococci, *Pseudomonas*, enteric flora	*Neisseria*, pyogenic bacteria	Streptococci, staphylococci, *Haemophilus, Neisseria meningitides*	Bacterial sepsis, especially *Salmonella typhi*	Similar to antibody deficiency, especially *N. meningitides*
Viruses			Enteroviruses	Cytomegalovirus, Epstein-Barr virus, varicella, chronic respiratory and intestinal viruses	All
Mycobacteria	Nontuberculous mycobacteria			Nontuberculous mycobacteria	
Fungi	*Candida, Nocardia, Aspergillus*		Severe intestinal giardiasis	*Candida*, *Pneumocystis, Histoplasma, Aspergillus*	Similar to T-cell defect, especially *Pneumocystis* and *Toxoplasma*
Special features			Recurrent sinopulmonary infections, sepsis, chronic meningitis	Aggressive disease with opportunistic pathogens, failure to clear infections	

TABLE 24-2 ■ Causes of Neutropenia

Pediatric patients	Neonatal sepsis Transient neonatal neutropenia (caused by maternal disease or drugs) Cyclic neutropenia (autosomal dominant genetic disorder) Kostmann's syndrome (autosomal recessive disorder of neutrophil maturation)
Adult patients	Acquired neutropenia (chemotherapy of cancer or HIV infection) Other drug side effects (gold salts, chloramphenicol, antithyroid mediations, analgesics, tricyclic antidepressants, phenothiazines) Autoimmune-related neutropenia (lupus, rheumatoid arthritis, Felty's syndrome) Lymphoma, other myeloproliferative diseases Severe liver disease with portal hypertension Sepsis Alcoholism HIV infection Chronic benign neutropenia

HIV, Human immunodeficiency virus.

TABLE 24-3 ■ Deficiencies of Complement System Components

Early components of the classic pathway: C1q, C1r, C2, C4	Autoimmune inflammatory disorders resembling lupus
Common pathway component C3	Usually fatal in utero
Terminal components C5-C8	Recurrent infection and rheumatic disease
C9 and components of the alternate pathway	Neisserial infection
Factor H deficiency	Familial relapsing hemolytic uremic syndrome
C1 inhibitor deficiency	Hereditary angioedema

TABLE 24-4 ■ Clinical Conditions Associated with Neutrophilia

DISORDER	MECHANISM
Infection, inflammation	Increased neutrophil production and marrow release of neutrophils
Stress, metabolic disorders (preeclampsia, diabetic ketoacidosis)	Increased neutrophil production
Steroid treatment	Demargination of neutrophils
Myeloproliferative disease	Increased marrow neutrophil release and demargination of neutrophils
Splenectomy	Decrease in splenic trapping of neutrophils

leukocytosis is associated with leukostasis which can produce splenic infarction or a decreased oxygen diffusion capacity in the lungs. The clinical features of moderate leukocytosis vary depending on the primary disease underlying the condition.

B. Asthma. Triggers for bronchospasm that are unrelated to the immune system such as exposure to cold, exercise, stress, or inhaled irritants produce *intrinsic* asthma and are considered part of innate immunity. Treatment consists of administration of β-agonists, anticholinergic drugs, corticosteroids, and leukotriene inhibitors.

III. MISDIRECTED INNATE IMMUNITY

A. Angioedema. Episodic edema of the skin and mucous membranes, or angioedema, may be hereditary or acquired.

1. **Hereditary Angioedema.** Most commonly, hereditary angioedema results from an autosomal dominant deficiency or dysfunction of C1 esterase inhibitor, which leads to a release of vasoactive mediators that increase vascular permeability and produce edema.
2. **Acquired Angioedema.** This occurs in some lymphoproliferative disorders because of antibodies to C1 inhibitor. Angiotensin-converting enzyme inhibitors also precipitate angioedema in about 0.5% of patients due to increased availability of bradykinin.
3. **Prophylaxis.** Patients experiencing recurrent angioedema, whether hereditary or acquired, require prophylaxis with danazol or stanozolol (anabolic steroids increase hepatic synthesis of e1 esterase inhibitor) before a stimulating procedure such as endotracheal intubation. Acute attacks should be treated with C1 inhibitor concentrate (25 units/kg) or fresh frozen plasma (2 to 4 units) to replace the deficient enzyme.
4. **Management of Anesthesia.** In patients with hereditary angioedema, consideration should be given to pretreatment before elective surgery in which airway manipulation, including laryngeal mask airway (LMA) placement, is anticipated. C1 inhibitor concentrates should be readily available. Catecholamines and antihistamines are not useful in the treatment of angioedema.
5. **Emergency Airway Management.** During an acute attack, emergency airway management includes administration of supplemental oxygen and endotracheal intubation, with standby personnel and equipment for emergency tracheostomy. Tracheostomy may be extremely difficult in the face of massive airway edema.

IV. INADEQUATE ADAPTIVE IMMUNITY

A. Defects of Antibody Production

1. **X-linked Agammaglobulinemia.** With this inherited defect in maturation of B cells, functional antibody is not produced. Affected boys have pyogenic infections during latter half of the first year of life. Treatment is intravenous immunoglobulin every 3 to 4 months. Most children survive to adulthood.
2. **Selective Immunoglobulin A (IgA) Deficiency.** Selective IgA deficiency occurs in 1 in every 600 to 800 adults. It is characterized by recurrent sinus and pulmonary infections. About 40% of patients produce IgA antibodies, and this subset may have life-threatening anaphylaxis if they receive blood products containing IgA. They therefore need blood components obtained from IgA-deficient donors.
3. **Waldenstrom's Macroglobulinemia.** Malignant plasma cell clone produces IgM, resulting in increased plasma viscosity. The bone marrow, liver, spleen, and lungs are infiltrated with malignant lymphocytes. Treatment is plasmapheresis and/or chemotherapy.
4. **Cold Autoimmune Diseases (Cryoglobulinemia, Cold Hemagglutinin Disease).** Cold autoimmune diseases are characterized by abnormal circulating proteins (IgM or IgA antibodies) that agglutinate in the presence of decreased body temperature (below 33° C).
5. **Amyloidosis.** Amyloidosis includes several disorders characterized by accumulation of insoluble fibrillar proteins (amyloid) in the heart, vascular smooth muscle, kidneys,

adrenal glands, gastrointestinal (GI) tract, peripheral nerves, and skin. Primary amyloidosis is a plasma cell disorder with accumulation of immunoglobulin light chains. Secondary amyloidosis is associated with multiple myeloma, rheumatoid arthritis, and prolonged antigen challenge (chronic infection). Treatment is symptomatic. Patients may be predisposed to hemorrhagic complications owing to trapping of factor X and increased fibrinolysis.

a. ***Macroglossia.*** Occurring in 20% of cases of amyloidosis, macroglossia may cause upper airway obstruction.

b. ***Cardiac Involvement.*** Cardiac effects include heart block, right-sided heart failure, and sudden death.

c. ***Kidney Involvement.*** Nephrotic syndrome may occur.

d. ***GI Involvement.*** GI involvement may cause malabsorption, ileus, delayed gastric emptying, and hepatomegaly.

e. ***Joint and Peripheral Nerve Involvement.*** Decreased range of motion and peripheral nerve entrapments may result.

B. Defects of T Lymphocytes

1. **DiGeorge's Syndrome (Thymic Hypoplasia).** DiGeorge's syndrome includes absent or diminished thymic development, hypoplasia of the thyroid and parathyroid glands, cardiac malformations, and facial dysmorphisms. Degree of immunocompromise correlates with the amount of thymus present, and complete absent of the thymus is associated with a severe combined immunodeficiency syndrome. Complete DiGeorge's syndrome is treated by thymus transplantation or infusion of mature T cells. Partial DiGeorge's syndrome requires no therapy.

2. **Combined Immune System Defects**

a. ***Severe Combined Immunodeficiency (SCI) Syndromes.*** SCI syndromes are caused by several genetic mutations. X-linked SCI accounts for about half of all cases. The only treatment is bone marrow or stem cell transplantation.

b. ***Adenosine Deaminase Deficiency.*** This accounts for 15% of combined immunodeficiency. T-cell death because toxic purine intermediates (normally controlled by adenosine deaminase) accumulate in the T cell. Treatment is bone marrow or stem cell transplantation, or enzyme replacement with bovine adenosine deaminase enzyme.

c. ***Ataxia Telangiectasia.*** Ataxia telangiectasia consists of cerebellar ataxia, oculocutaneous telangiectasias, chronic sinopulmonary disease, and immunodeficiency. Patients are predisposed to production of dysfunction lymphocytes and to malignancy, especially lymphoma or leukemia. Treatment is supportive and includes intravenous immunoglobulin.

V. EXCESSIVE ADAPTIVE IMMUNITY

A. Allergic Reactions. Allergic reactions are classified according to their mechanism. Type I allergic reactions (e.g., anaphylaxis) are IgE mediated and involve mast cells and basophils. Type II reactions mediate cytotoxicity with IgG, IgM, and complement. Type III reactions produce tissue damage via immune complex formation or deposition. Type IV reactions exhibit T lymphocyte–mediated delayed hypersensitivity. Anaphylactoid reactions appear to be caused by mediator release from mast cells and basophils through a *nonimmune* mechanism.

1. **Anaphylaxis.** Anaphylaxis is a life-threatening manifestation of antigen-antibody interaction in which previous exposure to antigens has evoked production of antigen-specific IgE antibodies. Vasoactive mediators released by degranulation of mast cells and basophils are responsible for the clinical manifestations of anaphylaxis (Table 24-5). Incidence of anaphylaxis during anesthesia is 1 in 5000 to 20,000 cases. Estimated mortality is 3% to 6%. Risk factors are history of asthma, longer-duration anesthesia, female sex, multiple past surgeries, and presence of other allergic conditions or systemic mastocytosis.

a. ***Diagnosis.*** Anaphylaxis can be suggested by the often dramatic nature of the clinical manifestations in close temporal relationship to exposure to a particular antigen (may

TABLE 24-5 ■ **Vasoactive Mediators Released During Anaphylaxis**

MEDIATOR	PHYSIOLOGIC EFFECT
Histamine	Increased capillary permeability, peripheral vasodilation, bronchoconstriction
Leukotrienes	Increased capillary permeability, intense bronchoconstriction, negative inotropy, coronary artery vasoconstriction
Prostaglandins	Bronchoconstriction
Eosinophil chemotactic factor	Attraction of eosinophils
Neutrophil chemotactic factor	Attraction of neutrophils
Platelet-activating factor	Platelet aggregation and release of vasoactive amines

mimic pulmonary embolism, acute myocardial infarction, aspiration, or vasovagal reaction).

i. ***Hypotension and Cardiovascular Collapse.*** These may be the only manifestations of anaphylaxis in patients under general anesthesia.
ii. ***Proof of Anaphylaxis.*** Proof lies in an increased plasma tryptase concentration within 1 to 2 hours of the suspected reaction. Plasma histamine concentration returns to baseline within 30 to 60 minutes of an anaphylactic reaction.
iii. ***Identification of the Offending Antigen.*** Identification can be provided by a positive intradermal test result (wheal and flare response), which confirms the presence of specific IgE antibodies.

b. ***Treatment.*** The immediate goals of treatment of anaphylaxis are reversal of hypotension and hypoxemia, replacement of intravascular volume, and inhibition of further cellular degranulation and release of vasoactive mediators (i.e., intravenous fluids; vasopressors such as epinephrine 10 to 100 mcg intravenously, doubled every 1 to 2 minutes until blood pressure increases; antihistamines; bronchodilators; corticosteroids; and support of oxygenation and ventilation) (Table 24-6).

2. **Drug Allergy.** Drug allergy has been implicated in 3.4% to 4.3% of anesthesia-related deaths. Regardless of the mechanism responsible for life-threatening allergic drug reactions, the manifestations and treatment are identical to those of anaphylaxis. Allergic drug reactions must be distinguished from drug intolerance, idiosyncratic reactions, and drug toxicity.

a. ***The Perioperative Period.*** Allergic drug reactions have been reported with most drugs that may be administered during anesthesia (Table 24-7), except possibly ketamine and benzodiazepines. Muscle relaxants are responsible for approximately 60% of perioperative drug-induced allergic reactions.

i. ***Cardiovascular Collapse.*** This is the predominant manifestation of a life-threatening allergic drug reaction in an anesthetized patient. Bronchospasm is present in fewer patients.
ii. ***Latex.*** Cardiovascular collapse during anesthesia and surgery may be caused by latex allergy. Onset is typically more than 30 minutes after exposure. Skin testing can confirm latex hypersensitivity. Questions about itching, conjunctivitis, rhinitis, rash, or wheezing after inflating toy balloons or wearing latex gloves or after dental or gynecologic examinations involving latex gloves may be helpful in identifying sensitized patients. Operating room personnel and patients with spina bifida have an increased incidence of latex allergy.

(a) ***Intraoperative Management.*** A latex-free environment must be maintained. Intravenous and bladder catheters, drains, anesthesia delivery tubing, ventilator bellows,

TABLE 24-6 ■ Management of Anaphylactic Reactions During Anesthesia

PRIMARY TREATMENT
General Measures
Inform the surgeon
Request immediate assistance
Stop administration of all drugs, colloids, blood products
Maintain airway with 100% oxygen
Elevate the legs, if practical
Epinephrine Administration
Titrate dose according to symptom severity and clinical response
Adults: 10 mcg to 1 mg by bolus, repeat every 1-2 min as needed
IV infusion starting at 0.05-1 mcg/kg/min
Children: 1-10 mcg/kg by bolus, repeat every 1-2 min as needed
Fluid Therapy
Crystalloid: normal saline 10-25 mL/kg over 20 min, more as needed
Colloid: 10 mL/kg over 20 min, more as needed
Anaphylaxis Resistant to Epinephrine
Glucagon: 1-5 mg bolus followed by 1-2.5 mg/hr IV infusion
Norepinephrine: 0.05-0.1 mcg/kg/min IV infusion
Vasopressin: 2-10 unit IV bolus followed by 0.01-0.1 unit/min IV infusion
SECONDARY TREATMENT
Bronchodilator
β_2-Agonist for symptomatic treatment of bronchospasm
Antihistamines
Histamine 1 antagonist: diphenhydramine 0.5-1 mg/kg IV
Histamine 2 antagonist: ranitidine 50 mg IV
Corticosteroids
Adults: hydrocortisone 250 mg IV or methylprednisolone 80 mg IV
Children: hydrocortisone 50-100 mg IV or methylprednisolone 2 mg/kg IV
AFTERCARE
Patient may experience relapse; admit for observation
Obtain blood samples for diagnostic testing
Arrange allergy testing at 6-8 wk postoperatively

Adapted from Mertes PM, Tajima K, Regnier-Kimmoun MA, et al. Perioperative anaphylaxis. *Med Clin North Am*. 2010;94:780.

endotracheal tubes, LMAs, nasogastric tubes, blood pressure cuffs, pulse oximeter probes, electrocardiogram pads, and syringes must be latex free.

iii. ***Antibiotics.*** The incidence of life-threatening allergic reactions after administration of cephalosporins is low (0.02%) and is only minimally increased in patients with a history of penicillin allergy.

iv. ***Blood and Plasma Volume Expanders.*** Allergic reactions to properly cross-matched blood occur in approximately 1% to 3% of patients. Synthetic colloid solutions have been implicated in anaphylactic and anaphylactoid reactions. Dextran may also activate the complement system.

TABLE 24-7 ■ **Perioperative Allergic Drug Reactions**

DRUG	ESTIMATED INCIDENCE (%)	MECHANISM(S)	COMMENTS
Muscle relaxants	50%-60%	Mostly IgE Nonspecific histamine release	Frequent cross-sensitization between drugs, mainly due to quaternary and tertiary ammonium ions
Latex	15%	IgE	Commonly occurs as a delayed clinical reaction
Antibiotics: β-lactam drugs, quinolones, sulfonamides, vancomycin	10%-15%	IgE, IgG Nonspecific histamine release	<1% cross-reactivity between penicillins and cephalosporins
Hypnotics: barbiturates, propofol	<3%	IgE	
Synthetic colloids: dextran, hydroxyethyl starch	<3%	IgE, IgG	
Opioids: morphine, codeine, fentanyl	<3%	IgE, Nonspecific histamine release	
Radiocontrast media	<2%	IgE, IgG Nonspecific histamine release	
Protamine, aprotinin	<2%	IgE, IgG	
Blood and blood products	<2%	IgA	
Local anesthetics (esters more than amides)	<2%	IgG	

Ig, Immunoglobulin.

v. ***Local Anesthetic-Induced Allergic Reactions.*** These reactions are rare. Ester-type local anesthetics are metabolized to the highly antigenic compound para-aminobenzoic acid and are more likely than amide-type local anesthetics that are not metabolized to this compound to evoke an allergic reaction. Anaphylaxis may also actually be caused by stimulation of antibody production by the preservative and not by the local anesthetic. It is acceptable to administer amide-based local anesthetics to patients with a history of allergy to ester-based local anesthetics.

vi. ***Protamine.*** Anaphylactic reactions after administration of protamine are more likely to occur in patients who are allergic to seafood (protamine is derived from salmon sperm) and in patients with diabetes mellitus who are being treated with protamine-containing insulin preparations.

vii. ***Radiocontrast Media.*** Contrast media evoke allergic reactions in approximately 5% of patients. Many of the allergic reactions to contrast media seem to be anaphylactoid and can be modified by pretreatment with corticosteroids and histamine antagonists and limitation of the iodine dose.

3. **Eosinophilia.** Defined as a sustained absolute eosinophil count of greater than 1000 to 1500/mm^3, eosinophilia is often seen with parasitic infections, systemic allergic disorders, collagen vascular disease, dermatitis, drug reactions, and tumors (Hodgkin's lymphoma). Hypereosinophilia (an eosinophil count >5000/mm^3) is associated with restrictive cardiomyopathy resulting from endomyocardial fibrosis. Hypereosinophilic patients need aggressive treatment with both corticosteroids and hydroxyurea. Leukapheresis may be helpful.

VI. MISDIRECTED ADAPTIVE IMMUNITY

A. Autoimmune Disorders (Table 24-8)

1. **Anesthetic Implications.** Implications of autoimmune disorders relate to the organ pathology specific to the particular autoimmune disorder, the consequences of therapy, and the risk of accelerated atherosclerosis and associated cardiovascular complications such as

TABLE 24-8 ■ **Examples of Autoimmune Diseases**

RHEUMATIC
Rheumatoid arthritis
Scleroderma
Sjögren's syndrome
Systemic lupus erythematosus
GASTROINTESTINAL
Chronic active hepatitis
Crohn's disease
Primary biliary cirrhosis
Ulcerative colitis
ENDOCRINE
Graves' disease
Hashimoto's thyroiditis
Type 1 diabetes mellitus
NEUROLOGIC
Multiple sclerosis
Myasthenia gravis
HEMATOLOGIC
Autoimmune hemolytic anemia
Idiopathic thrombocytopenic purpura
Pernicious anemia
RENAL
Goodpasture's syndrome
MULTIPLE ORGAN SYSTEM
Ankylosing spondylitis
Polymyositis
Psoriasis
Sarcoidosis
Vasculitis

heart disease and stroke (cardiovascular morbidity and mortality may be increased approximately eightfold by autoimmune diseases alone and 50-fold by autoimmune diseases treated with corticosteroids).

VII. ANESTHESIA AND IMMUNOCOMPETENCE

Many perioperative factors affect immunocompetence and may alter the incidence of infection or the body's response to cancer.

A. Transfusion-Related Immunomodulation (TRIM). TRIM effects include decreased natural killer (NK) cell and phagocytic function, impaired antigen presentation, and suppression of lymphocyte production. TRIM is likely to explain increased susceptibility to infection and promotion of tumor growth and also likely explains improved renal allograft survival after transplantation. Leukoreduction of stored blood appears to mitigate some TRIM effects.

B. Neuroendocrine Stress Response. Release of catecholamines, corticotropin, and cortisol perioperatively causes activation of receptors on monocytes, macrophages, and T cells, inducing immunosuppression through several mechanisms, such as release of cytokines. Acute pain suppresses NK cell activity and lymphocyte function. Hyperglycemia secondary to cortisol secretion promotes bacterial growth.

C. Effects of Anesthetics on the Immune Response. There is concern that exposure to surgery and anesthesia may promote tumor progression, via surgical disruption of the tumor, release of growth factors and suppression of antiangiogenic factors, and tissue injury–related suppression of cell-mediated immunity. Allogeneic red blood cell transfusions may increase risk of tumor recurrence. Anesthetics and analgesics affect the immune response; ketamine, thiopental, and all volatile agents suppress NK cell number and activity. Volatile agents suppress neutrophil function. Nitrous oxide impairs DNA and nucleotide synthesis. Recent interest has focused on propofol conjugates in the treatment of breast cancer, because they inhibit cellular adhesion and promote apoptosis of breast cancer cells. Opiate suppression of the immune response may be greater than nonopioid effects. The use of regional anesthesia for postoperative pain control is associated with measureable reduction in cancer recurrence perhaps because patients receive lesser amounts of general anesthetics or opioids. Local anesthetics may possess some antitumor activity. The benefit of regional anesthesia over general anesthesia in this regard is still unclear and may vary by tumor type.

CHAPTER 25

Psychiatric Disease, Substance Abuse, and Drug Overdose

MOOD DISORDERS

I. DEPRESSION

Depression is the most common psychiatric disorder, affecting 2% to 4% of the population. It is distinguished from normal sadness and grief by the severity and duration of the mood disturbance. Pathophysiologic causes of major depression are unknown, although abnormalities of amine neurotransmitter pathways are the most likely causative factors.

A. Diagnosis. Diagnosis is based on the persistent presence of at least five of the symptoms noted in Table 25-1 for a period of 2 weeks. Alcoholism and major depression often co-exist. Depression and dementia may be difficult to distinguish in elderly patients. All patients with depression should be evaluated for the potential to commit suicide. Interestingly, physicians have significantly higher suicide rates than the general population.

B. Treatment. Treatment involves antidepressant medications, psychotherapy, and/or electroconvulsive therapy (ECT). An estimated 70% to 80% of patients respond to pharmacologic therapy, and 50% or more who do not respond to antidepressant drugs respond favorably to ECT.

1. Antidepressant Drugs. Almost all antidepressants affect catecholamine and/or serotonin availability in the central nervous system (Table 25-2).

a. Selective Serotonin Reuptake Inhibitors (SSRIs). SSRIs block reuptake of serotonin at presynaptic membranes with relatively little effect on adrenergic, cholinergic, histaminergic, or other neurochemical systems. As a result, they are associated with few side effects.

i. Serotonin Syndrome. This is a potentially life-threatening adverse drug reaction that may occur with therapeutic drug use, overdose, or interaction between serotoninergic drugs. A large number of drugs have been associated with the serotonin syndrome (Table 25-3). Symptoms include agitation, delirium, autonomic hyperactivity, hyperreflexia, clonus, and hyperthermia. Additional syndromes to consider in the differential diagnosis of serotonin syndrome are listed in Table 25-4. Treatment includes supportive measures and control of autonomic instability, excess muscle activity, and hyperthermia. Cyproheptadine, an oral 5-HT_{2A} antagonist, can be used to bind serotonin receptors.

b. Tricyclic Antidepressants. These agents inhibit synaptic reuptake of norepinephrine and serotonin and affect other neurochemical systems, including histaminergic and cholinergic systems. They have a large range of side effects (postural hypotension, cardiac dysrhythmias, urinary retention). Tachydysrhythmias have been observed after administration of pancuronium to patients who were also receiving imipramine. Ketamine, meperidine, and epinephrine-containing local anesthetic solutions might produce similar adverse responses and are best avoided.

TABLE 25-1 ■ Characteristics of Severe Depression

Depressed mood
Markedly diminished interest or pleasure in almost all activities
Fluctuations in body weight and appetite
Insomnia or hypersomnia
Restlessness
Fatigue
Feelings of worthlessness or guilt
Decreased ability to concentrate
Suicidal ideation

TABLE 25-2 ■ Commonly Used Antidepressant Medications

DRUG CLASS	GENERIC NAME	TRADE NAME
SSRI	Fluoxetine	Prozac
	Paroxetine	Paxil
	Sertraline	Zoloft
	Fluvoxamine	Luvox
	Citalopram	Celexa
Tricyclics	Amitriptyline	Elavil
	Imipramine	Tofranil
	Protriptyline	Vivactil
	Doxepin	Sinequan
MAOIs	Phenelzine	Nardil
	Tranylcypromine	Parnate
Atypical antidepressants	Bupropion	Wellbutrin
	Trazodone	Desyrel
	Nefazodone	Serzone
	Venlafaxine	Effexor

MAOIs, Monoamine oxidase inhibitors; *SSRIs,* selective serotonin reuptake inhibitors.

c. ***Monoamine Oxidase Inhibitors (MAOIs).*** MAOIs change the concentration of neurotransmitters by preventing breakdown of norepinephrine and serotonin. Significant systemic hypertension can occur if patients ingest foods containing tyramine (cheeses, wines) or receive sympathomimetic drugs, because tyramine and sympathomimetic drugs are potent stimuli for norepinephrine release. Orthostatic hypotension is the most common side effect of MAOI therapy.

i. ***Management of Anesthesia in Patients on MAOIs*** *(Table 25-5)*

2. **Electroconvulsive Therapy.** The mechanism of the therapeutic effect of ECT remains unknown. ECT is indicated for treating patients who are unresponsive to drug therapy or who are suicidal.

a. ***Side Effects*** *(Table 25-6).* ECT produces significant cardiovascular and central nervous system effects that may be undesirable in patients with ischemic heart disease. Because of marked increases in cerebral blood flow and intracranial pressure, ECT is contraindicated in patients with known space-occupying lesions, cerebral aneurysms, or head injury.

b. ***Management of Anesthesia*** *(Table 25-7)*

TABLE 25-3 ■ Drug and Drug Interactions Associated with Serotonin Syndrome

DRUGS ASSOCIATED WITH SEROTONIN SYNDROME
SSRIs
Atypical and cyclic antidepressants
Monoamine oxidase inhibitors
Anticonvulsant drugs: valproate
Analgesics: meperidine, fentanyl, tramadol, pentazocine
Antiemetic drugs: ondansetron, granisetron, metoclopramide
Antimigraine drugs: sumatriptan
Bariatric medications: sibutramine
Antibiotics: linezolid, ritonavir
Over-the-counter cough medicine: dextromethorphan
Drugs of abuse: ecstasy, lysergic acid diethylamide (LSD), foxy methoxy, Syrian rue
Dietary supplements: St John's wort, ginseng
Other: lithium
DRUG INTERACTIONS ASSOCIATED WITH SEVERE SEROTONIN SYNDROME
Phenelzine and meperidine
Tranylcypromine and imipramine
Phenelzine and SSRIs
Paroxetine and buspirone
Linezolid and citalopram
Moclobemide and SSRIs
Tramadol, venlafaxine, and mirtazapine

Modified from Boyer EW, Shannon M. The serotonin syndrome. *N Engl J Med*. 2005;352:1112-1120.

SSRIs, Selective serotonin reuptake inhibitors.

II. BIPOLAR DISORDER

Bipolar disorder is characterized by marked mood swings from depressive episodes to manic episodes with normal behavior often seen in between these episodes (Table 25-8). The evaluation of mania must exclude the effects of substance abuse drugs, medications, and concomitant medical conditions.

A. Treatment. Lithium remains a mainstay of treatment, but antiepileptic drugs such as carbamazepine and valproate are often used. Olanzapine is another treatment option.

1. Lithium. Because of the drug's narrow therapeutic index, monitoring of serum lithium concentration is necessary to prevent toxicity.

a. Toxicity *(Table 25-9).* Toxicity occurs at serum lithium concentrations above 2 mEq/L. Thiazide diuretics trigger lithium reabsorption in the kidneys and should be avoided (loop diuretics are safe).

b. Management of Anesthesia. The patient should be evaluated for lithium toxicity, including recent serum lithium concentrations. Thiazide diuretics should be avoided. The electrocardiogram (ECG) should be monitored for evidence of lithium-induced conduction problems or dysrhythmias. The duration of all muscle relaxants may be prolonged in the presence of lithium.

III. SCHIZOPHRENIA

Schizophrenia is the major psychotic mental disorder and is characterized by abnormal reality testing or thought processes. Symptoms include delusions, hallucinations, flattened affect, apathy, social or occupational dysfunction including withdrawal, and changes in appearance and hygiene.

TABLE 25-4 ■ **Drug-Induced Hyperthermic Syndromes**

SYNDROME	TIME TO ONSET	CAUSATIVE DRUGS	OUTSTANDING FEATURES	TREATMENT
Malignant hyperthermia	Within minutes	Succinylcholine, inhalation anesthetics	Muscle rigidity, severe hypercarbia	Dantrolene, supportive care
Neuroleptic malignant syndrome	24-72 hr	Dopamine antagonist antipsychotic drugs	Muscle rigidity, stupor or coma, bradykinesia	Bromocriptine or dantrolene, supportive care
Serotonin syndrome	Up to 12 hr	Serotoninergic drugs including SSRIs, MAOIs, and atypical antidepressants	Clonus, hyperreflexia, agitation; may have muscle rigidity	Cyproheptadine, supportive care
Sympathomimetic syndrome	Up to 30 min	Cocaine, amphetamines	Agitation, hallucinations, myocardial ischemia, dysrhythmias, no rigidity	Vasodilators, α- and β-blockers, supportive care
Anticholinergic poisoning	Up to 12 hr	Atropine, belladonna	Toxidrome of hot, red, dry skin, dilated pupils, delirium, no rigidity	Physostigmine, supportive care
Cyclic antidepressant overdose	Up to 6 hr	Cyclic antidepressants	Hypotension, stupor or coma, wide-complex dysrhythmias, no rigidity	Serum alkalinization, magnesium

MAOIs, Monoamine oxidase inhibitors; *SSRIs,* selective serotonin reuptake inhibitors.

A. **Treatment.** Schizophrenia is likely the result of neurotransmitter dysfunction, specifically of the neurotransmitters dopamine and serotonin. Drugs that block dopamine receptors, especially D_2 and D_4 receptors, improve a variety of psychotic symptoms, especially delusions and hallucinations. Troubling side effects include tardive dyskinesia (choreoathetoid movements), akathisia (restlessness), acute dystonia (contraction of skeletal muscles of the neck, mouth, and tongue), and parkinsonism. Newer "atypical" antipsychotic drugs have variable effects on dopamine receptor subtypes and on serotonin receptors, especially the 5-HT_{2A} receptor, and appear to be effective in relieving the symptoms of schizophrenia with fewer extrapyramidal side effects than the classic drugs (Table 25-10).

1. **Anesthesia Considerations.** Important effects of antipsychotic medications include α-adrenergic blockade causing postural hypotension, prolongation of the QT interval potentially producing torsade de pointes, seizures, hepatic enzyme elevations, abnormal temperature regulation, and sedation. Drug-induced sedation may decrease anesthetic requirements.

TABLE 25-5 ■ Anesthesia Considerations in Patients Treated with Monoamine Oxidase Inhibitors (MAOIs)

Preoperative	Anesthesia can be managed safely without discontinuing MAOIs. Benzodiazepine premedication is acceptable.
Intraoperative	Anesthetic requirements may be increased. Most intravenous induction agents are safe. Fentanyl appears to be safe. Ketamine should be avoided. Succinylcholine dose should be reduced (serum cholinesterase activity may be reduced). Provide maintenance anesthesia with volatile agents with or without nitrous oxide. Regional anesthesia is acceptable but may have higher incidence of hypotension. Avoid epinephrine in local anesthetic solutions. Avoid light anesthesia, topical cocaine, and indirect-acting vasopressors (ephedrine). Treat hypotension with direct-acting vasopressors (phenylephrine).
Postoperative	Avoid meperidine (severe serotonin syndrome). Consider alternatives to opioid analgesics.

TABLE 25-6 ■ Side Effects of Electroconvulsive Therapy

Parasympathetic nervous system stimulation
- Bradycardia
- Hypotension

Sympathetic nervous system stimulation
- Tachycardia
- Hypertension

Dysrhythmias
Increased cerebral blood flow
Increased intracranial pressure
Increased intraocular pressure
Increased intragastric pressure

B. Neuroleptic Malignant Syndrome. This is a rare, potentially fatal complication of antipsychotic drug therapy. Clinical manifestations include hyperpyrexia, severe skeletal muscle rigidity, rhabdomyolysis, autonomic hyperactivity (tachycardia, hypertension, cardiac dysrhythmias), altered consciousness, and acidosis. Skeletal muscle spasm may be so severe that mechanical ventilation becomes necessary. Renal failure may occur owing to myoglobinuria and dehydration.

1. **Treatment.** Antipsychotic drug therapy is stopped immediately, and supportive therapy (ventilation, hydration, cooling) is initiated. Bromocriptine (5 mg orally every 6 hours) or dantrolene (up to 6 mg/kg daily as a continuous intravenous infusion) may decrease skeletal muscle rigidity Mortality rates approach 20% in untreated patients. At the present time there is no evidence of a pathophysiologic link between neuroleptic malignant syndrome and malignant hyperthermia.

TABLE 25-7 ■ Management of Anesthesia for Electroconvulsive Therapy (ECT)

Preoperative	Patient should be NPO. Preanesthesia sedation should be omitted to avoid prolonged emergence. Anticholinergic drugs (atropine, glycopyrrolate) decrease secretions and reduce the likelihood of bradycardia. Esmolol 1 mg/kg intravenously just before induction attenuates tachycardia and hypertension (nitroglycerin is an alternative treatment of hypertension). Pacer devices are usually shielded, but an external magnet should be available. Implantable defibrillators *must* be turned off before treatment and reactivated afterward.
Intraoperative	Induction is usually with methohexital 0.5-1.0 mg/kg. Propofol can be used but may shorten duration of seizure and reduce efficacy of ECT. Succinylcholine 0.3-0.5 mg/kg attenuates skeletal muscle contractions and risk of bone fractures from seizure activity. EEG is best monitor of seizure activity. A tourniquet placed on a limb and inflated to arterial pressure before administration of succinylcholine permits evaluation of tonic-clonic movement in that limb to signal seizure activity.
Postoperative	Support of ventilation and supplemental oxygen until recovered.

EEG, Electroencephalogram; *NPO,* nothing by mouth.

TABLE 25-8 ■ Manifestations of Mania

Expansive, euphoric mood
Inflated self-esteem
Decreased need for sleep
Flight of ideas
More talkative than usual
Distractibility
Psychomotor agitation

TABLE 25-9 ■ Signs of Lithium Toxicity

Skeletal muscle weakness
Ataxia
Sedation
Widening of the QRS complex
Heart block
Hypotension
Seizures

TABLE 25-10 ■ **Commonly Used Antipsychotic Medications**

CLASS	GENERIC NAME	TRADE NAME	EPSEs	SPECIAL SIDE EFFECTS
Traditional Drugs				
Phenothiazines	Chlorpromazine	Thorazine	Common	
	Perphenazine	Trilafon		
	Fluphenazine	Prolixin		
	Trifluoperazine	Stelazine		
	Thioridazine	Mellaril		
Butyrophenones	Haloperidol	Haldol	Common	Retinal pigmentation
Thioxanthenes	Thiothixene	Navane	Common	
Atypical Drugs				
	Risperidone	Risperdal	Uncommon	
	Clozapine	Clozaril	Rare	Agranulocytosis
	Quetiapine	Seroquel	Uncommon	Cataracts
	Olanzapine	Zyprexa	Uncommon	Neutropenia
	Ziprasidone	Geodon	Uncommon	Prolonged QT interval

EPSEs, Extrapyramidal side effects.

IV. ANXIETY DISORDERS

Anxiety disorders are associated with distressing symptoms such as nervousness, sleeplessness, hypochondriasis, and somatic complaints. There are two patterns: (1) chronic generalized anxiety and (2) episodic, often situation-dependent, anxiety. Anxiety resulting from identifiable stresses is usually self-limited and rarely requires pharmacologic treatment. Benzodiazepines can be helpful. Buspirone, a partial 5-HT_{2A} receptor antagonist, is a nonbenzodiazepine anxiolytic drug that is not sedating and does not produce tolerance but has a slow onset of action and requires multiple daily doses. β-Blockers are useful for performance anxiety ("stage fright"). Cognitive behavioral therapy, relaxation techniques, hypnosis, and psychotherapy may be useful. Panic disorders are qualitatively different from generalized anxiety and involve discrete periods of unprovoked intense fear, apprehension, and a sense of impending doom. SSRIs, benzodiazepines, cyclic antidepressants, and MAOIs are effective treatments.

V. EATING DISORDERS

Eating disorders typically occur in adolescent girls or young women, although 5% to 15% of cases of anorexia nervosa and bulimia and 40% of binge-eating disorder occur in boys and young men.

A. **Anorexia Nervosa.** Relatively rare, anorexia has a mortality rate of 5% to 10%. Approximately half of these deaths are via suicide.
   1. **Signs and Symptoms.** Signs include marked unexplained weight loss often associated with excessive physical activity in the obsessive pursuit of thinness. The most serious medical complications are caused by effects on the cardiovascular system, such as cardiomyopathy and ventricular dysrhythmias. Hyponatremia, hypochloremia, hypokalemia, and metabolic alkalosis result from vomiting and laxative and diuretic abuse. Other signs include amenorrhea, emaciation, decreased body temperature, orthostatic hypotension, decreased bone density, and impaired cognitive function. Anemia, neutropenia, and thrombocytopenia may be present.
   2. **Treatment.** Tricyclic antidepressants, lithium, antipsychotic drugs, and SSRIs may be administered.
   3. **Management of Anesthesia.** Management is based on the known pathophysiologic effects of starvation.

TABLE 25-11 ■ Characteristic Symptoms of Psychoactive Drug Dependence

Drug taken in higher doses or for longer periods than intended
Unsuccessful attempts to reduce use of the drug
Increased time spent obtaining the drug
Frequent intoxication or withdrawal symptoms
Restricted social or work activities because of drug use
Continued drug use despite social or physical problems related to drug use
Evidence of tolerance to the effects of the drug
Characteristic withdrawal symptoms
Drug use to avoid withdrawal symptoms

B. Bulimia Nervosa. This disorder is characterized by binge eating, purging, and dietary restriction.

1. **Signs and Symptoms.** Signs include dry skin, evidence of dehydration, and bilateral painless hypertrophy of the salivary glands. Resting bradycardia may occur. Increased serum amylase is the most common laboratory finding. Metabolic alkalosis can be seen, and dental damage (enamel loss) occurs due to repeated vomiting and exposure of the teeth to gastric acid.
2. **Treatment.** Treatment is best accomplished by cognitive-behavioral therapy. Tricyclic antidepressants and/or SSRIs maybe helpful. Potassium supplementation may be needed due to chronic hypokalemia.

C. Binge-Eating Disorder. Binge-eating disorder resembles bulimia nervosa, but without purging. Periods of dietary restriction are shorter. The diagnosis should be suspected in morbidly obese patients with continued weight gain or marked weight cycling. It is often accompanied by depression, anxiety, and personality disorders. Antidepressants may be helpful.

VI. SUBSTANCE ABUSE

Psychoactive drug dependence is diagnosed when patients manifest at least three of nine characteristic symptoms, with some of the symptoms having persisted for at least 1 month or having occurred repeatedly (Table 25-11). Substance abuse is often first discovered during the medical management of other conditions (hepatitis, acquired immunodeficiency syndrome [AIDS], pregnancy). Sociopathic characteristics (school dropout, criminal record, multiple drug abuse) seem to predispose to, rather than result from, drug addiction. Drug overdose is the leading cause of unconsciousness in patients in the emergency room. Treatment of overdose is similar regardless of the drug ingested. Airway considerations are addressed, then ventilation and circulation are secured. Decisions to attempt removal of the ingested drug (gastric lavage, forced diuresis, hemodialysis) depend on the drug involved.

A. Alcoholism. Alcoholism is defined as a primary chronic disease with genetic, psychosocial, and environmental factors that influence its development and manifestations. Up to one third of adult patients have medical problems related to alcohol (Table 25-12).

1. **Treatment.** Treatment of alcoholism mandates total abstinence from alcohol. Disulfiram, which produces unpleasant symptoms when alcohol is ingested (flushing, vertigo, diaphoresis, nausea, vomiting), may be administered as an adjunctive drug along with psychiatric counseling.
2. **Overdose.** In nonalcoholic patients, blood alcohol levels of 25 mg/dL are associated with impaired cognition and coordination. At blood alcohol concentrations greater than 100 mg/dL, signs of vestibular and cerebellar dysfunction (nystagmus, dysarthria, ataxia) are likely. Intoxication with alcohol is defined as a blood alcohol concentration above 80 to 100 mg/dL. Levels greater than 500 mg/dL are usually fatal as a result of respiratory depression. Treatment of life-threatening overdose is support of ventilation and treatment of hypoglycemia if needed.
3. **Alcohol Withdrawal Syndrome**(Table 25-13)

TABLE 25-12 ■ Medical Problems Related to Alcoholism

CENTRAL NERVOUS SYSTEM EFFECTS
Psychiatric disorders (depression, antisocial behavior)
Nutritional disorders (Wernicke-Korsakoff syndrome)
Withdrawal syndrome
Cerebellar degeneration
Cerebral atrophy
CARDIOVASCULAR EFFECTS
Cardiomyopathy
Cardiac dysrhythmias
Hypertension
GASTROINTESTINAL AND HEPATOBILIARY EFFECTS
Esophagitis
Gastritis
Pancreatitis
Hepatic cirrhosis
Portal hypertension
SKIN AND MUSCULOSKELETAL EFFECTS
Spider angiomata
Myopathy
Osteoporosis
ENDOCRINE AND METABOLIC EFFECTS
Decreased serum testosterone concentrations (impotence)
Decreased gluconeogenesis (hypoglycemia)
Ketoacidosis
Hypoalbuminemia
Hypomagnesemia
HEMATOLOGIC EFFECTS
Thrombocytopenia
Leukopenia
Anemia

4. **Wernicke-Korsakoff Syndrome.** This syndrome may accompany alcoholism and reflects a loss of neurons in the cerebellum (Wernicke's encephalopathy) and a loss of memory (Korsakoff's psychosis) caused by the lack of thiamine (vitamin B_1), which is required for the intermediary metabolism of carbohydrates. Signs include global confusion, drowsiness, nystagmus, orthostatic hypotension, and peripheral neuropathy. Treatment consists of intravenous thiamine, then oral intake when possible.
5. **Alcohol and Pregnancy.** Alcohol crosses the placenta and may result in decreased birth weight. High blood concentrations of alcohol (>150 mg/dL) may result in the fetal alcohol syndrome (craniofacial dysmorphology, growth retardation, mental retardation). There is increased risk of cardiac malformations (patent ductus arteriosus, septal defects).
6. **Management of Anesthesia.** The presence of disulfiram-induced sedation and hepatotoxicity should be suspected in alcoholic patients being treated with this drug. Acute, unexplained hypotension during general anesthesia could reflect inadequate stores of norepinephrine caused by disulfiram-induced inhibition of dopamine β-hydroxylase. Direct-acting sympathomimetics (phenylephrine) produce a more predictable response than indirect agents

TABLE 25-13 ■ **Alcohol Withdrawal Syndrome**

Early signs (6-8 hr after alcohol cessation, most pronounced in 24-36 hr)	Tremors Nightmares, hallucinations, insomnia, confusion Autonomic nervous system hyperreactivity (tachycardia, hypertension, cardiac dysrhythmias) Nausea, vomiting May be treated with benzodiazepines, β-receptor antagonists, or α_2-agonists
Delirium tremens (2-4 days after alcohol cessation) *Life-threatening!*	Hallucinations, combativeness Hyperthermia, tachycardia Hypertension or hypotension Seizures
TREATMENT OF DELIRIUM TREMENS	
	Diazepam 5-10 mg intravenously every 5 min until patient is calm β-Adrenergic antagonists (propranolol, esmolol) intravenously until heart rate <100 beats/min Correction of fluid and electrolyte disturbances Lidocaine for cardiac dysrhythmias Airway protection if consciousness is affected Physical restraint if necessary to prevent injury to self or others

(ephedrine). Use of regional anesthesia may be influenced by the presence of disulfiram-induced polyneuropathy. Alcohol-containing solutions, as used for skin cleansing, probably should be avoided in disulfiram-treated patients.

B. Cocaine. This drug produces sympathetic nervous system stimulation by blocking the presynaptic uptake of norepinephrine and dopamine, thereby increasing the postsynaptic concentrations of these neurotransmitters. Dopamine is present in high concentrations in synapses, producing the characteristic "cocaine high."

1. **Side Effects.** Acute cocaine administration can cause hypertension, tachycardia, coronary vasospasm, myocardial ischemia, myocardial infarction, and ventricular dysrhythmias, including ventricular fibrillation. Lung damage and pulmonary edema can occur in patients who smoke cocaine. Cocaine-abusing parturients are at higher risk of spontaneous abortion, abruptio placenta, and fetal malformations. Long-term abuse is associated with nasal septal atrophy, agitated behavior, paranoid thinking, and heightened reflexes. Symptoms associated with cocaine withdrawal include fatigue, depression, and increased appetite.
2. **Treatment.** Treatment of cocaine overdose may include nitroglycerin to manage myocardial ischemia and α-adrenergic blockade to treat coronary vasoconstriction. Intravenous benzodiazepines such as diazepam are effective in controlling seizures. Active cooling may be necessary for hyperthermia.
3. **Management of Anesthesia.** The vulnerability of patients acutely intoxicated with cocaine to myocardial ischemia and cardiac dysrhythmias must be considered. Nitroglycerin should be readily available. Thrombocytopenia associated with cocaine abuse may influence the selection of regional anesthesia. In the absence of acute intoxication, long-term abuse of cocaine has not been shown to be predictably associated with adverse anesthetic interactions.

C. Opioids. Numerous medical problems are encountered in opioid addicts, especially intravenous abusers (Table 25-14). Dependence rarely develops in the setting of opioid use to treat postoperative pain.

TABLE 25-14 ■ Medical Problems Associated with Chronic Opioid Abuse
Hepatitis
Cellulitis
Superficial skin abscesses
Septic thrombophlebitis
Endocarditis
Systemic septic emboli
Acquired immunodeficiency syndrome
Aspiration pneumonitis
Malnutrition
Tetanus
Transverse myelitis

1. **Overdose.** The most obvious sign of opioid overdose (usually heroin) is a slow breathing rate with a normal to increased tidal volume. Pupils are usually miotic. Central nervous system manifestations range from dysphoria to unconsciousness; seizures are unlikely. Pulmonary edema occurs in a large proportion of patients with heroin overdose. Naloxone is the specific opioid antagonist administered to maintain an acceptable respiratory rate.
2. **Withdrawal Syndrome.** Withdrawal from opioids is unpleasant but rarely life-threatening. Clonidine may also attenuate opioid withdrawal symptoms (diaphoresis, mydriasis, hypertension, tachycardia). Other symptoms include insomnia, abdominal cramps, diarrhea, hyperthermia, skeletal muscle spasms, and jerking of the legs. Rapid detoxification using high doses of an opioid antagonist (nalmefene) administered during general anesthesia followed by naltrexone maintenance has been proposed as a cost-effective alternative to conventional detoxification approaches.
3. **Treatment.** Pharmacotherapy for opioid dependence has included μ-agonists, such as methadone and levomethadyl, and partial agonists. Buprenorphine (Subutex) or buprenorphine in combination with naloxone (Suboxone) have been approved for treatment of opioid dependence.
4. **Management of Anesthesia.** Opioid addicts should have opioids or methadone maintained during the perioperative period. Opioid addicts often seem to experience exaggerated degrees of postoperative pain. For reasons that are not clear, satisfactory postoperative analgesia may be achieved when average doses of meperidine are administered in addition to the usual daily maintenance dose of methadone or other opioids. Alternative methods of postoperative pain relief include continuous regional anesthesia with local anesthetics, neuraxial opioids, and transcutaneous electrical nerve stimulation.

D. Barbiturates

1. **Overdose.** Central nervous system depression is the principal manifestation of barbiturate overdose. Treatment is supportive: maintenance of a patent airway, protection from aspiration, and support of ventilation using a cuffed endotracheal tube if necessary. Hypotension, hypothermia, acute renal failure, and rhabdomyolysis may occur. Forced diuresis and alkalinization of the urine promote elimination of phenobarbital but are of less value with many of the other barbiturates.
2. **Withdrawal Syndrome** (Table 25-15). In contrast to opiod withdrawal, the abrupt cessation of excessive barbiturate ingestion is associated with delayed but potentially life-threatening responses. Barbiturate withdrawal symptoms include anxiety, skeletal muscle tremors, hyperreflexia, diaphoresis, tachycardia, orthostatic hypotension, grand mal seizures, and cardiovascular collapse. Pentobarbital may be administered if evidence of barbiturate withdrawal manifests. Phenobarbital and diazepam may also be useful for suppressing signs of barbiturate withdrawal.

TABLE 25-15 ■ Time Course of Barbiturate Withdrawal Syndrome

	ONSET (hr)	PEAK INTENSITY (days)	DURATION (days)
Pentobarbital	12-24	2-3	7-10
Secobarbital	12-24	2-3	7-10
Phenobarbital	48-72	6-10	10+

3. **Management of Anesthesia.** There are no reports of increased anesthetic requirements (MAC) in chronic barbiturate abusers. Venous access is a likely problem in intravenous barbiturate abusers, as the alkalinity of the self-injected solutions is likely to sclerose veins.

E. **Benzodiazepines.** Addiction requires ingestion of large doses of drug. Symptoms of withdrawal generally occur later than with barbiturates and are less severe due to the prolonged elimination half-lives of most benzodiazepines and the fact that many of these drugs are metabolized to pharmacologically active metabolites that also have prolonged elimination half-lives. Anesthetic considerations in chronic benzodiazepine abusers are similar to those described for chronic barbiturate abusers.

1. **Acute Benzodiazepine Overdose.** Supportive treatment and flumazenil, a specific benzodiazepine antagonist, are used for severe or life-threatening overdose.

F. **Amphetamines.** These drugs stimulate the release of catecholamines, resulting in increased alertness, appetite suppression, and decreased need for sleep. Approved medical uses of amphetamines are treatment of narcolepsy, attention-deficit disorders, and hyperactivity associated with minimal brain dysfunction in children.

1. **Overdose.** Overdose causes anxiety, a psychotic state, progressive central nervous system irritability (hyperactivity, hyperreflexia, seizures), cardiovascular stimulation (hypertension, tachycardia, dysrhythmias), decreased gastrointestinal motility, mydriasis, diaphoresis, and hyperthermia.
   a. ***Treatment.*** Induced emesis or gastric lavage is performed, and activated charcoal and a cathartic are administered. Phenothiazine and diazepam may be useful. Acidification of the urine promotes elimination of amphetamines.
2. **Withdrawal Syndrome.** Abrupt cessation of excessive amphetamine use is accompanied by extreme lethargy, depression that may be suicidal, increased appetite, and weight gain.
3. **Management of Anesthesia.** Amphetamines administered chronically for medically indicated uses (narcolepsy, attention-deficit disorder) need not be discontinued before elective surgery. In the acutely intoxicated patient undergoing emergency surgery, effects from amphetamines may include hypertension, tachycardia, hyperthermia, increased requirements for volatile anesthetics, intracranial hypertension, and cardiac arrest. Direct-acting vasopressors, including phenylephrine and epinephrine, should be available to treat hypotension because the response to indirect-acting vasopressors such as ephedrine may be attenuated by the amphetamine-induced catecholamine depletion.

G. **Hallucinogens.** LSD, phencyclidine, and similar hallucinogens are usually ingested orally. There is no evidence of physical dependence or withdrawal symptoms. The effects of these drugs consist of visual, auditory, and tactile hallucinations and distortions of the surroundings and body image. Evidence of sympathetic nervous system stimulation includes mydriasis, increased body temperature, hypertension, and tachycardia.

1. **Overdose.** Overdose is usually not life-threatening. Patients should be placed in a calm, quiet environment with minimal external stimuli. Benzodiazepines may be useful. Supportive care (airway management, mechanical ventilation, treatment of seizures, control of the manifestations of sympathetic nervous system hyperactivity) may be required. Forced diuresis and acidification of the urine promotes elimination of

phencyclidine but increases the risk of fluid overload and electrolyte abnormalities, especially hypokalemia.

2. **Management of Anesthesia.** Perioperative management may be complicated by acute panic episodes and exaggerated responses to sympathomimetic drugs. Diazepam can be useful.

H. **Marijuana.** Marijuana abuse is associated with lethargy, sedation, tachycardia, orthostatic hypotension, and bronchitis (related to smoke ingestion). Pharmacologic effects of tetrahydrocannabinol (THC) occur within minutes of inhalation and last 2 to 3 hours.

1. **Management of Anesthesia.** The known effects of THC on the heart, lungs, and central nervous system are considered. Barbiturate and ketamine sleep times are prolonged in THC-treated animals, and opioid-induced respiratory depression may be potentiated.

I. **Substance Abuse as an Occupational Hazard in Anesthesiology.** Anesthesiologists are represented in addictive treatment programs at a rate three times higher than any other physician group.

1. **Characteristics and Demographics of the Addicted Anesthesiologist**
   - 50% are younger than 35 years of age.
   - Residents are overrepresented.
   - 67% to 88% are male, and 75% to 96% are white.
   - 76% to 90% use opiates as the drug of choice.
   - 33% to 50% are polydrug users.
   - 33% have a family history of addictive disease, most commonly alcohol.
   - 65% of anesthesiologists with a history of addiction are associated with academic departments.

2. **Commonly Abused Drugs.** Fentanyl and sufentanil are the most commonly abused drugs, followed by meperidine and morphine. Alcohol abuse occurs more often in anesthesia practitioners who have been out of residency for more than 5 years. Sevoflurane has been reported as the drug of choice among inhalational agents.

3. **Signs and Symptoms of Addictive Behavior.** Any unusual and persistent changes in behavior should be cause for alarm. Classically, these behaviors include mood swings, such as periods of depression, anger, and irritability alternating with periods of euphoria.
   - Denial is universal.
   - Symptoms at work are the last to appear (symptoms appear first in the community and then at home).
   - Detected addicts are often found comatose.
   - *Untreated addicts are often found dead!*

The most commonly overlooked symptoms of addictive behavior are:
   - The desire to work alone
   - Refusing lunch relief or breaks
   - Frequently relieving others
   - Volunteering for extra cases or calls
   - Patient pain needs in the postanesthetic care unit that are out of proportion to the narcotics recorded as given
   - Weight loss
   - Frequent bathroom breaks

4. **Associated Risks of Physician Drug Addiction**
   a. ***Physician.*** The relapse rate for anesthesiologists is the highest of all physicians and is greatest in the first 5 years after treatment. Death is the primary presenting sign of relapse.
   b. ***Patient.*** Impaired physicians (those who are actively abusing drugs) are at increased risk of malpractice suits.

5. **What to Do When Substance Abuse Is Suspected**
   a. ***Reporting and Intervention.*** Admission to an alcohol or drug addiction treatment program is not a reportable event to state or national agencies. After an individual has been

confronted and is awaiting final disposition, he or she should not be left alone because newly identified physician addicts are at increased risk of suicide.

b. ***Treatment.*** There is no cure for addiction, and recovery is a lifelong process. The most effective treatment programs are multidisciplinary in composition and can provide long-term follow-up for the impaired physician.

J. **Tricyclic Antidepressant Overdose.** Overdose of tricyclic antidepressants is a common cause of drug ingestion death. Signs include intense anticholinergic effects (delirium, fever, tachycardia, mydriasis, flushed dry skin, ileus, urinary retention) seizures, and cardiovascular toxicity (tachycardia; prolongation of the PR interval, QRS complex, and QT interval; ventricular dysrhythmias; myocardial depression). The risk of life-threatening cardiac dysrhythmias may persist for several days.

1. **Treatment.** Treatment of tricyclic antidepressant overdose in the presence of preserved upper airway reflexes includes gastric lavage and activated charcoal. Emesis should not be induced because of the risk of pulmonary aspiration. Serum alkalinization is the principal treatment and results in an increase of protein-bound drug, less free drug, and thereby less toxicity. Intravenous administration of sodium bicarbonate or hyperventilation to a pH of 7.45 to 7.55 should be accomplished to a clinical end point such as narrowing of the QRS or cessation of dysrhythmias. Lidocaine may be an additional treatment for cardiac dysrhythmias. If torsade de pointes is present, magnesium should be administered. Vasopressor or inotropic support may be needed. Diazepam is useful for seizure control. Hemodialysis is ineffective in removing cyclic antidepressants.

K. **Salicylic Acid Overdose.** Symptoms and signs include tinnitus, nausea and vomiting, fever, seizures, obtundation, hypoglycemia, low cerebrospinal fluid glucose concentration, coagulopathy, hepatic dysfunction, and direct stimulation of the respiratory center. Noncardiogenic pulmonary edema often occurs during the first 24 hours after aspirin overdose.

1. **Initial Treatment.** Initial treatment includes gastric lavage and activated charcoal, administration of dextrose to prevent low cerebrospinal fluid glucose concentrations, administration of sodium bicarbonate to increase arterial pH to 7.45 to 7.55 (alkalinizes the urine and dramatically increases renal clearance of salicylate), and hemodialysis for potentially lethal concentrations of salicylic acid (>100 mg/dL), refractory acidosis, coma, seizures, volume overload, or renal failure.

L. **Acetaminophen Overdose**

1. **Treatment.** Treatment is administration of activated charcoal to impede drug absorption. Four hours after drug ingestion, a plasma acetaminophen concentration is measured and plotted on the Rumack-Matthew nomogram, which stratifies the patient's risk of hepatotoxicity. All patients with possible or probable risk and anyone in whom the time of ingestion is not known are treated with *N*-acetylcysteine, which replenishes glutathione, combines directly with *N*-acetylbenzoquinone imine, and enhances sulfate conjugation of acetaminophen. *N*-acetylcysteine is virtually 100% effective in preventing hepatotoxicity when administered within 8 hours of drug ingestion.

POISONING

I. METHYL ALCOHOL

Methyl alcohol is found in paint remover, antifreeze, windshield washing fluid, and camper fuel. It is metabolized by alcohol dehydrogenase to formaldehyde and formic acid, resulting in an anion-gap metabolic acidosis. Toxicity occurs in the retina, the optic nerve, and the central nervous system.

A. **Treatment.** Treatment includes supportive care and a secure airway. Intravenous administration of ethyl alcohol will decrease the metabolism of methanol. Alternatively, the activity of alcohol dehydrogenase may be specifically inhibited by administration of fomepizole. Hemodialysis may be indicated for refractory acidosis or visual impairment.

TABLE 25-16 ■ **Signs of Organophosphate Poisoning**

MUSCARINIC EFFECTS
Copious secretions
Salivation
Tearing
Diaphoresis
Bronchorrhea
Rhinorrhea
Bronchospasm
Miosis
Hyperperistalsis
Bradycardia
NICOTINIC EFFECTS
Skeletal muscle fasciculations
Skeletal muscle weakness
Skeletal muscle paralysis
CENTRAL NERVOUS SYSTEM EFFECTS
Seizures
Coma
Central apnea

II. ETHYLENE GLYCOL

Ethylene glycol is found in antifreeze, de-icers, and industrial solvents.

A. Treatment. Treatment is similar to that described for methyl alcohol ingestion. Inhibition of formation of toxic metabolites can be accomplished by administration of ethyl alcohol or fomepizole. Thiamine, pyridoxine, and sufficient calcium to reverse hypocalcemia are also given. Urgent hemodialysis may be necessary.

III. ORGANOPHOSPHATE PESTICIDES, CARBAMATE PESTICIDES, AND ORGANOPHOSPHORUS COMPOUNDS

Organophosphate pesticides, carbamate pesticides, and organophosphorus compounds ("nerve agents" developed for chemical warfare and now used in terrorist attacks) all inhibit acetylcholinesterase, resulting in cholinergic overstimulation. The manifestations of pesticide and nerve agent poisoning are influenced by the route of absorption, with the most severe effects occurring after inhalation (Table 25-16).

A. Treatment. Three strategies are used: an anticholinergic drug to counteract the acute cholinergic crisis, an oxime drug to reactivate inhibited acetylcholinesterase, and an anticonvulsant drug to prevent or treat seizures (Table 25-17).

IV. CARBON MONOXIDE POISONING

A. Pathophysiology. Carbon monoxide (CO) competes with oxygen for binding to hemoglobin, shifts the oxygen-hemoglobin dissociation curve to the left, and impairs release of oxygen to tissues (Figure 25-1). CO also disrupts oxidative metabolism, increases nitric oxide concentrations, causes brain lipid peroxidation, generates oxygen free radicals, and produces other metabolic changes that may result in neurologic and cardiac toxicity. CO binds more tightly to fetal hemoglobin than adult hemoglobin, making infants particularly vulnerable to its effects.

TABLE 25-17 ■ Treatment in Organophosphate Poisoning

Reverse the acute cholinergic crisis created by the poison
Atropine 2 mg intravenously every 5-10 min as needed until ventilation improves
Reactivate the function of acetylcholinesterase
Pralidoxime 600 mg intravenously
Prevent and treat seizures
Diazepam or midazolam as needed
Supportive care

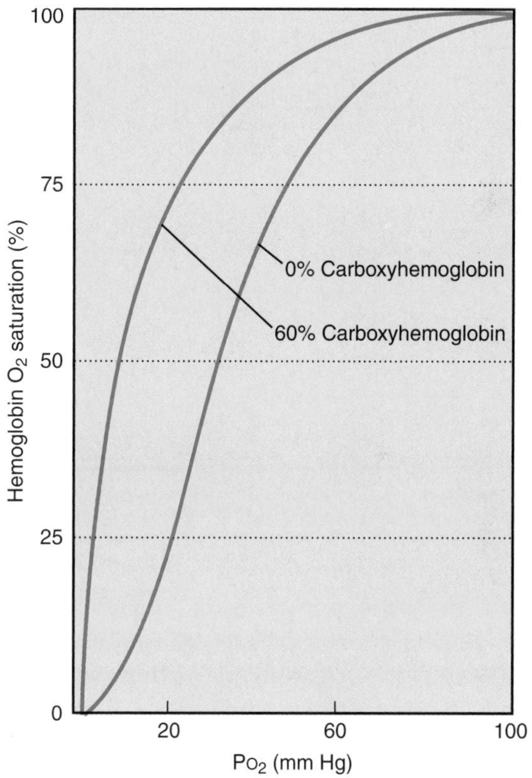

FIGURE 25-1 ■ Carboxyhemoglobin shifts the oxyhemoglobin dissociation curve to the left and changes it to a more hyperbolic shape. This results in decreased oxygen-carrying capacity and impaired release of oxygen at the tissue level. *(Adapted from Ernst A, Zibrak JD. Carbon monoxide poisoning.* N Engl J Med. *1998;339:1603-1608. Copyright 1998 Massachusetts Medical Society. All rights reserved.)*

B. Signs and Symptoms. Signs and symptoms include headache, nausea, vomiting, weakness, difficulty concentrating, confusion, syncope, and seizures. Angina pectoris, dysrhythmias, and pulmonary edema may result from the increased cardiac output necessitated by the hypoxemia. Persistent or delayed neurologic effects (cognitive dysfunction, memory loss, seizures, personality changes, parkinsonism, dementia, mutism, blindness, psychosis) may be seen after apparent recovery from the acute phase of CO intoxication.

C. Diagnosis. Serum carboxyhemoglobin concentrations should be obtained from patients suspected of CO exposure. Spo_2 values may be misleading.

D. **Treatment.** Treatment consists of removal of the individual from the source of the CO production, immediate administration of supplemental oxygen, and supportive care: airway management, blood pressure support, and cardiovascular stabilization. Oxygen therapy shortens the elimination half-life of CO by competing at the binding sites for hemoglobin and improves tissue oxygenation. Hyperbaric oxygen therapy accelerates the elimination of CO and may be indicated in selected patients who are comatose or neurologically impaired at presentation, who have carboxyhemoglobin concentrations greater than 40%, and who are pregnant and have carboxyhemoglobin concentrations above 15%.

CHAPTER 26

Pregnancy-Associated Diseases

I. PHYSIOLOGIC CHANGES ASSOCIATED WITH PREGNANCY

A. General Physiologic Changes (Table 26-1)

1. Cardiovascular

a. ***Decreased Systemic Vascular Resistance (SVR).*** SVR is decreased. Increased progesterone, nitric oxide, and prostacyclin and decreased response to norepinephrine and angiotensin cause renal artery and aortic dilatation.

b. ***Increased Cardiac Output.*** As a result of increased heart rate and renin activity, cardiac output is increased.

c. ***Increased Total Body Water.*** Owing to increased renin, total body water is increased (7 to 10 L). Volume increase begins at 4 weeks, is increased 10% to 15% by 6 to 12 weeks, and is increased 30% to 50% by 28 to 34 weeks.

d. ***Increased Blood Volume.*** Blood volume increases to 100 mL/kg at term.

e. ***Rapid Changes of Blood Volume During Labor.*** These occur when sympathetic stimulation and "autotransfusion" of blood from the contracting uterus cause an average increase in cardiac output of 20% in the first stage, 50% during the second stage, and 80% after placental delivery. Cardiac output falls to prelabor levels 24 to 48 hours later. Twin gestation results in an additional 20% increase in cardiac output over singleton gestation.

f. ***Ventricular Hypertrophy.*** Left ventricular mass increases 6%, and right ventricular mass 15% to 20%. Mild insufficiency of all cardiac valves except the aortic valve results from increased size and dilation of the cardiac chambers.

g. ***Electrocardiographic Changes.*** Elevation and rotation of the heart cause axis shift: deep S in lead I and Qs with negative T waves in III and aVF are common.

h. ***Obstruction of the Inferior Vena Cava.*** When the pregnant woman is in the supine position, obstruction of the inferior vena cava by the gravid uterus results in supine hypotension syndrome in about 15% of parturients. It can be minimized by positioning the patient in the lateral position or mechanically displacing the uterus to the left.

2. Respiratory

a. Relaxation of rib cage ligaments with horizontal displacement of the ribs, upward displacement of the diaphragm early in pregnancy before the uterus mechanically shifts abdominal contents.

b. Increased diameter of the chest (>5 cm), which increases lung volume up to 40% by term. Decreased expiratory reserve volume (25%), residual volume (15%), and functional residual capacity (FRC) (20%).

c. Respiratory stimulation by progesterone: increased tidal volume, respiratory rate, and minute ventilation (50%).

d. Blood gas changes: respiratory alkalosis (pH 7.44, $Paco_2$ 28 to 32 mm Hg, and HCO_3 20 mmol/L), Pao_2 increases to 104 to 108. These changes facilitate maternal-fetal gas exchange.

TABLE 26-1 ■ **Physiologic Changes Accompanying Pregnancy**

PARAMETER	AVERAGE CHANGE FROM NONPREGNANT VALUE (%)
Intravascular fluid volume	+35
Plasma volume	+45
Erythrocyte volume	+20
Cardiac output	+40
Stroke volume	+30
Heart rate	+15
Peripheral circulation	
Systolic blood pressure	No change
Systemic vascular resistance	−15
Diastolic blood pressure	−15
Central venous pressure	No change
Femoral venous pressure	+15
Minute ventilation	+50
Tidal volume	+40
Breathing rate	+10
Pa_{O_2}	+10 mm Hg
Pa_{CO_2}	−10 mm Hg
pHa	No change
Total lung capacity	No change
Vital capacity	No change
Functional residual capacity	−20
Expiratory reserve volume	−20
Residual volume	−20
Airway resistance	−35
Oxygen consumption	+20
Renal blood flow and glomerular filtration rate	−50
Serum cholinesterase activity	−25

e. Twenty percent increase in oxygen consumption, leading to more rapid desaturation during apnea (9 minutes in a fully preoxygenated healthy nonpregnant patient, versus 3 to 4 minutes in a healthy parturient, versus 98 seconds in an obese parturient).

f. Airway anatomy: edema and hyperemia of the oropharyngeal mucosa, glandular hyperactivity, and capillary engorgement resulting from estrogen, progesterone, and relaxin lead to upper airway narrowing. Failed intubation rates rise eightfold from those in nonpregnant patients.

3. **Hematologic**
   a. Patient becomes relative hypercoagulable: increased activity of factors I, VII, VIII, IX, X, XII, and activity of anticoagulants (protein S, activated protein C) is decreased.
   b. Fivefold increased risk of deep vein thrombosis (DVT).
   c. Activated fibrinolytic system: decreased activity of factors XI, XIII; relative deficiencies of factors XI, XIII.
   d. Predisposition to consumptive coagulopathy. Levels of D-dimers and fibrin degradation products increase.
4. **Gastrointestinal**
   a. Decreased lower esophageal sphincter tone resulting from upward displacement of the stomach and muscle relaxation from progestins.
   b. Increased bile secretion and composition of bile acids with increased rates of cholelithiasis.
5. **Endocrine**
   a. Insulin resistance resulting from increased progesterone, estrogen, cortisol, and placental lactogen. Fasting glucose is lower than in nonpregnant women.
   b. Elevation of total T_3 and T_4, although free T_3 and T_4 remain stable, resulting from increased levels of thyroxin-binding globulin.
6. **Miscellaneous**
   a. Increased pain threshold because of progesterone and endorphins. No increased sensitivity to the hypnotic effects of inhalational agents.
   b. Decreased cerebrospinal fluid (CSF), but stable intracranial pressure (ICP).
   c. Increased renal blood flow and glomerular filtration rate (GFR) (50%), with decreased serum blood urea nitrogen (BUN) and creatinine levels.

B. Anesthetic Considerations—Nonobstetric Surgery

1. **Induction and Emergence from Anesthesia.** These occur more rapidly than in the nonpregnant state because of increased minute ventilation, decreased FRC, and the decreased minimum alveolar concentration (MAC) of volatile agents.
   a. Local anesthetics have increased effects; regional block dosages should be reduced 25% to 30%. Local anesthetic cardiotoxicity occurs at lower serum levels.
2. **Teratogenicity.** Few, if any, studies support teratogenic effects of anesthetic or sedative medications in the doses used for anesthesia care in humans.
   a. ***Diazepam.*** Some studies have suggested a connection between high-dose diazepam in the first trimester and cleft palate; medicinal doses of benzodiazepine are safe when needed to treat perioperative anxiety.
   b. ***Nitrous Oxide.*** Teratogenesis has been seen only in animals under extreme conditions and is not likely to be reproduced in clinical care.
   c. ***Volatile Agents.*** Recent concerns have been raised regarding neural apoptosis in rats, but with questions about how that can be translated to humans.
3. **Avoid Intrauterine Fetal Asphyxia.** Maintain maternal Pao_2, $Paco_2$ (maternal alkalosis can cause uterine vasoconstriction and shift the oxyhemoglobin dissociation curve to the left, releasing less oxygen to the fetus), and uterine blood flow (avoid hypotension, alkalosis, uterine irritability).
4. **Preterm Labor.** During the intraoperative and postoperative periods, preterm labor can occur. For monitoring, at least preoperative and postoperative fetal heart rate (FHR) and uterine activity must be assessed.
5. **Timing of Surgery.** Elective surgery should be postponed until the patient has returned to her nonpregnant physiologic state (about 2 to 6 weeks), but surgery in the middle trimester lessens the theoretical risk of teratogenicity and preterm labor. There are no data to support one anesthetic technique over another for emergency surgery.

C. Obstetric Anesthesia Care

   a. ***Regional Analgesic Techniques During Labor and Delivery.*** During the first stage of labor, pain is visceral and supplied by spinal cord segments T10-L1. During the second stage of

TABLE 26-2 ■ **Epidural Labor Analgesia**

	INFUSION	
BOLUS (10 mL)	**LOCAL ANESTHETIC**	**OPIOID**
Bupivacaine 0.125% with hydromorphone 10 mcg/mL	Bupivacaine 0.0625%-0.125%	Hydromorphone 3 mcg/mL
Bupivacaine 0.125% with fentanyl 5 mcg/mL	Bupivacaine 0.0625%-0.125%	Fentanyl 2 mcg/mL
Bupivacaine 0.125% with sufentanil 1 mcg/mL	Bupivacaine 0.0625%-0.125%	Sufentanil 2 mcg/mL
(Ropivacaine 0.075% may be used with opioid as above)	(Ropivacaine 0.075%-0.125% may be used)	Any of the above

labor, pain is somatic from S2-4 spinal cord segments via the pudendal nerves. Neuraxial analgesia in early labor does not increase the incidence of cesarean delivery and may shorten labor when compared with systemic analgesia.

b. ***Lumbar Epidural Analgesia.*** See Table 26-2 for analgesic choices. It is important to confirm the absence of intravascular or subarachnoid placement of the epidural catheter. This is usually done by administering a test dose of a solution containing local anesthetic and epinephrine (15 mcg) through the catheter. Tachycardia and/or hypertension (HTN) alert the anesthesiologist to the possibility of an intravascular catheter. Rapid onset of analgesia suggests subarachnoid placement. Hypotension may require administration of small doses of ephedrine (5 to 10 mg intravenously [IV]) or phenylephrine (20 to 100 mcg IV).

c. ***Combined Spinal-Epidural Analgesia (CSE).*** Analgesia via CSE in labor is an alternative to epidural analgesia. Advantages include rapid onset of analgesia, increased reliability, effectiveness when instituted in a rapidly progressing labor, and minimal motor block. Subarachnoid administration of low doses of opioids (fentanyl 12.5 to 25 mcg, sufentanil 5 to 10 mcg) results in rapid (5 minutes), nearly complete pain relief during the first stage of labor. Disadvantages of CSE include increased technical complexity and the possible risk of post–dural puncture headache.

d. ***Anesthesia for Cesarean Delivery.*** Epidural analgesia for labor can be converted to a surgical anesthetic by changing the drug dose and concentration administered. Spinal anesthesia with hyperbaric bupivacaine solution provides reliable anesthesia, often with the addition of morphine or meperidine for postoperative analgesia. General anesthesia is reserved for the most emergent cases or when maternal condition contraindicates regional anesthesia.

   i. ***Availability.*** The American College of Obstetricians and Gynecologists/American Society of Anesthesiologists consensus is that hospitals should have the capability to begin a cesarean delivery within 30 minutes of the decision to operate, although not all indications for cesarean delivery require that 30-minute response time.

   ii. ***Maternal Risks for Anesthesia*** *(Table 26-3).* Pulmonary aspiration and failed intubation account for three fourths of all maternal deaths related to anesthesia care. Prevention includes premedication with H_2-blockers, the use of a nonparticulate antacid, and/or metoclopramide and/or famotidine. General anesthesia should be avoided whenever possible; cricoid pressure and an endotracheal tube should be used if general anesthesia is required. The incidence of failed intubation in the obstetric population is 10 times that in the general surgical population.

TABLE 26-3 ■ Factors That Increase Anesthetic Risk
Obesity
Facial and neck edema
Extremely short stature
Difficulty opening mouth
Arthritis of neck, short neck, small mandible
Abnormalities of face, mouth, or teeth
Large thyroid
Pulmonary disease
Cardiac disease

TABLE 26-4 ■ Criteria for Diagnosis of Preeclampsia
Systemic hypertension >139/89 mm Hg after 20 wk of gestation in a woman with previously normal blood pressure
Proteinuria ≥0.3 g protein in a 24-hr urine specimen

TABLE 26-5 ■ Diagnostic Features of Severe Preeclampsia
Blood pressure >159/109 mm Hg on two occasions at least 6 hr apart
≥5 g proteinuria over 24 hr or dipstick reading ≥3+ on two samples at least 4 hr apart
Oliguria (<500 mL in 24 hr)
Pulmonary edema or cyanosis
Abnormal liver function
Right upper quadrant pain or epigastric pain
Cerebral disturbances
Thrombocytopenia

II. HYPERTENSIVE DISORDERS OF PREGNANCY

Hypertensive disorders of pregnancy encompass a range of disorders that includes chronic HTN, chronic HTN with superimposed preeclampsia, gestational HTN (nonproteinuric HTN), preeclampsia (proteinuric HTN), and eclampsia.

A. Gestational Hypertension. Gestational HTN is characterized by the onset of systemic HTN (blood pressure [BP] >139/89), without proteinuria or edema, after the first 19 weeks of pregnancy or during the immediate postpartum period. It is defined as severe if BP exceeds 159/109 mm Hg for more than 6 hours.

B. Preeclampsia. A syndrome exhibited after 20 weeks of gestation, preeclampsia manifests as systemic HTN, proteinuria, and generalized edema. Diagnostic criteria for preeclampsia and severe preeclampsia are summarized in Tables 26-4 and 26-5, respectively.

1. **Etiology.** Preeclampsia is a syndrome that affects virtually all organ systems. It is associated with placental ischemia resulting from abnormal placentation-implantation. Shallow endovascular invasion prevents cytotrophoblastic-endothelium interaction, and decidual arteries are constricted, high-resistance vessels that fail to provide adequate oxygen and nutrients to the fetus. The placenta releases vasoactive substances, causing maternal endothelial dysfunction. Plasma concentrations of vasoconstrictive substances, markers of oxidative stress, and inflammatory cytokines are increased, and concentrations of vasodilators (nitric oxide, prostacyclin) are decreased. Antiangiogenic proteins cause endothelial

damage, especially in the kidney, liver, and brain. Sensitivity to angiotensin II, which is decreased in normal pregnancy, is increased in preeclampsia.

2. **Hypoalbuminemia.** Hypoalbuminemia and occasional impairment of synthetic liver function lead to low oncotic pressure, increased third spacing, and intravascular volume depletion.
3. **Risks for Development of Preeclampsia** (Table 26-6)
4. **Treatment** (Table 26-7). The definitive treatment is delivery. If the preeclampsia is mild and the patient remote from term, conservative management with bed rest and monitoring until 37 weeks of gestation or until the status of the mother or fetus deteriorates are

TABLE 26-6 ■ **Risks for Development of Preeclampsia**

FACTOR	RELATIVE RISK
Nulliparity	3
African American race	1.5
Age <15 yr or >35 yr	3
Multiple gestation	4
Family history of preeclampsia	5
Chronic hypertension	10
Chronic renal disease	20
Diabetes mellitus	2
Collagen vascular disease	2-3
Angiotensinogen T235 allele	
Homozygosity	20
Heterozygosity	4

TABLE 26-7 ■ **Treatment of Preeclampsia**

Maintain diastolic blood pressure <110 mm Hg
Hydralazine 5-10 mg IV every 20-30 min
Hydralazine 5-20 mg/hr IV as a continuous infusion following administration of 5 mg IV
Labetalol 50 mg IV or 100 mg PO
Labetalol 20-160 mg/hr IV as a continuous infusion
Nitroglycerin 10 mcg/min IV, titrated to response
Nitroprusside 0.25 mcg/kg/min IV, titrated to response
Fenoldopam 0.1 mcg/kg/min IV, increase by 0.05-0.2 mcg/kg/min until desired response reached; average dose 0.25-0.5 mcg/kg/min
Seizure prophylaxis
Magnesium 4-6 g IV followed by concentrations continuous infusion of 1-2 g/hr (goal is to maintain serum magnesium concentration of 2.0-3.5 mEq/L)
Monitor for magnesium toxicity
4.0-6.5 mEq/L associated with nausea, vomiting, diplopia, somnolence, loss of patellar reflex
6.5-7.5 mEq/L associated with skeletal muscle paralysis, apnea
≥10 mEq/L associated with cardiac arrest

IV, Intravenously; *PO*, by mouth.

recommended. In women with severe preeclampsia, the fetus should be delivered immediately regardless of gestational age. Management includes administration of magnesium sulfate to prevent seizures, antihypertensive therapy (hydralazine, labetalol, nifedipine), and fluid resuscitation Arterial and central venous pressure monitoring may be necessary. Treatment of HTN in women with mild preeclampsia is not necessary. Indications for antihypertensive treatment during pregnancy are chronic HTN, severe HTN during labor and delivery, and expectant management of preeclampsia. The goal of therapy is to maintain BP below 160/110 mm Hg.

5. **Prognosis**
   a. ***Maternal.*** Cerebral hemorrhage is a major cause of maternal death that results from preeclampsia and eclampsia (15% to 20% of maternal deaths). Patients may develop seizures or pulmonary edema within 24 to 48 hours after delivery; anticonvulsant therapy and antihypertensive therapy should continue for 48 hours or longer postpartum.
6. **Management of Anesthesia**
   a. ***Fluid Management.*** Preeclamptic patients are hypovolemic and prone to hypotension with the institution of neuraxial anesthesia, but they are also at risk of pulmonary edema. A 500- to 1000-mL crystalloid preload is appropriate before neuraxial analgesia is initiated. Invasive monitoring may be indicated if the patient develops either pulmonary edema or oliguria unresponsive to a fluid challenge. Intraarterial BP monitoring is indicated for refractory HTN, especially if an antihypertensive infusion is needed.
   b. ***Labor Analgesia.*** Vaginal delivery in the presence of preeclampsia and in the absence of fetal distress is acceptable. Epidural analgesia is the preferred technique for labor analgesia, if not contraindicated (reduces maternal catecholamine levels and facilitates BP control). Because of the hypersensitivity of the maternal vasculature to catecholamines, use of local anesthetic solutions without the addition of epinephrine should be considered.
   c. ***Anesthetic for Cesarean Delivery***
      i. ***Spinal Anesthesia.*** This is the anesthetic choice for patients with preeclampsia, unless contraindicated by hypocoagulation. In preeclamptic patients, HTN and vasoconstriction are the result of hyperactivity of angiotensin II receptors. Spinal anesthesia does not influence the angiotensin system and may therefore result in a lesser degree of hypotension in preeclamptic patients than healthy patients.
      ii. ***General Anesthesia.*** General anesthesia is indicated for preeclamptic patients undergoing cesarean section who refuse regional anesthesia or who are coagulopathic or septic. Risks include potentially difficult tracheal intubation, risk of aspiration, and exaggerated responses to sympathomimetics and methylergonovine. These patients have greater sensitivity to nondepolarizing muscle relaxants secondary to magnesium therapy. There is increased risk of uterine atony and peripartum hemorrhage resulting from magnesium therapy.

C. **HELLP Syndrome.** This severe form of preeclampsia is characterized by *H*emolysis, *E*levated *L*iver transaminase enzymes, and *L*ow *P*latelet counts. In addition to other signs of preeclampsia, HELLP syndrome patients may have epigastric pain, upper abdominal tenderness, and jaundice. Disseminated intravascular coagulation (DIC) is a risk, and maternal and perinatal mortality is increased.

1. **Treatment.** Definitive treatment of HELLP syndrome is the delivery of the fetus, often by cesarean section, regardless of gestational age.
   a. Seizure prophylaxis consists of magnesium sulfate.
   b. Correction of coagulopathy: dexamethasone may increase platelet count.
2. **Management of Anesthesia.**
   a. Regional techniques must often be avoided because of coagulation defects. The precise selection of drugs will be influenced by the presence of renal and hepatic dysfunction that could alter drug clearance, metabolism, and elimination.

D. Eclampsia. When seizures are superimposed on preeclampsia, eclampsia is present. The magnitude of HTN does not correlate with the risk of eclampsia. Eclampsia is associated with a maternal mortality of approximately 2%. Seizures occur more than 48 hours after delivery in 16% of cases. The obstetric and anesthetic management of the eclamptic patient is directed at controlling the seizures (airway support; oxygenation; antiseizure treatment with thiopental, a benzodiazepine, or magnesium) and protecting the patient from aspiration pneumonitis. Lateralizing neurologic signs after a seizure may be the first sign of intracranial hemorrhage. One third of patients develop respiratory failure, kidney failure, coagulopathy, CVA, or cardiac arrest. Fetal perinatal mortality is about 7%.

1. **Management of Anesthesia.** Eclampsia is not an indication for cesarean delivery. Anesthetic management of the patient proceeds as it would for a patient with preeclampsia, provided she is in stable condition after an eclamptic seizure.

III. OBSTETRIC COMPLICATIONS

Obstetric complications include hemorrhagic complications, amniotic fluid embolism, uterine rupture, vaginal birth after cesarean delivery (VBAC), abnormal presentations, and multiple births.

A. Obstetric Hemorrhage (Table 26-8)

1. **Placenta Previa.** This occurs in up to 1% of pregnancies and is characterized by painless vaginal bleeding. Placenta previa is classified as complete when the entire cervical os is covered by placental tissue, partial when the internal cervical os is covered by placental tissue when closed but not when fully dilated, and marginal when placental tissue encroaches on or extends to the margin of the internal cervical os. Parturients with a total or partial previa will deliver by cesarean section. Large-bore intravenous access should be established, and cross-matched blood should be immediately available.
2. **Placenta Accreta.** The condition in which the placenta is abnormally adherent to the myometrium is placenta accreta (placenta increta occurs when the placenta has invaded the myometrium). Massive hemorrhage may occur when removal of the placenta is attempted after delivery. The majority of cases require cesarean hysterectomy. Large-bore intravenous catheters should be placed, and blood should be immediately available. Recommendations

TABLE 26-8 ■ **Differential Diagnosis of Third-Trimester Bleeding**

PARAMETER	PLACENTA PREVIA	ABRUPTIO PLACENTAE	UTERINE RUPTURE
Signs and symptoms	Painless vaginal bleeding	Abdominal pain Bleeding partially or wholly concealed Uterine irritability Shock Acute renal failure Fetal distress	Abdominal pain Vaginal pain Recession of presenting part Disappearance of fetal heart tones, fetal bradycardia Hemodynamic instability
Predisposing conditions	Advanced age Multiple parity	Advanced parity Advanced age, Cigarette smoker Cocaine abuse Trauma Uterine anomalies Compression of the inferior vena cava Chronic systemic hypertension	Previous uterine incision Rapid spontaneous delivery Excessive uterine stimulation Cephalopelvic disproportion Multiple parity Polyhydramnios

include that 4 units of red blood cells (RBCs) and 4 units of fresh frozen plasma (FFP) be available; in complex cases, available blood should include 10 units of RBCs, 10 units of FFP, and 10 units of platelets. Ketamine and etomidate may be preferred anesthetic agents if emergency delivery is necessitated by hemorrhage and general anesthesia is selected. Although hysterectomy used to be a traditional expectation at the time of cesarean section, now uterine-sparing techniques such as arterial embolization may be attempted.

a. ***Management of Blood Loss.*** Hemorrhagic shock occurs in more than 50% of patients who undergo emergency postpartum hysterectomy, and coagulopathy or DIC occurs in 25%.
b. ***Salvaged Autologous "Cell Saver" Blood.*** There is scant evidence about use in parturient patients, but the possibility of amniotic fluid contamination and risk of severe hypotension should be considered.
c. ***Damage Control Resuscitation.*** This involves matching packed RBCs (PRBCs) in a 1:1:1 ratio with FFP and platelets. Colloid and crystalloid administration is minimized. Studies in the military suggested that mortality decreases dramatically (65% to 19%), but extrapolation to pregnant women should be done with caution, because coagulation effects of trauma are different from coagulation changes of pregnancy.
d. ***Fibrinogen.*** A higher fibrinogen level may be needed in postpartum hemorrhage for adequate hemostasis (2 to 3 g/L versus 1 g/L). Factor XIII activity should be kept above 50% to 60%. Early transfusion of cryoprecipitate is recommended.
e. ***Factor VII.*** Administration of 80 to 95 mcg/kg may reduce hemorrhage without increasing risk of thromboembolic events.
f. ***Monitoring.*** Partial thromboplastin time (PTT), prothrombin time (PT), platelet count, and fibrinogen level should be measured at baseline and hourly to guide therapy. Thromboelastography may provide goal-directed therapy. Plasma electrolytes should be measured at baseline and hourly for assessment of hyperkalemia, hypomagnesemia, hypocalcemia, and hyperchloremia.

3. **Abruptio Placentae.** Separation of the placenta from the uterus after 20 weeks of gestation, or abruptio placentae, can cause severe blood loss, fetal distress or demise, clotting abnormalities, and acute renal failure. Abdominal pain is always present, but bleeding may not be obvious owing to sequestration in the uterus. Definitive treatment is delivery of the fetus and placenta, often by cesarean section. Anesthetic management is similar to that employed with placenta previa. Blood and blood products should be readily available because of the risk of bleeding and DIC. Perinatal mortality is 25-fold higher in cases of abruption.
4. **Postpartum Hemorrhage**
   a. ***Uterine Atony.*** Treatment is with intravenous oxytocin resulting in contraction of the uterus. Intravenous or intramuscular methylergonovine or intramuscular or intrauterine carboprost tromethamine (misoprostol) may also be used. Rarely, it may be necessary to perform an emergency hysterectomy.
   b. ***Retained Placenta.*** Manual removal of the retained placenta may be attempted with the patient under epidural or spinal anesthesia. Low doses (40-mcg boluses, as needed) of intravenous nitroglycerin are used to relax the uterus for placental removal when indicated.

B. Trial of Labor After Cesarean Section (TOLAC). The risk of uterine rupture increases with the number of previous uterine incisions. Both the American College of Obstetricians and Gynecologists and the American Society of Anesthesiologists recommend that personnel, including the obstetrician, anesthetist, and operating room personnel, be immediately available at all times to perform an emergency cesarean delivery when VBAC is being attempted. Risks for failed TOLAC or uterine rupture during VBAC are summarized in Table 26-9.

1. **Anesthetic Management.** Epidural analgesia is an ideal technique for pain control in parturients attempting a VBAC. Approximately 60% to 80% of patients undergoing a trial for VBAC ultimately have a cesarean delivery, and epidural analgesia can be quickly converted to surgical anesthesia in these patients.

TABLE 26-9 ■ Risks Associated with Trial of Labor After Cesarean Section

Risks for failed labor	African American or Hispanic ethnicity Advanced maternal age Single motherhood <12 yr of maternal education Delivery at low-volume hospital Maternal comorbidities: HTN, diabetes, asthma, seizure disorder, renal disease, heart disease, obesity Induction of labor Fetal gestational age >40 weeks Fetal weight >4000 g Poor cervical dilation
Risks for uterine rupture	Classic uterine scar Induction of labor Fetal gestational age >40 wk Two or more previous cesarean deliveries Maternal obesity Fetal weight >4000 g Delivery at low-volume hospital Interdelivery interval <18 months Single layer closure during previous cesarean section

HTN, Hypertension.

2. **Uterine Rupture.** Presenting signs and symptoms may include severe abdominal pain (often referred to the shoulder), maternal hypotension, and disappearance of fetal heart tones. Ultrasound examination may be useful in uncertain cases. Treatment is immediate laparotomy, delivery, and surgical repair of the uterus or hysterectomy. Although maternal mortality is rare, fetal mortality is about 35%.

C. **Amniotic Fluid Embolism.** This is a rare catastrophic and life-threatening complication of pregnancy heralded by abrupt onset of dyspnea, arterial hypoxemia, cyanosis, seizures, loss of consciousness, and hypotension disproportionate to blood loss. Fetal distress is present at the same time. Coagulopathy resembling DIC with associated bleeding may be the only presenting sign. Presence of amniotic fluid material (fetal squamous cells, fat, mucin) in the parturient's blood may ultimately confirm diagnosis. Treatment includes tracheal intubation, mechanical ventilation with 100% oxygen, inotropic support, and correction of coagulopathy. Even with aggressive treatment, mortality from amniotic fluid embolism is greater than 80%.

D. **Abnormal Presentations and Multiple Births**

1. **Breech Presentation.** Breech vaginal deliveries result in increased maternal morbidity (cervical lacerations, perineal injury, retained placenta, shock caused by hemorrhage) and neonatal morbidity and mortality. Preferred delivery is by elective cesarean section. Dense perineal anesthesia is needed if vaginal instrumentation is anticipated and must be administered rapidly (3% 2-chloroprocaine epidurally or by the induction of general anesthesia).

2. **Multiple Gestations.** All triplet and higher-order gestations are delivered by cesarean section. For twin gestations, presentation of the twins is considered when determining mode of delivery. If both are vertex, vaginal delivery is appropriate. If twin A is breech, cesarean delivery is recommended.

   a. ***Anesthetic Concerns.*** Worsened FRC, worsened supine hypotension syndrome, and increased risk of postpartum hemorrhage are concerns.

TABLE 26-10 ■ Risk Factors for Cardiac Events in Pregnancy and Labor

- History of previous cardiac arrest
- Baseline New York Heart Association Class II
- Cyanosis
- Left heart obstruction (mitral valve area ≤2 cm^2, aortic valve area <1.5 cm^2, peak LV outflow tract gradient >30 mm Hg by echocardiography)
- Reduced systemic ventricular systolic function (EF <40%)

One point assigned per risk factor. Risk estimate = 5% with no points, 27% with 1 point, and 75% for ≥2 points.

EF, Ejection fraction; *LV,* left ventricular.

TABLE 26-11 ■ Multivariable Model for the Composite End Points of Cardiac and Neonatal Complications Corrected for Maternal Age and Parity

	ODDS RATIO	*P* VALUE
History of arrhythmia	4.3	.0011
Cardiac medication use before pregnancy	4.2	<.0001
NYHA functional class	2.2	.0298
Left-sided heart obstruction (peak gradient >50 mm Hg, aortic valve area <1.0 cm^2)	12.9	<.0001
Moderate to severe AI	2.0	.0427
Moderate to severe PI	2.3	.0287
Mechanical prosthetic valve	74.7	.0014
Cyanotic heart disease (corrected or not)	3.0	<.0001
NEONATAL COMPLICATIONS		
Twin or multiple gestation	5.4	.0014
Smoking during pregnancy	1.7	.0070
Cyanotic heart disease (corrected or not)	2.0	.0003
Mechanical prosthetic valve	13.9	.0331
Cardiac medication use before pregnancy	2.2	.0009

Adapted from ZAHARA investigators. Predictors of pregnancy complications in women with congenital heart disease. *Eur Heart J.* 2010;31(17):2124-2132. Epub Jun 28, 2010.

AI, Aortic insufficiency; *NYHA,* New York Heart Association; *PI,* pulmonary insufficiency.

IV. CO-EXISTING MEDICAL DISEASES

A. Heart Disease

1. **Circulatory Changes and Co-existing Heart Disease.** Pregnancy and labor may lead to cardiovascular decompensation of an already diseased cardiovascular system because of pregnancy-induced and labor-induced increases in cardiac output.
2. **Risks of Cardiac Events During Pregnancy and Labor.** Risks can be estimated using a scale based on the presence of certain risk factors (Table 26-10). Additional risks include pulmonary HTN (patients are usually advised against pregnancy), arrhythmia, use of cardiac medications before pregnancy, moderate or severe mitral or tricuspid regurgitation, and presence of a mechanical valve. A summary of risks and odds ratios for cardiac events is found in Table 26-11.

TABLE 26-12 ■ **White's Classification of Diabetes During Pregnancy**

CLASS	DEFINITION
A_1	Diet-controlled gestational DM
A_2	Gestational DM requiring insulin
B	Preexisting DM without complications (duration <10 yr or age at onset >20 yr)
C	Preexisting DM without complications (duration 10-19 yr or age at onset 10-19 yr)
D	Preexisting DM (duration >20 yr or age at onset <10 yr)
F	Preexisting DM with nephropathy
R	Preexisting DM with retinopathy
T	Preexisting DM S/P renal transplant
H	Preexisting DM with heart disease

DM, Diabetes mellitus; *S/P,* postoperative status.

3. **Cardiomyopathy of Pregnancy.** Left ventricular failure late in the course of pregnancy or during the first 6 weeks postpartum is cardiomyopathy of pregnancy. The precise cause remains unknown. Medical treatment of peripartum cardiomyopathy is similar to that of other dilated cardiomyopathies, except that angiotensin-converting enzyme inhibitors, which are routinely used for afterload reduction in nonpregnant patients, are contraindicated during pregnancy. Nitroglycerin or nitroprusside can be used for afterload reduction. In about 50% of patients, heart failure is transient and resolves within 6 months of delivery. In the remaining patients, idiopathic cardiomyopathy persists and mortality is 25% to 50%.
   a. ***Anesthetic Management.*** Invasive hemodynamic monitoring is usually needed. Cardiac decompensation during labor can be treated with intravenous nitroglycerin or nitroprusside (preload, afterload reduction) and dopamine or dobutamine (inotropic support). Early epidural labor analgesia minimizes the cardiac stress associated with the pain of labor. If cesarean delivery is required, epidural or spinal anesthetic may be used, with fluid management guided by the use of the invasive monitors. If general anesthesia is required, a high-dose opioid technique is often preferred; neonatal depression from the opioid is expected, and personnel for neonatal resuscitation must be available.

B. **Diabetes Mellitus.** Pregnancy is a state of progressive insulin resistance. Women who cannot produce enough insulin to compensate for this develop gestational diabetes. Patients with diabetes before pregnancy have increased insulin requirements in pregnancy. Diabetic ketoacidosis occurs at lower glucose levels in pregnancy.
   1. **Diagnosis.** If results of the routine 1-hour glucose tolerance test are abnormal, a 3-hour glucose tolerance test is administered; if these results are abnormal, this establishes the diagnosis of gestational diabetes (Table 26-12).
   2. **Treatment.** Glycemic control (blood sugar 60 to 120 mg/dL) is the goal. Management of diabetic ketoacidosis is similar to that for nonpregnant patients. In patients with gestational diabetes, dietary control is used initially. If glycemic control cannot be achieved, insulin therapy is initiated.
   3. **Antenatal Surveillance.** This begins in the third trimester with twice-weekly nonstress tests beginning at 28 weeks. A nonreactive nonstress test result leads to a biophysical profile to determine timing and route of delivery. Elective induction of labor is commonly chosen to avoid neonatal risks associated with maternal diabetes.
   4. **Fetal Effects of Diabetes.** These include a greater risk of fetal anomalies, intrauterine fetal death including stillbirth, macrosomia, greater incidence of cesarean delivery, shoulder dystocia, and birth trauma. Neonates are at risk for hypoglycemia and respiratory distress.

5. **Anesthetic Management.** Patients with autonomic dysfunction are especially prone to hypotension with epidural analgesia, and thus hypervigilance and rapid treatment are indicated. Epidural analgesia may be preferred to CSE, as the catheter should be known to be functioning to minimize the need for general anesthesia in the event of a cesarean section.

C. **Myasthenia Gravis.** This disorder is characterized by skeletal muscle fatigability and weakness caused by autoantibody destruction or blockade of postsynaptic nicotinic acetylcholine receptors. Exacerbations are most likely during the first trimester or within 10 days postpartum. Anticholinesterase drugs should be continued during pregnancy and labor. Epidural analgesia is acceptable for labor and vaginal delivery. Regional anesthesia can be used safely for cesarean section, but co-existing skeletal muscle weakness may lead to hypoventilation during anesthesia. General anesthesia considerations include the possibility of prolonged effects from nondepolarizing muscle relaxants, and the potential of reversal of nondepolarizing muscle relaxants to cause cholinergic crisis. Neonatal myasthenia gravis occurs transiently in 20% to 30% of babies born to mothers with myasthenia. Anticholinesterase therapy is usually necessary in neonates for approximately 21 days after birth.

D. **Obesity.** Obesity is associated with increased risk of hypertensive disorders, including chronic HTN and preeclampsia, gestational diabetes, thromboembolic disease, abnormal labor, cesarean delivery, dystocia, maternal death, infection, and anesthesia-associated airway difficulties. Perinatal risks include increased incidence of macrosomia, birth trauma, shoulder dystocia, meconium aspiration, neural tube defects, and other congenital abnormalities.

1. **Anesthetic Management.** Epidural analgesia is a reasonable choice for labor analgesia and surgical anesthesia. The sitting, rather than the lateral, position may facilitate successful identification of the epidural space. The incidence of cesarean delivery is increased in obese patients and is complicated by longer surgical duration and increased blood loss in obese patients. Regional anesthesia is preferred whenever possible for the obese parturient but may be associated with exaggerated spread of local anesthetic in these patients (high spinal).

E. **Advanced Maternal Age.** Age greater than 35 years is independently associated with higher rates of maternal morbidities, including gestational diabetes, preeclampsia, placental abruption, and cesarean delivery. Advanced maternal age is also independently associated with an increased likelihood of cesarean delivery because of comorbidities and an increased rate of requested cesarean delivery. Anesthesia considerations are directed toward management of comorbidities.

F. **Substance Abuse**

1. **Alcohol Abuse.** Fetal alcohol syndrome (neurobehavioral deficit, intrauterine growth retardation, congenital abnormalities) occurs in approximately one third of infants born to mothers who drink more than 3 ounces of alcohol per day during pregnancy. Anesthetic care of the pregnant alcohol abuser is the same as in the nonpregnant patient.
2. **Tobacco Abuse.** Tobacco abuse is strongly associated with low birth rate, abruptio placentae, impaired respiratory function in newborns, and sudden infant death syndrome. Anesthetic considerations for care of the tobacco-abusing parturient are similar to those considerations in the nonpregnant patient.
3. **Opioid Abuse.** Complications include human immunodeficiency virus (HIV) infection, hepatitis, abscesses, endocarditis, and thrombophlebitis. A pregnant patient admitted on chronic opioid therapy should be maintained on that therapy during her pregnancy and into the postpartum period. Neonates should be observed and treated for withdrawal symptoms as necessary.
4. **Cocaine Abuse.** In parturients, cocaine abuse is associated with maternal cardiovascular, respiratory, neurologic, and hematologic complications similar to those seen in the nonpregnant patient. An increased incidence of significant obstetric complications (spontaneous abortion, stillbirth, preterm labor, abruptio placentae) occurs in parturients who abuse cocaine during pregnancy (Table 26-13). Fetal complications include decreased birth weight, intrauterine growth retardation, microcephaly, and prematurity.

TABLE 26-13 ■ Obstetric Complications Associated with Cocaine Abuse During Pregnancy
Spontaneous abortion
Preterm labor
Premature rupture of membranes
Abruptio placentae
Precipitous delivery
Stillbirth
Maternal hypertension
Meconium aspiration
Low Apgar scores at birth

a. ***Anesthetic Considerations.*** Cocaine-induced thrombocytopenia must be excluded before regional anesthesia. Phenylephrine, because of its direct actions, is a better choice for treatment of hypotension than ephedrine. Cocaine-induced thrombocytopenia may be present and must be excluded if regional anesthesia is contemplated. Body temperature increases and sympathomimetic effects associated with cocaine toxicity may mimic malignant hyperthermia.

V. FETAL ASSESSMENT AND NEONATAL PROBLEMS

A. **Electronic Fetal Monitoring** A three-tiered system for categorizing the tracings obtained in FHR monitoring is summarized in Table 26-14.

1. **Fetal Heart Rate**

a. ***Baseline Heart Rate.*** Normally this is 110 to 160 beats/min; bradycardia is defined as less than 110 beats/min for longer than 10 minutes, and tachycardia as more than 160 beats/min for longer than 10 minutes.

b. ***Beat-to-Beat Variability.*** The FHR varies 5 to 20 beats/min (normal heart rate is 120 to 160 beats/min). Fetal distress caused by arterial hypoxemia, acidosis, or central nervous system damage is associated with minimal to absent beat-to-beat variability. Drugs most commonly associated with loss of beat-to-beat variability are benzodiazepines, opioids, barbiturates, anticholinergics, and local anesthetics used for continuous lumbar epidural analgesia. Terms describing FHR variability are as follows:

- Absent: variability undetectable
- Minimal: 5 beats/min or less
- Moderate: 6 to 25 beats/min
- Marked: more than 25 beats/min

c. ***Accelerations.*** Visually apparent abrupt increases in FHR are accelerations. Prolonged accelerations last longer than 2 minutes but less than 10 minutes. An acceleration lasting longer than 10 minutes constitutes a change in baseline.

d. ***Decelerations***

i. ***Early Decelerations.*** This pattern is characterized by the slowing of the FHR that begins with the onset of uterine contractions, is at its maximum at the peak of the contraction, and returns to near baseline at its termination. This FHR pattern is not associated with fetal distress. Decreases are usually not more than 20 beats/min and seldom below an absolute rate of 100 beats/min.

ii. ***Late Decelerations.*** This pattern is characterized by slowing of the FHR that begins 10 to 30 seconds after the onset of uterine contractions and maximizes after the peak intensity of the contractions. Mild slowing is a decrease of less than 20 beats/min, whereas profound slowing is a decrease of 40 beats/min or more. Late decelerations

TABLE 26-14 ■ Three-Tiered System for Interpretation of Electronic Fetal Heart Rate (FHR) Monitoring

CATEGORY	CHARACTERISTICS
Category I (Must include all characteristics listed)	**Rate:** 110-160 beats/min **Variability:** moderate **Late or variable decelerations:** absent **Early decelerations:** present or absent **Accelerations:** present or absent
Category II (All FHR tracings not classified as category I or III; must include all characteristics listed)	**Baseline rate** Bradycardia not accompanied by absence of variability Tachycardia **Baseline FHR variability** Minimal variability Absence of variability not accompanied by recurrent decelerations Marked baseline variability **Accelerations** Absence of induced accelerations after fetal stimulation **Periodic or episodic decelerations** Recurrent variable decelerations accompanied by minimal or moderate baseline variability Prolonged deceleration of ≥2 min but <10 min Recurrent late decelerations with moderate baseline variability Variable decelerations with other characteristics, such as slow return to baseline, overshoots, or "shoulders"
Category III (Includes either of the characteristics listed)	**Absence of baseline FHR variability *and* any of the following:** Recurrent late decelerations Recurrent variable decelerations Bradycardia **Sinusoidal pattern**

are associated with fetal distress, most likely reflecting myocardial hypoxia secondary to uteroplacental insufficiency. Treatment involves left uterine displacement, intravenous fluids, and, if maternal hypotension is present, ephedrine administration.

iii. ***Variable Decelerations.*** These represent the most common pattern of fetal heart changes observed during the intrapartum period. Decelerations are variable in magnitude, duration, and time of onset relative to uterine contractions. Severe variable deceleration patterns that persist for 15 to 30 minutes are associated with fetal acidosis. Variable decelerations are caused by umbilical cord compression, and delivery may become necessary if variable decelerations persist or worsen.

iv. ***Prolonged Decelerations.*** Prolonged decelerations are decreases in FHR of greater than 15 beats/min that last longer than 2 minutes but less than 10 minutes. A deceleration lasting longer than 10 minutes is considered a change in baseline.

v. ***Sinusoidal Pattern.*** This is a visually smooth, undulating sine wave pattern with a cyclic frequency of 3 to 5 minutes, persisting for 20 minutes or longer.

2. **Fetal Scalp Sampling.** This technique may be used to evaluate a fetus with an abnormal FHR tracing. Fetal hypoxia may be confirmed, establishing a need for urgent delivery. A pH of less than 7.20 suggests fetal compromise necessitating immediate delivery.

TABLE 26-15 ■ Evaluation of Neonates Using the Apgar Score

PARAMETER	0	1	2
Heart rate (beats/min)	Absent	<100	>100
Respiratory effort	Absent	Slow Irregular	Crying
Reflex irritability	No response	Grimace	Crying
Muscle tone	Limp	Flexion of extremities	Active
Color	Pale Cyanotic	Body pink Extremities cyanotic	Pink

3. **Fetal Pulse Oximetry.** This technique provides continuous fetal arterial oxygen saturation readings when the sensor is placed through the cervix to lie alongside the fetal cheek or temple. Normal fetal oxygen saturations range from 30% to 70%. Saturations less than 30% suggest fetal acidosis.
4. **Ultrasound Examination.** Ultrasound examination of the fetus when the mother is in labor may be useful to determine the fetal presenting part, to confirm intrauterine fetal health or demise, and to diagnose placental abruption and placenta previa.

B. Evaluation of the Neonate

1. **Apgar Score.** A numeric value is assigned to five vital signs measured or observed in neonates 1 minute and 5 minutes after delivery (Table 26-15). Apgar scores correlate well with acid-base measurements performed immediately after birth. When scores are higher than 7, neonates have either normal blood gases or mild respiratory acidosis. Infants with scores of 4 to 6 are moderately depressed; those with scores of 3 or lower have combined metabolic and respiratory acidosis. Mildly to moderately depressed infants (Apgar scores of 3 to 7) often improve in response to oxygen administered by face mask, with or without positive-pressure ventilation. Tracheal intubation and perhaps external cardiac massage are indicated when Apgar scores are less than 3.
2. **Oxygenation and Ventilation.** Immediately after delivery with clamping of the umbilical cord, SVR increases, left atrial pressure increases, and flow through the foramen ovale ceases. Pulmonary vascular resistance drops with expansion of the lungs, and right ventricular output is diverted to the lungs. Increase in Pao_2 to more than 60 mm Hg leads to functional closure of the ductus arteriosus. When oxygenation and ventilation are inadequate after delivery, a fetal circulation pattern persists (increased pulmonary vascular resistance and decreased pulmonary blood flow) and the ductus arteriosus and foramen ovale remain open, resulting in large right-to-left intracardiac shunts with associated arterial hypoxemia and acidosis.
3. **Abnormalities Present at or Shortly After Delivery**
   a. ***Hypovolemia.*** In newborns with mean arterial pressures higher than 50 mm Hg at birth, hypovolemia is likely. Hypovolemia often follows intrauterine fetal distress, during which larger than normal portions of fetal blood are shunted to the placenta and remain there after delivery and clamping of the umbilical cord.
   b. ***Hypoglycemia.*** Hypoglycemia can manifest as hypotension, tremors, and seizures. Infants with intrauterine growth retardation and those born to diabetic mothers or after severe intrauterine fetal distress are vulnerable to hypoglycemia.
   c. ***Meconium Aspiration.*** Meconium may be present in the major airways and is distributed to the lung periphery with the onset of spontaneous breathing. Obstruction of small airways causes ventilation-to-perfusion mismatching. In severe cases, pulmonary HTN and

right-to-left shunting through the patent foramen ovale and ductus arteriosus (persistent fetal circulation) lead to severe arterial hypoxemia. Routine oropharyngeal suctioning is recommended at the time of delivery. Infants with low Apgar scores or who are clinically obstructed with meconium require active resuscitation, including tracheal intubation and attempts to remove meconium via suctioning.

d. ***Choanal Stenosis and Atresia.*** Nasal obstruction should be suspected in neonates who have good breathing efforts but become cyanotic when forced to breathe with their mouths closed. Unilateral or bilateral choanal stenosis is diagnosed based on the failure to pass a small catheter through each naris; such failure may reflect congenital (anatomic) obstruction or functional atresia caused by blood, mucus, or meconium. An oral airway may be necessary for anatomic obstruction until surgical correction can be accomplished. Functional choanal atresia is treated by nasal suctioning.

e. ***Diaphragmatic Hernia.*** This condition is characterized by severe respiratory distress at birth, associated with cyanosis and a scaphoid abdomen. Initial treatment is tracheal intubation and ventilation with oxygen.

f. ***Tracheoesophageal Fistula.*** Tracheoesophageal fistula should be suspected when polyhydramnios is present (see Chapter 27). An initial diagnosis in the delivery room is suggested when a catheter is inserted into the esophagus but cannot be passed into the stomach. Copious amounts of oropharyngeal secretions are usually present. Chest radiographs with the catheter in place confirm the diagnosis.

g. ***Laryngeal Anomalies and Subglottic Stenosis.*** These conditions manifest at birth as stridor. Insertion of a tube into the trachea beyond the obstruction alleviates the symptoms.

CHAPTER 27

Pediatric Diseases

I. UNIQUE CONSIDERATIONS IN PEDIATRIC PATIENTS

A. Psychology. Perianesthesia anxiety (Table 27-1) is common in pediatric patients and their parents. Perianesthetic programs including play and simulation of induction, videos, or separate preanesthetic visits ahead of time can help alleviate anxiety. Allowing parental visits in the postanesthesia care unit (PACU) can contribute to a positive experience for patients and parents.

II. ANATOMY AND PHYSIOLOGY

A. Body Size and Thermoregulation. Shivering contributes little to heat production in neonates, whose primary mechanism of heat production is nonshivering thermogenesis mediated by brown fat. "Neutral temperature" is defined as the ambient temperature that results in the least oxygen consumption. "Critical temperature" is the ambient temperature below which an unclothed, unanesthetized person cannot maintain a normal core body temperature (Table 27-2). Most operating rooms are below the critical temperature of a term neonate. Steps aimed at decreasing loss of body heat include transporting neonates in heated modules; increasing the ambient temperature of operating rooms; using a heating mattress, radiant warmer, and forced-air warming devices; and humidifying and warming inspired gases.

B. Central Nervous System. A newborn's brain constitutes about 10% of body weight; an adult brain constitutes 2% of total body weight. The brain achieves 75% of its adult size by age 2. Myelinization and synaptic connections are complete at around age 3 or 4. The spinal cord extends to L3 at birth but is at L1 or L2 by the third year of life.

C. Airway Anatomy. The large head and tongue, mobile epiglottis, and anterior position of the larynx characteristic of neonates make tracheal intubation easier with the neonate's head at a neutral or slightly flexed position than with the neck hyperextended. The cricoid cartilage (as opposed to the vocal cords in adults) is the narrowest portion of the larynx and necessitates the use of tracheal tubes that minimize risks of trauma to the airway and subsequent development of subglottic edema.

D. Respiratory System (Table 27-3). The single most important difference in pediatric patients is that oxygen consumption and alveolar ventilation are significantly higher (in neonates, about double those of adults per kilogram).

E. Cardiovascular System. Fetal circulation has high pulmonary vascular resistance, low systemic vascular resistance (placenta), and right-to-left shunting of blood through the foramen ovale and patent ductus arteriosus (PDA). At birth, pulmonary vascular resistance drops and pulmonary blood flow increases. The foramen ovale and PDA functionally close with increased left atrial pressure and increased arterial oxygen saturation, respectively. Anatomic closure of the foramen ovale occurs between 3 months and 1 year of age, and of the PDA within 4 to 6 weeks after birth. Neonates are highly dependent on heart rate to maintain cardiac output and systemic blood pressure.

TABLE 27-1 ■ Age-Related Perianesthetic Anxiety

AGE GROUP	PSYCHOLOGICAL ASSESSMENT
Neonate (0-30 days of life)	Parental anxiety may be extreme
Infant (1-12 mo)	Separation anxiety begins at 8-10 mo
Toddler (1-3 yr)	Loss of control
Child (4-12 yr)	Preschool age: concrete thoughts School age: desire to meet adults' expectations
Teenager or adolescent (13-19 yr)	Fears death, hides emotions

TABLE 27-2 ■ Neutral and Critical Temperatures

PATIENT AGE	NEUTRAL TEMPERATURE (°C)	CRITICAL TEMPERATURE (°C)
Preterm neonate	34	28
Term neonate	32	23
Adult	28	1

TABLE 27-3 ■ Mean Pulmonary Function Values

PARAMETER	NEONATES (3 kg)	ADULTS (70 kg)
Oxygen consumption (mL/kg/min)	6.4	3.5
Alveolar ventilation (mL/kg/min)	130	60
Carbon dioxide production (mL/kg/min)	6	3
Tidal volume (mL/kg)	6	6
Breathing frequency (min)	35	15
Vital capacity (mL/kg)	35	70
Functional residual capacity (mL/kg)	30	35
Tracheal length (cm)	5.5	12
Pa_{O_2} (room air, mm Hg)	65-85	85-95
Pa_{CO_2} (room air, mm Hg)	30-36	36-44
pH	7.34-7.40	7.36-7.44

F. **Fluids and Renal System.** Total body water content and extracellular fluid (ECF) volume are increased in neonates. The increased metabolic rate in neonates results in accelerated turnover of ECF and dictates meticulous attention to intraoperative fluid replacement (Table 27-4). Newborns and young infants require glucose supplementation, with maintenance requirements for newborns being 6 to 8 mg/kg/min. Table 27-5 summarizes calorie, water, and fluid maintenance requirements. Glomerular filtration rate is greatly decreased in term neonates but increases nearly fourfold by 3 to 5 weeks. Blood loss is generally replaced 3:1 per milliliter of blood loss with isotonic crystalloid.

G. **Hepatic.** Neonatal liver glycogen stores are at least equivalent to those of an adult. Vitamin K levels are 50% of adult levels but do not cause excess bleeding in newborns.

H. **Fetal Hemoglobin (FHb).** Fetal hemoglobin (FHb) has higher oxygen affinity than adult hemoglobin (Hb), with decreased delivery of oxygen to tissues and compensatory increased Hb concentrations in neonates. At 4 to 6 months, the oxyhemoglobin dissociation curve approximates that of adults. Calculation of the estimated erythrocyte mass and the acceptable erythrocyte loss provides a useful guide for intraoperative blood replacement (Table 27-6). Routine preoperative Hb determinations in children younger than 1 year of age rarely influence management of anesthesia or cause delays in planned surgery.

TABLE 27-4 ■ Intraoperative Fluid Therapy for Pediatric Patients

	NORMAL SALINE OR LACTATED RINGER'S SOLUTION (mL/kg/hr)		
PROCEDURE	**MAINTENANCE**	**REPLACEMENT**	**TOTAL**
Minor surgery (herniorrhaphy)	4	2	6
Moderate surgery (pyloromyotomy)	4	4	8
Extensive s urgery (bowel resection)	4	6	10

TABLE 27-5 ■ Holliday-Segar Formula for Caloric Expenditure

WEIGHT	CALORIC EXPENDITURE	WATER REQUIREMENT	FLUID MAINTENANCE*
0-10 kg	100 kcal/kg/day	100 mL/kg/day	4 mL/kg/hr (for first 10 kg)
11-20 kg	50 kcal/kg/day	50 mL/kg/day	2 mL/kg/hr (for second 10 kg)
>20 kg	20 kcal/kg/day	20 mL/kg/day	1 mL/kg/hr (for each additional kg above 20 kg)

*Fluid maintenance rates are additive. For example, a 25-kg child requires 4 mL/kg/hr for the first 10 kg (40 mL/hr) plus 2 mL/kg/hr for the second 10 kg (20 mL/hr) plus 1 mL/kg/hr for each additional kg above 20 kg (5 mL/hr), for a total of 65 mL/hr (40 + 20 + 5) for the hourly fluid maintenance rate.

TABLE 27-6 ■ Estimation of Acceptable Blood Loss*

A 3.2-kg term neonate is scheduled for intraabdominal surgery. The preoperative hematocrit is 50%. What is the acceptable intraoperative blood loss for the hematocrit to be maintained at 40%?

PARAMETER	CALCULATION
Estimated blood volume	85 mL/kg × 3.2 kg = 272 mL
Estimated erythrocyte mass	272 mL × 0.5 = 136 mL
Estimated erythrocyte mass for hematocrit to be maintained at 40%	272 mL × 0.4 = 109 mL
Acceptable intraoperative erythrocyte loss	136 mL – 109 mL = 27 mL
Acceptable intraoperative blood loss for hematocrit to be maintained at 40%	27 × 2† = 54 mL

*These calculations are only guidelines and do not consider the potential impact of intravenous infusion of crystalloid or colloid solutions on the hematocrit.
†Factor to correct the original hematocrit to 50%.

I. Pharmacologic Responses

1. **Anesthetic Requirements.** Minimum alveolar concentration (MAC) is 25% less in neonates than in infants, and MAC in preterm infants is even lower. MAC increases until 2 to 3 months of age and steadily declines with age thereafter. The MAC of sevoflurane is unique and does not decline with advancing age in childhood. It remains constant at 2.5%.
2. **Muscle Relaxants.** The infant's diaphragm is paralyzed by muscle relaxants simultaneously with peripheral muscles (as opposed to later in adults). Initial doses, however, are similar on a weight basis to adult doses. Antagonism of neuromuscular blockade appears reliable in infants. Neonates and infants require more succinylcholine per kilogram than older children (probably because of increased ECF volumes and a larger volume of distribution of succinylcholine). Adverse side effects of succinylcholine (myoglobinuria, malignant hyperthermia [MH], hyperkalemia) limit the use of this drug in children (especially younger than age 5) to rapid securing of the airway and treatment of laryngospasm.
3. **Pharmacokinetics.** Uptake of inhaled anesthetics is more rapid in infants than in older children or adults, and infants are more sensitive to barbiturates and opioids. Neonates require higher doses of propofol than adults, and children from 5 to 15 years of age require higher doses of thiopental than do adults. Decreased hepatic and renal clearance of drugs in neonates leads to prolonged drug effects. Clearance rates increase to adult levels by 5 to 6 months of age.
4. **Monitoring.** Monitoring should include assessment of blood pressure with a cuff of appropriate size, temperature, and end-tidal CO_2 (because of high inspired gas flows, which may be falsely low in neonates and infants). If arterial catheterization is considered, blood sampled from an artery distal to a ductus arteriosus (left radial artery, umbilical artery, posterior tibial artery) may not accurately reflect the Pao_2 delivered to the retina or brain in the presence of a PDA.

J. Pediatric Cardiac Arrest During Anesthesia. Incidence is reported in infants at 15 per 10,000 anesthetics. Overall rates are 3.3 per 10,000 anesthetics in children, and 0 to 4.3 per 10,000 in all pediatric age groups.

1. **Causes.** Medication accounted in one study for 37% of all arrests, the most common of which was cardiovascular depression from volatile anesthetic agents. Other medication-related arrests resulted from syringe swaps, succinylcholine-related hyperkalemia, accidental intravenous injection of local anesthetic, and toxicity from local anesthetic overdose.
2. **Management.** Initial management is directed by the same principles as for any pediatric cardiac arrest. Certification in pediatric advanced life support (PALS) is recommended for anesthesiologists regularly caring for infants and children.

III. DISEASES OF NEONATES

Infants are "premature" if born before 37 weeks of gestation (Table 27-7).

A. Respiratory Distress Syndrome. Respiratory distress syndrome (RDS) or hyaline membrane disease is progressive impairment of gas exchange at the alveolar level because of deficient production and secretion of surfactant. Mature levels of surfactant are not present until 35 weeks of gestation.

TABLE 27-7 ■ **Classification of Prematurity**

DEGREE OF PREMATURITY	GESTATIONAL AGE
Borderline	36-37 wk
Moderate	31-36 wk
Severe	24-30 wk

1. **Signs and Symptoms.** Signs of RDS are usually apparent within minutes of birth (tachypnea, prominent grunting, intercostal and subcostal retractions, nasal flaring, duskiness). Apnea and irregular respirations are ominous signs.
2. **Diagnosis.** The diagnosis is established by clinical course, chest radiograph (fine reticular granularity, air bronchograms), and blood gas analysis (progressive hypoxemia, hypercarbia, variable metabolic acidosis).
3. **Treatment.** Surfactant is now administered to preterm newborns. Surfactant treatment has not decreased the need for high inspired O_2 concentrations, nor has it decreased the incidence of subsequent chronic lung disease or bronchopulmonary dysplasia (BPD). Additional treatment includes nasal continuous positive airway pressure (CPAP). If CPAP fails, intubation may be required.
4. **Management of Anesthesia.** An intraarterial catheter is useful to assess oxygenation, avoid hyperoxia, and prevent respiratory and metabolic acidosis. Pneumothorax secondary to barotrauma should be considered if oxygenation deteriorates abruptly. Administration of albumin (1 g/kg intravenously [IV]) to premature neonates with RDS will likely increase the blood volume and glomerular filtration rate. Keeping the neonate's hematocrit near 40% optimizes tissue oxygen delivery. Excessive hydration may reopen the ductus arteriosus and should be avoided.

B. Bronchopulmonary Dysplasia. A chronic disease of lung parenchyma and small airways, BPD usually results from lung injury in premature infants requiring prolonged mechanical ventilation.

1. **Signs and Symptoms.** Signs are persistent respiratory distress characterized by increased airway reactivity and resistance, decreased pulmonary compliance, ventilation-to-perfusion mismatch, hypoxemia, hypercarbia, tachypnea, and, in severe cases, right-sided heart failure.
2. **Diagnosis.** BPD is a clinical diagnosis defined as oxygen dependence at 36 weeks of postconceptual age with oxygen requirements (to maintain Pa_{O_2} >50 mm Hg) beyond 28 days of life in infants with birth weights less than 1500 g.
3. **Treatment.** Maintenance of adequate oxygenation (with Pa_{O_2} >55 mm Hg and Sp_{O_2} >94%) is necessary to prevent cor pulmonale and to promote growth of lung tissue and remodeling of the pulmonary vascular bed. Reactive airway bronchoconstriction is treated with bronchodilators. Fluid restriction and diuretics may be needed to decrease pulmonary edema and improve gas exchange.
4. **Management of Anesthesia.** Desaturation may be rapid during apnea. Subglottic stenosis, tracheomalacia, and bronchomalacia may be present. Increased risk of bronchospasm warrants establishing a deep level of anesthesia before instrumenting the airway. High airway pressures required during mechanical ventilation may cause pneumothorax. Fluid administration should be monitored and minimized to avoid pulmonary edema.

C. Laryngomalacia and Bronchomalacia. Laryngomalacia is an acquired condition of excessive flaccidity of the laryngeal structures, especially the epiglottis and arytenoids, accounting for more than 70% of all persistent stridor in neonates and young infants. It may be caused by lack of neural control. Bronchomalacia is seen in infants with a prolonged stay in the intensive care unit (ICU). With time and good nutrition, both laryngomalacia and bronchomalacia usually resolve.

D. Retinopathy of Prematurity. Retinopathy of prematurity (ROP) or retrolental fibroplasia, is a vasoproliferative retinopathy occurring almost exclusively in preterm infants. The risk is inversely related to birth weight and gestational age. Risk factors are not fully known but include hyperoxia, sepsis, congenital infections, congenital heart disease, mechanical ventilation, RDS, blood transfusions, intraventricular hemorrhage (IVH), hypoxia, hypercapnia and hypocapnia, asphyxia, and vitamin E deficiency.

1. **Signs and Symptoms.** Signs range from mild, transient changes to severe progressive extraretinal vasoproliferation (over the surface of the retina as well as into the vitreous humor), cicatrization, and subsequent retinal detachment (the primary cause of visual impairment and blindness in ROP).

2. **Diagnosis.** Ophthalmologic examination at 6 weeks of chronologic age or at 32 weeks of postconceptual age is recommended in infants weighing less than 1500 g at birth and those born before 28 weeks of gestation.
3. **Treatment.** Transscleral cryotherapy or laser photocoagulation destroys the peripheral avascular areas of the retina, resulting in slowing or reversing the abnormal growth of blood vessels and reducing risk of retinal detachment. Central vision is measured at the expense of some peripheral vision.
4. **Prognosis.** Approximately 80% to 90% of cases spontaneously regress with few effects or visual disability. Infants who develop ROP are at higher risk of developing ophthalmologic problems later in life (retinal tears, retinal detachment, myopia, strabismus, amblyopia, glaucoma).
5. **Management of Anesthesia.** The dilemma of minimizing oxygen administration to a group of neonates susceptible to arterial hypoxemia must be considered. The use of supplemental oxygen at pulse oximetry saturations of 96% to 99% has not been shown to worsen preexisting ROP. There is also no published evidence to indicate that high oxygen saturation increases ROP after 32 weeks of postconceptual age. Efforts should be made to maintain Pao_2 at 50 to 80 mm Hg, $Paco_2$ at 35 to 45 mm Hg, and oxygen saturation at a pulse oximetry target of 89% to 94%. Infants undergoing peripheral retinal ablation have an increased incidence of apnea and bradycardia during the procedure and for up to 3 days afterward.

E. **Apnea of Prematurity (AOP).** *Apnea of prematurity* (AOP) is defined as a cessation of breathing that is accompanied by cyanosis and bradycardia or that lasts longer than 20 seconds. Periodic breathing and apnea in preterm infants is usually caused by idiopathic AOP but may also be a sign of other neonatal diseases. Idiopathic AOP is a disorder of respiratory control and may be obstructive, central, or mixed.

1. **Signs and Symptoms.** In central apnea, there is complete cessation of airflow and respiratory efforts. In obstructive apnea, airflow is absent despite chest wall movements. The majority (50% to 75%) of apnea episodes in preterm neonates are of mixed cause.
2. **Treatment.** Apnea monitors should be used on infants at risk of apnea.
   a. ***Transfusion*** of infants with low HCT
   b. ***Nasal CPAP Therapy,*** and in severe cases, mechanical ventilation
   c. ***Methylxanthines***
3. **Prognosis.** AOP usually resolves by 36 weeks of postconceptual age. In the absence of significant life-threatening events, monitoring can often be discontinued at 44 to 45 weeks of postconceptual age.
4. **Management of Anesthesia.** Life-threatening apnea has occurred in former preterm infants after even minor surgeries. The risk is increased in infants with anemia (hematocrit <30) and after exposure to inhaled and injected anesthetics. Infants who were born prematurely should be admitted and monitored with pulse oximetry and apnea monitors for at least 12 hours after surgery. The risk of postoperative apnea appears to be significantly decreased after 50 to 52 weeks of gestational age. Elective surgery should be postponed if possible until that time.

F. **Hypoglycemia.** Hypoglycemia is the most common metabolic problem occurring in newborn infants. The risk is highest in small-for-gestational-age infants. Causes include alterations in maternal metabolism, intrinsic neonatal problems, and endocrine or metabolic disorders (Table 27-8).

1. **Signs and Symptoms.** Signs are irritability, apnea, cyanotic spells, seizures, hypotonia, lethargy, and difficulty feeding. Many clinical manifestations are subtle or nonspecific, and a high index of suspicion is necessary.
2. **Diagnosis.** Signs of hypoglycemia occur when serum glucose concentrations are less than 20 mg/dL in premature infants, less than 30 mg/dL in term infants during the first 72 hours, and less than 40 mg/dL thereafter.
3. **Treatment.** Infants with symptoms other than seizures should receive an intravenous bolus of 2 mL of 10% dextrose per kilogram (4 mL/kg if seizures occur) followed by an infusion at 8 mg/kg per minute titrated to maintain the serum glucose at more than 40 mg/dL.

TABLE 27-8 ■ Causes of Neonatal Hypoglycemia

Maternal factors	Intrapartum administration of glucose
	Drug treatment
	β-Adrenergic blocking agents (terbutaline, ritodrine, propranolol)
	  Oral hypoglycemic agents
	  Salicylates
	Maternal diabetes, gestational diabetes

Neonatal factors	Depleted glycogen stores
	  Asphyxia
	  Perinatal stress
	Increased glucose usage (metabolic demands)
	  Sepsis
	  Polycythemia
	  Hypothermia
	  Respiratory distress syndrome
	Congestive heart failure (cyanotic congenital heart disease)
	Limited glycogen stores
	  Intrauterine growth retardation
	  Prematurity
	Hyperinsulinism or endocrine disorders
	  Infants of diabetic mothers
	  Erythroblastosis fetalis, fetal hydrops
	  Insulinomas
	  Beckwith-Wiedemann syndrome
	  Panhypopituitarism
	Decreased glycogenolysis, gluconeogenesis, or usage of alternate fuels
	  Inborn errors of metabolism
	  Adrenal insufficiency

4. **Prognosis.** The prognosis is good in asymptomatic neonates with transient hypoglycemia. The prognosis is more guarded in symptomatic infants, particularly low-birth-weight infants, those with persistent hyperinsulinemic hypoglycemia, and infants of diabetic mothers.
5. **Management of Anesthesia.** Signs of hypoglycemia may be masked by anesthetic drugs, supporting the concept of intraoperative blood glucose monitoring and supplemental glucose administration (e.g., 5% dextrose and 0.2 normal saline at 4 mL/kg/hr). Serum glucose concentrations of 125 mg/dL can cause osmotic diuresis, subsequent dehydration, and further release of insulin with rebound hypoglycemia.

G. **Hypocalcemia.** Infants with intrauterine growth retardation, infants of insulin-dependent diabetics, and infants with birth asphyxia during prolonged, difficult deliveries are at risk. Late neonatal hypocalcemia occurring 5 to 10 days after birth is usually caused by ingestion of cow's milk, which contains high levels of phosphorus. Other notable causes of hypocalcemia in the newborn include maternal hypercalcemia and DiGeorge's syndrome.

1. **Signs and Symptoms.** Signs are irritability, seizures, increased skeletal muscle tone, twitching, tremors, and hypotension. Additional nonspecific symptoms of neonatal hypocalcemia such as poor feeding, vomiting, and lethargy often prompt investigation for sepsis, intracranial hemorrhages, and meningitis.
2. **Diagnosis.** The laboratory definition of hypocalcemia depends on the specific range of normal values at each institution. Hypoalbuminemia may falsely suggest hypocalcemia because the total serum calcium is low even though the ionized calcium concentration remains normal. The ionized calcium concentration, rather than the total calcium, is low in true hypocalcemia.
3. **Treatment.** Calcium is administered. Correction of hypomagnesemia and other metabolic or acid-base disorders is also necessary. Calcium gluconate 10% is given as 100 to 200 mg/kg (1 to

2 mL/kg) repeated every 6 to 8 hours until the calcium level has stabilized. Cardiac monitoring is mandatory, and atropine should be available to treat possible bradycardia. Other potential complications of treatment include soft-tissue necrosis caused by extravasation of drug, precipitation in intravenous tubing and small veins when administered concomitantly with bicarbonate, and digitalis toxicity in patients on digoxin.

4. **Prognosis.** Early neonatal hypocalcemia usually resolves within a few days without treatment in asymptomatic newborns. Serum calcium levels typically normalize within 1 to 3 days with treatment in symptomatic early neonatal hypocalcemia.
5. **Management of Anesthesia.** Hypocalcemia should be corrected preoperatively. Events that precipitate hypocalcemia (alkalosis, sodium bicarbonate administration, or rapid infusion of albumin and citrated blood products) should be avoided.

IV. NEONATAL SURGICAL DISEASES

A. Congenital Diaphragmatic Hernia. This condition is usually associated with pulmonary hypoplasia caused by in utero compression of the developing lungs by the herniated viscera.

1. **Signs and Symptoms.** Signs are scaphoid abdomen, barrel-shaped chest, detection of bowel sounds in the chest, and profound arterial hypoxemia. Chest radiographs show loops of intestine in the thorax and mediastinal shift to the opposite side. Arterial hypoxemia is caused by right-to-left shunting through a PDA resulting from persistent fetal circulation. There is a high incidence of congenital heart disease and intestinal malrotation.
2. **Diagnosis.** The diagnosis is now commonly made prenatally because of routine ultrasonography. Prenatal findings that correlate with poor prognosis are polyhydramnios, displacement of the stomach above the diaphragm, and diagnosis made before 20 weeks of gestation.
3. **Treatment.** Immediate treatment includes decompression of the stomach with an orogastric or nasogastric tube and administration of supplemental oxygen. Positive-pressure mask ventilation should be avoided (gas inflation of the stomach further compromises pulmonary function). Positive airway pressures should not exceed 25 to 30 cm H_2O (excessive airway pressures can damage the neonate's normal lung). Sedation, skeletal muscle paralysis, mechanical ventilation of the lungs (including high frequency oscillatory ventilation [HFOV]), or extracorporeal membrane oxygenation (ECMO) before surgery may decrease the mortality rate among unstable patients. Permissive hypercapnia (P_{CO_2} <60 mm Hg) with gentle ventilation to minimize airway inflation pressures and barotrauma is associated with improved survival. Inhaled nitric oxide does not improve survival with the pulmonary hypertension associated with congenital diaphragmatic hernia.
4. **Prognosis.** Survival ranges from 42% to 75% and is related to the degree of pulmonary hypoplasia and associated anomalies.
5. **Management of Anesthesia.** Anesthesia begins with awake tracheal intubation after preoxygenation. Preductal arterial cannulation is useful, or, if the neonate already has an umbilical arterial line, a pulse oximeter is applied to the right hand. Venous access should be avoided in the lower extremities (venous return may be limited because of compression of the inferior vena cava after reduction of the hernia). Nitrous oxide should be avoided (bowel distention compromises pulmonary function). Airway pressures should be maintained at less than 25 to 30 cm H_2O to minimize the risk of pneumothorax. A sudden decrease in lung compliance or deterioration in oxygenation or blood pressure suggests a pneumothorax. Hypothermia must be avoided (increased pulmonary vascular resistance with right-to-left shunting). After reduction of the hernia, inflation of the hypoplastic lung is not recommended. It is unlikely to expand, and contralateral lung damage may result.
6. **Postoperative Course.** The postoperative course may include rapid improvement followed by sudden deterioration with arterial hypoxemia, hypercapnia, and acidosis (because of reappearance of fetal circulatory patterns and right-to-left shunting through the foramen

ovale and PDA) and possibly death. Sedation is necessary (stressful stimuli can further elevate pulmonary pressures, increasing shunt).

B. Esophageal Atresia and Tracheoesophageal Fistula. More than 90% of affected individuals with esophageal atresia (EA) also have a tracheoesophageal fistula (TEF). The most common form of EA is a blind upper esophageal pouch plus a distal esophagus that forms a TEF (Figure 27-1). Approximately 50% of infants with EA have other anomalies, most often VATER (*v*ertebral defects, imperforate *a*nus, *t*racheo*e*sophageal fistula, *r*enal dysplasia) or VACTERL (VATER plus *c*ardiac and *l*imb anomalies). Survival of neonates with EA and no associated defects approaches 100%.

1. **Signs and Symptoms.** The neonate with EA manifests respiratory distress (coughing, cyanosis, and frothing at the mouth and nose). Feeding exacerbates these symptoms and causes regurgitation.
2. **Diagnosis.** Prenatally, EA is suspected if maternal polyhydramnios is present. EA is usually diagnosed after birth when an oral catheter cannot be passed into the stomach or when the neonate exhibits cyanosis, coughing, and choking during oral feedings. Pure EA may manifest as an airless, scaphoid abdomen.

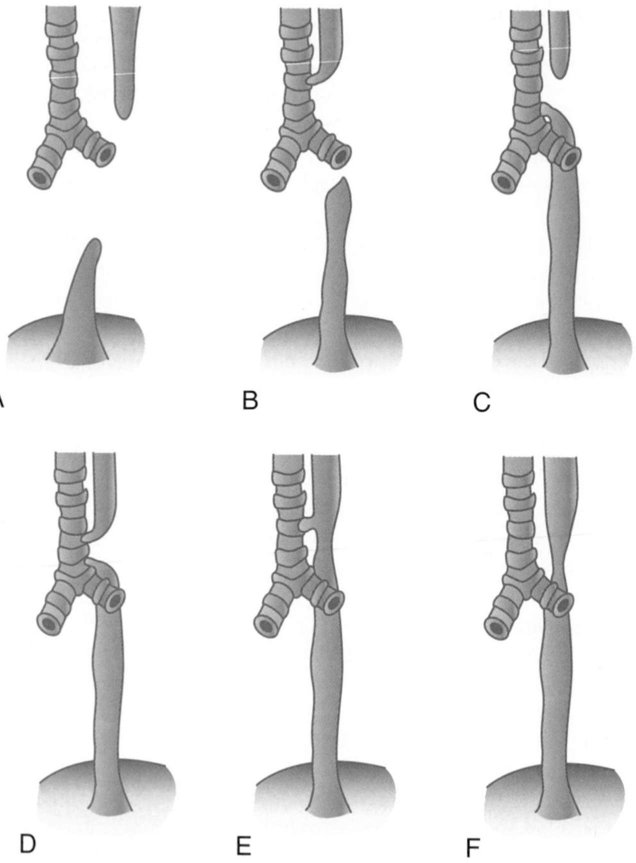

FIGURE 27-1 ■ Types of esophageal atresia (EA). **A,** Pure EA; **B,** proximal fistula; **C,** EA, distal fistula; **D,** proximal and distal fistula; **E,** pure tracheoesophageal fistula. **F,** Esophageal stenosis. *(Adapted from Ravitch MM, et al, eds.* Pediatric Surgery, *Vol 1. 3rd ed. Chicago: Year Book Medical Publishers; 1979; and Smith BM, Matthes-Kofidis C, Golianu B, Hammer GB: Pediatric general surgery. In Jaffe RA, Samuels SI, eds:* Anesthesiologist's Manual of Surgical Procedures. *3rd ed. Philadelphia: Lippincott Williams & Wilkins; 2004:1019.)*

3. **Treatment.** Treatment includes maintaining a patent airway, preventing aspiration, ceasing feedings, and placing the infant in a head-up position to minimize regurgitation. Endotracheal intubation is avoided, if possible, because of the potential to worsen distention of the stomach. One-lung ventilation may be necessary if life-threatening gastric distention occurs. Surgical repair of TEF is urgent. However, some neonates will require a staged surgical approach with an initial gastrostomy and later definitive repair.
4. **Prognosis.** Tracheal collapse after extubation and esophageal stricture are not uncommon. Chronic gastroesophageal reflux and dysphagia can predispose children to recurrent aspiration pneumonitis. Early deaths are caused by cardiac or chromosomal abnormalities, and later deaths are usually the result of respiratory complications.
5. **Management of Anesthesia.** Ideally, awake intubation with spontaneous ventilation allows the appropriate positioning of the endotracheal tube while minimizing the risk of ventilatory impairment from gastric distention caused by positive-pressure ventilation. However, awake intubation may be difficult and traumatic in a vigorous infant. Inhalation induction allows spontaneous ventilation. If inhalational induction is chosen, peak inspiratory pressure (PIP) must be minimized during ventilation to avoid inflation of the stomach. Proper placement of the tracheal tube is critical (above the carina but below the TEF). A peripheral arterial catheter permits continuous monitoring of systemic blood pressure and measurement of arterial blood gases. Intraoperative insensible and third-space fluid losses should be replaced with crystalloid (6 to 8 mL/kg/hr). Blood loss may be replaced with 5% albumin and blood to maintain a hematocrit above 35%. Lung retraction may impair ventilation, surgical manipulation of the trachea may cause airway obstruction, and blood and secretions can obstruct the endotracheal tube, necessitating frequent suctioning or even replacement of the tube. Extubation of term infants at the end of surgery is preferable, although continued intubation and ventilation are necessary if cardiac or pulmonary complications arise intraoperatively or if the adequacy of ventilation is in question. Excessive neck extension and reintubation can compromise the new anastomosis.

C. **Abdominal Wall Defects: Omphalocele and Gastroschisis.** Omphalocele is external herniation of abdominal viscera through the base of the umbilical cord. Gastroschisis is external herniation of abdominal viscera through a small (usually <5 cm) defect in the anterior abdominal wall (Table 27-9).

TABLE 27-9 ■ Comparison of Omphalocele and Gastroschisis

	OMPHALOCELE	GASTROSCHISIS
Cause	Failure of midgut migration from yolk sac into abdomen	Abnormal development of right omphalomesenteric artery or umbilical vein with ischemia to right paraumbilical area
Location	Within umbilical cord	Periumbilical (usually to right of cord)
Covering	Membranous sac	None (exposed viscera)
Associated conditions	Beckwith-Wiedemann syndrome Congenital heart disease Trisomies 13, 18, 21 Malrotation of gastrointestinal tract Pentalogy of Cantrell Exstrophy of bladder	Malrotation of gastrointestinal tract, prematurity, intestinal atresia

Adapted from Roberts JD Jr, Cronin JH, Todres ID. Neonatal emergencies. In: Cote CJ, Todres ID, Goudsouzian NG, Ryan JF, eds. *A Practice of Anesthesia for Infants and Children*. 3rd ed. Philadelphia: Saunders; 2001.

1. **Diagnosis.** Omphalocele and gastroschisis can be diagnosed prenatally by fetal ultrasonography.
2. **Treatment.** Gastroschisis requires urgent repair. Placing the infant's lower body and exposed intestine immediately after delivery into a plastic drawstring bowel bag reduces evaporative fluid and heat loss from the large surface area of exposed bowel. Although omphalocele also requires urgent corrective surgery, the association of cardiac anomalies warrants preoperative cardiology evaluation and echocardiography.
3. **Prognosis.** The survival rate for gastroschisis is 90% or more. Survival rates for omphalocele range from 70% to 95%. Mortality is related to associated cardiac and chromosomal abnormalities.
4. **Preoperative Management.** The primary concerns are prevention of infections and minimization of fluid and heat loss from exposed abdominal viscera. The stomach should be decompressed with an orogastric tube to decrease the risk of aspiration. Fluid requirements are two to four times daily maintenance requirements (≥8 to 16 mL/kg/hr). To maintain normal oncotic pressures, protein-containing solutions (5% albumin) should constitute 25% of the replacement fluids.
5. **Management of Anesthesia.** Important concerns are preservation of body temperature and fluid replacement. Primary closure may require the ability to ventilate the patient with high PIPs into the postoperative period. If inspiratory pressures are greater than 25 to 30 cm H_2O or intravesical or intragastric pressures are greater than 20 cm H_2O, primary closure is not recommended. The viscera should be covered with a prosthetic silo and the abdominal viscera allowed to slowly reduce over a period of several days to 1 week. Repair of a large defect will require maximal relaxation intraoperatively and during the initial postoperative period. Nitrous oxide is avoided because of bowel distention. Tight surgical abdominal closure can result in compression of the inferior vena cava and decreased diaphragmatic excursion, resulting in impaired abdominal organ perfusion and decreased pulmonary compliance. Evidence of unacceptable intraabdominal pressure necessitates removal of fascial sutures and closure of only the skin or addition of a prosthesis. Intensive intraoperative and postoperative monitoring is recommended. Direct monitoring of arterial blood gases and pH is helpful for guiding fluid therapy. Intraoperative fluid requirements of at least 25% of estimated blood volume are expected during surgical repair of large abdominal defects. Mechanical ventilation may be needed for 24 to 48 hours postoperatively.

D. **Hirschsprung's Disease.** Congenital aganglionic megacolon, or Hirschsprung's disease, is the most common cause of lower intestinal obstruction in full-term neonates; it is characterized by the absence of parasympathetic ganglion cells in the large bowel.

1. **Signs and Symptoms.** Signs include constipation, dilation of the proximal bowel, and abdominal distention. Progressive bowel distention causes increasing intraluminal pressure, decreased blood flow, and deterioration of the mucosal barrier. Persistent intestinal stasis promotes bacterial proliferation, leading to enterocolitis (abdominal distention, fever, explosive diarrhea).
2. **Diagnosis.** Hirschsprung's disease is suspected in any full-term neonate with delayed passage of stool. A classic radiographic finding after a contrast enema is the presence of a transition zone between normal dilated proximal colon and a narrow, spastic distal colon segment caused by nonrelaxation of the aganglionic bowel. Rectal biopsy is the diagnostic gold standard, confirming the absence of ganglion cells and the presence of hypertrophied nerve bundles that stain positively for acetylcholinesterase.
3. **Treatment.** Treatment is surgical, bringing ganglionated bowel down to the anus.
4. **Prognosis.** Most patients attain fecal continence. Patients with retained or acquired aganglionosis, severe strictures, dysfunctional bowel, and intestinal neuronal dysplasia may require reoperation.
5. **Management of Anesthesia.** Intraoperative blood loss is usually mild, but third-space fluid losses can be significant. Patients may require an initial bolus of 10 to 20 mL of crystalloid

per kilogram IV to offset the volume deficit resulting from bowel preparation and fasting. Epidural anesthesia provides intraoperative and postoperative analgesia in patients undergoing open abdominal procedures. Extubation at the end of surgery is routine.

E. Anorectal Malformations. These include a spectrum of defects, most of which involve a fistula between the lower intestinal tract and genitourinary structures. Imperforate anus without fistula occurs in a small number of patients, especially in association with Down's syndrome. Spinal and vertebral anomalies occur in up to 50% of patients with anorectal malformations. Cardiovascular anomalies (atrial septal defect, PDA, tetralogy of Fallot, ventricular septal defect [VSD]) are present in one third of patients with imperforate anus.

1. **Signs and Symptoms.** Inspection of the perineum reveals an anorectal malformation. The neonate may fail to pass meconium in the first 24 to 48 hours of life.
2. **Diagnosis.** Meconium seen on the neonate's perineum is evidence of a rectoperineal fistula. Meconium in the urine indicates a rectourinary fistula. Rectovaginal fistula in female neonates and rectourethral fistula in male neonates are the most common presentations.
3. **Treatment.** Preliminary treatment for high lesions is a diverting colostomy followed later by a definitive procedure. Low lesions (perineal fistulas) may be repaired during the neonatal period without a protective colostomy.
4. **Prognosis.** The greater the degree of sacral malformation, the greater the likelihood of fecal and urinary incontinence. Most patients with perineal fistula and rectal atresia are expected to be fully continent after repair.
5. **Management of Anesthesia.** Electrical muscle stimulation is used during the procedure to identify muscle structures and to define the anterior and posterior limits of the new anus. Blood loss and third-space fluid losses are usually moderate. Intravenous catheters should be placed in upper extremities because surgical positioning of the legs may impede venous flow or limit access to the intravenous site. Patients are usually extubated at the end of surgery.

F. Pyloric Stenosis. This is a common cause of gastric outlet obstruction in infants. Idiopathic hypertrophy of the circular muscle of the pylorus results in compression and narrowing of the pyloric channel.

1. **Signs and Symptoms.** Signs include nonbilious projectile vomiting at 2 to 5 weeks of age. Jaundice may occur in some infants, possibly because of hepatic glucuronyl transferase deficiency associated with starvation. The most common metabolic presentation is hypokalemic, hypochloremic primary metabolic alkalosis with secondary respiratory acidosis.
2. **Diagnosis.** An olivelike mass can usually be palpated in the epigastrium. After feeding, a gastric peristaltic wave may be seen progressing across the abdomen from left to right. Confirmation of the diagnosis is by abdominal ultrasonography.
3. **Treatment.** Pyloromyotomy (either open or laparoscopic) is performed. Severely dehydrated infants require fluid resuscitation before surgery, which should be guided by measurement of serum electrolyte concentrations (essential for estimating the degree of dehydration, alkalosis, and metabolic derangements). Feedings can usually be initiated within 4 to 6 hours after surgery.
4. **Management of Anesthesia.** Pulmonary aspiration of gastric fluid is a definite risk in infants with gastric outlet obstruction. The stomach should be emptied with a large-bore orogastric catheter after premedication with atropine and before induction of anesthesia. Awake tracheal intubation is indicated if a difficult intubation is anticipated. Otherwise, rapid-sequence induction is recommended. Skeletal muscle relaxation is usually not needed. Infiltration of the incision sites with local anesthetics usually provides sufficient postoperative analgesia. Postoperative depression of ventilation of unknown cause often occurs, and apnea monitoring for 12 hours after surgery is indicated. Hypoglycemia may occur 2 to 3 hours after surgical correction of pyloric stenosis, most likely because of inadequate liver glycogen stores and cessation of intravenous dextrose infusions.

G. Necrotizing Enterocolitis. Characterized by various degrees of mucosal or transmural necrosis of the intestine, necrotizing enterocolitis (NEC) is the most common neonatal surgical emergency and is associated with substantial perinatal morbidity and mortality. Although the greatest risk factor for NEC is prematurity, other risk factors include perinatal asphyxia, systemic infections, umbilical artery catheterization, exchange blood transfusions, hypotension, RDS, PDA, cyanotic congenital heart disease, and aggressive hyperosmolar formula feeding.

1. **Signs and Symptoms.** Signs include recurrent apnea, lethargy, temperature instability, glucose instability, and shock. More specific signs of NEC are abdominal distention, high gastric residuals after feeding, and bloody or mucoid diarrhea. Metabolic acidosis, neutropenia, and thrombocytopenia are common.
2. **Diagnosis.** Diagnosis is by clinical correlation with plain abdominal x-ray findings. Pneumatosis intestinalis, or air in the intestinal wall, is diagnostic of NEC in newborns.
3. **Treatment.** Medical treatment (cessation of feeding, gastric decompression, intravenous fluids, antibiotics) is often successful. Mechanical ventilation, fluid resuscitation, transfusion, and inotropic support may be indicated. Surgery is reserved for neonates in whom medical management fails (50% of infants with NEC).
4. **Prognosis.** The prognosis is worse in the presence of pneumatosis intestinalis (20% fail medical management, 25% die). Short bowel syndrome, central venous catheter complications, and cholestatic jaundice may follow surgery.
5. **Management of Anesthesia.** Management includes fluid resuscitation and transfusion if needed. Arterial pressure and blood gas monitoring is helpful. Rapid fluid administration in preterm infants may cause intracranial hemorrhage or reopening of the ductus arteriosus. Full stomach precautions are needed. High intraabdominal pressures and decreased pulmonary compliance are likely during surgery. Inotropes may be required to maintain adequate cardiac output and bowel perfusion. Fluids and the operating room should be appropriately warmed to maintain normothermia. Postoperative mechanical ventilation is usually required because of abdominal distention and co-existing RDS. Because of bacteremia, neuraxial anesthesia and analgesia are not recommended.

H. Biliary Atresia. Biliary atresia is characterized by obliteration or discontinuity of the extrahepatic bile duct system with resultant biliary obstruction. Associated abnormalities include intestinal malrotation, situs inversus, and polysplenia.

1. **Signs and Symptoms.** Signs include persistent jaundice in the early weeks after birth, accompanied by dark urine and acholic stool. Any term infant who has been jaundiced for longer than 14 days should be evaluated. Mixed unconjugated and conjugated hyperbilirubinemia is present.
2. **Diagnosis.** Diagnosis is by laboratory testing (bilirubin, transaminase levels, liver synthetic function tests, γ-glutamyltransferase level) and ultrasonography. Endoscopic retrograde cholangiopancreatography (ERCP) and magnetic resonance imaging (MRI) are occasionally performed. Liver biopsy is diagnostic.
3. **Treatment.** Kasai's operation (portoenterostomy) and liver transplantation are the primary treatment.
4. **Prognosis.** Left untreated, biliary atresia results in liver cirrhosis and death by 2 years of age.
5. **Management of Anesthesia.** Preoperative correction of coagulopathy is important. Rapid sequence induction is indicated in the presence of ascites. Central venous access may be needed. Peripheral arterial catheterization is recommended for hemodynamic monitoring and frequent blood draws. Nitrous oxide should be avoided. Temperature maintenance is key. Severe, sudden hypotension can occur if the inferior vena cava (IVC) is compressed by surgical manipulation. Postoperative ICU care is needed. Epidural analgesia can be considered if coagulopathy is not present.

I. Congenital Lobar Emphysema. This is a rare cause of respiratory distress in neonates that results from localized bronchial obstruction, air trapping, and lobar overexpansion. Acquired lobar emphysema may result from barotrauma associated with the treatment of BPD. There is an increased incidence of congenital heart disease (VSD, PDA).

1. **Signs and Symptoms.** Signs range from mild tachypnea and wheezing to severe dyspnea and cyanosis.
2. **Diagnosis.** Diagnosis is made by chest radiography, computed tomography (CT), and ventilation/perfusion scan.
3. **Treatment.** Treatment is resection of the diseased lobe. Some infants with only very mild symptoms and without evidence of progression may not require surgery.
4. **Prognosis.** Long-term pulmonary growth and function are excellent after lobectomy.

J. **Congenital Cystic Adenomatoid Malformations.** These are congenital cystic pockets that communicate with the tracheobronchial tree and may become overdistended owing to air trapping. Up to 80% of affected infants have respiratory distress in the newborn period because of compression of normal lung tissue. Signs and symptoms are similar to congenital lobar emphysema, and the x-ray appearance may mimic congenital diaphragmatic hernia. Treatment is surgical resection of the abnormal lobe, and prognosis depends on the amount and health of remaining lung tissue.

1. **Anesthesia Management.** Inhalation induction is recommended to avoid positive pressure ventilation before the chest is opened and to decrease air trapping. Maintenance of spontaneous breathing is recommended, as is avoidance of nitrous oxide. The surgeon should be present at induction, because sudden cardiopulmonary decompensation may necessitate urgent thoracotomy. A peripheral arterial catheter should be placed for frequent blood gas sampling. Possible one-lung ventilation should be anticipated, which is accomplished in these small patients by endobronchial intubation or placement of a bronchial blocker. Patients can usually be extubated postoperatively. Postoperative analgesia can be via intravenous medication or neuraxial technique.

V. CENTRAL NERVOUS SYSTEM DISORDERS

A. **Cerebral Palsy.** A symptom complex rather than a specific disease, cerebral palsy (CP) comprises a group of nonprogressive motor impairment syndromes secondary to lesions or anomalies of the developing brain. CP is classified according to the extremity involved (monoplegia, hemiplegia, diplegia, quadriplegia) and the characteristics of the neurologic dysfunction (spastic, hypotonic, dystonic, athetotic). There is a high frequency of association of CP with epilepsy and cognitive disorders. The cause of most cases is unknown.

1. **Signs and Symptoms.** The most common manifestation is skeletal muscle spasticity. Extrapyramidal CP is associated with choreoathetosis, and atonic CP is characterized by dystonia and cerebellar ataxia. Varying degrees of mental retardation and speech defects may accompany CP.
2. **Treatment.**
   a. ***Surgical Treatment.*** These children often undergo elective orthopedic corrective procedures (Achilles tendon lengthening, hip adductor and iliopsoas release, derotational osteotomy of the femur, correction of scoliosis); stereotactic surgery to decrease skeletal muscle rigidity, spasticity, and dyskinesia; and dental restorations, requiring general anesthesia and antireflux operations owing to increased incidence of reflux disease.
   b. ***Medications.*** Medications to relieve muscle spasm include dantrolene, botulinum neurotoxin (Botox) injections, and baclofen. Baclofen should not be discontinued abruptly in the perioperative period because of potential withdrawal symptoms (seizures, hallucinations, delirium, pruritus), which may persist up to 72 hours. Valproic acid is associated with hepatotoxicity, bone marrow suppression, and platelet dysfunction.
3. **Management of Anesthesia.** Tracheal intubation is recommended (risk of aspiration because of reflux). Succinylcholine does not produce abnormal potassium release. Children on anticonvulsants may be resistant to nondepolarizing muscle relaxants because of hepatic

enzyme induction. Emergence from anesthesia may be slow. Tracheal extubation should be delayed until these children are fully awake and body temperature is near normal.

B. Hydrocephalus. This is a congenital or acquired increase in cerebrospinal fluid (CSF) resulting in enlarged cerebral ventricles. Hydrocephalus can be caused by obstruction to the flow of CSF (e.g., tumor), as well as overproduction or decreased absorption of CSF. Patients with hydrocephalus usually have an increase in intracranial pressure (ICP).

1. **Signs and Symptoms.** Signs depend on the age of the child and the presence of increased ICP. Congenital hydrocephalus manifests at birth or soon thereafter with an enlarged head; separation of cranial sutures; inferiorly deviated eyes ("sunsetting eyes"); dilated scalp veins; and thin; shiny skin. Normal pressure hydrocephalus is triad of abnormal gait, dementia, and urinary incontinence.
2. **Diagnosis.** Serial head circumference measurements, skull radiographs, and CT confirm the diagnosis.
3. **Treatment.** Treatment depends on the cause of the hydrocephalus. When surgical excision of obstructive lesions is not feasible or is unsuccessful, a shunting procedure (ventriculoperitoneal [VP], ventriculoatrial, ventriculopleural) is necessary. The most common of these is the VP shunt. VP shunts often require revisions or replacement because of infections involving the shunt or shunt malfunction (80% at the proximal end of the shunt). In patients with increased ICP secondary to shunt malfunction, the ICP may be lowered acutely by tapping the proximal reservoir.
4. **Management of Anesthesia**
   a. ***Preoperative.*** Inhalation induction may be acceptable in the absence of clinical or radiographic evidence of severe intracranial hypertension.
   b. ***Intraoperative.*** Arterial catheterization is reserved for the patient with uncontrolled ICP and hemodynamic instability. Atropine premedication is recommended in infants because of the immaturity of the sympathetic autonomic system. Laryngoscopy may cause significant increases in ICP, and the benefit of lidocaine administration before laryngoscopy in preventing such increases has not been demonstrated in infants and small children. Sudden cardiac arrest in infants receiving 1.0 to 1.5 mg of intravenous lidocaine per kilogram at time of induction has been reported. Mild hypocapnia (32 to 35 mm Hg) may prevent further elevation of the ICP. Normocapnia should be maintained in patients with normal ICP. Intraoperative spontaneous ventilation is not recommended because of the risk of air embolism and (in ventriculopleural shunts) the risk of pneumothorax. Nitrous oxide is not recommended because it increases cerebral blood flow and volume (raises ICP), and it is associated with nausea and emesis that may confuse evaluation of the patient postoperatively. Ketamine is contraindicated because it can precipitate sudden rises in ICP. Ventricular shunt procedures usually do not result in significant blood or third-space losses. Hypothermia can occur because of the large body surface areas exposed during surgical preparation. Positional changes are important: extreme positions of the head can cause further displacement of a structural abnormality (Chiari's malformation) and impair venous drainage, with resultant increase in ICP. Patients should be awake before extubation.

C. Cerebrovascular Abnormalities. Cerebrovascular abnormalities are uncommon in the pediatric population but are an important cause of stroke and hemorrhage. Stroke is among the top 10 causes of death in children. Vascular malformations (arteriovenous malformation [AVM], cavernous malformations, and aneurysms) are important causes of hemorrhagic stroke in children. Cerebrovascular arteriopathy such as moyamoya disease is a major cause of ischemic stroke in children.

1. **Anesthesia Management.** Goals are to minimize risk of intracranial bleeding and prevent cerebral ischemia. A trend of baseline blood pressure in sleep and awake states can help determine the lower tolerable blood pressure for the patient. Prolonged fasting and subsequent dehydration should be avoided. Preoperative anxiolysis is helpful; hypocapnia from crying and hyperventilation increase the possibility of cerebral ischemia. Arterial

catheterization for monitoring and blood draws is indicated. In cases of AVMs, hypertension must be avoided, and large-bore intravenous access is needed. Extubation should be performed as soon as possible to allow neurologic evaluation.

D. Spina Bifida and Myelomeningocele. Failure of the canal end of the neural tube to close during development can result in spina bifida, or saclike herniation of the meninges (meningocele), or herniation containing neural elements (myelomeningocele).

1. **Signs and Symptoms.** Children with meningoceles are usually born without neurologic deficits; those with myelomeningoceles usually have varying degrees of motor and sensory deficits, including flaccid paraplegia, loss of sensation to pinprick, and loss of anal and bladder-sphincter tone. Associated congenital conditions include clubfoot, hydrocephalus, dislocation of the hips, exstrophy of the bladder, prolapsed uterus, Klippel-Feil syndrome, and congenital cardiac defects. Patients are prone to recurrent urinary tract infections (UTIs), gram-negative sepsis, and scoliosis.
2. **Diagnosis.** These defects may be found at birth (Arnold-Chiari II malformation) or incidentally (spina bifida) when plain films are obtained for other reasons. MRI is the most useful radiographic test to confirm the presence of neural tube defects and/or spinal cord anomalies.
3. **Treatment.** Early neurosurgical repair of a myelomeningocele will lead to restoration of a more normal configuration of the spine. The more severe anomalies will be detected at birth and will require surgical intervention within the first 24 hours of life to reduce the risk of infection of exposed central nervous system (CNS) tissue.
4. **Management of Anesthesia**
   a. ***Preoperative.*** Infants requiring repair of a meningomyelocele defect rarely have increased ICP. Neonates with a myelomeningocele may have an abnormal ventilatory response to hypoxia and hypercarbia, gastroesophageal reflux, and abnormal vocal cord mobility. Intraoperative blood loss can be insidious, especially if the sac is large. Invasive monitoring is indicated for patients with large defects, such as a multilevel myelomeningocele in which significant cutaneous undermining will be needed. Hypothermia is common during these procedures, considering the surface area of tissue exposed and the age of the patients.
   b. ***Intraoperative.*** If general anesthesia is selected, awake tracheal intubation may be performed with these children in the lateral decubitus position (to avoid pressure on the meningocele sac) or in the supine position with the meningocele sac protected by elevating it on a doughnut-shaped support. Long-acting nondepolarizing muscle relaxants are avoided, as the surgeon may use a nerve stimulator to identify functional neural elements. Succinylcholine does not elicit a hyperkalemic response in these patients. Children with a myelomeningocele may have an increased incidence of sensitivity to latex because of chronic exposure to indwelling latex catheters.

E. Craniosynostosis. This is a condition in which one or more cranial sutures fuse prematurely, leading to focal or global growth delay of the skull, which can result in esthetic abnormalities as well as functional problems (increased ICP, hydrocephalus, developmental delay, amblyopia).

1. **Diagnosis.** The condition is suspected in the presence of abnormal head circumference and head shape, fontanel size, and palpable bony ridges along affected sutures. The diagnosis is confirmed with plain radiographs, ultrasonography, CT, and/or MRI.
2. **Treatment.** Surgical intervention is performed early in infancy to prevent further progression of the deformity and potential complications associated with increased ICP.
3. **Anesthetic Management.** ICP may be elevated in syndromic children, and airway management may be challenging (upper airway obstruction) because of other concomitant craniofacial anomalies. Alternative airway management techniques (e.g., laryngeal mask airway [LMA], fiberoptic bronchoscope) should be available. In the presence of increased ICP, specific anesthetic measures must be considered (avoiding hypercapnia, hypoxemia, arterial hypotension). Large-bore intravenous access is required, and an arterial

indwelling catheter is recommended to allow for real-time blood pressure measurements and repeated blood sampling. Techniques to reduce allogeneic blood transfusions include cell saver, preoperative acute normovolemic hemodilution, and controlled arterial hypotension. Hypotensive anesthesia can be achieved by using volatile anesthetics, opioids, and/or adrenergic receptor–blocking drugs. Arterial hypotension should not be used in patients with increased ICP. A precordial Doppler ultrasound probe may be indicated to detect intraoperative venous air embolism. A long central venous catheter may be placed to evacuate air from the right side of the heart in case of significant air embolism. Because air embolism is common, nitrous oxide should be avoided. Facial swelling related to surgery can be quite pronounced (particularly when the surgery extends below the orbital ridge) and necessitates postoperative mechanical ventilation.

F. Craniofacial Abnormalities

1. **Cleft Lip and Palate.** These are among the most common congenital anomalies. The clefting may be an isolated anomaly or be part of a syndrome (e.g., Pierre Robin syndrome, Treacher Collins syndrome).
   a. ***Signs and Symptoms.*** Signs may include airway obstruction, feeding problems, aspiration, failure to thrive, and chronic otitis media.
   b. ***Diagnosis.*** Most commonly the diagnosis is made postnatally, sometimes requiring meticulous inspection and palpation of the hard and soft palates.
   c. ***Treatment.*** Treatment is surgical correction, preferably before the development of speech.
   d. ***Prognosis.*** The prognosis is excellent, although several corrective surgeries may be required.
   e. ***Management of Anesthesia.*** In infants with nonsyndromic clefting, an inhalational induction is usually preferred, and after establishment of venous access, a small dose of neuromuscular blocker and opioid (fentanyl or morphine) is administered, followed by oral endotracheal intubation. In infants with syndromic clefting, spontaneous ventilation should be maintained until the airway has been secured. Local anesthetics should be used to minimize pain intraoperatively and postoperatively. The patient may be extubated once fully awake and after confirming that any throat pack inserted during surgery has been removed. Cool mist in the postoperative period may help keep these children comfortable and prevent airway complications.
2. **Mandibular Hypoplasia.** Upper airway obstruction and difficult tracheal intubation are likely.
   a. ***Pierre Robin Sequence.*** The Pierre Robin sequence consists of micrognathia usually accompanied by glossoptosis (posterior displacement of the tongue) and cleft palate. Acute upper airway obstruction, feeding problems, failure to thrive, and cyanotic episodes are early complications. Associated congenital heart disease is common.
   b. ***Hemifacial Microsomia.*** This condition is second to cleft lip and palate as one of the most common facial anomalies. It typically involves the lower face. *Goldenhar's syndrome* is unilateral mandibular hypoplasia. Associated anomalies include eye, ear, and vertebral abnormalities on the affected side. Ease of tracheal intubation is highly variable.
   c. ***Treacher Collins Syndrome.*** The most common of the mandibulofacial dysostoses, Treacher Collins syndrome results in early airway problems similar to those experienced by infants with Pierre Robin syndrome. Congenital heart disease (VSD) often accompanies this syndrome. Other features include malar hypoplasia, colobomas (notching of the lower eyelids), and an antimongoloid slant of the palpebral fissures. Tracheal intubation, as in infants with Pierre Robin syndrome, is difficult and sometimes impossible.
   d. **Anesthesia Concerns**
      i. ***Preoperative.*** Evaluation includes airway evaluation, plans for intubation, and assessment of the cardiovascular system and the Hb concentration. Opioids and other ventilatory depressants are usually avoided in the preoperative medication.
      ii. ***Intraoperative.*** Equipment for emergency bronchoscopy, cricothyrotomy, or tracheostomy should be available. Preoxygenation should occur before initiation of direct

laryngoscopy. Use of muscle relaxants is not recommended until the airway has been secured. Awake tracheal intubation is a consideration, but more often, fiberoptic tracheal intubation is accomplished after inhalation induction of anesthesia with volatile anesthetics. Use of LMAs is an alternative to tracheal intubation in selected patients or when tracheal intubation proves impossible. Tracheostomy under local anesthesia may be required when all other attempts to maintain the airway have failed. Tracheal extubation after surgery should occur when the patient is fully awake and alert. Equipment for urgent tracheal reintubation must be immediately available.

3. **Midface Hypoplasia and Hypertelorism.** Midface hypoplasia and hypertelorism (an increased distance between the eyes) are associated with many craniofacial anomalies.
   a. ***Apert's Syndrome.*** This is a rare autosomal dominant disorder characterized by acrocephalosyndactyly: craniosynostosis, midface hypoplasia, and symmetric syndactyly of the extremities. Choanal atresia, tracheal stenosis, cervical spine fusion, congenital heart defects, genitourinary anomalies, and developmental delay can be present. Obstructive sleep apnea (OSA) is common, and cor pulmonale can develop. Proptosis and exophthalmos can predispose to corneal injury, amblyopia, strabismus, and optic nerve atrophy.
   b. ***Crouzon's Syndrome.*** Crouzon's syndrome shares clinical features with Apert's syndrome. Mental delay is not intrinsic to Crouzon's syndrome but may develop in the presence of high ICP. Conductive hearing loss is common. Acanthosis nigricans occurs in 5% of patients.
   c. ***Treatment.*** Treatment is complex surgical correction, preferably before ossification of the facial bones occurs.
   d. ***Management of Anesthesia.*** Tracheal intubation may be difficult. Corneal abrasions are likely; eye ointment should be used, and the eyelids sutured closed. High ICP should be suspected if there is a history of nausea and vomiting. Intravenous access may be difficult owing to syndactyly.

VI. DISORDERS OF THE UPPER AIRWAY

A. Acute Epiglottitis (Supraglottitis). Acute epiglottitis is a short-lived disease seen most often in children 2 to 6 years of age. The most common pathogen is *Haemophilus influenzae* type B. Acute epiglottitis may be difficult to differentiate from laryngotracheobronchitis (croup) (Table 27-10).

1. **Signs and Symptoms.** Signs of acute epiglottitis are acute difficulty swallowing, high fever, and inspiratory stridor, typically developing in less than 24 hours. Patients display a characteristic posture of sitting upright and leaning forward with the chin up and mouth open. The classic presentation is with "the 4 Ds": dysphagia, dysphonia, dyspnea, and drooling. Pulmonary edema, pericarditis, meningitis, and septic arthritis may accompany acute epiglottitis.
2. **Diagnosis.** Acute epiglottitis is a medical emergency (can be fatal in 6 to 12 hours), with diagnosis based on clinical signs. The history is quickly obtained and the child examined for signs of upper airway obstruction. No attempts to directly visualize the epiglottis should be made, because any instrumentation, even a tongue blade, may provoke laryngospasm.
3. **Treatment.** Physicians skilled in airway management must accompany these children at all times. Definitive treatment of acute epiglottitis includes prompt establishment of a secure airway and administration of antibiotics effective against *H. influenzae,* once blood and throat cultures have been obtained.
4. **Prognosis.** Up to 6% of children with epiglottitis without an artificial airway (endotracheal tube or tracheostomy) die. Because the response to antibiotics is rapid, extubation may be achieved within 2 to 3 days in most cases.

TABLE 27-10 ■ Clinical Features of Acute Epiglottitis and Laryngotracheobronchitis

PARAMETER	ACUTE EPIGLOTTITIS	LARYNGOTRACHEOBRONCHITIS
Age group affected	2-7 yr	<2 yr
Incidence	Accounts for 5% of children with stridor	Accounts for about 80% of children with stridor
Etiologic agent	Bacterial *(Haemophilus influenzae)*	Viral
Onset	Rapid over 24 hr	Gradual over 24-72 hr
Signs and symptoms	Inspiratory stridor, pharyngitis, drooling, fever (often >39° C), lethargic to restless, insists on sitting up and leaning forward, tachypnea, cyanosis	Inspiratory stridor, "barking" cough, rhinorrhea, fever (rarely >39° C)
Laboratory	Neutrophilia	Lymphocytosis
Lateral radiographs of the neck	Swollen epiglottis	Narrowing of the subglottic area
Treatment	Oxygen, urgent tracheal intubation or tracheostomy during general anesthesia, fluids, antibiotics, corticosteroids (?)	Oxygen, aerosolized racemic epinephrine, humidity, fluids, corticosteroids, tracheal intubation for severe airway obstruction

5. **Management of Anesthesia.** An otolaryngologist should be present at the time of induction and tracheal intubation, which are accomplished with the child in the sitting position, breathing the volatile anesthetic sevoflurane in oxygen. Before induction of anesthesia, the care team should be completely prepared to carry out emergency cricothyrotomy or tracheostomy. An intravenous line is placed after adequate depth of anesthesia has been established. Direct laryngoscopy and intubation (with a styletted endotracheal tube that is one half-size smaller than would ordinarily be selected) are performed. Postoperative ICU care is mandatory. Tracheal extubation may be considered when the child's fever and other signs of infection have waned and an air leak develops around the endotracheal tube. The airway is examined by direct laryngoscopy or flexible fiberoptic laryngoscopy during sedation or general anesthesia to confirm that inflammation of the epiglottis and other supraglottic tissues has resolved before the trachea is extubated.

B. **Laryngotracheobronchitis (Croup).** Croup is a viral infection of the upper respiratory tract that typically affects children 6 months to 6 years of age (see Table 27-10).

1. **Signs and Symptoms.** Croup has a gradual onset over 24 to 72 hours, with signs of upper respiratory tract infection (rhinorrhea, pharyngitis, low-grade fever, "barking" cough, hoarse voice, inspiratory stridor). Leukocyte counts are normal or only slightly increased with lymphocytosis. Patients have a characteristic "barking" cough, hoarse voice, and inspiratory stridor.
2. **Diagnosis.** Diagnosis is made clinically. Neck radiographs may show a characteristic subglottic narrowing or "steeple sign" on the anteroposterior view.
3. **Treatment.** Treatment of mild to moderate laryngotracheobronchitis is administration of supplemental oxygen and cool mist. In cases of severe respiratory distress with cyanosis and retractions, nebulized racemic epinephrine (0.05 mL/kg up to 0.5 mL of 2.25% epinephrine solution in 3 mL normal saline) in addition to oxygen may help relieve airway obstruction. Patients often require repeated treatments 1 to 4 hours apart and may experience a rebound

obstruction after an initial state of improvement. Administration of corticosteroids, such as dexamethasone (0.5 to 1.0 mg/kg IV) or inhaled budesonide, decreases edema in the laryngeal mucosa. Increasing $Paco_2$ is an indication for tracheal intubation. The trachea should be intubated with a smaller than normal tube to minimize the edema associated with intubation.

4. **Prognosis.** Most patients, especially older children, with croup experience only stridor and mild dyspnea before recovering. The infection is usually self-limiting and lasts approximately 72 hours.
5. **Management of Anesthesia.** When intubation is necessary, the procedure should be performed in the operating room as for a child with epiglottitis. A surgeon should be present in case a tracheostomy becomes necessary.

C. Postintubation Laryngeal Edema. This is a potential complication of tracheal intubation in all children, but the incidence is highest in children 1 to 4 years old.

1. **Symptoms and Signs.** Signs are stridor, a "barking" or "brassy" cough, hoarseness, retractions, flaring of the ala nasi, hypoxemia, and mental status changes and generally occur within 1 hour of extubation, with peak intensity within 4 hours and resolution of stridor within 24 hours.
2. **Diagnosis.** Inspiratory stridor suggests airway obstruction at or above the level of the vocal cords, whereas expiratory stridor suggests airway obstruction below the level of the vocal cords.
3. **Treatment.** Treatment of postintubation laryngeal edema may include hourly administration of aerosolized racemic epinephrine (0.05 mL/kg [maximum 0.5 mL] in 3.0 mL of saline) until symptoms subside. In severe cases of postintubation laryngeal edema, helium and oxygen mixtures have proven to be useful. Steroids do not reliably prevent postintubation laryngeal edema, although the progression of airway edema may be prevented. In severe cases, treatment with heliox (helium-oxygen mixture) can be tried.
4. **Prognosis.** In most cases, postintubation laryngeal edema is self-limited. For patients requiring racemic epinephrine, one or two treatments usually produce significant improvement.
5. **Management of Anesthesia.** The use of uncuffed endotracheal tubes has traditionally been recommended in children younger than 8 years old because of concerns that cuffed endotracheal tubes might contribute to the risk of subglottic edema. Extubation is considered when a leak around the endotracheal tube is demonstrated, indicating adequate improvement in the laryngeal edema.

D. Subglottic Stenosis. This is a congenital or acquired narrowing of the subglottic airway at the level of the cricoid ring. It is defined as a luminal diameter less than 4 mm in the full-term neonate and less than 3 mm in those born prematurely.

1. **Clinical Signs and Symptoms.** Signs depend on the severity of airway narrowing and can range from stridor to complete obstruction. The diagnosis should be considered in neonates and infants in whom multiple extubation attempts have failed.
2. **Diagnosis.** The diagnosis is made by endoscopic examination. Severity is graded I (<50% luminal obstruction), II (50% to 70% obstruction), III (71% to 91% obstruction), or IV (no discernible lumen).
3. **Treatment.** Grade I and II stenosis do not generally require surgical treatment and may be treated with antiinflammatory and vasoconstrictive agents (corticosteroid and nebulized epinephrine). Stenosis requiring surgical intervention may require only steroid injection, serial dilations, and CO_2 laser ablation with or without topical mitomycin C. Severe stenosis may require an open procedure, such as anterior cricoid split, laryngotracheoplasty with cartilage graft, and tracheostomy.
4. **Management of Anesthesia.** A leak should always be demonstrable around an endotracheal tube at a pressure of 25 cm H_2O. During airway procedures, the risk of fire in the setting of laser use and electrocautery should always be kept in mind.

E. **Foreign Body Aspiration.** Foreign body aspiration into the airways can produce a wide range of responses, from mild symptoms that are barely noticeable to death from asphyxiation. Children aged 1 to 3 represent the overwhelming majority of patients with aspiration.

1. **Signs and Symptoms.** Signs are cough, wheezing, and decreased air entry into the affected lung. The most common site of aspiration is the right mainstem bronchus. The type of foreign body aspirated influences the clinical course. For example, nuts and certain vegetable materials are highly irritating to the bronchial mucosa.
2. **Diagnosis.** Choking or coughing episodes accompanied by wheezing in a previously normal child are highly suggestive of an airway foreign body. Chest radiography provides direct evidence (radiopaque objects) or indirect evidence (hyperinflation of the affected lung [caused by air trapping] and shifting of the mediastinum toward the opposite side on expiratory chest radiograph). Laryngeal foreign bodies manifest with complete obstruction and asphyxiation unless promptly relieved, or with partial obstruction and croup, hoarseness, cough, stridor, and dyspnea. Tracheal foreign bodies most commonly manifest with choking, stridor, and wheezing.
3. **Treatment.** Treatment requires endoscopic removal using direct laryngoscopy and/or rigid bronchoscopy.
4. **Prognosis.** Fragmentation of the foreign body during the course of removal is extremely dangerous and can result in death if the pieces occlude both mainstem bronchi and prevent ventilation. Objects small enough to pass through the vocal cords rarely occlude the trachea.
5. **Management of Anesthesia.** When a laryngeal foreign body or airway obstruction is present, induction of anesthesia using only volatile anesthetics such as sevoflurane in oxygen is useful. Induction of anesthesia with intravenous drugs followed by inhalation of volatile anesthetics is acceptable if the airway is less tenuous. Spraying the larynx with a lidocaine solution is effective in preventing laryngospasm. Administration of atropine (10 to 20 mcg/kg IV) or glycopyrrolate (3 to 5 mcg/kg IV) decreases the likelihood of bradycardia from vagal stimulation during endoscopy. Positive airway pressures could contribute to distal migration of foreign bodies, complicating their extraction. Spontaneous ventilation is desirable until the nature and location of the foreign body have been identified by bronchoscopy. After completion of bronchoscopy, the patient is intubated with an endotracheal tube and extubated when appropriate criteria have been met. Dexamethasone is often given prophylactically to decrease subglottic edema. Nebulized racemic epinephrine is useful for postintubation croup. Chest radiographs should be obtained after bronchoscopy to detect atelectasis or pneumothorax. Postural drainage and chest percussion enhance clearance of secretions and decrease the subsequent risk of infection.

F. **Laryngeal Papillomatosis.** This is the most common benign laryngeal neoplasm in children. The most likely cause is a tissue response to human papillomavirus.

1. **Signs and Symptoms.** A change in the character of the child's voice is the most common initial symptom. Children have hoarseness, and infants may have an altered cry and sometimes stridor.
2. **Diagnosis.** Diagnosis is confirmed by microlaryngoscopy and biopsy of lesions.
3. **Treatment.** Treatment includes surgical excision, cryosurgery, topical 5-fluorouracil, exogenous interferon, and laser ablation. Tracheostomy can be life-saving and is usually reserved for cases with rapid recurrence and airway obstruction.
4. **Prognosis.** Distal involvement of the lower tracheobronchial tree represents an aggressive variant that may be fatal. Malignant degeneration of juvenile papillomas is rare but can occur in older children. Papillomas usually regress spontaneously at puberty.
5. **Management of Anesthesia.** Spontaneous ventilation is recommended until the extent and nature of airway obstruction is determined. Awake tracheal intubation is recommended for severe airway obstruction but is not always feasible. Intubating the trachea after inducing anesthesia with sevoflurane in oxygen is usually a safe approach. Skeletal muscle paralysis

or deep anesthesia is required to immobilize the vocal cords during treatment. The usual safety precautions concerning laser use should be observed. The tracheal tube should be removed only when the child is fully awake and laryngeal bleeding has ceased. After tracheal extubation, inhalation of aerosolized racemic epinephrine and intravenous administration of dexamethasone may decrease subglottic edema.

G. **Laryngeal Clefts.** A group of rare congenital abnormalities in the separation between the posterior laryngotracheal wall and the adjacent esophagus, laryngeal clefts cause varying degrees of communication among the larynx, trachea, and esophagus. The incidence is about 1 in 10,000 to 20,000 live births, with a slight male predominance.

1. **Signs and Symptoms.** Signs depend on the cleft severity. Stridor, choking, and regurgitation are all typical. Recurrent croup or aspiration may occur.
2. **Diagnosis.** Diagnosis requires a high index of suspicion and should be entertained for any child with a history of feeding problems associated with respiratory complaints. Microlaryngoscopic exam is the gold standard.
3. **Treatment.** Treatment is surgical; only minimally invasive surgery may be required. Severe clefts may require median sternotomy or lateral pharyngotomy.
4. **Anesthesia Management.** Procedures are performed during spontaneous ventilation under general anesthesia, to allow spontaneous movement of the vocal cords and surrounding structures to be maintained. Tubeless procedures allow best visualization of the area of concern. Postoperative monitoring should occur initially in the ICU.

H. **Macroglossia.** Macroglossia is true enlargement of the tongue, which can be focal or generalized. Speech, breathing, and swallowing may all be affected. Prognathism, bite deformities, malocclusion, temporomandibular joint pain, drooling, speech impairment, failure to thrive, and stridor can all occur. Surgical reduction aims at restoring normal functions. Anesthesia management is focused on difficult airway management. Spontaneous ventilation is essential until a definitive airway has been established.

I. **Adenotonsillar Hypertrophy and Sleep-Disordered Breathing.** Adenotonsillar hypertrophy is the most common cause of snoring in children. Sleep-disordered breathing may range from inconsequential snoring to complete OSA.

1. **Signs and Symptoms.** Signs include mouth breathing, snoring, and symptoms of obstructive sleep disorder, such as behavioral difficulties, hyperactivity, and learning disabilities. Children may have a history of chronic rhinorrhea, allergic rhinitis, and poor appetite.
2. **Diagnosis.** Tonsillar hypertrophy is graded on a scale: 0 (normal) to 4 (tonsils obstruct at least 75% of the lateral oropharyngeal dimension). Polysomnography is the gold standard for diagnosing OSA. OSA is defined as cessation of airflow despite continued respiratory effort for at least two breaths or 10 seconds. Hypopnea is at least a 50% reduction in airflow with respiratory effort for at least two breaths, or a 3% or greater decrease in oxygen saturation.
3. **Treatment.** In general, adenotonsillectomy relieves obstruction and improves quality of life.
4. **Management of Anesthesia.** Perioperative anxiolytic medication should be avoided. Inhalation induction is followed by tracheal intubation with a cuffed endotracheal tube to minimize aspiration of blood. Nonsteroidal antiinflammatory drugs for postoperative pain are controversial. Intravenous acetaminophen may be preferred owing to lack of effects on bleeding and respiration. High-dose dexamethasone (1 mg/kg, max 25 mg) reduces swelling and nausea and vomiting.

J. **Upper Respiratory Tract Infection.** The tradition of postponing elective surgery for 1 to 2 weeks in children with mild upper respiratory infection (URI) and 4 to 6 weeks for those with more severe symptoms may be too conservative. Urgency and type of surgery should be considered. General anesthesia via mask or LMA is preferable to intubation. Regional anesthesia should also be considered. A smaller than normal endotracheal tube should be used owing to increased risk of postintubation laryngeal edema. Dexamethasone can be given to reduce postintubation croup.

TABLE 27-11 ■ **Grading of Vesicoureteral Reflux**

GRADE	DESCRIPTION
1	Urine refluxes into the ureter only.
2	Urine refluxes into the ureter, renal pelvis, and calyces.
3	Urine refluxes into the ureter and collecting system. There is mild dilation of the ureter and renal pelvis, and the calyces are mildly blunted.
4	Urine refluxes into the ureter and collecting system. There is moderate dilation of the ureter and renal pelvis. The calyces are moderately blunted.
5	Urine refluxes into the ureter and collecting system. The pelvis is severely dilated, the ureters are tortuous, and the calyces are severely blunted.

Adapted from Holzman RS. Urogenital system. In: Holzman RS, Mancuso TJ, Polaner DM. *A Practical Approach to Pediatric Anesthesia*. Philadelphia: Lippincott Williams & Wilkins; 2008:449.

VII. GENITOURINARY DISORDERS

A. **Vesicoureteral Reflux.** Vesicoureteral reflux (VUR) is abnormal reflux of the urine from the bladder into the upper urinary tract. It is the most common urologic disorder in children.
   1. **Signs and Symptoms.** Workup for VUR should be performed for any child who has recurrent UTIs, any male child with a single UTI, any child younger than 5 years with a febrile UTI, and any child with significant renal abnormalities.
   2. **Diagnosis.** Diagnosis is usually based on contrast voiding cystourethrography. VUR is graded on five levels of severity (Table 27-11).
   3. **Treatment.** Antibiotic prophylaxis is administered. A majority of children with mild VUR (80%) will experience spontaneous resolution by 5 years of age. Favorable prognostic factors are younger age at presentation and unilateral disease. Severe VUR rarely resolves without surgery.
   4. **Management of Anesthesia.** Children with VUR may require repeat procedures and have severe anxiety. Preoperative evaluation should take into account the possibility of renal dysfunction, chronic renal disease, and hypertension. Although procedures are short, a deep plane of anesthesia is needed to minimize risk of laryngospasm during the procedure. Postoperative epidural analgesia is recommended for reimplantation procedures.

B. **Posterior Urethral Valve**
   1. **Signs and Symptoms.** The condition usually manifests antenatally during ultrasound with megaureter and hydronephrosis. Pulmonary insufficiency, dysuria, abnormal urinary stream, diurnal enuresis, UTI, abdominal mass (distended bladder), VUR, renal failure, and uremic symptoms may all be part of the postnatal picture. One third of patients will progress to renal failure.
   2. **Treatment.** Bladder outlet obstruction is treated with urinary catheterization. The obstructive valves can be incised in the first few days of life. Direct vesicocutaneous or ureterocutaneous urinary diversion may be required.
   3. **Management of Anesthesia.** Principles are the same as for patients with advanced renal insufficiency. Attention to fluid and electrolyte balance is key.

C. **Cryptorchidism.** Cryptorchidism is the congenital absence of one or both testes in the scrotum resulting from incomplete testicular descent. Undescended testes present the risk of malignant transformation, concurrent hernia with risks of incarceration, and increased risks of infertility and testicular torsion.
   1. **Signs and Symptoms.** Signs include inability to palpate the testis or palpation of a malpositioned testis.

2. **Diagnosis.** Palpation must be performed in a warm room to prevent testicular retraction. Nonpalpable testes occur in 20% of cases. In 40% of cases the testis is intraabdominal, in 40% it is in a high inguinal location, and in the remainder the testis is atrophied or congenitally absent. Most testes do not descend after 9 months of age.
3. **Treatment.** Treatment is surgical orchiopexy.
4. **Management of Anesthesia.** Owing to a high incidence of postoperative nausea and vomiting, prophylactic antiemetic treatment should be routinely given. Caudal analgesia is highly recommended.

D. Hypospadias. Hypospadias is a congenital malpositioning of the urethral meatus on the ventral aspect of the penis.

1. **Diagnosis.** Diagnosis is via physical exam at birth. The abnormal opening can occur anywhere from the glans penis to the penile shaft, and even down to the scrotum and perineum. Chordee, an abnormal ventral curvature of the penis, is common.
2. **Treatment.** Treatment is surgical repair, usually between the ages of 4 and 18 months of age.
3. **Management of Anesthesia.** General anesthesia supplemented with caudal analgesia is preferred.

VIII. ORTHOPEDIC-MUSCULOSKELETAL DISORDERS

A. Clubfoot (Talipes Equinovarus). Clubfoot is caused by malalignment of the calcaneotalar-navicular complex, resulting in plantar flexion, medially deviated forefoot, and inward-facing sole. Bilateral involvement occurs in 30% to 50% of cases.

1. **Signs and Symptoms.** Clubfoot is evident at birth.
2. **Treatment.** Nonoperative treatment includes taping and serial casting for positional clubfoot. There is a high rate of recurrence, and surgical Achilles tenotomy is often needed. Ponseti's method involves weekly stretching and casting, Achilles tenotomy, long leg casting, and a bracing program for 3 to 5 years. Rigid deformities require surgical realignment.
3. **Management of Anesthesia.** Continuous epidural analgesia is highly recommended because of significant postoperative pain.

B. Slipped Capital Femoral Epiphysis. This condition results from a fracture in the femoral growth plate.

1. **Signs and Symptoms.** This is a disorder of adolescence but is seen at increasingly earlier ages, possibly because of the increase in childhood obesity. It usually manifests at age 10 to 16, in boys more than in girls. Risk factors are obesity, Down's syndrome, endocrinopathies, and renal osteodystrophy. Groin, thigh, and knee pain are often present, and the hip is held in external rotation. Gait and weight bearing are affected; 20% of cases are bilateral.
2. **Diagnosis.** Diagnosis is from physical examination and radiographs.
3. **Treatment.** Surgical pinning of the growth plate is performed.
4. **Management of Anesthesia.** In general, management of anesthesia is related to comorbid conditions and the urgency of the case (full-stomach considerations).

C. Blount's Disease. Blount's disease is abnormal cartilage growth at the proximal tibial growth plate resulting in genu varum (bowleg) deformity.

1. **Signs and Symptoms.** Two forms exist: infantile and adolescent. The infantile form manifests before age 3, with 80% of cases bilateral. The adolescent form can be unilateral. Risk factors are walking at an early age, African descent, and obesity. Physical exam may reveal a nontender prominence on the medial side of the proximal tibia.
2. **Diagnosis.** Diagnosis is via radiography. It is important to distinguish Blount's disease from other causes of genu varum (e.g., physiologic genu varum in children younger than 2 years, rickets), because treatment is different.
3. **Treatment.** The infantile form is often amenable to corrective bracing. The adolescent form generally requires surgical therapy. Complications of surgery include nonunion, neurovascular injury, and compartment syndrome.

4. **Management of Anesthesia.** Although postoperative pain is significant, surgeons often oppose regional and neuraxial analgesia to avoid masking symptoms of nerve injury and compartment syndrome.

D. **Developmental Dysplasia of the Hip.** Developmental dysplasia of the hip (DDH) is abnormal growth of the hip caused by joint laxity and acetabular dysplasia with dislocation.

1. **Signs and Symptoms.** Leg-length discrepancy and gluteal fold asymmetry are clues to DDH. Untreated, DDH can lead to repetitive and chronic dislocations. DDH is associated with Ehlers-Danlos syndrome.
2. **Diagnosis.** Diagnosis and monitoring can be accomplished using the Barlow (hip adduction with posterior pressure) and Ortolani (abduction and anterior pressure on the greater trochanter) maneuvers. Ultrasound is the primary diagnostic modality until 5 months of age, after which radiographs are used.
3. **Treatment.** Treatment is with bracing (Pavlik's harness) and body casting. Children who manifest the condition after 2 years of age need open reduction.

E. **Thoracic Insufficiency Syndrome.** Thoracic insufficiency syndrome is an inability of the thorax to support postnatal lung growth and respiratory function. This can arise from a spectrum of thoracospinal abnormalities including fused ribs, spinal deformities such as scoliosis, or shortened and narrow thorax as in Jarcho-Levin syndrome and Jeune's syndrome.

1. **Signs and Symptoms.** Signs are those of restrictive lung disease and chronic respiratory failure. Intermittent nocturnal hypercarbia and hypoxemia are early signs. Other signs include recurrent lower respiratory tract infections, poor nutritional status caused by high metabolic demands, and cardiovascular disease, such as pulmonary hypertension and cor pulmonale.
2. **Diagnosis.** Diagnosis is via lung perfusion scans and measurements of spinal deformity (Cobb's angle).
3. **Treatment.** Treatment includes medical therapy (noninvasive ventilation and chest percussion) and surgical correction of deformities.
4. **Management of Anesthesia.** Management is based on considerations for restrictive pulmonary disease. Preoperative evaluation of cardiac function may be necessary. Surgery should be postponed in the presence of any acute respiratory illness. Postoperative ICU care is needed.

F. **Juvenile Idiopathic Arthritis.** Juvenile idiopathic arthritis (JIA) includes all types of juvenile arthritis, including what was formerly known as *juvenile rheumatoid arthritis.* JIA is the most common autoimmune disease of childhood.

1. **Signs and Symptoms.** JIA is defined as joint pain, stiffness, and swelling that last longer than 6 weeks and has an onset earlier than 16 years of age.
   a. ***Oligoarticular JIA.*** This type of JIA accounts for 50% of all cases, peaks around 2 years of age, and involves four or fewer joints after 6 months of illness. Knees are commonly involved, and 75% of patients test positive for antinuclear antibodies (ANAs). Joint destruction is rare.
   b. ***Polyarticular JIA.*** Polyarticular JIA involves more than four joints after 6 months of illness (30% to 40% of cases) and peaks at 3 years of age. Small joints of the hand are often involved. Less than half of patients are positive for ANAs, and only 10% are positive for rheumatoid factor (RF).
   c. ***Still's Disease.*** Still's disease represents the smallest subset (10% to 15% of cases). It manifests with symmetric polyarthritis, intermittent fever, macular rash, hematopoietic abnormalities (leukocytosis, thrombocytopenia, lymphadenopathy, hepatosplenomegaly), and systemic complaints (uveitis, pleuritis, pericarditis). It can manifest after 16 years of age, when it is called *adult onset Still's disease.*
2. **Management of Anesthesia.** Consideration is given to possible difficult airway, temporomandibular joint arthritis and cervical spine involvement, systemic issues such as pleuritis and pericarditis, and the implications of immunosuppressive medications.

IX. CHILDHOOD MALIGNANCIES

A. Wilms's Tumor (Nephroblastoma). Wilms's tumor is the most common malignant renal tumor and the most common malignant abdominal tumor in children. Median age at onset is 3 years, and 95% of these tumors occur before age 10. Nephroblastoma is associated with WAGR syndrome (Wilms's tumor, aniridia, genitourinary malformations, and mental retardation), Beckwith-Wiedemann syndrome (hemihypertrophy, visceromegaly, macroglossia, and hyperinsulinemic hypoglycemia), Denys-Drash syndrome (pseudohermaphroditism, progressive glomerulopathy, and Wilms's tumor), fetal gigantism, Soto's syndrome (cerebral gigantism), and isolated hemihypertrophy.

1. **Signs and Symptoms.** Nephroblastoma is usually found accidentally as an asymptomatic flank mass. Pain, fever, and hematuria are late manifestations. These children may exhibit malaise, weight loss, anemia, disturbed micturition, vomiting, or constipation. Systemic hypertension (mild to severe, caused by renin release directly or as an indirect effect of the tumor) may occur, particularly if the tumor involves both kidneys. Increases in systemic blood pressure are usually mild, but on rare occasions hypertension is so severe that encephalopathy and congestive heart failure develop. Secondary hyperaldosteronism and hypokalemia may be present. Acquired von Willebrand's disease is seen in 8% of cases.
2. **Diagnosis.** Diagnosis is via radiography, including intravenous pyelography (to examine the renal collecting system and assess the contralateral kidney), inferior vena cavagram (to examine tumor invasion), arteriogram, and chest radiographs or liver scans (to look for metastases).
3. **Treatment.** Nephrectomy is performed, with or without subsequent radiation and chemotherapy. Preoperative chemotherapy is administered to patients with bilateral tumors who will undergo parenchyma-sparing procedures, patients with extensive intravascular (inferior vena caval) tumor extension, or those with inoperable tumors. Radiation therapy may be given initially to shrink the tumor, followed by surgery. Surgical treatment of bilateral disease may consist of bilateral partial nephrectomy or bilateral total nephrectomy followed by dialysis and eventually renal transplantation.
4. **Prognosis.** Tumor size, stage, and histology are major prognostic factors. Survival rate approaches 90% in patients with favorable histology and stage, and is more than 60% across all stages.
5. **Management of Anesthesia.** Anemia and adverse effects of chemotherapy (e.g., cardiomyopathy as a result of doxorubicin) are considerations. Blood loss during surgery may be significant. Electrolyte and fluid abnormalities may exist secondary to diarrhea. Invasive monitoring with an arterial catheter and central venous catheter may be needed, and a Foley catheter should be placed to monitor urine output. Lower-extremity venous catheters should be avoided, as it may be necessary to ligate or partially resect the inferior vena cava. Measurement of central venous pressure is helpful for evaluating intravascular fluid volume and the adequacy of fluid replacement. Tumor extension into the suprahepatic vena cava and right atrium may necessitate cardiopulmonary bypass. Epidural analgesia should be avoided in these patients because of potential complications associated with full heparinization but is recommended if heparinization is not needed. Manipulation of the inferior vena cava containing a metastatic tumor can result in a tumor embolism to the heart or pulmonary artery.

B. Hepatoblastoma. Hepatoblastoma is the most common pediatric hepatic malignancy.

1. **Signs and Symptoms.** Median age at presentation is 1 year. It is more common in boys, Caucasians, and premature children with low birth weight. Associated disorders are Beckwith-Wiedemann syndrome (see Wilms's tumor), hemihypertrophy, and familial adenomatous polyposis. Signs are abdominal mass, anorexia, and penile and testicular enlargement (caused by tumor secretion of β–human chorionic gonadotropin); 10% of patients have metastases at presentation, with lungs being the most common site.
2. **Diagnosis.** Diagnosis is via tissue biopsy, and regular monitoring of α-fetoprotein is important in assessing disease progression.
3. **Prognosis.** The prognosis is dependent on histologic features and the completeness of tumor resection.

4. **Treatment.** Treatment is chemotherapy (cisplatin and doxorubicin), surgical resection of tumor, and liver transplantation in some cases.
5. **Management of Anesthesia.** Management is dependent on the general health of the patient undergoing surgery. Assessment of hepatic and metabolic functions is important. Major blood loss can occur, and blood component therapy should be planned. Invasive arterial monitoring is recommended, as is large-bore intravenous access. Hypothermia is a risk because of the large areas of surgical exposure. In the absence of preoperative coagulation abnormalities, epidural analgesia should be considered.

C. **Neuroblastoma.** Neuroblastoma is the most common extracranial solid tumor in infants and children, resulting from malignant proliferation of sympathetic ganglion cell precursors. Neuroblastoma may metastasize by direct invasion into surrounding structures, lymphatic infiltration, or hematogenous spread.

1. **Signs and Symptoms.** Children typically have protuberant abdomens. Neuroblastomas are large, firm, nodular, sometimes painful flank masses that are usually fixed to surrounding structures. Paraspinal neuroblastomas may extend into the epidural space, producing paraplegia. Neuroblastomas may secrete vasoactive intestinal peptide causing persistent watery diarrhea with loss of fluid and electrolytes. Frequent metastatic involvement of bone and bone marrow cause bone pain. Orbital involvement can manifest as orbital ecchymosis and proptosis. Opsoclonus-myoclonus-ataxia is a paraneoplastic syndrome seen in 2% of cases (random eye movements and myoclonic jerks). A subtype of tumor (stage 4S) with a favorable prognosis is seen in infants under age 6 months and consists of a small primary tumor with metastases to the liver and skin.
2. **Diagnosis.** Median age at diagnosis is 2 years, and 90% of cases are diagnosed by 5 years of age. Ultrasonography, CT, and MRI are the primary diagnostic procedures. Urinary excretion of vanillylmandelic acid is increased in most children with neuroblastomas, reflecting the metabolism of catecholamines produced by these tumors (hypertension is rare).
3. **Treatment.** Treatment includes surgical removal, radiation therapy, and chemotherapy (cyclophosphamide, doxorubicin, cisplatin, vincristine).
4. **Prognosis.** The prognosis depends on molecular markers and degree of tumor differentiation, patient age, and tumor stage. Infants younger than 1 year old at diagnosis have a significantly improved outcome across all tumor stages. *MYCN* status (amplification of the N-Myc protooncogene) predicts poor outcome.
5. **Management of Anesthesia.** For resection of neuroblastoma, management is as described for children with nephroblastoma. Cardiac evaluation should be considered in patients who have received doxorubicin chemotherapy. Adequate intravenous access is essential because neuroblastomas are quite vascular and often adhere to or surround the great vessels, creating the potential for significant blood loss. Despite potential catecholamine release, intraoperative hypertension is uncommon. Epidural analgesia is a beneficial adjunct as long as the tumor does not involve the spine.

D. **Ewing's Sarcoma.** This is the second most common primary bone malignancy in children and adolescents, after osteosarcoma.

1. **Signs and Symptoms.** Primarily a disease of adolescence, 30% of Ewing's sarcoma cases occur in children younger than 10 years of age, and 10% manifest at age 20 and older. Lesions often involve long bones of the lower extremities, followed by the pelvis and then long bones of the upper extremities. Patients have localized pain (exacerbated by exercise and worse at night), often a palpable mass, and pathologic fractures (15% of cases). Systemic symptoms are uncommon, but when they occur they tend to be associated with metastatic disease.
2. **Diagnosis.** Diagnosis is based on tissue biopsy. Plain radiography, CT, MRI, and positron emission tomography (PET) scanning may be helpful.
3. **Treatment.** Treatment is neoadjuvant chemotherapy (vincristine, cyclophosphamide, doxorubicin, Ifosfamide, and etoposide) followed by surgical resection. Radiotherapy may be used in unresectable disease.

4. **Prognosis.** Five-year survival with localized disease is 70%, compared with 30% with metastatic disease.
5. **Management of Anesthesia.** The most important consideration is pain control. Regional and neuraxial analgesia should be strongly considered. Possible prior doxorubicin therapy (and cardiac effects) should be borne in mind.

X. TUMORS OF THE CENTRAL NERVOUS SYSTEM

CNS malignancies are a major proportion of all solid tumors in children younger than 15 years of age. They are the second most common cancer in childhood after leukemia. Among children aged 1 to 10 years, infratentorial tumors dominate.

A. **Clinical Presentation.** The presentation depends on tumor location, effects on ICP, and age of the child. Tumors obstructing flow of CSF may cause behavioral changes, headache, nausea and vomiting, visual disturbances, and nystagmus, and increased head size in children whose cranial sutures have not yet closed. Supratentorial tumors cause sensorimotor deficits, speech disorders and seizures. Tumors of the suprasellar region and third ventricle often cause neuroendocrine abnormalities. Brainstem tumors may cause cranial nerve palsies and hyperreflexia. Tumors of the spinal cord cause back pain, motor and sensory deficits, and bowel and bladder dysfunction. Diagnosis is via imaging, with MRI the gold standard. Laboratory testing to assess neuroendocrine function is sometimes needed.

B. **Tumor Types**
   1. **Astrocytomas.** Accounting for 40% of CNS tumors, astrocytomas often have an indolent course and have a favorable survival rate (80% to 100% overall) if complete surgical resection can be achieved. Aggressive subtypes (glioblastomas) are rare in children.
   2. **Medulloblastomas.** These are a form of primitive neuroectodermal tumors (which overall account for 25% of CNS tumors). Peak incidence is age 5 to 7 years. Signs and symptoms related to high ICP and cerebellar dysfunction are common.
   3. **Ependymomas.** Ependymomas account for 10% of CNS tumors, the majority in the posterior fossa. Surgery, the primary treatment, is rarely curative without adjuvant chemotherapy. Overall survival is 40%.
   4. **Craniopharyngiomas.** These are the most common nonglial tumors and are almost always suprasellar. They are usually benign but are associated with significant morbidities owing to proximity to the hypothalamus, pituitary gland, optic chiasm, ventricular system, and carotid arteries. Surgical resection often leaves the child with serious neuroendocrine and visual complications. Radiation, brachytherapy, and chemotherapy are also employed.
   5. **Choroid Plexus Tumors.** Choroid plexus tumors are the most common CNS tumor of infancy but are rare. Clinical signs are related to high ICP. Virtually 100% of choroid papillomas are curable by resection, but choroid carcinoma has a survival rate of only about 40%.

C. **Management of Anesthesia.** Anesthetic concerns are of two general types: those related to high ICP (see discussion of management of hydrocephalus), and those related to neuroendocrine disturbance as they affect perioperative fluid and electrolyte management.
   1. **Diabetes Insipidus**
      a. ***Diagnosis.*** Diagnosis is based on a rising serum sodium concentration (>145 mg/dL) in the setting of copious dilute urine production (specific gravity <1.005).
      b. ***Intraoperative Management.*** Vasopressin therapy if already initiated must be maintained. Isotonic fluid administration should continue at two thirds the maintenance rate. Blood and evaporative losses must also be replaced. Vasopressin infusion can be started at 0.5 milliunits/kg/hr and increased in increments of 0.5 milliunits/kg/hr until urine osmolality is twice serum osmolality or urine output is less than 2 mL/kg/hr. Desmopressin (DDAVP) can also be used (0.4 to 4 mcg IV as a single dose every 8 to 12 hours).

XI. ANTERIOR MEDIASTINAL MASS (MAY BE CAUSED BY MANY TYPES OF TUMORS: LYMPHOMA, LYMPHANGIOMA, TERATOMA, NEUROBLASTOMA)

A. **Signs and Symptoms.** Cardiovascular and respiratory symptoms depend on the size and location of the tumor. Tachypnea, orthopnea, and nocturnal dyspnea suggest airway compression. The patient's respiratory status may be normal in the sitting, decubitus, or prone position but poor in the supine position. Cardiovascular structures can be compressed or constricted by an enlarging mediastinal tumor. Superior vena cava (SVC) syndrome causes facial and periorbital edema, shortness of breath, engorgement of jugular veins, and CNS symptoms (headache and visual disturbances) that worsen in the supine position.

B. **Diagnosis.** Chest radiographs, computed axial tomography scans, and MRI images are static pictures of airway compression and may not accurately quantitate the degree of compression. Flow volume loops sitting and supine may give a dynamic assessment of the airway, as may flexible fiberoptic bronchoscopy under local anesthesia or sedation. Echocardiography may help delineate cardiac compromise. Definitive tumor diagnosis is based on tissue biopsy.

C. **Treatment.** Procedures that may need general anesthesia or sedation include computed axial tomography scan, biopsy of cervical nodes, and central venous catheter placement. Before surgical removal of tumor, preoperative chemotherapy, radiation therapy, and steroid therapy should be considered, to shrink tumor mass. Decreasing the size of the tumor before surgery is often beneficial.

D. **Management of Anesthesia**

1. **Preoperative.** Limitations in respiratory and cardiovascular reserves must be evaluated, and further deterioration anticipated. Children with hematologic malignancies may have coagulation abnormalities.
2. **Intraoperative.** Premedication should be avoided and intravenous access established before induction, preferably in a lower extremity if SVC obstruction is present. Inhalation or intravenous induction with maintenance of spontaneous ventilation at all times (intravenous ketamine and/or dexmedetomidine 1 to 3 mcg/kg/hr with or without a loading dose of 1 mcg/kg over 10 minutes) and avoidance of all muscle relaxants are recommended. Nitrous oxide should be avoided. If the child's condition deteriorates during induction, turning him or her into the left lateral decubitus or prone position may improve cardiorespiratory function. Another option if collapse of the airway occurs is rigid bronchoscopy. Cardiopulmonary bypass (femorofemoral bypass) or venovenous bypass may be necessary if either complete airway obstruction or vessel occlusion is anticipated. A helium and oxygen mixture may be used to improve oxygenation in patients with airway compression caused by mediastinal tumors (lower density than oxygen, decreased airway resistance). Extubation is best when the patient is awake, ensuring adequate return of airway reflexes and prevention of laryngospasm.
3. **Postoperative.** Recovery room personnel must be notified of the effect of position on the patient's cardiorespiratory status. Children with significant tracheomalacia may manifest tracheal obstruction and respiratory difficulties in recovery, necessitating reintubation. Unilateral pulmonary edema may be associated with lung reexpansion after mediastinal tumor removal.

XII. DOWN'S SYNDROME (TRISOMY 21)

Down's syndrome is the most common human chromosomal syndrome. It is usually recognized at birth or soon thereafter because of a constellation of characteristic dysmorphic features. It is the most common form of intellectual disability, with most patients having mild-to-moderate impairment.

A. **Signs and Symptoms.** Common features affect the head (brachycephaly, a flat occiput, dysplastic ears, epicanthal folds with typical up-slanting of the palpebral folds [mongoloid slanting] and strabismus, and Brushfield spots on the iris). The tongue is normal at birth but later becomes enlarged because of hypertrophy of the papillae. Midface hypoplasia, a high-arched palate, and micrognathia complicate this problem. Skeletal anomalies may include short stature and a short, broad neck with occipitoatlantoaxial instability (approximately 20% of patients). The hands are usually short and broad with a simian crease, and the middle phalanx of the fifth finger is often hypoplastic. Muscle tone is reduced, and the joints are hypermobile. A floppy soft palate, enlarged tonsils, laryngotracheal or subglottic stenosis, OSA, and recurrent pulmonary infections can cause respiratory problems. Cardiac defects are common (atrial septal defect, VSD [25%], endocardial cushion defect [50%], PDA, or tetralogy of Fallot). Pulmonary hypertension should be suspected and may even lead to Eisenmenger's complex. Visceral anomalies include gastroesophageal reflux, duodenal atresia, imperforate anus, and Hirschsprung's disease.

B. **Diagnosis.** The diagnosis can be established antenatally by chorionic villous sampling or by amniocentesis. Postnatally, the diagnosis is based on the typical clinical features and confirmed by karyotyping.

C. **Prognosis.** There is a tenfold to twentyfold increased risk of leukemia (acute myelocytic leukemia or acute lymphocytic leukemia). Hypothyroidism, early onset dementia, and conductive hearing loss are other common problems.

D. **Management of Anesthesia.** Preoperative assessment includes evaluation of the current respiratory and cardiac status. Airway management can be difficult (macroglossia, micrognathia, narrow hypopharynx, muscular hypotonia). The risk of spinal cord compression resulting from occipitoatlantoaxial instability should be kept in mind during intubation or positioning for surgical procedures (neck radiographs do not reliably predict this). A history of gait anomalies, a preference for the sitting position, hyperreflexia, and signs of clonus could all be suggestive of spinal canal stenosis or cord compression. A smaller than normal endotracheal tube should be used because of a predisposition to postoperative croup. The anesthetic risk is increased in the presence of cardiac disease. Vascular access can be challenging secondary to xerodermia, atopic dermatitis, and obesity. Narrowing of the trachea (subglottic stenosis) is common and may necessitate use of a smaller endotracheal tube than expected. These patients have reduced immune competence and require strict asepsis with all invasive procedures. Airway abnormalities increase the risk of OSA and mandate close monitoring in the early postoperative period.

XIII. MALIGNANT HYPERTHERMIA

Susceptible patients (estimated to be 1 in 3000 to 1 in 15,000 children) have a genetic predisposition for the development of this disorder when they are exposed to triggering pharmacologic agents (all volatile inhalation anesthetic agents and succinylcholine) or stressful environmental factors. MH represents a spectrum of reactions from minor reactions to rapid temperature increase, muscle rigidity, acidosis, arrhythmias, and death. Some reactions may not occur until the postoperative period.

A. **Signs and Symptoms** (Table 27-12)

B. **Diagnosis.** Without hypercapnia and acidosis, the diagnosis of MH is questionable. If sufficiently sensitive measuring equipment is used, jaw stiffness after administration of succinylcholine can be detected in most patients but is often more pronounced in children. Children in whom masseter muscle rigidity (MMR) develops have a 50% incidence of susceptibility to MH. Skeletal muscle biopsies are positive for MH susceptibility in all patients in whom plasma creatinine kinase concentrations exceed 20,000 units/L after succinylcholine-induced masseter spasm. Findings that support the diagnosis of MH include myoglobinuria, elevated serum creatinine kinase, fever, hypoxemia, hypercarbia, respiratory and metabolic acidosis, hyperkalemia, and marked central venous oxygen desaturation. Late complications of untreated MH include disseminated intravascular coagulation, pulmonary edema, and acute renal failure. CNS damage may manifest as blindness, seizures, coma, or paralysis.

C. **Differential Diagnosis** (Table 27-13)

TABLE 27-12 ■ Clinical Features of Malignant Hyperthermia

TIMING	CLINICAL SIGNS	CHANGES IN MONITORED VARIABLES	BIOCHEMICAL CHANGES
Early	Masseter spasm		
	Tachypnea	Increased minute ventilation	
	Rapid exhaustion of soda lime	Increasing end-tidal carbon dioxide concentration	Increased $Paco_2$
	Warm soda lime canister		
	Tachycardia		Acidosis
	Irregular heart rate	Cardiac dysrhythmias, peaked T waves on ECG	Hyperkalemia
Intermediate	Patient warm to touch	Increasing core body temperature	
	Cyanosis	Decreasing oxygen saturation	
	Dark blood in surgical site		
	Irregular heart rate	Cardiac dysrhythmias, peaked T waves on ECG	Hyperkalemia
Late	Generalized skeletal muscle rigidity		Increased creatine kinase concentrations
	Prolonged bleeding		
	Dark urine		Myoglobinuria
	Irregular heart rate	Cardiac dysrhythmias, peaked T waves on ECG	Hyperkalemia

Adapted from Hopkins PM. Malignant hyperthermia: advances in clinical management and diagnosis. *Br J Anaesth*. 2000;85:118-128.
ECG, Electrocardiogram.

D. Treatment of an Acute Episode (Table 27-14)

1. **Intravenous Dantrolene.** Dantrolene (2 to 3 mg/kg IV repeated every 5 to 10 minutes to a maximum dose of 10 mg/kg) is the only drug that is reliably effective treatment for MH. The patient should respond to treatment within 45 minutes. Recrudescence may occur in 25% of patients, usually within 4 to 8 hours but can occur as late as 36 hours. Dantrolene should probably be repeated, even if the initial episode is under control, at a dose of 1 to 2 mg/kg IV every 6 hours for a 24-hour period. Some recommend continuing oral dantrolene 1 mg/kg every 4 to 8 hours for 48 hours.
2. **Supportive and Resuscitative Measures.** Measures are performed to address hypermetabolic consequences; see Table 27-14.

E. Prognosis. After recovery from acute episodes of MH, patients should be closely monitored in an ICU for up to 72 hours. Urine output, arterial blood gases, pH, and serum electrolyte concentrations should be determined frequently.

F. Identification of Susceptible Patients. Detailed medical and family anesthetic histories should be obtained. MH appears to be linked with central core disease (most have mutation at the RYR1 locus). Skeletal muscle biopsies with in vitro contracture testing provide definitive confirmation of susceptibility to MH but are not appropriate in children younger than 6 years or those who weigh less than 20 kg, because of the amount of muscle needed for the test. It

TABLE 27-13 ■ Differential Diagnosis of Malignant Hyperthermia (MH)

DIAGNOSIS	DISTINGUISHING TRAITS
Hyperthyroidism	Symptoms and physical findings often present; blood gas abnormalities increase gradually
Sepsis	Usually normal blood gases
Pheochromocytoma	Similar to MH except marked blood pressure swings
Metastatic carcinoid	Same as pheochromocytoma
Cocaine intoxication	Fever, rigidity, rhabdomyolysis similar to that of neuroleptic malignant syndrome
Heat stroke	Similar to MH except that the patient is outside the operating room
Masseter spasm (MMR)	May progress to MH; total body spasm more likely than isolated MMR
Neuroleptic malignant syndrome	Similar to MH; usually associated with the use of dopamine antagonist antipsychotic drugs
Serotonin syndrome	Similar to MH and neuroleptic malignant syndrome; associated with the administration of serotoninergic drugs

Adapted from Bissonnette B, Ryan JF. Temperature regulation: Normal and abnormal (malignant hyperthermia). In: Cote CJ, Todres ID, Goudsouzian NG, Ryan JF, eds: *A Practice of Anesthesia for Infants and Children*. 3rd ed. Philadelphia: Saunders; 2001:621.

TABLE 27-14 ■ Treatment of Malignant Hyperthermia

TREATMENT OF CAUSE
Administer dantrolene (2-3 mg/kg IV) as an initial bolus; follow with repeat doses every 5-10 min until symptoms are controlled (rarely need total dose 10 mg/kg). Prevent recrudescence (dantrolene 1 mg/kg IV every 6 hours for 72 hours).
TREATMENT OF HYPERMETABOLIC STATE
Immediately discontinue inhaled anesthetics and conclude surgery as soon as possible. Hyperventilate the lungs with 100% oxygen. Initiate active cooling (iced saline 15 mL/kg IV every 10 min; gastric and bladder lavage with iced saline; surface cooling). Correct metabolic acidosis (sodium bicarbonate 1-2 mEq/kg IV based on arterial pH). Maintain urine output (hydration, mannitol 0.25 g/kg IV, furosemide 1 mg/kg IV). Treat cardiac dysrhythmias (procainamide 15 mg/kg IV). Monitor in an intensive care unit (urine output, arterial blood gases, pH, electrolytes).

IV, Intravenously.

is preferable to take a biopsy sample from the patient with MMR before testing other family members. Follow-up of patients who have had MMR is summarized in Table 27-15.

G. **Anesthesia-Induced Rhabdomyolysis.** This is a clinical syndrome associated with hypermetabolic signs seen in patients with dystrophinopathies (Duchenne's and Becker's muscular dystrophy). It was previously thought that these patients are susceptible to MH, but the condition is now known to occur through a different mechanism: instability of the sarcolemma. The role of dantrolene in treatment is unknown, but it is unlikely to have significant efficacy.

TABLE 27-15 ■ Follow-Up of Patients with Masseter Muscle Rigidity

MedicAlert bracelet or other conspicuous form of identification must be worn. The patient and first-degree relatives must be assumed to have malignant hyperthermia susceptibility (MHS) unless the patient is subsequently shown to have a negative caffeine halothane contracture test.
Refer the patient to MHS sites, Malignant Hyperthermia Association of the United States (MHAUS) (800-98MHAUS; www.mhaus.org). MHAUS can refer the patient to a malignant hyperthermia diagnostic center.
Review the family history for adverse anesthetic events or suggestion of heritable myopathy.
Consider evaluation for temporomandibular joint disorder.
Consider neurologic consultation to evaluate for a potential myotonic disorder; if rhabdomyolysis is severe, consider evaluation for a muscular dystrophy (e.g., Duchenne's or Becker's muscular dystrophy) or a heritable metabolic disorder (e.g., carnitine palmitoyltransferase II deficiency or McArdle's disease).

TABLE 27-16 ■ Nontriggering Drugs for Malignant Hyperthermia

Barbiturates
Propofol
Etomidate
Benzodiazepines
Opioids
Droperidol
Nitrous oxide
Nondepolarizing muscle relaxants
Anticholinesterases
Anticholinergics
Sympathomimetics
Local anesthetics (esters and amides)
α_2-Agonists
Clonidine
Dexmedetomidine

H. Management of Anesthesia

1. **Dantrolene Prophylaxis.** This is unnecessary if one adheres to a nontriggering technique. If a severe MH reaction has previously occurred, dantrolene 2 to 4 mg/kg IV may be administered over 10 to 30 minutes just before induction of anesthesia, and one half the dose is repeated in 6 hours. Diuresis may accompany intravenous administration of dantrolene (caused by mannitol in the powder), and patients should have a urinary catheter placed. Dantrolene may cause nausea, diarrhea, blurred vision, and skeletal muscle weakness. Patients should have anxiolytic therapy before surgery.
2. **Drug Selections** (Table 27-16). Drugs that can trigger MH include volatile anesthetics and succinylcholine. Administration of calcium entry-blocking drugs in the presence of dantrolene has been associated with hyperkalemia and myocardial depression. Antagonism of nondepolarizing muscle relaxants has not been shown to trigger MH.
3. **Anesthesia Machine.** A conventional anesthesia machine can be used with a disposable anesthesia breathing circuit and fresh gas outlet hoses, fresh carbon dioxide absorbent, no vaporizers (removed or taped), and a continuous flow of oxygen at 10 L/min for 10 to 100 minutes (see manufacturer's recommendations) before the machine is used with patients susceptible to MH.

4. **Regional Anesthesia.** Regional anesthesia is acceptable in MH-susceptible patients. Both ester- and amide-based local anesthetics are now considered safe for regional or local anesthesia.
5. **Postoperative Discharge Home.** It is acceptable to perform surgery in ambulatory centers on patients susceptible to MH as long as they are monitored for at least 1 hour (and preferably 4 hours) after use of a nontriggering anesthetic.

CHAPTER 28

Geriatric Disorders

The elderly population (>65 years of age) represented 17% of the U.S. population in 2010 (47 million persons). It is estimated that the number of people 65 years of age and older will be 80 million by 2030. Those over age 80 will increase from 9.3 million in 2000 to 19.5 million in 2030. The combined cost of Medicare and Social Security is predicted to grow to be 11.2% of the gross national product by 2030 (Figure 28-1). The aging of the U.S. population will result in significant growth in the demand for surgical services, and anesthesiologists will need to develop strategies to address this increased demand while maintaining quality of care for senior patients.

I. PHYSIOLOGY OF AGING (TABLE 28-1)

II. GERIATRIC SYNDROMES

A. Skeletal Changes

1. **Osteoporosis.** Osteoporosis is characterized by microarchitectural deterioration and decreased bone density, with increased bone fragility and susceptibility to fracture. Complications of hip fracture account for 37,000 deaths annually in the United States. Prevention is key; weight-bearing exercises and adequate calcium and vitamin D intake are essential.

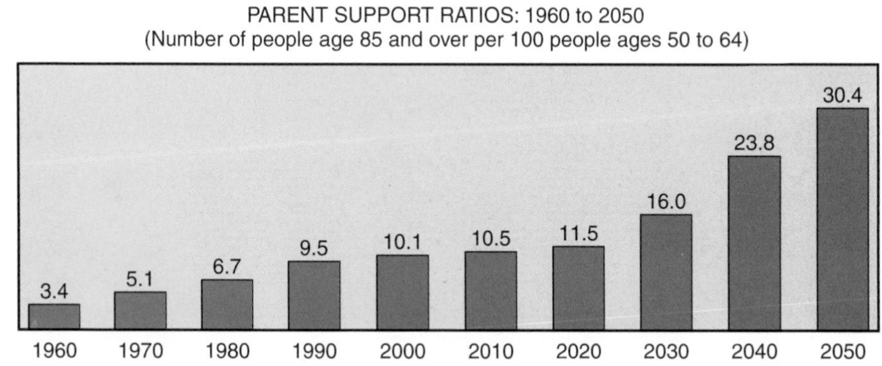

FIGURE 28-1 ■ As more and more people live long enough to experience multiple chronic illnesses and/or disability, there will be more and more relatives in their 50s and 60s who will be facing the concern and expense of caring for them. *(Data from the U.S. Bureau of the Census.)*

2. **Osteoarthritis.** The most common joint disease, osteoarthritis is characterized by degeneration of articular cartilage primarily of the weight-bearing joints. Diagnosis is based on clinical assessment of the affected joints and positive radiographic findings. Weight loss, physical therapy, occupational therapy, reduction of joint stress, acetaminophen, nonsteroidal antiinflammatory drugs, and selective use of muscle relaxants to relieve muscle

TABLE 28-1 ■ Organ System Function and Aging

Nervous system	Loss in neurons, reduced cerebral blood flow, diminished neurotransmitters Cerebral atherosclerosis, Parkinson's disease, depression, dementia, Alzheimer's disease, delirium all more prevalent Parasympathetic function declines, sympathetic outflow increases (increase in hypothermia, heat stroke, orthostatic hypotension, syncope) Reduced anesthetic requirement Increased postoperative cognitive dysfunction
Cardiovascular system	Reduced exercise tolerance Loss of vascular elasticity (HTN) Decreased baroreceptor activity Higher incidence of coronary and valvular heart disease
Respiratory system	Decreased protective mechanisms (coughing, swallowing) Loss of alveolar surface area Decreased responsiveness to hypercapnia and hypoxemia Work of breathing increased (reduced chest wall elasticity, reduced FEV_1, and FVC, increased RV) Decreased mean arterial oxygen tension from 95 mm Hg at age 20 to 70 mm Hg at age 80
Hepatic, GI, renal systems	Decreased hepatic synthetic activity Changes in drug clearance Decreased renal blood flow Reduced glomerular function (50% reduction by age 80)
Pharmacodynamic and pharmacokinetic changes	Increased volume of distribution for lipid-soluble drugs, reduced plasma volume, reduced plasma protein binding, slower hepatic conjugation, diminished renal elimination
Endocrine system	Diabetes, hypothyroidism, impotence, osteoporosis more common Basal metabolic rate declines 1% per year after age 30
Hematology, oncology, immune function	Reduced production of bone marrow elements Compromised cellular immunity Increased rate of cancer Increased prevalence of autoantibodies

FEV_1, Forced expiratory volume in 1 second; *FVC*, forced vital capacity; *GI*, gastrointestinal; *HTN*, hypertension; *RV*, residual volume.

TABLE 28-2 ■ **Comparison of Different Central Nervous System Disorders**

DIAGNOSIS	DISTINGUISHING FEATURE	SYMPTOMS	COURSE
Dementia	Memory impairment	Disorientation, agitation	Slow onset, progressive, chronic
Delirium	Decreased attention, fluctuating levels of consciousness	Disorientation, visual hallucination, agitation, withdrawal, memory and attention impairment	Acute; most cases remit with correction of underlying medical condition
Psychotic disorders	Deficit in reality testing	Social withdrawal, apathy	Slow onset with prodromal syndrome; chronic with exacerbations
Depression	Decreased pleasure in usual activities Sadness, loss of interest	Disturbances of sleep, appetite, concentration; suicidal ideation, decreased energy; feelings of hopelessness	Single episode, or recurrent episodes; may be chronic

spasm constitute the primary therapy. Intraarticular glucocorticoid injections, narcotics, and arthroplasty are reserved for patients with the most severe pain.

a. ***Cervical Spinal Mobility and Stability.*** These factors carry special implications for the anesthesiologist when laryngoscopy and tracheal intubation are planned.

B. Parkinson's Disease. Parkinson's disease is a disorder of the extrapyramidal system. Age is the most consistent risk factor, with Parkinson's disease affecting approximately 3% of the population older than 66 years of age. Over 50% of individuals over age 85 have symptoms of Parkinson's disease.

1. **Characteristics.** Progressive depletion of dopaminergic neurons of the substantia nigra of the basal ganglia is characteristic of Parkinson's disease. Clinical presentation is the classic triad of rigidity, resting tremor, and bradykinesia.
2. **Treatment.** Treatment is directed at allowing the patient to pursue normal daily activities using L-dopa or dopamine receptor agonists. Surgical treatments include subthalamic deep brain stimulation and fetal mesencephalic tissue implantation.
3. **Anesthetic Management.** Management includes aspiration prophylaxis and close monitoring of adequate perioperative respiratory function. The patient's regimen of anti-parkinsonian drugs should be continued as close to the regular schedule as possible. Phenothiazines, butyrophenones, and metoclopramide should be avoided. Diphenhydramine may be effective if extrapyramidal signs develop.

C. Dementia. Intellectual decline is one of the early hallmarks of dementia. Mental status is often a barometer of health in the patient with dementia, and abrupt changes necessitate a search for additional superimposed problems that may be occurring (Table 28-2). Causes of reversible dementia include drug intoxication, vitamin deficiencies, subdural hematoma, major depression, normal pressure hydrocephalus, and hypothyroidism.

1. **Treatment.** Treatment is aimed at behavioral and sleep problems. Those treatments include vitamin E, nonsteroidal antiinflammatory drugs, estrogen replacement, and centrally acting acetylcholinesterase inhibitors.
2. **Informed Consent.** Consent may be an issue.

TABLE 28-3 ■ **Special Considerations in Anesthesia Management of Geriatric Patients**

PROBLEM	STRATEGY
Increased comorbidities in individuals over age 70: · 60% have hepertension · 22% have diabetes · 20% have ischemic heart disease · 17% have renal impairment · 14% have cerebrovascular disease · 8% have lung disease Two thirds of patients over age 70 have ASA score of 3 or higher	Take a thorough history and perform a thorough physical examination. Undirected or routine testing does not result in improvement of care. Tests should be directed toward the type of surgical procedure or known co-existing disease(s) or should be based on history and physical examination findings. ECG and baseline Hct and Hgb are commonly useful. Functional capacity is the best predictor of postoperative function.
Sensory impairments	Be prepared for impaired vision and hearing.
Age-related alterations in drug clearance	Be aware of adverse drug effects and polypharmacy with increased risks.
Integumentary system issues	Avoid tape on thin, delicate skin, and protect bony prominences.
Fluid status problems	Monitor for increased risk of dehydration due to diminished thirst sensation.
Diastolic dysfunction	Be aware of increased risk of hypotension and congestive heart failure.
Increased risk of hypothermia	Use warming devices.
Prolonged clearance of anesthetic agents and decreased MAC with age	Patients are slower to awaken; lower anesthetic drug doses are needed. Short-acting agents may be advantageous.
Postoperative cognitive dysfunction	Regional anesthesia may be advantageous.
Postoperative respiratory complications are common	Postoperative supplemental oxygen, pulse oximetry monitoring, and capnography may be useful.
Thromboembolic events	Use compression stockings. Encourage early ambulation.

ASA, American Society of Anesthesiologists; *ECG,* electrocardiogram; *Hct,* hematocrit; *Hgb,* hemoglobin; *MAC,* minimum alveolar concentration.

III. GERIATRIC ANESTHESIA STRATEGIES (TABLE 28-3)

A. Preoperative Evaluation. Undirected or routine testing does not improve quality of care. Tests should be directed toward the type of surgery, known co-existing disease, and findings on history and physical examination. Electrocardiogram (ECG), hematocrit (Hct), and hemoglobin (Hgb) are often the most useful tests. Preoperative functional status is the best predictor of postoperative function.

1. **Cardiac.** Major indicators of cardiovascular risk are unstable coronary syndrome, decompensated heart failure, significant or unstable dysrhythmias, and severe or critical valvular disease, especially aortic stenosis. Cardiac testing should be reserved for patients undergoing intermediate- or high-risk surgery who cannot achieve 4 metabolic equivalents (METs) of activity and have three or more additional risk factors for significant coronary artery disease.

2. **Pulmonary.** Referral to an internist or pulmonologist may be indicated if the patient has signs and symptoms of undiagnosed or decompensated lung dysfunction. Risk factors for postoperative pneumonia include inability to carry out the activities of daily living, weight loss of 10% or more in the previous 6 months, history of stroke, impaired sensorium, ingestion of two or more alcoholic drinks per day, long-term steroid use, smoking, and underlying lung disease.
3. **Renal.** It is prudent to obtain serum electrolyte levels and creatinine concentration before procedures that carry a significant risk of renal failure (e.g., cardiopulmonary bypass, aortic aneurysm resection, or surgeries in which large fluid shifts or significant blood loss are anticipated).
4. **Hepatic.** Baseline liver function tests may be reasonable before surgeries that involve significant liver manipulation.
5. **Diabetes Mellitus.** Diabetes is an independent predictor of long-term problems after surgery. Poor glucose control (blood sugar higher than 200 mg/dL) is associated with aspiration, poor wound healing, infection, cardiac and cerebral events, and autonomic dysfunction. Whenever possible, control of serum glucose to levels of 120 to 180 mg/dL is desirable before surgery.
6. **Malnutrition.** This is an independent predictor of 30-day and 1-year postoperative mortality. A serum albumin below 3 g/dL with hypocholesterolemia and low body mass index are indicative of malnutrition.

B. **Pharmacokinetics and Pharmacodynamics.** There is no evidence that any specific inhaled or injected anesthetic agent is preferable in elderly patients. Changes in body composition can affect the distribution, metabolism, and clearance of drugs.

1. **Total Body Water.** Total body water is decreased, leading to a higher plasma concentration of hydrophilic drugs for a given dose.
2. **Adipose to Lean Muscle Ratio.** The ratio is increased, and the volume of distribution of lipophilic drugs is greater, facilitating accumulation of drug and prolongation of effects. This is even more pronounced in the face of impaired hepatic or renal function.
3. **Circulation Levels of Drug-Binding Proteins.** Levels decrease, leading to increased free drug and drug effects.
4. **Decreased Cardiac Output.** This may prolong circulation time and may result in more rapid uptake of volatile agents.
5. **Muscle Relaxant Effects.** Decreased muscle blood flow delays onset of action. Reduced clearance by liver and kidneys may prolong the action of some relaxants.
6. **Multiple Drug Prescriptions.** Commonly, elderly patients are taking multiple medications, which may lead to undesirable drug effects or drug interactions.
7. **Minimum Alveolar Concentration (MAC) of Volatile Agents.** MAC decreases with age, about 4% per decade after 40 years of age.

C. **Anesthetic Plan.** Anesthetic management for elderly patients requires consideration of many details (see Table 28-3).

1. **Anesthetic Technique.** Retrospective and prospective studies have failed to show a benefit of regional versus general anesthesia. Technique should be based on patient choice, the anesthesiologist's experience with the technique, American Society of Anesthesiologists (ASA) status of the patient, and the planned operation.
2. **Monitoring.** Monitoring should be based on potential risks and benefits, the potential for large blood loss or fluid shifts, the ASA status and comorbidities, and the planned surgery.
3. **Optimal Analgesia.** Treatment of analgesia may be challenging due to pharmacokinetic and pharmacodynamic changes and to the side effects of analgesic drugs. Dementia, delirium, and problems with hearing and vision can complicate pain assessment. The physiologic consequence of inadequate analgesia (tachycardia, hypertension, agitation) may be poorly tolerated.

D. **Postoperative Delirium and Cognitive Dysfunction**

1. **Delirium**
   a. ***Characteristics.*** Table 28-4 lists the characteristics of delirium.
   b. ***Risk Factors.*** Advanced age (>70), underlying dementia, various comorbidities, drugs (narcotics and benzodiazepines), alcohol abuse, previous episodes of delirium, visual

TABLE 28-4 ■ Components of Delirium

For a diagnosis of delirium to be established, a patient must show each of the following features:
- Disturbance of consciousness (i.e., reduced clarity of awareness about the environment) with reduced ability to focus, sustain, or shift attention
- Change in cognition (e.g., memory deficit, disorientation, language disturbance) or development of a perceptual disturbance that is not better accounted for by a preexisting, established, or evolving dementia
- Development over a short period (usually hours to days); tends to fluctuate during the course of the day
- Evidence from the history, physical examination, or laboratory findings indicating that the disturbance is caused by direct physiologic consequences of a general medical condition

TABLE 28-5 ■ Factors That Can Precipitate Delirium

Drug use (especially when the dose is changed)
Electrolyte and physiologic abnormalities (hypoxemia, hyponatremia)
Lack of drugs (withdrawal)
Infection (especially urinary tract or respiratory infection)
Reduced sensory input (blindness, deafness, darkness, unfamiliar surroundings)
Intracranial problems (stroke, bleeding, meningitis, postictal state)
Urinary retention (presence of a urinary catheter) and fecal impaction
Myocardial problems (myocardial infarction, heart failure, dysrhythmia)

impairment, certain types of injuries (e.g., hip fracture), and elevated blood urea nitrogen (BUN) are risk factors.

c. ***Precipitating Factors.*** Almost any acute illness, or an exacerbation of any chronic illness, may precipitate delirium (Table 28-5).

d. ***Outcomes.*** Hospitalized patients with delirium demonstrate up to a tenfold higher risk of developing other medical complications (including death), longer hospitalization, higher hospital costs, and increased need for long-term care after discharge.

e. ***Treatment.*** Orient the patient, stimulate cognition, promote nutritional and fluid intake, and promote exercise. Treat underlying disorders. For acute control of delirium, 0.25 to 2 mg of oral haloperidol is the preferred treatment, but diazepam, droperidol, and chlorpromazine are also often used with good results.

2. **Postoperative Cognitive Dysfunction (POCD)**

a. ***Characteristics.*** Persistent deterioration of cognitive performance after surgery is characteristic. Most POCD is mild and resolves within 3 months of surgery. Severe POCD can affect overall functional capacity and can have an adverse impact on 1-year mortality.

b. ***Risk Factors.*** Risk factors include cardiac surgery, underlying cerebrovascular disease, advanced age, lower educational level, poor ability to perform activities of daily living at baseline, and preexisting dementia. There is a possible association with duration of anesthesia.

IV. ETHICAL CHALLENGES IN GERIATRIC ANESTHESIA AND PALLIATIVE CARE

A. **Autonomy and Consent.** The ultimate decision of what medical therapy is to be employed rests with the patient. Essential criteria for informed consent include sufficient information,

TABLE 28-6 ■ Definition of *Palliative Care* by the World Health Organization

Affirms life and regards dying as a normal process
Neither hastens nor postpones death
Provides relief from pain and other distressing symptoms
Integrates the psychologic and spiritual aspects of patient care
Offers a support system to help the family cope during the patient's illness and their own bereavement

patient competence, and voluntary decision making. Patients with possible dementia may need referral for competency evaluations to assess mental function and decision-making capacity. Surrogate decision makers may be designated by living will or durable powers of attorney. Each state has a legal hierarchy to appoint a proxy decision maker if these documents are not available to guide the process.

B. **"Do-Not-Resuscitate" Orders in the Operating Room.** Informed consent for or informed refusal of medical intervention is guided by the same moral principles as during end-of-life care, regardless of location. Institutional protocols and policies regarding do-not-resuscitate status in the operating room and postanesthetic care unit should be consulted.

C. **Palliative Care.** This type of care is defined as the all-inclusive care of patients whose disease is not responsive to curative treatment (Table 28-6). It requires a multidisciplinary approach to treat symptoms, control pain, and address the psychologic, social, and spiritual needs of the patient and his or her family. By training, anesthesiologists are invaluable experts at pharmacologic and procedural pain management.

INDEX

Page numbers followed by "b" indicate boxes; "f" figures; "t" tables.

D

N

R

T

U